COST CONTAINMENT AND DRGs

A GUIDE TO PROSPECTIVE PAYMENT

COST CONTAINMENT AND DRGs

A GUIDE TO PROSPECTIVE PAYMENT

By
Allen D. Spiegel, Ph.D.
and
Florence Kavaler, MD

Foreword by
Walter McNerney

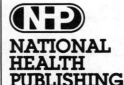

NATIONAL HEALTH PUBLISHING

Copyright © 1986 by
Rynd Communications
99 Painters Mill Road
Owings Mills, MD 21117

Printed in the United States of America
First Printing
ISBN: 0-932500-44-7
LC: 86-61800

CONTENTS

PART I

FEDERAL AND STATE PROSPECTIVE PAYMENT SYSTEMS

CHAPTER 1

LIST OF EXHIBITS

ACKNOWLEDGMENTS

Clearly, we had a great deal of assistance with this book. The Library staff at Downstate Medical Center, with patience and diligence, went out of their way to help us to find and secure the burgeoning body of literature on the subject. Our research associates, Shari Claude, Barry Freedman, M.D. and Andrea M. Spiegel, played a major role in digesting that tremendous volume of relevant literature into chewable bites to fit into our classification framework. Portions of the book were reviewed by Pascal J. Imperato, M.D., Donald J. Scherl, M.D., Isaac Topor, R.R.A., and Benjamin Wainfeld, M.D., all of whom made pertinent suggestions for enhancing the material. Jack Lubowsky, Ph.D. and Matthew Avitable, Ph.D. helped us come to terms with the computer. Finally, the efforts of Phyllis Alexander, Kay Dobson, Constance Jones, Molly Kessert, Joan Kruger, Cheryl Moore, and Maureen Roaldsen joined together to get the frequently illegible, scribbled words translated into the typed and duplicated manuscript pages. Without the combined energy of all these people, this book would still be in the talking stage.

Allen D. Spiegel, Ph.D., M.P.H.
Florence Kavaler, M.D., M.P.H.

ABOUT THE AUTHORS

Allen D. Spiegel, Ph.D., M.P.H.

Dr. Allen D. Spiegel is a Professor of Preventive Medicine and Community Health, State University of New York, Health Science Center at Brooklyn, College of Medicine, Brooklyn, New York. His experiences include a wide range of activities in medical and health care services, comprehensive health planning, public health education, and health and medical communications. Formerly, Dr. Spiegel was with the New York City Health Department and The Medical Foundation, Inc. of Boston. He was also a Special Research Fellow at Brandeis University. His services as a consultant have been sought on numerous health and welfare projects by an assortment of private and governmental agencies. He has authored and coauthored more than 100 articles, reports, and mass media material on health care. His books include the following: *Perspectives in Community Mental Health; Medicaid: Lessons for National Health Insurance; Basic Health Planning Methods; The Medicaid Experience; Curing and Caring; Medical Technology, Health Care and the Consumer; Rehabilitating People with Disabilities into the Mainstream of Society; and Home Health Care: Home Birthing to Hospice.*

Florence Kavaler, M.D., M.P.H.

Florence Kavaler, M.D., M.P.H., is a professor of preventive medicine at the State University of New York, Health Science Center at Brooklyn, Brooklyn, New York. She was formerly Assistant Surgeon General and director of the U.S. Public Health Service Hospital at Staten Island, New York, study director for the Milbank Memorial Fund Commission for the Study of Higher Education for Public Health, and assistant commissioner for Health and Medical Insurance Programs of the New York City Health Department.

Dr. Kavaler was educated at Barnard College, Downstate Medical Center, SUNY and Columbia University School of Public Health and Administrative Medicine. Her consultation skills capitalize on extensive experience in hospital administration and ambulatory care services—both hospital based and satellite. Wide experience in long-term care stems from her role as medical director of a combined skilled nursing/intermediate care facility.

Her many publications address the areas of medical care evaluation in multiple settings, administrative public policy dynamics, and research activities in drug addiction, hospital cost control, aging, long-term care, and public health. Recent books include *Computers in Medical Administration, Higher Education for Public Health, Foster-Child Health Care.*

FOREWORD

In the last two years, "DRG" has become the most frequently used abbreviation in the health field. More than any other health care catchword, it symbolizes a period of major, almost audacious, changes in the financing and delivery of health services. DRGs have become the subject of innumerable articles, endless speculation, strong commendations, and barbed criticisms. It is time for a comprehensive and thoroughly researched book on DRGs. In *Cost Containment and DRGs: A Guide to Prospective Payment*, we have such a book, coauthored by two well-known and respected experts in health care management, Allen D. Spiegel, Ph.D. and Florence Kavaler, M.D., reflecting broad experience in medicine, public health, and management.

Of course, the focus of this book is on diagnosis related groups, a form of prospective payment under the Medicare program for inpatient hospital care. Specifically, the authors put DRGs in historical perspective, both as a payment policy and as a part of an overall strategy of cost containment. In this context, the authors elaborate on unresolved issues, alternative remedies, and speculations on future public policy.

From both a practical and conceptual point of view, this book will be invaluable to trustees, managers, professionals, and public policy experts. No one can afford to overlook the current and future consequences of DRG strategies. Medicare pays from 20 percent to more than 50 percent of the bill for inpatient services in acute, general hospitals, and it sets the pace for other payers. Some private payers, such as Blue Cross, are already using DRGs or similar methods of payment.

In 1983, DRGs arrived on the scene with far less forewarning than such major changes usually entail, reflecting an urgency on the federal government's part to contain costs. This feeling of urgency was shared by private payers who were by then convinced that paying costs and charges was "a bottomless pit." Such widespread implementation of a new and bold payment scheme, with relatively little testing, was bound to result in mixed reactions. While Senator Heinz was highlighting problems with the quality of care under Medicare, the Inspector General and HHS reported that hospital profit margins on Medicare operations were triple the average profit margins for all patients in recent years, up 14 percent in 1984. In either case, let no one deny that DRGs caught everyone's attention and helped focus the nation's concern on efficiency and effectiveness better than most other programs introduced in recent years.

As in most instances in health financing, the evaluation of DRGs is handicapped by a lack of data. Because of this, opinions about their worth and their future vary considerably. There appears to be reasonably broad consensus among students of the health field that DRGs have made a strong impact on admissions, intensity of services, and length of stay, but opinions vary widely on the nature and favorability of the impact.

Evaluation is made more difficult by the fact that the prospective payment system and DRGs make up only one of several factors affecting utilization. Others include a maturing market, increasing regulation, more aggressive use of deductibles and copayments, availability of benefits to cover alternate site services, and tougher utilization review programs in both the public and private sectors. Further, the complexity of market and regulatory interactions is such that several years' experience will be needed to pin down what are now largely conjectures. However, it is safe to say, that DRGs are *associated* with a changing use of inpatient services, increased care on an ambulatory basis, vertical and horizontal integration of services, renewed interest in HMOs and greater attention in health systems to strategic planning, Management Information Systems (MIS), human resource planning, and marketing.

Spiegel and Kavaler have gathered most of the relevant data bearing on the issues, added generous references to expert opinions, and organized the material around the major subjects of contention. For example, the question of how DRGs affect quality of care is addressed. Are patients being discharged sicker than previously? Is the fiduciary responsibility of the physician to the patient being compromised by management now armed with incentive payment tools? With limited resources, who rations care? Can the Office of Management and Budget (OMB) be trusted to measure benefits as well as costs? Weighing experience to date, the authors raise a series of important tactical questions: how can DRG cells be made more homogeneous, how and when should DRG payments be made for new areas, such as ambulatory care, psychiatric long-term care, preventive care, and physicians' services, what exceptions should be allowed, and what changes are needed in the wage index? Important strategic issues are raised as well: for example, what role should DRGs play in financing care for the underprivileged, medical education, new technology and for privately insured people.

Another major issue arises: can a prospective payment system built on averages and meant to provide broad incentives survive? If DRGs were to be totally "fair," HCFA would be forced to set payment rates for each hospital individually. Otherwise, the number of DRG categories would have to increase and the database used would require considerable expansion. And, of course, it is patently unfair to burden DRGs with public policy issues such as payment for the indigent and medical education. DRGs were conceived of and are being used essentially as cost containment tools. Resolutions on public policy issues are needed at a higher level, in a broader context involving both OMB and HHS.

Given the real and potential limitations of DRGs, the authors wisely address the next generation of prospective payment and conclude that capitation is the most likely successor, aided and abetted by quality assurance programs and backed implicitly by public decisions regarding major policy issues. In looking ahead, the authors reflect the feelings of many they interviewed or quoted, who all conclude that given the number of contradictory forces at play, very few generalizations can be made with confidence. If one generalization can be made, it is that very likely cost reimbursement is dead and all payments will entail some form of incentives. Over the next 10 years both competition and regulation will be fostered, and no one method of financing or delivery of care will be employed. As in the past, the dominant themes will be pluralism and pragmatism.

None of the above is meant to imply that the debate over PPS/DRGs will not be heated. As pointed out in the book, DRGs and PPS in general are surrogates for a growing concern over whether health can be viewed as an economic good among other goods and services or as a social good, requiring widespread interventions and props, and based heavily on professional versus managerial initiatives. This book sharpens the debate considerably in the interest of health care institutions, professionals, and the community.

Walter J. McNerney
Herman Smith Professor
J.L. Kellogg Graduate
School of Management Program in Hospital
and Health Services Management
Northwestern University
Evanston, Illinois

INTRODUCTION

DRG, which stands for Diagnosis Related Groups, is the prospective reimbursement mechanism currently in force for those people who are covered by the federal government's Medicare program for inpatient hospital expenditures. However, certain population groups have suggested other meanings for DRG—an indication of their respective opinions of this change in the reimbursement procedure:

Hospital administrators feel that it means Disastrous Regulations Galore[1] or that the Difficulty Rate is Growing,[2] or that De Revenue's Gone.[3]

Physicians complain about the Deluge of Regulatory Garbage[4] and the Doctor Regulating Government;[5] the Dismal, Ridiculous, and Godforsaken;[6] the Dirty Rotten Government[7] and the Denials, Refusals, and Gibberish.[8]

Legislators may consider it Divine Redeeming Grace[9] as a solution to a problem.

Consumers may feel that it aims to Do Right and Good[10] in their best interests.

A pertinent comment was made at the 1983 annual meeting of the Association of University Programs in Health Administration. What made the comment particularly relevant was the fact that the speaker was a member of the original Yale University team that developed the DRG concept. He told the audience:

Now we come to figure out how the Feds are going to screw it up, because you know they are going to screw it up. It's just (a matter of) trying to figure out when.[11]

Such reactions reflect the complexity of issues in a system that is proposed as a cost-containment device to resolve runaway health care expenditures. Specifically, DRGs are intended to contain inflationary increases in available Medicare funds that provide benefits for the elderly receiving care in hospitals.

Health care professionals and consumers are instinctively suspicious of the country's health care system. The DRG program has been a catalyst for serious questioning and discussion about that system's intentions. The following statements have long been considered the basic tenets of our health care system, though they have not been unanimously accepted as true by every segment of the population—and now the DRG issue has brought these premises under public scrutiny again:

Health care is a right.

A hospital is a provider of services (not a business).

Quality health care means high technology medical care.

A hospital is the hub of health care.[12]

If health care is *not* a right, if a hospital *is* a business, if high technology is *not* used, and if the hospital is *not* the hub of care—then what are the contrary basic principles of the U.S. health care system? Scholars have suggested that health care be rationed;[13] that for-profit hospitals have an edge;[14] that high technology will be restricted;[15] and that outpatient care will increase dramatically.[16] While we have only cited a few references, there are many other articles that echo those suggestions time and again. Is this a backlash against the DRG system?

Even before considering the possible changes in the generally held basic beliefs about health care in America or the backlash against DRGs, there are still unresolved issues for all concerned within the proposed DRG mechanism. This book concentrates on those issues.

From a management/business viewpoint, DRGs effectively have forced hospitals into scrutinizing profit centers, with an eye toward the "winners" and "losers" under the DRG system. Medical record departments have leapfrogged into the top managerial levels, becoming the solid right arm of the administrators and the trustees to insure against red ink on the balance sheet.

Institutions excluded from the initial DRG package such as long-term care facilities, psychiatric centers, and ambulatory care providers are to be included in future reimbursement programs. New acronyms crop up frequently; investigators speak of RUGs (Resource Utilization Groups) and AVGs (Ambulatory Visit Groups). Considerations of the intensity of services provided by ancillary health care personnel to improve the patient's ability to handle Activities of Daily Living (ADL) constitute a major emphasis in these reimbursement calculations.

Health care providers, particularly physicians, have varied reactions to the DRG system and its impact upon their professional actions and their ethical decisions. Partly they are concerned with the quality of patient care at the bedside. A number of professional journals have devoted entire issues to the examination of the impact of the DRG scheme upon their members and the medical profession.

Not much attention has been given to the warm bodies that occupy the hospital beds—the patients/consumers. Is there any effect upon the people who eventually pay the bill? Are there financial losses incurred by the patients and/or their families? Does the quality of care suffer and result in greater mortality or morbidity? What do the consumers think about the DRG plan? What input do consumers have in the DRG system? At this time, few consumer groups have actively been involved with the emerging DRG implementation efforts. Some have testified at Congressional hearings and held seminars for the elderly but generally the consumer front has been quiet.

Exhibit A   On Paying Hospitals

Reagan, beware.
La Belle Dame au DRG[1,2]
Thee hath in thrall.

Fettered to a system so arcane,
Which wiser men might craftily disdain,
Yale's[3,4] researchers devised a novel way
To pay bills by disease and not by day.

The money spent in building DRGs
Alone could bring our system to its knees.
Would prospective reimbursement of research
Have also left our country in the lurch?

Gentles, question not how we should pay,
Whether by disease or length of stay,
Or yet to pay with cheer ahead of time,
Or with a grumble late, but on the dime.

Question rather where lie the controls
To pare the costs of our insurance rolls?
Question who should foot the growing bill:
The government, the insurors, or the ill?

Should government have sway o'er but a part,
It then would rule the shell, but not the heart;
And so the costs of sickness still would soar,
While the ill and the insurors would pay more.

The sons of Eli no solution gave
To cure a system only law can save.
For clipping costs, alas, the answer lies
With public rule, or else the patient dies.

ANNE-MARIE FOLTZ
New York University
March 1983

1. J.K. Iglehart, "The new era of prospective payment for hospitals," *New England Journal of Medicine* 307, (1982):1288–92.
2. J.K. Iglehart, "New Jersey's experiment with DRG-based hospital reimbursement," *New England Journal of Medicine* 307, (1982):1655–1660.
3. R. Mills, R.B. Fetter, D.B. Riedel, R. Averill, "AUTOGRP: an interactive computer system for the analysis of health care data," *Medical Care* 14, (1976):603–615.
4. R.B. Fetter, Y. Shin, J.L. Freeman, R.F. Averill, J.D. Thompson, "Case mix by diagnosis-related groups," *Medical Care* 18 (Feb. supplement), (1980).

In addition to taking on the unresolved issues, we have included a chapter that deals with the events leading up to the DRG legislation. Events in the states that conducted experimental programs, with a concentration on New Jersey, are also covered in some detail. However, we do not wish to duplicate existing how-to-do-it books that explain in detail the complicated accounting DRG system. Rather, our purpose is to provide a solid resource volume by gathering together a multiplicity of references for those who wish to know more about the future of reimbursement policies and procedures in the United States. We hope that hospital administrators, trustees, physicians, nurses, other health care providers, and other institutional administrators will find the data they need in this book.

Two exhibits (Exhibits A and B) illustrate clearly and humorously the current situation regarding DRGs. As you read this book, the exhibits will be elucidated more directly in regard to the issues at hand. We recommend rereading both exhibits after completion of the book for enhanced enjoyment of their contents.

Exhibit B   DRG Awareness Test

Since December 1982, when Health and Human Services Secretary Schweiker made his recommendation to the Congress for a prospective payment system based on DRGs, it seems that virtually anyone who had flown over Trenton, New Jersey in the preceding five years became an "Instant DRG Expert." Over the course of the last year, we've seen a great deal of information and misinformation about DRGs. We have also been pleasantly surprised to find many knowledgeable and proactive providers to be thoroughly familiar with the subject.

The test that follows contains 10 multiple choice questions to help you diagnose your level of DRG awareness. While the test is not comprehensive, completing the test and scoring your answers should help you to raise the quality of your social conversation on the subject. We hope that you will find the test as enjoyable to complete and score as we did to prepare.

1. DRG is
   a. Diagnostic-related groupings
   b. Dr. Richard Goldstein
   c. Diagnosis-related groups
   d. All of the above
   e. None of the above

2. GROUPER is
   a. A tasty freshwater fish
   b. Software used for grouping patients based on clinical characteristics
   c. One who chases rock groups
   d. All of the above
   e. None of the above.

3. ICD means
   a. Intensive Care Department
   b. 1 Certificate of Deposit
   c. International Classification of Diseases
   d. All of the above
   e. None of the above

4. TIA stands for
   a. Transient ischemic attacks
   b. Teacher's Insurance Annuities
   c. Terribly indecent approach
   d. All of the above
   e. None of the above

5. "DRG Creep" is
   a. The Yalie who invented GROUPER
   b. Coding and sequencing diagnoses to obtain maximum payment for services
   c. A contagious disease
   d. All of the above
   e. None of the above

6. CC is an abbreviation for
   a. Comorbidity and complications
   b. Carbon copy
   c. Correlation coefficient
   d. All of the above
   e. None of the above

7. RIMs are
   a. An RVU system for nursing services
   b. Nursing relative intensity measures
   c. A statistic being used to allocate nursing costs to DRGs
   d. All of the above
   e. None of the above

8. MDC is an abbreviation for
   a. Major Diagnostic Category
   b. Major Disease Classification
   c. Medical Disease Coding
   d. All of the above
   e. None of the above

9. There are
   a. 83 MDCs and 383 DRGs
   b. 23 MDCs and 470 DRGs
   c. 23 MDCs and 467 DRGs
   d. All of the above
   e. None of the above

10. Chapter 83, laws of New Jersey
    a. Assures the financial viability of hospitals
    b. Establishes an all-payor rate setting system
    c. Is the principal difference between Medicare's Prospective Payment System and New Jersey's rate-setting system
    d. All of the above
    e. None of the above.

DRG Awareness Test—Answers

1. (d) Although diagnostic related groupings is not technically correct, much of the health care literature persists in using the term. Dr. Richard Goldstein is New Jersey's Commissioner of Health.

2. (b) And there are nearly as many varieties of the GROUPER software as there are species of grouper, a bland but nutritious salt water fish.

3. (c) However, if you think you're going to prosper under Medicare's Prospective Payment System, you might be better off liquidating the hospital's assets and investing them in Certificates of Deposit. Otherwise, "budget neutrality" may lead to your being admitted to intensive care.

4. (a) DRG 15—it includes everything from fainting spells to acute ischemic episodes. Some wags have suggested that DRGs are a terrible indecent approach to hospital rate setting and that CFOs who are eligible should cash in their Teacher's Insurance Annuities and retire before they wind up as a DRG 15 patient.

5. (b) In many instances the term is used interchangeably with "coding up", which medical record professionals will tell you is unethical. We fully expect that the phenomenon will spread rapidly in the 46 nonwaiver states and you could argue that (c), "a contagious disease" also is correct.

6. (a) Presence of comorbidity or complications will, for many patients, assure that patient will be assigned to a DRG with a higher prospective payment rate. Statisticians will tell you that you should not expect a high degree of correlation between DRGs and actual resource consumption. Anyone who tells you that Medicare's Prospective Payment System is a carbon copy of New Jersey's DRG system hasn't looked at the two systems very closely.

7. (d) Nursing relative intensity measures (RIMs) have been developed based on an extensive study of nursing services delivered to 3,336 patients in eight New Jersey hospitals during 1979 (prior to DRG implementation). Nursing service directors generally agree that, while RIMs are not perfect, they do represent a better way of assigning nursing costs to patients than do average nursing costs per patient day. Accordingly, New Jersey will be evaluating the relative merits of the RIMs methodology in 20 New Jersey hospitals during 1984. RVU stands for Relative Value Unit.

8. (a) In both Medicare's and New Jersey's system, patients are first grouped into 23 major diagnostic categories (MDCs), which are organized mainly by organ system, from the ICD-9-CM code for the principal diagnosis.

9. (d) All of the above. New York State's prospective hospital reimbursement methodology (NYPHRM) utilizes a "seed cluster" grouping methodology that incorporates case mix measures based on the old DRGs (83 MDCs, 383 DRGs). New Jersey's systems has 467 DRGs plus outliers; Medicare added three more:

   ● DRG 468—a discharge showing an operating room procedure that is unrelated to the assigned MDC

   ● DRG 469—a discharge with a diagnosis that is valid in the principal diagnosis field, but not acceptable as a principal diagnosis for purposes of DRG assignment.

   ● DRG 470—a discharge with invalid data.

10. (d) All of the above. Medicare adopted DRGs as a payment mechanism, but ignored Chapter 83 and stuck with Medicare's less generous principles of reimbursement.

Results

9–10 correct. Consider yourself a genuine DRG expert. Accordingly, you may wish to move from your job in Trenton to a position with HCFA.

6–8 correct. You are sufficiently qualified to carry on an intelligent conversation about DRGs with your peers.

3–5 correct. You are generally aware that something's been happening, but need to attend a good seminar on the subject before indulging in serious cocktail hour conversation.

0–2 correct. If you're currently involved in health care delivery and scored this low, you may wish to consider a career change.

Exhibit A is a poem—with references. This poem refers to the Yale researchers with a prominent name hidden in the wording. Comments about costs, length of stay, cost by disease, an all-payer scheme, and legislative actions all highlight the complex considerations embodied within the DRG proposal.

Exhibit B is a DRG Awareness Test devised for a seminar in New Jersey. Questions 1 and 10 are specific for New Jersey, but you can guess on those. In any event, the correct answers will explain those idiosyncrasies. We invite you to take the exam as a pre-test and later as a post-test.

If the volume of literature dealing with DRGs is an indication of professional interest, then this book needs no further introduction. Obviously, those directly connected with the U.S. health care system feel that the DRG scheme merits their immediate and intensive attention. We feel that this book will provide an effective means to channel that attention.

References

1. S. Porter, "How Ohio hospitals are Coping With DRGs," *Ohio State Medical Journal* 80, no. 4 (1984): 263-265.

2. The DRG Maze. *Unravelling the Mysteries of Hospital Reimbursement in New Jersey* (Princeton, NJ: New Jersey Hospital Association, 1979).

3. K. Mitchell, "DRGs: De Revenue's Gone!!" *Pediatric Nursing* 10, no. 5 (1984): 317.

4. "House Adopts Resolutions on DRGs," *American Medical News* 26, no. 25 (July 1-8, 1983):23.

5. *The DRG Maze: Unravelling the Mysteries*, New Jersey Hospital Association.

6. A. Lurvey, "DRG: Letters That Could Make or Break a Hospital," *Private Practice* 16, no. 11 (1984): 28-29.

7. Ibid.

8. Ibid.

9. Porter, "How Ohio Hospitals are Coping."

10. *The DRG Maze: Unravelling the Mysteries*, New jersey Hospital Association.

11. P. C. Smith, "Use of His Research Tool Worries Yale Professor," *Medical Tribune* September 28, 1983.

12. E. Scharder, "Will DRGs Change Our Ideas About What Health Care Means?" *AORN Journal* 38, no. 5 (1984): 752-754.

13. H. J. Aaron and W. B. Schwartz, *The Painful Prescription: Rationing Hospital Care* (Washington, DC: The Brookings Institution, 1984).

14. M. Nathanson, "Comprehensive Cost Accounting Systems Give Chains and Edge," *Modern Health care* 14, no. 3 (February 15, 1984): 122, 124, 128.

15. U.S. Congress, Office of Technology Assessment. *Diagnosis Related Groups (DRGs) and the Medicare Program: Implications for Medical Technology. A Technical memorandum*. Washington, DC, July, 1983.

16. "Prospective Payment—The Regulator's View; An Interview with Mr. Larry A. Oday," *DRG Monitor* 1, no. 2 (1983): 1-8.

PART I
FEDERAL AND STATE PROSPECTIVE PAYMENT SYSTEMS

CHAPTER 1
PPS and DRGs:
a Primer

A prospective payment system (PPS) using diagnosis related groups (DRGs) as a reimbursement mechanism may completely alter the health care delivery system in the United States. For that reason, the amount of literature explaining PPS and DRGs has been voluminous. Articles in primer style appear in a variety of professional medical society journals,[1-7] in hospital association magazines,[8-12] in professional nursing journals,[13-17] in medical records and other professional journals,[18-24] in health industry trade association reports,[25] in governmental publications,[26-33] in professional school reports,[34] in local newspapers,[35] in books for everyone concerned,[36-41] in insurance sponsored journals,[42] and in reports by commercial companies engaged in the health care business.[43-48] Furthermore, this listing is merely illustrative and certainly not comprehensive. More articles appear regularly as specific groups catch up with their memberships' need to learn about the basic workings of PPS and DRGs.

Although we assume that most people who buy this book will have some knowledge of PPS and DRGs, we are including a brief primer on the new system for those who need to brush up or want to refresh their memories. The following material outlining the basics about PPS and DRGs was adapted from a 1985 update by the Congressional Research Service of the Library of Congress.[49]

Background

Medicare is a nationwide, federally-funded health insurance program for the aged, certain disabled persons, and certain individuals who need kidney transplantation or dialysis. It consists of two parts: Medicare Hospital Insurance (Part A) helps pay for inpatient hospital services, skilled nursing facility services, home health services, and hospice care; and Supplementary Medical Insurance (Part B) helps pay for the services of independent practitioners (primarily physicians), and outpatient hospital services, laboratory services, and other medical and related services.

3

Before the passage of P.L. 98-21 (the Social Security Amendments of 1983), Medicare reimbursed hospitals according to the reasonable costs incurred in providing services to Medicare beneficiaries. Because actual reasonable costs could not be determined until after the hospital provided the services, this method of reimbursement was known as "retrospective cost-based reimbursement."

Critics argued that retrospective cost-based reimbursement provided few incentives for hospitals to be efficient or cost-conscious. The more they spent for Medicare allowable costs, the more they were reimbursed. Rising Medicare expenditures for hosptial care led to interest in alternative methods of Medicare hospital reimbursement and to limits on the existing cost-based method of reimbursement.

Under authority provided by Section 222 of the Social Security Amendments of 1972 (P.L. 92-603), the Department of Health and Human Services (HHS) funded experiments and demonstration projects to determine the advantages and disadvantages of a "prospective payment system" (PPS) with fixed payment rates determined in advance of the provision of the hospital services.

Section 223 of the 1972 Amendments authorized the Secretary to set prospective limits on costs that were recognized as reasonable by Medicare. Under this authority, limits have been set on Medicare reimbursement to hospitals annually since 1974. In addition, the Tax Equity and Fiscal Responsibility Act of 1982 (P.L. 97-248, or TEFRA) established a new three-year Medicare ceiling (or target rate) on the allowable annual rate of increase in operating costs per case for inpatient hospital services.

Despite these actions, concern over rising Medicare hospital expenditures (which reached a high of 22 percent in 1981) and projected depletion of the Medicare Hospital Insurance Trust Fund (expected to be exhausted by the mid-1990s) renewed efforts to change the Medicare cost-based hospital reimbursement system. TEFRA provisions required HHS to develop legislative proposals for the prospective reimbursement of hospitals (and other providers) by Medicare to be reported to Congress by December 31, 1982. Legislation was introduced in Congress, amended, approved, and signed into law on April 20, 1983, as Title VI of P.L. 98-21, the Social Security Amendments of 1983. This new method of Medicare payment for hospitals began on or after October 1, 1983. Final regulations were issued January 3, 1984. Several modifications to the prospective payment system were included in P.L. 98-369, the Deficit Reduction Act of 1984 (July 18, 1984). On August 31, 1984, HHS issued final rules modifying the prospective payment system and describing the methodology for determining the payment rates in FY 1985.

Major Provisions of the Medicare Prospective Payment System: General Summary

Medicare payment for hospital inpatient services is now made according to a prospective payment system. Payments are made at predetermined, fixed rates representing the average cost, nationwide, of treating a Medicare patient according to his or her diagnosis. The classification system used to group hospital inpatients according to their diagnoses is known as Diagnosis Related Groups (DRGs). Separate DRG rates apply depending on whether a hospital is located in an urban or rural area of the country. During a transition period, a declining portion of the total prospective payment to a hospital is based on the hospital's historical reasonable costs and an increasing portion is based on a combination of regional and national DRG rates. In the fourth year of the program, Medicare payments are determined totally under a national DRG payment methodology.

If a hospital can treat a patient for less than the DRG payment amount, it can keep the savings. If the treatment costs more, the hospital must absorb the loss. A hospital is prohibited from charging Medicare beneficiaries for any difference between the hospital's cost of providing covered care and the Medicare DRG payment amount. Exceptions include deductible and coinsurance amounts, services not covered by Medicare, and services furnished to beneficiaries who elect to stay in the hospital when such services have been determined to be medically unnecessary or to be custodial care.

Certain hospital costs are excluded and are paid for on a reasonable cost basis. In addition, certain hospitals are excluded from the system and are reimbursed on a reasonable cost basis, subject to the rate of increase limits provided for in TEFRA. Authority is provided for states to establish their own Medicare hospital payment systems if they meet certain federal requirements.

Prospective Payments

Unless excluded from PPS, all Medicare participating hospitals are paid a specific amount for inpatient services provided to Medicare beneficiaries based on the patient's classification into one of 470 DRGs (see Exhibit 1-1, and Exhibit 1-2). Separate DRG rates apply to hospitals located in urban or rural areas of the country as determined by Metropolitan Statistical Areas (urban rates are higher than rural rates). Hospitals located in areas reclassified from urban to rural are allowed a two-year transition to the rural rates. DRG rates are adjusted by a wage index for area differences in hospital wage levels compared to the national average hospital wage level.

Exhibit 1-1   List of Diagnosis Related Groups (DRGs) by Major Diagnostic Category, Medical or Surgical Procedure, Title, Relative Weighting Factors, Arithmetic and Geometric Mean Length of Stay, and Length of Stay Outlier Cutoff Points Used in the Prospective Payment System

DRG	MDC	Title	Relative Weights	Arithmetic Mean LOS	Geometric Mean LOS	Outlier Threshold
1	1 SURG	Craniotomy Age > 17 Except for Trauma	3.5632	21.4	16.2	33
2	1 SURG	Craniotomy for Trauma Age >17	3.8117	19.7	13.4	30
3	1 SURG	Craniotomy Age <18*	2.9183		12.7	30
4	1 SURG	Spinal Procedures	2.7300	20.2	15.0	32
5	1 SURG	Extracranial Vascular Procedures	1.6510	9.7	8.0	25
6	1 SURG	Carpal Tunnel Release	.4072	2.8	2.3	7
7	1 SURG	Periph + Cranial Nerve + Other Nerv Syst Proc Age >69 +/or C.C.	1.3867	11.5	6.1	23
8	1 SURG	Periph + Cranial Nerve + Other Nerv Syst Proc Age <70 w/o C.C.	.7466	5.6	3.7	19
9	1 MED	Spinal Disorders + Injuries	1.4237	14.4	8.4	25
10	1 MED	Nervous System Neoplasms Age >69 and/or C.C.	1.1324	11.6	7.8	25
11	1 MED	Nervous System Neoplasms Age <70 w/o C.C.	.9338	10.2	6.1	23
12	1 MED	Degenerative Nervous System Disorders	1.0016	11.4	7.8	25
13	1 MED	Multiple Sclerosis + Cerebellar Ataxia	.9789	10.9	7.7	25
14	1 MED	Specific Cerebrovascular Disorders Except TIA	1.3144	12.6	8.5	26
15	1 MED	Transient Ischemic Attack and Precerebral Occlusions	.6241	6.1	4.7	19
16	1 MED	Nonspecific Cerebrovascular Disorders with C.C.	.9044	8.9	6.8	24
17	1 MED	Nonspecific Cerebrovascular Disorders w/o C.C.	.6803	7.8	5.6	23
18	1 MED	Cranial + Peripheral Nerve Disorders Age >69 and/or C.C.	.7567	8.2	6.1	23
19	1 MED	Cranial + Peripheral Nerve Disorders Age <70 w/o C.C.	.6548	7.2	5.3	22
20	1 MED	Nervous System Infection Except Viral Meningitis	1.4090	11.5	7.8	25
21	1 MED	Viral Meningitis	1.3144	10.6	7.9	25
22	1 MED	Hypertensive Encephalopathy	.7087	6.5	5.0	20
23	1 MED	Nontraumatic Stupor + Coma	1.1242	8.5	5.2	22
24	1 MED	Seizure + Headache Age >69 and/or C.C.	.7644	6.8	5.0	22
25	1 MED	Seizure + Headache Age 18–69 w/o C.C.	.5522	5.5	4.0	18
26	1 MED	Seizure + Headache Age 0–17	.6255	3.9	2.7	14

DRG	MDC	Type	Description	Weight	Arith. Mean	Geom. Mean	Outlier
27	1	MED	Traumatic Stupor + Coma, Coma >1 Hr	1.5648	9.8	4.7	22
28	1	MED	Traumatic Stupor + Coma, Coma <1 Hr Age>69 and/or C.C.	.9422	8.5	5.0	22
29	1	MED	Traumatic Stupor + Coma <1 Hr Age 18-69 w/o C.C.	.6462	6.0	3.6	21
30	1	MED	Traumatic Stupor + Coma <1 Hr Age 0-17*	.3539		2.0	8
31	1	MED	Concussion Age >69 and/or C.C.	.5383	5.7	3.9	20
32	1	MED	Concussion Age 18-69 w/o C.C.	.4064	4.1	2.9	14
33	1	MED	Concussion Age 0-17*	.2457		1.6	5
34	1	MED	Other Disorders of Nervous System Age >69 and/or C.C.	.9777	8.9	6.1	23
35	1	MED	Other Disorders of Nervous System Age <70 w/o C.C.	.7384	7.6	4.9	22
36	2	SURG	Retinal Procedures	.7103	4.7	4.1	12
37	2	SURG	Orbital Procedures	.6688	4.2	3.2	12
38	2	SURG	Primary Iris Procedures	.3990	3.1	2.4	8
39	2	SURG	Lens Procedures with or without Vitrectomy	.5721	2.3	2.1	4
40	2	SURG	Extraocular Procedures Except Orbit Age >17	.4129	2.5	2.1	6
41	2	SURG	Extraocular Procedures Except Orbit Age 0-17*	.3657		1.6	4
42	2	SURG	Intraocular Procedures Except Retina, Iris + Lens	.6543	3.7	3.0	10
43	2	MED	Hyphema	.3462	4.6	3.7	13
44	2	MED	Acute Major Eye Infections	.6397	7.3	5.9	21
45	2	MED	Neurological Eye Disorders	.5409	4.7	3.6	14
46	2	MED	Other Disorders of the Eye Age >17 with C.C.	.6010	5.6	3.7	21
47	2	MED	Other Disorders of the Eye Age >17 w/o C.C.	.4192	3.6	2.5	11
48	2	MED	Other Disorders of the Eye Age 0-17*	.4018		2.9	13
49	3	SURG	Major Head + Neck Procedures	2.8745	17.1	13.1	30
50	3	SURG	Sialoadenectomy	.7034	4.4	3.7	11
51	3	SURG	Salivary Gland Procedures Except Sialoadenectomy	.5887	4.0	3.3	10
52	3	SURG	Cleft Lip + Palate Repair	.6956	4.4	3.5	13
53	3	SURG	Sinus + Mastoid Procedures Age >17	.6176	3.8	3.0	10
54	3	SURG	Sinus + Mastoid Procedures Age 0-17*	.6889		3.2	11
55	3	SURG	Miscellaneous Ear, Nose + Throat Procedures	.4342	2.6	2.1	6

* Medicare data have been supplemented by data from Maryland and Michigan for low volume DRGs.

** DRGs 469 and 470 contain cases which could not be assigned to valid DRGs.

Note: Geometric mean is used only to determine payment for outlier cases.
Note: Relative weights are based on Medicare patient data and may not be appropriate for other patients.
Note: Arithmetic mean included for comparative purposes. It is not used for payment.

Exhibit 1-1 *(Continued)*

DRG	MDC		Title	Relative Weights	Arithmetic Mean LOS	Geometric Mean LOS	Outlier Threshold
56	3	SURG	Rhinoplasty	.4358	2.8	2.3	7
57	3	SURG	T + A Proc Except Tonsillectomy +/or Adenoidectomy Only, Age >17	.7718	5.7	3.7	20
58	3	SURG	T + A Proc Except Tonsillectomy +/or Adenoidectomy Only, Age 0–17*	.3097		1.5	3
59	3	SURG	Tonsillectomy and/or Adenoidectomy Only Age >17	.4132	2.9	2.3	7
60	3	SURG	Tonsillectomy and/or Adenoidectomy Only Age 0–17*	.2616		1.5	3
61	3	SURG	Myringotomy with Tube Insertion Age >17	.4274	2.9	2.0	8
62	3	SURG	Myringotomy with Tube Insertion Age 0–17*	.3089		1.3	3
63	3	SURG	Other Ear, Nose + Throat O.R. Procedures	1.1619	8.1	5.1	22
64	3	MED	Ear, Nose + Throat Malignancy	.9769	8.5	4.8	22
65	3	MED	Dysequilibrium	.4499	4.8	3.8	14
66	3	MED	Epistaxis	.4146	4.3	3.3	13
67	3	MED	Epiglottitis	.9364	6.5	4.8	21
68	3	MED	Otitis Media + URI Age >69 and/or C.C.	.6092	6.3	5.1	17
69	3	MED	Otitis Media + URI Age 18–69 w/o C.C.	.5040	5.1	4.1	14
70	3	MED	Otitis Media + URI Age 0–17	.5251	4.2	3.3	12
71	3	MED	Laryngotracheitis	.6594	5.8	4.6	18
72	3	MED	Nasal Trauma + Deformity	.5217	5.2	3.5	19
73	3	MED	Other Ear, Nose + Throat Diagnoses Age >17	.6049	5.1	3.4	18
74	3	MED	Other Ear, Nose + Throat Diagnoses Age 0–17*	.3427		2.1	9
75	4	SURG	Major Chest Procedures	2.9780	16.2	13.4	30
76	4	SURG	Respiratory System O.R. Procedures with C.C.	2.5667	14.9	10.3	27
77	4	SURG	Respiratory System O.R. Procedures w/o C.C.	1.6735	11.5	7.0	24
78	4	MED	Pulmonary Embolism	1.4802	11.7	9.5	27
79	4	MED	Respiratory Infections + Inflammations Age >69 and/or C.C.	1.9546	13.0	9.6	27
80	4	MED	Respiratory Infections + Inflammations Age 18–69 w/o C.C.	1.4403	12.2	8.5	26
81	4	MED	Respiratory Infections + Inflammations Age 0–17*	.8652		6.1	23
82	4	MED	Respiratory Neoplasms	1.1259	9.9	6.6	24

DRG	MDC		Description				
83	4	MED	Major Chest Trauma >69 and/or C.C.	.8398	8.6	6.6	24
84	4	MED	Major Chest Trauma Age <70 w/o C.C.	.5921	6.0	4.6	19
85	4	MED	Pleural Effusion Age >69 and/or C.C.	1.1198	9.9	7.2	24
86	4	MED	Pleural Effusion Age <70 w/o C.C.	.9761	8.8	5.9	23
87	4	MED	Pulmonary Edema + Respiratory Failure	1.8078	10.2	7.0	24
88	4	MED	Chronic Obstructive Pulmonary Disease	1.0769	8.5	6.6	24
89	4	MED	Simple Pneumonia + Pleurisy Age >69 and/or C.C.	1.1768	9.6	7.5	25
90	4	MED	Simple Pneumonia + Pleurisy Age 18–69 w/o C.C.	.8800	7.7	6.2	22
91	4	MED	Simple Pneumonia + Pleurisy 0–17	.8216	5.7	4.4	19
92	4	MED	Interstitial Lung Disease Age >69 and/or C.C.	1.1117	9.0	6.8	24
93	4	MED	Interstitial Lung Disease Age <70 w/o C.C.	.8642	7.5	5.4	22
94	4	MED	Pneumothorax Age >69 and/or C.C.	1.3044	10.1	7.6	25
95	4	MED	Pneumothorax Age <70 w/o C.C.	.8797	7.8	5.9	23
96	4	MED	Bronchitis + Asthma Age >69 and/or C.C.	.8448	7.3	6.0	20
97	4	MED	Bronchitis + Asthma Age 18–69 w/o C.C.	.7092	6.2	5.1	17
98	4	MED	Bronchitis + Asthma Age 0–17	.7202	4.5	3.8	12
99	4	MED	Respiratory Signs + Symptoms age >69 and/or C.C.	.8078	6.4	4.6	22
100	4	MED	Respiratory Signs + Symptoms Age <70 w/o C.C.	.6255	5.0	3.6	16
101	4	MED	Other Respiratory System Diagnoses Age>69 and/or C.C.	.8461	7.5	5.5	23
102	4	MED	Other Respiratory System Diagnoses Age<70 w/o C.C.	.6843	6.1	4.3	21
103	5	SURG	Heart Transplant	.0000			
104	5	SURG	Cardiac Valve Procedure with Pump + with Cardiac Cath	7.3161	21.0	18.0	35
105	5	SURG	Cardiac Valve Procedure with Pump + w/o Cardiac Cath	6.3400	18.2	15.0	32
106	5	SURG	Coronary Bypass with Cardiac Cath	5.3332	16.3	14.7	32
107	5	SURG	Coronary Bypass w/o Cardiac Cath	4.6614	14.5	12.7	30
108	5	SURG	Other Cardiovascular or Thoracic Proc, with Pump	4.7810	14.7	10.6	28
109	5	SURG	Cardiothoracic Procedures w/o Pump	4.3597	14.7	9.0	26

*   Medicare data have been supplemented by data from Maryland and Michigan for low volume DRGs.

**   DRGs 469 and 470 contain cases which could not be assigned to valid DRGs.

Note: Geometric mean is used only to determine payment for outlier cases.
Note: Relative weights are based on Medicare patient data and may not be appropriate for other patients.
Note: Arithmetic mean included for comparative purposes. It is not used for payment.

Exhibit 1-1 (Continued)

DRG	MDC	Title	Relative Weights	Arithmetic Mean LOS	Geometric Mean LOS	Outlier Threshold
110	5 SURG	Major Reconstructive Vascular Proc w/o Pump Age >69 and/or C.C.	3.3215	16.4	13.1	30
111	5 SURG	Major Reconstructive Vascular Proc w/o Pump age <70 w/o C.C.	2.4581	13.1	11.2	28
112	5 SURG	Vascular Procedures Except Major Reconstruction w/o Pump	2.2239	11.8	8.1	25
113	5 SURG	Amputation For Circ System Disorders Except Upper Limb+Toe	2.5406	21.8	17.2	34
114	5 SURG	Upper Limb + Toe Amputation For Circ System Disorders	1.8946	17.2	12.4	29
115	5 SURG	Perm Cardiac Pacemaker Implant with AMI, Heart Failure or Shock	4.1634	16.6	13.9	31
116	5 SURG	Perm Cardiac Pacemaker Implant w/o AMI, Heart Failure or Shock	2.9709	9.6	7.8	25
117	5 SURG	Cardiac Pacemaker Replace + Revis Exc Pulse Gen Repl Only	1.4684	6.5	4.8	20
118	5 SURG	Cardiac Pacemaker Pulse Generator Replacement Only	1.8784	4.7	3.4	14
119	5 SURG	Vein Ligation + Stripping	.9165	7.7	5.6	23
120	5 SURG	Other Circulatory System O.R. Procedures	2.2580	17.0	11.4	28
121	5 MED	Circulatory Disorders with AMI + C.V. Comp. Disch. Alive	1.7694	12.4	10.3	27
122	5 MED	Circulatory Disorders w/o AMI + C.V. Comp. Disch. Alive	1.3270	10.6	8.8	26
123	5 MED	Circulatory Disorders with AMI, Expired	1.3525	5.6	3.0	20
124	5 MED	Circulatory Disorders Exc AMI, with Card Cath + Complex Diag	1.2553	7.1	5.0	22
125	5 MED	Circulatory Disorders Exc AMI, with Card Cath w/o Complex Diag	.7266	3.8	2.8	11
126	5 MED	Acute + Subacute Endocarditis	2.9840	23.8	18.1	35
127	5 MED	Heart Failure + Shock	1.0100	8.9	6.8	24
128	5 MED	Deep Vein Thrombophlebitis	.8456	9.9	8.6	24
129	5 MED	Cardiac Arrest, Unexplained	1.7200	7.9	3.8	21
130	5 MED	Peripheral Vascular Disorders Age >69 and/or C.C.	.8254	8.3	5.7	23
131	5 MED	Peripheral Vascular Disorders Age <70 w/o C.C.	.6712	6.7	4.5	22
132	5 MED	Atherosclerosis Age >69 and/or C.C.	.8040	7.0	5.3	22
133	5 MED	Atherosclerosis Age <70 w/o C.C.	.7050	5.2	3.8	16

DRG	MDC	Type	Description	Weight			
134	5	MED	Hypertension	.6365	6.6	5.1	20
135	5	MED	Cardiac Congenital + Valvular Disorders Age >69 and/or C.C.	.8936	7.3	5.3	22
136	5	MED	Cardiac Congenital + Valvular Disorders Age 18–69 w/o C.C.	.7526	5.6	3.8	18
137	5	MED	Cardiac Congenital + Valvular Disorders Age 0–17*	.6315		3.3	20
138	5	MED	Cardiac Arrhythmia + Conduction Disorders Age >69 and/or C.C.	.8138	6.5	4.9	21
139	5	MED	Cardiac Arrhythmia + Conduction Disorders Age <70 w/o C.C.	.6517	5.1	3.9	16
140	5	MED	Angina Pectoris	.6895	5.7	4.6	16
141	5	MED	Syncope + Collapse Age >69 and/or C.C.	.6188	5.7	4.4	18
142	5	MED	Syncope + Collapse Age <70 w/o C.C.	.5335	4.7	3.6	14
143	5	MED	Chest Pain	.5895	4.5	3.5	13
144	5	MED	Other Circulatory Diagnoses with C.C.	1.1158	8.4	6.2	23
145	5	MED	Other Circulatory Diagnoses w/o C.C.	.8477	7.1	5.0	22
146	6	SURG	Rectal Resection Age >69 and/or C.C.	3.0755	18.9	16.6	34
147	6	SURG	Rectal Resection Age <70 w/o C.C.	2.2737	15.6	14.0	31
148	6	SURG	Major Small + Large Bowel Procedure Age >69 and/or C.C.	2.9407	17.8	15.3	32
149	6	SURG	Major Small + Large Bowel Procedure Age <70 w/o C.C.	2.1072	14.3	12.6	30
150	6	SURG	Peritoneal Adhesiolysis Age >69 and/or C.C.	2.3428	14.9	12.8	30
151	6	SURG	Peritoneal Adhesiolysis Age <70 w/o C.C.	1.5902	11.5	10.1	27
152	6	SURG	Minor Small + Large Bowel Procedures Age >69 and/or C.C.	1.4069	10.8	8.6	26
153	6	SURG	Minor Small + Large Bowel Procedures Age <70 w/o C.C.	1.0993	9.1	7.3	24
154	6	SURG	Stomach, Esophageal + Duodenal Procedures Age >69 +/or C.C.	2.6880	15.1	11.5	25
155	6	SURG	Stomach, Esophageal + Duodenal Procedures Age 18–69 w/o C.C.	1.7906	11.7	8.9	26
156	6	SURG	Stomach, Esophageal + Duodenal Procedures Age 0–17*	.8382		6.0	20
157	6	SURG	Anal and Stomal Procedures Age >69 and/or C.C.	.7302	6.4	4.8	21
158	6	SURG	Anal and Stomal Procedures Age <70 w/o C.C.	.5513	4.9	3.9	14
159	6	SURG	Hernia Procedures Except Inguinal + Femoral Age >69 and/or C.C.	1.0000	7.8	6.3	22

* Medicare data have been supplemented by data from Maryland and Michigan for low volume DRGs.

** DRGs 469 and 470 contain cases which could not be assigned to valid DRGs.

Note: Geometric mean is used only to determine payment for outlier cases.

Note: Relative weights are based on Medicare patient data and may not be appropriate for other patients.

Note: Arithmetic mean included for comparative purposes. It is not used for payment.

Exhibit 1-1 *(Continued)*

DRG	MDC	Title	Relative Weights	Arithmetic Mean LOS	Geometric Mean LOS	Outlier Threshold
160	6 SURG	Hernia Procedures Except Inguinal + Femoral Age 18–69 w/o C.C.	.7457	5.9	5.0	16
161	6 SURG	Inguinal + Femoral Hernia Procedures Age >69 and/or C.C.	.6538	5.3	4.4	14
162	6 SURG	Inguinal + Femoral Hernia Procedures Age 18–69 w/o C.C.	.5264	4.1	3.6	10
163	6 SURG	Hernia Procedures Age 0–17	.9648	5.6	4.2	18
164	6 SURG	Appendectomy with Complicated Princ. Diag Age >69 +/or C.C.	2.0649	12.2	10.7	28
165	6 SURG	Appendectomy with Complicated Princ. Diag Age <70 w/o C.C.	1.4379	9.2	8.4	19
166	6 SURG	Appendectomy w/o Complicated Princ. Diag Age >69 +/or C.C.	1.3606	9.0	7.5	23
167	6 SURG	Appendectomy w/o Complicated Princ. Diag Age <70 w/o C.C.	.8855	6.0	5.3	13
168	6 SURG	Mouth Procedures Age >69 and/or C.C.	.9188	6.2	4.0	21
169	6 SURG	Mouth Procedures Age <70 w/o C.C.	.6585	4.0	3.0	12
170	6 SURG	Other Digestive System O.R. Procedures Age >69 and/or C.C.	2.7615	17.6	12.3	29
171	6 SURG	Other Digestive System O.R. Procedures Age <70 w/o C.C.	2.3305	15.4	9.8	27
172	6 MED	Digestive Malignancy Age >69 and/or C.C.	1.0749	10.4	6.7	24
173	6 MED	Digestive Malignancy Age <70 w/o C.C.	.9604	9.3	5.4	22
174	6 MED	G.I. Hemorrhage Age >69 and/or C.C.	.9075	7.5	5.8	23
175	6 MED	G.I. Hemorrhage Age <70 w/o C.C.	.7069	6.0	4.7	18
176	6 MED	Complicated Peptic Ulcer	.9318	8.3	6.3	23
177	6 MED	Uncomplicated Peptic Ulcer >69 and/or C.C.	.6617	6.6	5.4	18
178	6 MED	Uncomplicated Peptic Ulcer <70 w/o C.C.	.5556	5.5	4.6	15
179	6 MED	Inflammatory Bowel Disease	.9877	9.6	7.1	24
180	6 MED	G.I. Obstruction Age >69 and/or C.C.	.7584	7.4	5.4	22
181	6 MED	G.I. Obstruction Age <70 w/o C.C.	.5828	5.8	4.5	18
182	6 MED	Esophagitis, Gastroent. + Misc. Digest. Dis Age >69 and/or C.C.	.6034	6.1	4.8	18
183	6 MED	Esophagitis, Gastroent. + Misc. Digest. Dis Age 18–69 w/o C.C.	.5107	5.0	4.0	15
184	6 MED	Esophagitis, Grastroenteritis + Misc. Digest. Disorders Age 0–17	.4828	3.7	2.6	12
185	6 MED	Dental + Oral Dis. Exc Extractions + Restorations, Age >17	.7147	6.6	4.3	21
186	6 MED	Dental + Oral Dis. Exc Extractions + Restorations, Age 0–17*	.4112		2.9	11
187	6 MED	Dental Extractions + Restorations	.4211	2.9	2.3	7

DRG	MDC	Type	Description	Weight	Arith. Mean	Geom. Mean	Days
188	6	MED	Other Digestive System Diagnoses Age >69 and/or C.C.	.7173	6.4	4.3	21
189	6	MED	Other Digestive System Diagnoses Age 18–69 w/o C.C.	.5272	4.8	3.3	17
190	6	MED	Other Digestive System Diagnoses Age 0–17	.9178	6.1	4.3	21
191	7	SURG	Major Pancreas, Liver + Shunt Procedures	4.4608	22.0	18.1	35
192	7	SURG	Minor Pancreas, Liver + Shunt Procedures	4.0442	21.7	16.7	34
193	7	SURG	Biliary Tract Proc Exc Tot Cholecystectomy Age >69 +/or C.C.	2.8120	18.4	15.7	33
194	7	SURG	Biliary Tract Proc Exc Tot Cholecystectomy Age <70 w/o C.C.	2.1206	15.0	12.3	29
195	7	SURG	Total Cholecystectomy with C.D.E. Age >69 and/or C.C.	2.2727	14.6	13.1	30
196	7	SURG	Total Cholecystectomy with C.D.E. Age <70 w/o C.C.	1.5976	11.2	10.3	22
197	7	SURG	Total Cholecystectomy w/o C.D.E. Age >69 and/or C.C.	1.7058	11.9	10.5	27
198	7	SURG	Total Cholescystectomy w/o C.D.E. Age <70 w/o C.C.	1.1400	8.7	8.0	17
199	7	SURG	Hepatobiliary Diagnostic Procedure for Malignancy	2.3378	17.4	14.2	31
200	7	SURG	Hepatobiliary Diagnostic Procedure for Non–Malignancy	2.6286	15.8	10.9	28
201	7	SURG	Other Hepatobiliary or Pancreas O.R. Procedures	2.7130	16.1	10.4	27
202	7	MED	Cirrhosis + Alcoholic Hepatitis	1.1665	10.8	7.8	25
203	7	MED	Malignancy of Hepatobiliary System or Pancreas	1.0339	10.1	6.9	24
204	7	MED	Disorders of Pancreas Except Malignancy	.9703	8.2	6.5	24
205	7	MED	Disorders of Liver Exc Malig. Cirr, Alc Hepa Age >69 and/or C.C.	1.0720	9.5	6.7	24
206	7	MED	Disorders of Liver Exc Malig. Cirr, Alc Hepa Age <70 w/o C.C.	.7735	7.5	5.0	22
207	7	MED	Disorders of the Biliary Tract Age >69 and/or C.C.	.7775	7.0	5.4	22
208	7	MED	Disorders of the Biliary Tract Age <70 w/o C.C.	.5794	5.2	4.0	16
209	8	SURG	Major Joint and Limb Reattachment Procedures	2.3930	15.8	14.4	31
210	8	SURG	Hip + Femur Procedures Except Major Joint Age >69 and/or C.C.	2.0320	16.9	14.6	32
211	8	SURG	Hip + Femur Procedures Except Major Joint Age 18–69 w/o C.C.	1.7867	15.0	12.7	30
212	8	SURG	Hip + Femur Procedures Except Major Joint Age 0–17	1.6609	9.7	8.3	23

*   Medicare data have been supplemented by data from Maryland and Michigan for low volume DRGs.

**   DRGs 469 and 470 contain cases which could not be assigned to valid DRGs.

Note: Geometric mean is used only to determine payment for outlier cases.
Note: Relative weights are based on Medicare patient data and may not be appropriate for other patients.
Note: Arithmetic mean included for comparative purposes. It is not used for payment.

Exhibit 1-1 (*Continued*)

DRG	MDC		Title	Relative Weights	Arithmetic Mean LOS	Geometric Mean LOS	Outlier Threshold
213	8	SURG	Amputations for Musculoskeletal System + Conn. Tissue Disorders	1.9753	17.1	12.1	29
214	8	SURG	Back + Neck Procedures Age >69 and/or C.C.	1.8776	15.6	13.1	30
215	8	SURG	Back + Neck Procedures Age <70 w/o C.C.	1.4281	12.0	10.2	27
216	8	SURG	Biopsies of Musculoskeletal System + Connective Tissue	1.5566	13.7	8.9	26
217	8	SURG	Wnd Debrid + Skin Graft Hand, for Musculoskeletal + Connective Tissue Dis	2.3100	18.8	11.2	28
218	8	SURG	Lower Extrem + Humer Proc Exc Hip, Foot, Femur Age >69 and/or C.C.	1.3798	11.2	8.9	26
219	8	SURG	Lower Extrem + Humer Proc Exc Hip, Foot, Femur Age 18-69 w/o C.C.	1.0437	8.1	6.7	22
220	8	SURG	Lower Extrem + Humer Proc Exc Hip, Foot, Femur Age 0-17*	.9242	7.0	5.3	22
221	8	SURG	Knee Procedures Age >69 and/or C.C.	.9758	4.7	4.7	22
222	8	SURG	Knee Procedures Age <70 w/o C.C.	.7113	4.7	3.4	15
223	8	SURG	Upper Extremity Proc Exc Humerus + Hand Age >69 and/or C.C.	.9853	7.1	5.3	22
224	8	SURG	Upper Extremity Proc Exc Humerus + Hand Age <70 w/o C.C.	.7891	5.2	4.1	15
225	8	SURG	Foot Procedures	.6520	4.8	3.9	13
226	8	SURG	Soft Tissue Procedures Age >69 and/or C.C.	.9811	8.1	5.4	22
227	8	SURG	Soft Tissue Procedures Age <70 w/o C.C.	.6872	5.2	3.8	17
228	8	SURG	Ganglion (Hand) Procedures	.3661	2.3	1.9	5
229	8	SURG	Hand Procedures Except Ganglion	.6212	4.0	2.9	12
230	8	SURG	Local Excision + Removal of Int Fix Devices of Hip + Femur	1.0555	9.2	6.1	23
231	8	SURG	Local Excision + Removal of Int Fix Devices Except Hip + Femur	.7516	5.6	3.8	19
232	8	SURG	Arthroscopy	.6706	4.6	3.2	14
233	8	SURG	Other Musculoskeletal Sys + Conn Tiss O.R. Proc Age >69 and/or C.C.	1.3723	11.5	8.1	25
234	8	SURG	Other Musculoskelet Sys + Conn Tiss O.R. Proc Age <70 w/o C.C.	.9457	7.5	5.3	22
235	8	MED	Fractures of Femur	1.4137	17.9	10.1	27
236	8	MED	Fractures of Hip + Pelvis	1.0714	13.1	8.8	26

DRG	MDC	Type	Description	Weight	Arith Mean	Geom Mean	
237	8	MED	Sprains, Strains + Dislocations of Hip, Pelvis + Thigh	.6049	7.4	5.4	22
238	8	MED	Osteomyelitis	1.6470	15.8	11.1	28
239	8	MED	Pathological Fractures + Musculoskeletal + Conn Tiss. Malignancy	.9272	10.6	8.0	25
240	8	MED	Connective Tissue Disorders Age >69 and/or C.C.	.9049	9.5	7.3	24
241	8	MED	Connective Tissue Disorders <70 w/o C.C.	.7492	8.2	6.2	23
242	8	MED	Septic Arthritis	1.4562	13.5	9.7	27
243	8	MED	Medical Back Problems	.6843	8.0	6.2	23
244	8	MED	Bone Diseases + Specific Arthropathies Age >69 and/or C.C.	.6748	7.9	6.1	23
245	8	MED	Bone Diseases + Specific Arthropathies Age <70 w/o C.C.	.6407	6.7	5.1	22
246	8	MED	Non-Specific Arthropathies	.5936	6.9	5.4	21
247	8	MED	Signs + Symptoms of Musculoskeletal System + Conn Tissue	.5797	6.4	4.7	21
248	8	MED	Tendonitis, Myositis + Bursitis	.5892	6.3	4.8	20
249	8	MED	Aftercare, Musculoskeletal System + Connective Tissue	.7899	8.8	5.6	23
250	8	MED	Fx, Sprns, Strns + Disl of Forearm, Hand Foot Age >69 +/or C.C.	.5162	5.6	3.8	20
251	8	MED	Fx, Sprns, Strns + Disl of Forearm, Hand, Foot Age 18-69 w/o C.C.	.4004	3.5	2.5	11
252	8	MED	Fx, Sprns, Strns + Disl of Forearm, Hand, Foot Age 0-17*	.3496		1.8	7
253	8	MED	Fx, Sprns, Strns + Disl of Uparm, Lowleg Ex Foot Age >69 +/or C.C.	.6323	7.8	5.4	22
254	8	MED	Fx, Sprns, Strns + Disl of Uparm, Lowleg Ex Foot Age 18-69 w/o C.C.	.4931	5.8	4.0	20
255	8	MED	Fx, Sprns, Strns + Disl of Uparm, Lowleg Ex Foot Age 0-17*	.4638		2.9	15
256	8	MED	Other Diagnoses of Musculoskeletal System + Connective Tissue	.6993	7.2	4.9	22
257	9	SURG	Total Mastectomy for Malignancy Age >69 and/or C.C.	1.0634	8.7	7.8	19
258	9	SURG	Total Mastectomy for Malignancy Age <70 w/o C.C.	.9698	7.6	6.9	16
259	9	SURG	Subtotal Mastectomy for Malignancy Age >69 and/or C.C.	.8605	7.0	4.9	22
260	9	SURG	Subtotal Mastectomy for Malignancy Age <70 w/o C.C.	.6661	4.8	3.5	15
261	9	SURG	Breast Proc for Non-Malig Except Biopsy + Loc Exc	.6104	4.1	3.3	11
262	9	SURG	Breast Biopsy + Local Excision for Non-Malignancy	.4252	2.8	2.3	6

* Medicare data have been supplemented by data from Maryland and Michigan for low volume DRGs.

** DRGs 469 and 470 contain cases which could not be assigned to valid DRGs.

Note: Geometric mean is used only to determine payment for outlier cases.

Note: Relative weights are based on Medicare patient data and may not be appropriate for other patients.

Note: Arithmetic mean is included for comparative purposes. It is not used for payment.

Exhibit 1-1 *(Continued)*

DRG	MDC		Title	Relative Weights	Arithmetic Mean LOS	Geometric Mean LOS	Outlier Threshold
263	9	SURG	Skin–Grafts for Skin Ulcer or Cellulitis Age >69 and/or C.C.	2.4177	22.1	16.1	33
264	9	SURG	Skin–Grafts for Skin Ulcer or Cellulitis Age <70 w/o C.C.	2.1802	21.7	14.9	32
265	9	SURG	Skin–Grafts Except for Skin Ulcer or Cellulitis with C.C.	1.3993	11.6	7.6	25
266	9	SURG	Skin–Grafts Except for Skin Ulcer or Cellulitis w/o C.C.	.7313	6.1	4.0	21
267	9	SURG	Perianal + Pilonidal Procedures	.6362	5.4	4.0	17
268	9	SURG	Skin, Subcutaneous Tissue + Breast Plastic Procedures	.5690	3.9	2.8	12
269	9	SURG	Other Skin, Subcut Tiss + Breast O.R. Proc Age >69 +/or C.C.	1.1338	9.6	5.5	23
270	9	SURG	Other Skin, Subcut Tiss + Breast O.R. Proc Age <70 w/o C.C.	.7623	6.3	3.8	21
271	9	MED	Skin Ulcers	1.2609	14.1	10.1	27
272	9	MED	Major Skin Disorders Age >69 and/or C.C.	.8523	9.5	7.2	24
273	9	MED	Major Skin Disorders Age <70 w/o C.C.	.7972	9.4	6.5	24
274	9	MED	Malignant Breast Disorders Age >69 and/or C.C.	1.0368	10.9	7.0	24
275	9	MED	Malignant Breast Disorders Age <70 w/o C.C.	.9882	10.4	5.8	23
276	9	MED	Non-Malignant Breast Disorders	.5676	5.4	3.4	19
277	9	MED	Cellulitis Age >69 and/or C.C.	.8866	9.2	7.3	24
278	9	MED	Cellulitis Age 18–69 w/o C.C.	.7594	7.9	6.2	23
279	9	MED	Cellulitis Age 0–17*	.4739		4.2	13
280	9	MED	Trauma to the Skin, Subcut Tiss + Breast Age >69 and/or C.C.	.5417	6.4	4.6	22
281	9	MED	Trauma to the Skin, Subcut Tiss + Breast Age 18–69 w/o C.C.	.4468	4.8	3.4	16
282	9	MED	Trauma to the Skin, Subcut Tiss + Breast Age 0–17*	.3424		2.2	9
283	9	MED	Minor Skin Disorders Age >69 and/or C.C.	.6368	7.0	5.0	22
284	9	MED	Minor Skin Disorders Age <70 w/o C.C.	.5172	5.3	3.7	18
285	10	SURG	Amp of Lower limb for Endocrine, Nutritional + Metabolic Dis	3.2724	28.0	21.5	39
286	10	SURG	Adrenal + Pituitary Procedures	2.6731	15.8	13.3	30
287	10	SURG	Skin Grafts + Wound Debride for Endoc, Nutrit + Metab Dis	2.3781	21.5	15.7	33
288	10	SURG	O.R. Procedures for Obesity	2.1130	12.4	9.7	27
289	10	SURG	Parathyroid Procedures	1.3308	8.8	6.9	24
290	10	SURG	Thyroid Procedures	.8563	5.9	5.0	14
291	10	SURG	Thyroglossal Procedures	.6073	4.2	3.4	11

#	MDC	Type	Description	Rel. Wt.	Arith.	Geom.	Outlier
292	10	SURG	Other Endocrine, Nutrit + Metab O.R. Proc Age >69 +/or C.C.	2.3131	16.7	11.3	28
293	10	SURG	Other Endocrine, Nutrit + Metab O.R. Proc Age <70 w/o C.C.	1.7962	14.0	8.2	25
294	10	MED	Diabetes Age =>36	.7454	8.3	6.7	24
295	10	MED	Diabetes Age 0–35	.7886	6.7	5.0	22
296	10	MED	Nutritional + Misc Metabolic Disorders Age >69 and/or C.C.	.8271	8.3	6.1	23
297	10	MED	Nutritional + Misc Metabolic Disorders Age 18–69 w/o C.C.	.6998	7.0	4.9	22
298	10	MED	Nutritional + Misc Metabolic Disorders Age 0–17	.7202	5.3	3.3	18
299	10	MED	Inborn Errors of Metabolism	.8080	7.7	5.3	22
300	10	MED	Endocrine Disorders Age >69 and/or C.C.	.9349	9.2	6.9	24
301	10	MED	Endocrine Disorders Age <70 w/o C.C.	.6882	6.9	5.1	22
302	11	SURG	Kidney Transplant	4.6273	24.6	21.3	38
303	11	SURG	Kidney, Ureter + Major Bladder Procedure for Neoplasm	2.7610	16.6	14.2	31
304	11	SURG	Kidney, Ureter + Maj Bldr Proc for Non-Neopl Age >69 and/or C.C.	2.0323	13.5	10.8	28
305	11	SURG	Kidney, Ureter + Maj Bldr Proc for Non-Neopl Age <70 w/o C.C.	1.4894	10.4	8.4	25
306	11	SURG	Prostatectomy Age >69 and/or C.C.	1.2595	9.8	8.1	25
307	11	SURG	Prostatectomy Age <70 w/o C.C.	.9587	7.7	6.5	19
308	11	SURG	Minor Bladder Procedures Age >69 and/or C.C.	1.1490	8.8	6.1	23
309	11	SURG	Minor Bladder Procedures Age <70 w/o C.C.	.8665	6.7	4.7	22
310	11	SURG	Transurethral Procedures Age >69 and/or C.C.	.7266	5.6	4.3	17
311	11	SURG	Transurethral Procedures Age <70 w/o C.C.	.5563	4.1	3.3	11
312	11	SURG	Urethral Procedures, Age >69 and/or C.C.	.7308	5.8	4.4	18
313	11	SURG	Urethral Procedures, Age 18–69 w/o C.C.	.5936	4.7	3.5	14
314	11	SURG	Urethral Procedures, Age 0–17*	.4323		2.3	11
315	11	SURG	Other Kidney + Urinary Tract O.R. Procedures	2.7760	15.4	9.8	27
316	11	MED	Renal Failure	1.3212	10.0	6.4	23
317	11	MED	Admit for Renal Dialysis	.4907	3.4	2.3	10
318	11	MED	Kidney + Urinary Tract Neoplasms Age >69 and/or C.C.	.9231	8.8	5.5	23

* Medicare data have been supplemented by data from Maryland and Michigan for low volume DRGs.

** DRGs 469 and 470 contain cases which could not be assigned to valid DRGs.

Note: Geometric mean is used only to determine payment for outlier cases.
Note: Relative weights are based on Medicare patient data and may not be appropriate for other patients.
Note: Arithmetic mean included for comparative purposes. It is not used for payment.

Exhibit 1-1 *(Continued)*

DRG	MDC	Title	Relative Weights	Arithmetic Mean LOS	Geometric Mean LOS	Outlier Threshold
319	11 MED	Kidney + Urinary Tract Neoplasms Age <70 w/o C.C.	.7418	6.6	3.8	21
320	11 MED	Kidney + Urinary Tract Infections Age >69 and/or C.C.	.8629	8.2	6.5	24
321	11 MED	Kidney + Urinary Tract Infections Age 18–69 w/o C.C.	.6753	6.4	5.1	19
322	11 MED	Kidney + Urinary Tract Infections Age 0–17	.6998	6.4	5.2	19
323	11 MED	Urinary Stones Age >69 and/or C.C.	.5863	5.1	3.7	17
324	11 MED	Urinary Stones Age <70 w/o C.C.	.4098	3.6	2.8	11
325	11 MED	Kidney + Urinary Tract Signs + Symptoms Age >69 and/or C.C.	.6504	6.5	4.6	22
326	11 MED	Kidney + Urinary Tract Signs + Symptoms Age 18–69 w/o C.C.	.5159	4.9	3.5	16
327	11 MED	Kidney + Urinary Tract Signs + Symptoms Age 0–17	.5511	28.6	3.3	20
328	11 MED	Urethral Stricture Age >69 and/or C.C.	.5939	5.4	4.0	18
329	11 MED	Urethral Stricture Age 18–69 w/o C.C.	.4870	4.1	3.0	12
330	11 MED	Urethral Stricture Age 0–17*	.2788		1.6	5
331	11 MED	Other Kidney + Urinary Tract Diagnoses Age >69 and/or C.C.	.8333	7.6	5.4	22
332	11 MED	Other Kidney + Urinary Tract Diagnoses Age 18–69 w/o C.C.	.6740	6.0	4.1	21
333	11 MED	Other Kidney + Urinary Tract Diagnoses Age 0–17	.7915	5.9	3.7	21
334	12 SURG	Major Male Pelvic Procedures with C.C.	1.8038	13.5	12.3	28
335	12 SURG	Major Male Pelvic Procedures w/o C.C.	1.4644	11.9	11.0	23
336	12 SURG	Transurethral Prostatectomy Age >69 and/or C.C.	.9871	7.9	7.0	18
337	12 SURG	Transurethral Prostatectomy Age <70 w/o C.C.	.7788	6.3	5.8	12
338	12 SURG	Testes Procedures for Malignancy	.8907	7.3	4.9	22
339	12 SURG	Testes Procedures, Non–Malignant Age >17	.5766	4.4	3.4	12
340	12 SURG	Testes Procedures, Non–Malignant Age 0–17*	.4355		2.4	7
341	12 SURG	Penis Procedures	.9974	6.4	5.3	16
342	12 SURG	Circumcision Age >17	.4266	3.0	2.4	8
343	12 SURG	Circumcision Age 0–17*	.3788		1.7	4
344	12 SURG	Other Male Reproductive System O.R. Procedures for Malignancy	1.1216	8.3	6.3	23
345	12 SURG	Other Male Reproductive System O.R. Proc Except for Malig	.8196	6.5	4.8	22
346	12 MED	Malignancy, Male Reproductive System, Age >69 and/or C.C.	.8569	8.5	5.6	23

347	12	MED	Malignancy, Male Reproductive System, Age <70 w/o C.C.	.6441	5.9	3.7	21
348	12	MED	Benign Prostatic Hypertrophy Age >69 and/or C.C.	.6260	5.6	3.9	19
349	12	MED	Benign Prostatic Hypertrophy Age <70 w/o C.C.	.4854	3.9	2.9	12
350	12	MED	Inflammation of the Male Reproductive System	.6270	5.9	4.8	17
351	12	MED	Sterilization, Male	.3334	1.9	1.6	5
352	12	MED	Other Male Reproductive System Diagnoses	.5388	4.8	3.3	16
353	13	SURG	Pelvic Evisceration, Radical Hysterectomy + Vulvectomy	1.8818	14.0	10.8	28
354	13	SURG	Non-Radical Hysterectomy Age >69 and/or C.C.	1.2338	9.7	8.8	19
355	13	SURG	Non-Radical Hysterectomy Age <70 w/o C.C.	.9767	7.8	7.4	13
356	13	SURG	Female Reproductive System Reconstructive Procedures	.8511	7.7	7.0	15
357	13	SURG	Uterus + Adnexa Procedures for Malignancy	2.1101	14.9	12.3	29
358	13	SURG	Uterus + Adnexa Proc for Non-Malignancy Except Tubal Interrupt	1.1185	8.6	6.9	24
359	13	SURG	Incisional Tubal Interruption for Non-Malignancy	.5044	3.3	2.7	9
360	13	SURG	Vagina, Cervix + Vulva Procedures	.6055	4.8	3.4	16
361	13	SURG	Laparoscopy + Endoscopy (Female) Except Tubal Interruption	.7063	4.8	3.2	17
362	13	SURG	Laparoscopic Tubal Interruption	.3596	2.0	1.8	4
363	13	SURG	D+C, Conization + Radio-Implant, for Malignancy	.6176	4.9	3.6	15
364	13	SURG	D+C, Conization Except for Malignancy	.3922	2.8	2.3	7
365	13	SURG	Other Female Reproductive System O.R. Procedures	1.9086	14.0	10.9	28
366	13	MED	Malignancy, Female Reproductive System Age >69 and/or C.C.	.8626	8.4	4.9	22
367	13	MED	Malignancy, Female Reproductive System Age <70 w/o C.C.	.5354	4.7	2.8	16
368	13	MED	Infections, Female Reproductive System	.7610	7.8	5.9	23
369	13	MED	Menstrual + Other Female Reproductive System Disorders	.5498	5.6	3.9	20
370	14	SURG	Cesarean Section with C.C.	1.0856	7.9	7.1	16
371	14	SURG	Cesarean Section w/o C.C.	.7670	6.2	5.6	12
372	14	MED	Vaginal Delivery with Complicating Diagnoses	.5945	5.2	4.0	14
373	14	MED	Vaginal Delivery w/o Complicating Diagnoses	.3538	3.1	2.8	7
374	14	SURG	Vaginal Delivery with Sterilization and/or D+C	.5755	3.7	3.3	8

*   Medicare data have been supplemented by data from Maryland and Michigan for low volume DRGs.
** DRGs 469 and 470 contain cases which could not be assigned to valid DRGs.

Note: Geometric mean is used only to determine payment for outlier cases.
Note: Relative weights are based on Medicare patient data and may not be appropriate for other patients.
Note: Arithmetic mean included for comparative purposes. It is not used for payment.

Exhibit 1-1 (*Continued*)

DRG	MDC		Title	Relative Weights	Arithmetic Mean LOS	Geometric Mean LOS	Outlier Threshold
375	14	SURG	Vaginal Delivery with O.R. Proc Except Steril and/or D+C	.6817	4.9	4.4	15
376	14	MED	Postpartum + Postabortion Diagnoses w/o O.R. Procedure	.4523	4.3	3.3	16
377	14	SURG	Postpartum + Postabortion Diagnoses with O.R. Procedure	.7886	5.2	3.3	15
378	14	MED	Ectopic Pregnancy	.7358	2.6	4.3	14
379	14	MED	Threatened Abortion	.2409	2.8	1.9	8
380	14	MED	Abortion w/o D+C	.3609	2.8	1.9	9
381	14	MED	Abortion with D+C, Aspiration Curettage, or Hysterotomy	.3783	2.1	1.7	5
382	14	MED	False Labor	.1137	1.5	1.2	3
383	14	MED	Other Antepartum Diagnoses with Medical Complications	.4453	4.8	3.4	16
384	14	MED	Other Antepartum Diagnoses w/o Medical Complications	.4586	4.4	2.6	16
385	15		Neonates, Died or Transferred*	.6811		1.8	14
386	15		Extreme Immaturity or Respiratory Distress Syndrome, Neonate*	3.6480		17.9	35
387	15		Prematurity with Major Problems*	1.8267		13.3	30
388	15		Prematurity w/o Major Problems*	1.1571		8.6	26
389	15		Full Term Neonate with Major Problems*	.5425		4.7	16
390	15		Neonates with Other Significant Problems*	.3486		3.4	9
391	15		Normal Newborns*	.2218		3.1	7
392	16	SURG	Splenectomy Age >17	3.2494	17.3	13.7	31
393	16	SURG	Splenectomy Age 0-17*	1.5206		9.1	26
394	16	SURG	Other O.R. Procedures of Blood + Blood Forming Organs	1.0891	8.0	5.0	22
395	16	MED	Red Blood Cell Disorders Age >17	.7153	6.7	4.7	22
396	16	MED	Red Blood Cell Disorders Age 0-17	.2952	1.7	1.3	4
397	16	MED	Coagulation Disorders	.9971	8.4	5.9	23
398	16	MED	Reticuloendothelial + Immunity Disorders Age >69 and/or C.C.	.9753	8.1	5.5	23
399	16	MED	Reticuloendothelial + Immunity Disorders Age >70 w/o C.C.	.7247	6.4	4.2	21
400	17	SURG	Lymphoma or Leukemia with Major O.R. Procedure	2.6646	16.7	12.8	30
401	17	SURG	Lymphoma or Leukemia with Other O.R. Proc Age >69 and/or C.C.	1.5902	12.3	8.2	25

DRG	MDC	Type	Description	Rel. Wt.	Arith. Mean	Geom. Mean	Days
402	17	SURG	Lymphoma or Leukemia with Other O.R. Procedure Age <70 w/o C.C.	1.0555	8.2	5.6	23
403	17	MED	Lymphoma or Leukemia Age >69 and/or C.C.	1.3279	10.7	6.7	24
404	17	MED	Lymphoma or Leukemia Age 18–69 w/o C.C.	1.0449	8.4	5.0	22
405	17	MED	Lymphoma or Leukemia Age 0–17*	1.0407		4.9	22
406	17	SURG	Myeloprolif Disord or Poorly Diff Neopl W Maj O.R. Proc + C.C.	2.5307	16.8	12.9	30
407	17	SURG	Myeloprolif Disord or Poorly Diff Neopl W Maj O.R. Proc w/o C.C.	1.7127	13.0	8.6	26
408	17	SURG	Myeloprolif Disord or Poorly Diff Neopl W Other O.R. Proc	1.0502	8.3	5.3	22
409	17	MED	Radiotherapy	.9856	10.9	7.0	24
410	17	MED	Chemotherapy	.4285	3.1	2.4	9
411	17	MED	History of Malignancy w/o Endoscopy	.5907	5.9	3.8	21
412	17	MED	History of Malignancy with Endoscopy	.3389	2.4	1.9	6
413	17	MED	Othr Myeloprolif Disord or Poorly Diff Neopl DX Age >69 +/or C.C.	1.0457	10.7	6.9	24
414	17	MED	Othr Myeloprolif Disord or Poorly Diff Neopl DX Age <70 w/o C.C.	.8984	9.2	5.4	22
415	18	SURG	O.R. Procedure for Infectious + Parasitic Diseases	3.3292	20.5	14.7	32
416	18	MED	Septicemia Age >17	1.6183	11.7	8.3	25
417	18	MED	Septicemia Age 0–17*	1.1532	7.6	5.4	22
418	18	MED	Postoperative + Post–Traumatic Infections	1.0026	9.8	7.5	25
419	18	MED	Fever of Unknown Origin Age >69 and/or C.C.	.9306	8.4	6.1	23
420	18	MED	Fever of Unknown Origin Age 18–69 w/o C.C.	.8319	7.5	5.5	23
421	18	MED	Viral Illness Age >17	.5674	5.8	4.6	16
422	18	MED	Viral Illness + Fever of Unknown Origin Age 0–17	.6582	5.2	3.6	18
423	18	MED	Other Infectious + Parasitic Diseases Diagnoses	1.3207	11.0	8.0	25
424	18	MED	O.R. Procedures with Principal Diagnosis of Mental Illness	2.2112	22.1	15.0	32
425	19	MED	Acute Adjust React + Disturbances of Psychosocial Dysfunction	.6097	7.6	4.8	22
426	19	MED	Depressive Neuroses	.8330	11.8	7.8	25

*   Medicare data have been supplemented by data from Maryland and Michigan for low volume DRGs.

** DRGs 469 and 470 contain cases which could not be assigned to valid DRGs.

Note: Geometric mean is used only to determine payment for outlier cases.

Note: Relative weights are based on Medicare patient data and may not be appropriate for other patients.

Note: Arithmetic mean: included for comparative purposes. It is not used for payment.

Exhibit 1-1 *(Continued)*

DRG	MDC	Title	Relative Weights	Arithmetic Mean LOS	Geometric Mean LOS	Outlier Threshold
427	19 MED	Neuroses Except Depressive	.7019	9.8	6.4	23
428	19 MED	Disorders of Personality + Impulse Control	.8513	11.9	7.4	24
429	19 MED	Organic Disturbances + Mental Retardation	.8424	11.0	7.6	25
430	19 MED	Psychoses	1.0762	15.5	10.5	28
431	19 MED	Childhood Mental Disorders	.8495	10.4	5.6	24
432	19 MED	Other Diagnoses of Mental Disorders	.6969	8.1	4.9	22
433	20	Substance Use and Induced Organic Mental Disord, Left AMA	.3906	4.4	2.9	16
434	20	Subst Abuse, Intox Induce Mntl Syn Exc Depend and/or Other Sympt Trt	.7098	8.2	5.4	22
435	20	Subst Dependence, Detox +/or Other Symptomatic Treatment	.7980	10.2	6.7	24
436	20	Subst Dependence with Rehabilitation Therapy	1.0166	14.2	9.8	27
437	20	Subst Dependence, Combined Rehab and Detox Therapy	1.3276	19.0	14.6	32
438	20	No Longer Valid	.0000			
439	21 SURG	Skin Grafts for Injuries	1.7930	15.4	9.0	26
440	21 SURG	Wound Debridements for Injuries	2.0315	15.8	9.3	26
441	21 SURG	Hand Procedures for Injuries	.7305	4.6	2.7	16
442	21 SURG	Other O.R. Procedures for Injuries Age >69 and/or C.C.	1.8156	10.5	6.1	23
443	21 SURG	Other O.R. Procedures for Injuries <70 w/o C.C.	1.4872	9.4	5.6	23
444	21 MED	Multiple Trauma Age >69 and/or C.C.	.7074	7.7	5.4	22
445	21 MED	Multiple Trauma Age 18–69 w/o C.C.	.6015	6.2	4.1	21
446	21 MED	Multiple Trauma Age 0–17*	.4796		2.4	21
447	21 MED	Allergic Reactions Age >17	.4471	4.1	2.9	10
448	21 MED	Allergic Reactions Age 0–17*	.3470		2.9	14
449	21 MED	Poisoning and Toxic Effects of Drugs Age >69 and/or C.C.	.6954	6.5	4.7	9
450	21 MED	Poisoning and Toxic Effects of Drugs Age 18–69 w/o C.C.	.5422	5.1	3.3	22
451	21 MED	Poisoning and Toxic Effects of Drugs Age 0–17*	.5498	5.0	3.4	18
452	21 MED	Complications of Treatment Age >69 and/or C.C.	.8080	7.0	4.7	20
453	21 MED	Complications of Treatment Age >69 and/or C.C.	.7505	6.5	4.3	22
454	21 MED	Other Injuries, Poisonings + Toxic Eff Diag Age >69 +/or C.C.	.8098	7.5	4.6	21

DRG	MDC	Type	Description	Weight	Arith. Mean	Geom. Mean	Days
455	21	MED	Other Injuries, Poisonings + Toxic Eff Diag Age <70 w/o C.C.	.6003	6.0	3.5	21
456	22		Burns, Transferred to Another Acute Care Facility	1.8156	11.9	5.5	23
457	22		Extensive Burns	7.5688	22.0	8.8	26
458	22	SURG	Non-Extensive Burns with Skin Grafts	3.9455	26.0	18.9	36
459	22	SURG	Non-Extensive Burns with Wound Debridement + Other O.R. Proc	3.2662	20.8	13.5	31
460	22	MED	Non-Extensive Burns w/or O.R. Procedure	1.1595	11.2	7.5	25
461	23	SURG	O.R. Proc with Diag of other Contact with Health Services	1.3572	10.2	5.3	22
462	23	MED	Rehabilitation	2.1408	24.2	18.0	35
463	23	MED	Signs + Symptoms with C.C.	.7951	8.0	5.9	23
464	23	MED	Signs + Symptoms w/o C.C.	.6948	7.8	5.0	22
465	23	MED	Aftercare with History of Malignancy as Secondary DX	.2882	2.1	1.7	5
466	23	MED	Aftercare w/o History of Malignancy as Secondary DX	.4153	4.5	2.7	16
467	23	MED	Other Factors Influencing Health Status	.7223	7.9	3.9	21
468			Unrelated O.R. Procedure	2.4542	17.1	11.7	29
469			PDX Invalid as Discharge Diagnosis**	.0000			
470			Ungroupable**	.0000			
471	8	SURG	Bilat or Mult Maj Joint Procedures of the Lower Extremities	3.8994	23.5	20.9	38

* Medicare data have been supplemented by data from Maryland and Michigan for low volume DRGs.

** DRGs 469 and 470 contain cases which could not be assigned to valid DRGs.

Note: Geometric mean is used only to determine payment for outlier cases.

Note: Relative weights are based on Medicare patient data and may not be appropriate for other patients.

Note: Arithmetic mean included for comparative purposes. It is not used for payment.

Source: Federal Register. *Part III. Medicare Program; Changes to the Inpatient Hospital Prospective Payment System and Fiscal Year 1986 Rates; Final Rule.* 50(170): 35722–35735 (September 3), 1985.

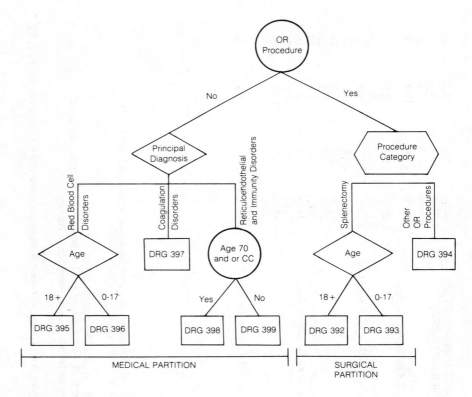

CC = Comorbidity and/or Complication

Exhibit 1-2   Example of Variables Used in DRG Assignment, i.e. Medical or Surgical Procedure/Age/Comorbidity and/or Complication

Major Diagnostic Category 16: Diseases and Disorders of the Blood and Blood-Forming Organs and Immunological Disorders

Source: New Jersey State Department of Health Decision Trees.

Effective Date and Transition Period

Application of the DRG payment rates (urban and rural) are phased in over a three-year transition period, starting with each hospital's first cost reporting period. During the transition period, a hospital's payment rate is a combination of the federal DRG payment rates and a hospital's historical costs. In addition, during the transition, the federal DRG portion of the rate is based on a combination of national rates and regional rates for each of the nine census regions of the country. During the first year of the program (FY 1984), 25 percent of the prospective payment is based on federal DRG rates and 75 percent is based on

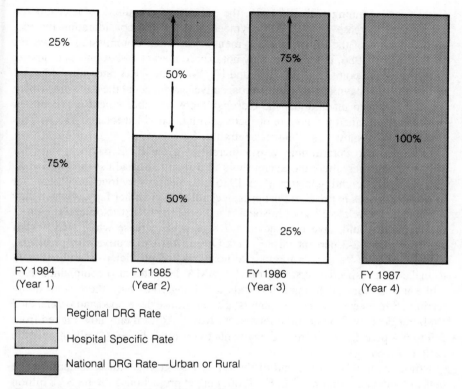

FY 1984 (Year 1)   FY 1985 (Year 2)   FY 1986 (Year 3)   FY 1987 (Year 4)

☐ Regional DRG Rate

▨ Hospital Specific Rate

▨ National DRG Rate—Urban or Rural

Exhibit 1-3 Transition Period for DRG Rates

each hospital's cost base. In year two (FY 1985), 50 percent of the payment is based on a combination of DRG rates and 50 percent is based on each hospital's cost base. In year three (FY 1986), 75 percent of the payment is based on federal DRG rates and 25 percent is based on each hospital's cost base. In year four (FY 1987), 100 percent of the payment is determined under the national DRG payment methodology (see Exhibit 1-3).

DRG Payment Levels and Updating

Payment rates for each DRG are derived from an average of historical (1981) Medicare cost data for each hospital. Rates were updated through FY 1983 by the estimated actual rate of increase in hospital costs nationally. By law, the rates were increased for FY 1984 by the estimated annual increase in a market basket index representing the cost of goods and services purchased by hospitals, plus one percentage point. For FY 1985, the rate of increase is by law the increase in the market basket plus one-quarter of a percentage point. For each fiscal year beginning with FY 1986, the Secretary is required to determine an appropriate increase in the DRG payments, taking into consideration the recommendations of the Prospective Payment Assessment Commission. However, by law, in FY 1986, the increase may not exceed market basket plus one-quarter of a percentage point. For FY 1984 and FY 1985, the DRG rates were adjusted so that the total payments under the prospective system equal the payments which would have been made under the reasonable cost reimbursement provisions of prior law, as limited by the rate of increase limits provided for in TEFRA. This requirement is known as "budget neutrality."

In addition to determining yearly increases in the DRG payment rates for FY 1986 and thereafter, the Secretary is also required to adjust the DRG classification and weighting factors in FY 1986 and at least every four years thereafter to reflect changes in treatment patterns, technology, and other factors which may not change the relative use of hospital resources. Using a strict interpretation of the formula would have resulted in a 7-8 percent increase while HCFA staff contemplated a 2-3 percent raise.[50] Jack Owen, AHA executive vice president, called the move "a slap in the face to hospitals and physicians who have tried to make the prospective system work."[51] AMA delegates also complained even while it was noted that some hospitals are doing fine, but others were doing terribly.[52] In reacting to the complaints, a compromise developed and was labeled "a fairer decision" by hospital representatives.[53] Adjustments now ranged from 5.9 to 6.4 percent and increased payments to hospitals by $300 million over the earlier percentages.[54]

However, this is not the end of the furor. Congress is still considering huge cuts in Medicare spending.[55] In FY 1986, budget projections look for $2.8 billion in Medicare reductions.[56] To counter these drastic measures, the AHA mobilized a coalition of 39 diverse groups representing hospitals, physicians, the elderly, labor, business, and local governments. Every member of Congress will be alerted to the severe cost containment proposals and urged to hold the line on the programs to avoid sacrifices.[57] These sacrifices could affect specific populations and services such as intensive care units (ICUs),[58-60] clincial laboratories,[61-62] burn centers,[63] and anesthesia services.[64] Even patients could be affected financially. Court decisions required a man treated for two days for a migraine headache in a New Jersey hospital to pay the full DRG price of $1,400 rather than the actual cost of $1,100.[65]

Governmental efforts to contain costs even further are bolstered by studies such as a U.S. Government Accounting Office (GAO) investigation of respiratory therapy reimbursement rates. This 1984 study of 33 hospitals found that unallowable and inappropriate costs were included in the initial DRG rate calculation and added about $2.5 million in overstated costs. As the study notes, "As a result, the average DRG rates are inflated and hospitals are being paid more than intended under the prospective payment methodology. Furthermore, they will continue to be overpaid until appropriate adjustments are made."[66]

Additional Payment Amounts

In addition to the prospective payment rates per discharge, additional Medicare payments will be made for the following items or services.

Outliers

Extra monies will be paid to hospitals for atypical cases (known as "outliers") which have either extremely long lengths of stay or extraordinarily high costs compared to most discharges classified in the same DRG. Legislation requires that total outlier payments to all hospitals represent no less than 5 percent and no more than 6 percent of the total estimated Medicare prospective payments for the fiscal year. The Health Care Financing Administration (HCFA) has reduced the amount of funds available for outlier payments from 6 percent of total hospital payments in FY 1984 to 5 percent in FY 1985. Effective with discharges occurring on or after October 1, 1984, a transferring hospital may qualify for an additional payment for extraordinary high cost cases meeting the criteria for cost outliers.

Hospitals report that outlier payments do not prevent some of them from incurring tremendous losses under PPS. Hillcrest Medical Center, Tulsa, Oklahoma, detailed eight cases in which the net loss per case was more than $45,000. This occurred during the hospital's initial six months under the federal PPS.[67] Dallas-Fort Worth Medical Center, Grand Prairie, Texas, had the largest single loss under the DRG program in 1984. A 71-year-old man attempted suicide after being told that he had bladder cancer. After performing a splenectomy necessitated by the gunshot wound, five additional operations took place with the patient spending 65 days in the ICU and dying of pneumonia after 71 days at the hospital. Charges for care amounted to $165,000 and Medicare reimbursed the hospital $8,900—a total loss of $156,100. A HCFA analyst "knows of no contingencies in the PPS that could have prevented such a large loss." Ironically, an autopsy proved that the patient did not have bladder cancer.[68]

Hughes cites two cases: one cost the rural hospital $96,353.18 and the other $9,620,69. Both patients had comorbid conditions and suffered unanticipated complications. Nevertheless the DRG payment left the hospital with more than $100,000 in losses.[69]

According to an expert in hospital administration, "Illinois hospitals will lose $200 million a year after Medicare reimbursement based on standard national rates is fully implemented in October 1986."[70]

Obviously these examples could be repeated and gathered for both losers and winners. However, pessimistic predictors appear to outweigh optimists. Eli Ginzberg, a noted economist, projected that "over the next decade, 40 to 50 percent of the hospitals in this country are going to disappear." He made that statement at a December 1982 symposium sponsored by Blue Cross and Blue Shield of Illinois.[71]

In response to the threat of losses from the Medicare PPS, Lloyds of London began to offer DRG outlier insurance to U.S. hospitals on January 1, 1985. Only outliers are covered and the policy seeks "to help a hospital protect its budget, its profitability, and its balance sheet."[72] A Minneapolis company, NorthStar/BeneCorp, Inc., also joined in offering DRG insurance later in the year.[73]

Indirect Medical Education Costs

Hospitals secure additional payments for the indirect costs attributable to approved medical education programs. These indirect costs may be due to a variety of factors, including the extra demands placed on the hospital staff as a result of the teaching activity or additional tests and procedures that may be ordered by residents. Indirect medical education payments also account for factors not necessarily related to medical education which may increase costs in teaching hospitals. Under PPS, the additional payment to a hospital equals twice the factor used to adjust the cost of limits which were applied under Medicare's former cost-based method of reimbursement to hospitals. This results in an 11.59 percent increase to the federal portion of the hospital's DRG payments for each 0.1 increase (above zero) in the ratio of the hospital's number of full-time equivalent interns and residents to its number of beds.

Payments on Reasonable Cost

Costs for certain items are excluded from the prospective payment system rates. Medicare will pay for its share of the following such costs separately from the DRG payment system using the former reasonable cost-based system.

Capital-related costs.   Capital-related costs (including depreciation, leases and rentals, interest, and a return on equity for proprietary hospitals) are excluded until October 1, 1986, and are paid for on a reasonable cost basis. The Secretary is required to report to Congress within 18 months of enactment on methods and proprosals by which capital costs can be included in the prospective payment rates. This report has not yet been submitted. Medicare payment for capital costs is prohibited after September 30, 1986, unless a state has a capital expenditure review agreement with the Secretary (under Section 1122 of the Social Security Act) and the state has recommended approval of the specific expenditure.

Direct medical education costs.   Direct costs of approved medical education programs (such as salaries for residents and teachers, classroom costs) are reimbursed on a reasonable cost basis. Such programs include the training of physicians, nurses, and paraprofessionals. They may not include on-the-job training, patient education, community health awareness programs, or the costs of interns and residents hired to replace anesthetists.

Physicians in teaching hospitals. If a teaching hospital so elects, the direct medical and surgical services of physicians in such hospitals will be excluded from the prospective payment system and paid for on the basis of reasonable costs.

Kidney acquisition costs. Estimated net expenses associated with kidney acquisition in certified renal transplantation centers are excluded. Prospective payments to a hospital are adjusted in each reporting period to compensate for the reasonable expenses of kidney acquisition.

Services of hospital-employed nonphysician anesthetists. For the cost reporting period beginning on or after October 1, 1984, and before October 1, 1987, the costs of anesthesia services provided by qualified nonphysician anesthetists employed by the hospital or obtained under arrangements are excluded and are paid for on the basis of reasonable costs.

Bad debts of Medicare beneficiaries. An additional payment is made to hospitals for bad debts attributable to deductible and coinsurance amounts related to covered services received by Medicare beneficiaries.

ESRD beneficiary discharges. Effective with cost reporting periods beginning on or after October 1, 1984, additional payments are made to hospitals for inpatient dialysis provided to End Stage Renal Disease (ESRD) beneficiary discharges. A hospital meeting the criteria is paid an additional payment for each ESRD beneficiary discharge based on the estimated weekly cost of dialysis and the average length of stay of ESRD beneficiaries for the hospital.

Special Treatment of Certain Facilities

Certain exceptions and adjustments to the prospective payment rates are provided as follows:

Sole Community Hospitals (SCHs)

A special payment formula applies to hospitals that are the sole source of inpatient services reasonably available in a geographic area (by reason of factors such as isolated location, weather conditions, travel conditions, or absence of other hospitals). SCHs will be paid indefinitely on the same basis as all other hospitals are paid in the first year of the transition period: 25 percent of the payment will be based on regional DRG rates and 75 percent on each hospital's cost base.

During the transition period, SCHs may also receive an additional payment amount if, due to circumstances beyond their control, they experience a decrease of more than 5 percent in their number of inpatient cases.

Cancer Hospitals

Provisions are made for exceptions and adjustments to the prospective payment amounts appropriate for hospitals involved extensively in treatment for and research on cancer. Regulations define a cancer hospital as one which (1) was recognized by the National Cancer Institute as a comprehensive cancer center or a clinical cancer research center as of April 20, 1983; (2) demonstrates that the entire facility is organized primarily for treatment of and research on cancer; and (3) has a patient population such that at least 50 percent of the hospital's total discharges have a principal diagnosis that reflects a finding of neoplastic disease. Cancer hospitals meeting these criteria will be paid on a reasonable cost basis.

Regional and National Referral Centers

Provisions are made for exceptions and adjustments appropriate for regional and national referral centers (including those with 500 or more beds located in rural areas). Regulations define such hospitals as: (1) rural hospitals having 500 or more beds; (2) hospitals having at least 50 percent of their Medicare patients referred from other hospitals or from physicians not on the hospital's staff, at least 60 percent of their Medicare patients residing more than 25 miles from the hospital, and at least 60 percent of the services furnished to Medicare beneficiaries who live 25 miles or more from the hospital; or (3) for hospital discharges occurring on or after October 1, 1984, rural hospitals meeting the following criteria: (a) a case-mix index threshold (for example, at least 1.03 in 1981) and (b) a minimum number of discharges (for example, 6,000 for the hospital's cost reporting period ending in 1981). In addition to criteria (3) (a) and (b), hospitals must meet at least one of the following three criteria: (c) more than 50 percent of the hospital's medical staff are specialists; (d) at least 60 percent of discharges are for inpatients who reside more than 25 miles from the hospital; or (e) at least 40 percent of inpatients treated at the hospital have been referred either from physicians not on the hospital's staff or from other hospitals. Hospitals meeting criterion (1) will be paid prospective payments based on the applicable urban payment rates rather than the rural rates, as adjusted by the hospital's area wage index. Beginning with cost reporting periods after October 1, 1984, rural hospitals meeting criterion (2) and hospitals meeting criterion (3) will also be paid prospective payments based on the applicable urban payment rates, as adjusted by the hospital's wage index.

Public or Other Hospitals with Many Low Income Patients or Medicare Beneficiaries

Authorizations provide for exceptions and adjustments to the prospective payment rates to take into account the needs of hospitals that serve a significantly disproportionate number of low-income patients or Medicare beneficiaries. Currently, HCFA has not provided for such an adjustment. Prior to December 31, 1984, the Secretary is required to define and identify such hospitals.

Rural and Urban Facility Differentials

Beginning with the assumption that labor and supplies cost less in rural areas than in urban areas, the federal government designated lower DRG reimbursement rates on that basis. Exhibit 1-4 indicates the nine geographic regions for the United States and the states in each region. Then, each of the nine regions has a designated labor-related and nonlabor-related DRG rate broken down by urban and rural designations. In addition, a national rate is also listed since the PPS is to use only that national rate after the four year phase-in period. In each instance, the rural reimbursement rate is lower.[74]

With the inception of the urban/rural classification, the American Hospital Association warned that geographic anomalies resulted in unfair treatment for many hospitals.[75] Even before the initiation of the federal PPS, Wennberg explored the geographic inequities that resulted in ignoring local hospital markets in cost containment activities. In the state of Massachusetts, Wennberg found 69 hospital markets but only 14 counties geographically identified. On top of that, the boundaries differed greatly with most counties containing multiple hospital markets. For example, Boston and Cambridge hospital markets are contiguous but are geographically separated by the Charles River and are in different counties. Actual per capita expenditures for Medicare inpatient hospital care in 1976 was estimated at $746 in Cambridge (Middlesex County) and at $923 in Boston (Suffolk County). Using a countywide reimbursement rate, Cambridge would get $680 ($-$66) and Boston $916 ($-$7). Using a statewide reimbursement rate of $657, Cambridge would get $89 less than the per capita estimate while Boston would get $266 less. Considering that residents of either hospital market simply could walk across a bridge, the geographic reimbursement inequity clearly shows that low cost market areas may subsidize high cost hospital market areas.[76] As the chairman of the American Small and Rural Hospital Association remarked, "Something is wrong with the idea that just because we're in a rural setting we should get less money."[77]

At a 1984 annual meeting of the AMA, Free, a physician from Indiana, claimed that "arbitrary discrimination against rural hospitals could force many to close."[78] A call was made to collect data and to seek regulatory changes to insure that

Exhibit 1-4   Adjusted Standardized Labor/Nonlabor DRG Rates by Urban/Rural
Designations

Region	Urban		Rural	
	Labor related	Nonlabor related	Labor related	Nonlabor related
1. New England (CT, ME, MA, NH, RI, VT)......................	2361.23	668.56	2132.35	507.22
2. Middle Atlantic (PA, NJ, NY)....	2217.30	660.71	2166.25	514.40
3. South Atlantic (DE, DC, FL, GA, MD, NC, SC, VA, WV)	2354.76	612.14	1987.52	427.03
4. East North Central (IL, IN, MI, OH, WI)......................	2435.73	712.68	1971.73	478.79
5. East South Central (AL, KY, MS, TN).........................	2235.04	544.16	1977.12	399.85
6. West North Central (IA, KS, MN, MO, NB, ND, SD)	2260.57	633.09	1836.34	410.83
7. West South Central (AR, LA, OK, TX)......................	2307.62	599.67	1853.44	398.47
8. Mountain (AZ, CO, ID, MT, NV, NM, UT, WY)	2203.70	634.49	1819.46	445.73
9. Pacific (AK, CA, HI, OR, WA)...	2208.57	745.34	1828.74	521.49
10. National.....................	2308.29	664.16	1920.46	437.97

Source: Federal Register. *Part III. Medicare Program. Changes to Inpatient Hospital Prospective Payment System and Fiscal Year 1986 Rates; Final Rule.* 50(170): 35715 (September 3), 1985.

DRG payments are based on "true differences in the costs of providing services by those hospitals rather than an arbitrary geographic criteria."[79] An article in the *Ohio State Medical Journal* noted that more than a third of the hospitals in Ohio—72 institutions—lie in designated rural counties, which definitely creates an urban/rural problem. One hospital, just 300 yards away from an urban designation, estimates receiving an average of $1,000 less per DRG when the national urban/rural rates are phased in in 1987—a total of $3 million less due to the rural classification.[80] In Iowa, urban hospitals get 5 percent more for labor costs and 54 percent more for nonlabor costs than rural hospitals.[81] Albert Speth, president of Lock Haven Hospital (PA) put it succinctly, "If I had a jack, and could move my hospital seven miles, I could get $600 more a case."[82]

In response to the criticisms of the urban/rural differentials, HHS proposed to study the situation in mid-1984 and to recommend adjustments. Wage indexes were to include attention to full- and part-time employees in recalculations. Secretary Heckler noted that 49 counties changed from urban to rural as a result of the 1980 census.[83] Almost a year later to the day, HHS released a study on urban/rural labor costs, but without recommendations.[84] Although the report is considered favorable to rural hospitals, many urban hospitals would be losers.

About half of the rural hospitals should be getting more money while the other half should remain constant. Since the report was ordered by Congress in the Deficit Reduction Act of 1984 and specified retroactivity to October 1, 1983, there could be a considerable financial impact on many hospitals. Incidentally, the HHS report was eight months overdue.[85]

Rural and urban classification lawsuit.   On February 17, 1984, eleven hospitals in Ohio sued the federal government seeking to redress the undue penalty imposed upon rural hospitals by PPS classifications. Taking legal action in U.S. District Court, the hospitals charged that the urban/rural classifications are "arbitrary and bear no rational relationship to health care or to health care costs."[86] Furthermore, the suing hospitals argue that the government's procedures are unconstitutional and invalid. Lawyers contend that the PPS regulations "violate the Fifth Amendment to the U.S. Constitution because the boundary classifications amount to the taking of private property without just compensation."[87]

In late September 1984, the federal court decided that jurisdiction exists and ruled that the Ohio hospitals had no basis to challenge the constitutionality of the urban/rural classification system. In fact, the court held that Congress did have a reasonable basis for the setting up of the distinction.[88] An appeal will be made by the Ohio hospitals. An AHA official found importance in the jurisdictional and constitutional issues: "If the appellate court upholds the decision that federal court jurisdiction exists over PPS-related constitutional matters, providers will have a direct avenue for judicial review and no longer will hospitals need to exhaust the administrative appeals process in similar matters."[89]

Congressional pressure.   Members of Congress, particularly those members with a large rural population, have been receiving reports about the inequities of the urban/rural designations. At one hearing in early 1984, Representative Marty Russo (D-IL) urged that data be collected to justify repairing the PPS.[90] Representative Robert Matsui (D-CA) proposed a one-year delay in the transition phasing to consider refinements.[91] Both a senator and a representative from Indiana were persuaded to introduce bills to remedy the plight of rural hospitals.[92] In March 1985, the *Congressional Record* reported on rural hospitals getting the short end of the DRG stick. Legislators from Iowa, Kansas, Nebraska, and Texas told Congress about the letters from their constituents complaining about DRG payments to rural hospitals. At least 22 Congressmen also blasted HCFA for stalling on the adjustment of rural labor-related wage indexes. As noted earlier, HCFA released its report two months after the Congressional call for it.

Continuing the political pressure, the Select Committee on Aging's Task Force on the Rural Elderly held hearings on February 26, 1985. Earlier, the U.S. GAO conducted studies for Congress that found early discharges and a lack of aftercare services in rural areas.[93] In addition to "horror stories," the Task Force heard first-hand about the problems of rural hospitals. Ben C. White, administrator of a 42-bed hospital in Purcell, Oklahoma, told the legislators that his hospital does good, but finds "it increasingly difficult to do well."[94] He also stated that personnel and supplies don't cost less in rural areas and may even cost more. In closing, White said, "It is difficult to comprehend how lower payment to the rural provider can be justified unless the intent is to force the demise of the rural hospital." Several Congressmen also "complained that HCFA had targeted rural hospitals for extinction."[95] An HCFA official responded: "Medicare's swing-bed provisions and special DRG rules for sole community and rural referral hospitals protected rural communities."[96]

In keeping with the inequities theme and the need to rectify the situation, the Select Committee on Aging released a study of 39 ombudsmen in a state-by-state survey on long-term care for the elderly. Their report concluded: "It is clear that rural areas have more severe problems than urban settings."[97]

Hospitals Excluded from the Prospective Payment System

By law, the following hospitals are excluded from the prospective payment system and will be paid on the basis of reasonable costs, subject to the TEFRA rate of increase limits:

- Psychiatric hospitals

- Rehabilitation hospitals

- Psychiatric or rehabilitation units which are distinct parts of a hospital

- Alcohol and drug hospitals or distinct units of hospitals, until October 1, 1986

- Children's hospitals with patients averaging under 18 years of age

- Long-term hospitals with an average inpatient length of stay greater than 25 days

- Hospitals outside the 50 states and the District of Columbia.

Hospitals reimbursed under approved state cost control systems are also excluded from the prospective rates. In addition, the regulations indicate that there are special cases where the prospective payment system is inappropriate and will not be applied, such as for emergency services provided to Medicare beneficiaries in hospitals not participating in Medicare, and in Veterans Administration hospital services provided to Medicare beneficiaries who belong to health maintenance organizations or competitive medical plans. Such organizations may choose to have the Secretary pay hospitals directly for such services or may negotiate their own rates with hospitals.

Administrative and Judicial Review

Administrative and judicial appeals are allowed under procedures and authorities already established under the Medicare program. However, P.L. 98-21 precludes administrative and judicial review of the "budget neutrality" adjustment, and the DRG payment amounts, including the establishment of DRGs, the methodology for classifying discharges within DRGs, and the DRG weighting factors.

Review Activities

P.L. 97-248, (TEFRA) replaced existing Professional Standards Review Organizations (PSRO) with a utilization and quality control peer review program. HHS was required to enter into performance-based contracts with physician-sponsored or physician-access organizations known as peer review organizations (PROs) by late 1984. As a condition of receiving payments under the new prospective payment system, P.L. 98-21 required hospitals to enter into an agreement with a PRO under which the PRO will review the validity of diagnostic information provided by the hospitals; the completeness, adequacy, and quality of care provided; the appropriateness of admissions and discharges; and the appropriateness of care provided to patients designated by hospitals as outliers. Final regulations firmly set the regulatory power of PROs.

In addition, a super PRO will review the work of the state PROs. In addition to the PRO activities, HCFA was required by TEFRA to establish a hospital admissions pattern monitoring plan. If HCFA or a PRO determine that a hospital is engaged in unacceptable admissions, medical, or other practices, HCFA may deny Medicare payments to the hospital or may require the hospital to take corrective action.

Nonphysician Services Furnished to Hospital Inpatients

Prior to P.L. 98-21, payments for nonphysician services (in such areas as radiology, laboratory, physical therapy, prosthetics) were made sometimes to the hospital under Part A of Medicare on a reasonable cost basis and sometimes to an outside supplier of the service under Part B on the basis of reasonable charges. This practice of billing for services provided to hospital inpatients has been known as the "unbundling" of Part A services. P.L. 98-21 provides that all hospitals participating in the Medicare program (including those under prospective payment, excluded hospitals, and those reimbursed as demonstrations or state cost control systems) will be paid for all nonphysician services provided to hospital inpatients only as hospital services under Part A.

HHS has authority to waive this requirement during the transition period to allow billing under Part B for hospitals that had such extensive billings under Part B prior to October 1, 1982 that compliance with the new requirement would threaten the stability of patient care. The January 3, 1984 regulations provided for an exception to the "unbundling" requirement for the inpatient hospital services of anesthetists, such as certified registered nurse anesthetists (CRNAs). For hospital cost reporting periods beginning before October 1, 1986, if a physician (usually an anesthesiologist) employed CRNAs on the last day of the hospital's most recent cost reporting period ending before September 1, 1983, then the physician could continue to bill the Medicare program for the CRNAs' services under Part B of Medicare. If the physician chooses to continue such Part B billing during the transition period, the hospital may not add the costs of the CRNAs' services to its base period costs for purposes of determining the hospital-specific portion of its DRG system rates. In addition, effective with cost reporting periods beginning October 1, 1984, and before October 1, 1987, the costs of anesthesia services provided by qualified nonphysician anesthetists (CRNAs and anesthesiology assistants) employed by hospitals or obtained under arrangements are removed from the prospective payments, to be reimbursed on the basis of reasonable costs.

State Waivers

Section 1886(c) of the Social Security Act (as added by TEFRA) authorized discretion to the HHS Secretary to reimburse hospitals in a state according to the state's hospital reimbursement control system, rather than according to Medicare's prospective payment system, if the state requests this change and if HHS determines that the state system meets certain requirements. Four states had waivers to operate their own systems: Maryland, Massachusetts, New Jersey, and New York. Both New York and Massachusetts now come under the federal plan, leaving only two states with waivers.

P.L. 98-21 added several more requirements for state systems: provisions related to reimbursement of health maintenance organizations or competitive medical plans, charges to Medicare beneficiaries for payment amounts denied by the Medicare program because of improper hospital admissions or medical practices, and nonphysician services provided to hospital inpatients from payment under Part B of Medicare. HHS Secretary is prohibited from denying a state waiver because the state's system is based on a payment methodology other than

DRGs or from requiring that Medicare expenditures under the state's system be less than the expenditures which would have been made under the federal prospective payment system. The Secretary is *required* to approve any state system which meets certain requirements in addition to the conditions mentioned above. The Secretary is required to respond within 60 days to waiver requests from states meeting all requirements.

P.L. 98-369 (the Deficit Reduction Act of 1984) requires proposed regulations implementing Section 1886(c) to be published by July 1, 1984, and final regulations by October 1, 1984. Regulations were published in May 1985.

Prospective Payment Assessment Commission

P.L. 98-21 requires the director of the Congressional Office of Technology Assessment (OTA) to appoint by April 1, 1984 a commission of 15 independent experts, known as the Prospective Payment Assessment Commission. The commission is required to review the percentage increase used to update the DRG payment rates for FY 1984 and FY 1985 and make recommendations to the Secretary on the appropriate percentage change for fiscal years beginning with FY 1986. In addition, the commission must: (1) consult with and make recommendations to the Secretary on the need for adjustments to the DRG classifications, the methodology for classifying specific hospital discharges within the DRGs, and weighting factors for the DRGs, and (2) report to Congress its evaluation of any adjustments which the Secretary makes.

Fifteen ProPAC members are appointed by the Director of the Congressional Office of Technology Assessment and the commission is considered part of the OTA. Dr. Stuart H. Altman, Dean of the Florence Heller School for Advanced Studies in Social Welfare, Brandeis University, was chosen to chair ProPAC. Other members included experts from hospital administration, nursing, a state rate setting agency, an insurance company, private practice physicians, a proprietary hospital chain, organized labor, medical schools, and a hospital supply firm. These experts are skilled in technological and scientific research, biomedical investigation, and health care system development.[98]

It is apparent that ProPAC will need to collect a great deal of data to evaluate "the safety, efficiency and cost effectiveness of new and existing medical and surgical procedures."[99] This task appears overwhelming and ProPAC will need the cooperation of all concerned parties to do its job.

In addition, it is important to understand that "the Secretary is not bound" by the recommendations of ProPAC.[100] However, on a practical basis, ProPAC is an extension of Congress under jurisdiction of OTA and the Secretary will obviously weigh ProPAC's advice carefully.

ProPAC held its first meeting on December 19, 1983 and the commission met an additional seven times over the next year. In an appearance before ProPAC, Dr. Carolyne Davis, HCFA Administrator, stated that her agency would work closely with ProPAC. She also predicted that ProPAC would be "the most watched—and probably the most lobbied—group in town."[101] Dr. Altman's comments are also enlightening: "I want to see DRGs work: they represent an important and needed change, but it's a payment approach that needs to be administered with a degree of flexibility and wisdom or it will end up being worse than the existing system."[102]

Dr. Altman's remarks reflect the Congressional intent to appraise the workings of the DRG system in the real world and to suggest adjustments that need to be made. However, Dr. David Banta, a physician OTA staff person, viewed ProPAC "as a tool for considering social goals and use of technology."[103] In either case, Dr. Altman repeatedly urged all interested parties to submit objective data to the Commission.[104,105] He stated, "My role isn't to be anti or pro (health care) industry."[106]

In an interview in *Hospitals,* Dr. Altman emphasized that ProPAC had no final authority and only recommends to the Secretary. After receiving the commission's charges, Dr. Altman commented that "the most important thing we have to do is to be a truly honest broker."[107] He then goes on to explain that ProPAC needs to operate as a "surrogate for the competitive marketplace,"[108] reacting to the ups and downs and keeping the health care system in tune with the changes. A headline in an article cited Altman as saying that PPS needs an overhaul to survive.[109]

To attack the tasks, three subcommittees were appointed to investigate specific issues. Each committee met separately and did their own research into the matters. Subcommittees covered the following areas:

- Data Development and Research

- Hospital Productivity and Cost Effectiveness

- Diagnostic and Therapeutic Practices

In February 1984, ProPAC appointed Dr. Donald Young as the executive director of the statutory limit of a 25-member staff. Prior to this, Dr. Young, a physician, was deputy director of the Bureau of Eligibility, Reimbursement and Coverage for HCFA. In an interview in *Hospitals,* Dr. Young reiterated Pro-PAC's tasks and noted that early recommendations would probably stress incremental change. He also stated that the first year will concentrate on defining the questions and investigations to undertake in future years. Interestingly, Young remarked that there is a consensus on the Commission that is opposed to moving back to a cost-based reimbursement system.[110] Supporting this hesitation to make recommendations, ProPAC members concluded that the database is inadequate to make major decisions about DRG price revisions. "It may be premature to recommend fundamental changes in the system," according to Young.[111] Nevertheless, ProPAC's Hospital Productivity Subcommittee "voted to establish separate hospital market baskets" and approved a plan that would use a blend of hospital and nonhospital wage data to calculate the labor measures.[112] However, Altman warned that pushing toward regional hospital rates moved toward cost-based reimbursement and "could undermine ProPAC's impact on Congress."[113] In yet another example, an American Hospital Association study influenced a ProPAC subcommittee to recommend that HHS adjust Medicare payments to reflect the "disproportionate share" of low-income patients treated in specific hospitals.[114]

First ProPAC Report

On April 1, 1985, ProPAC sent its first report and recommendations to the Secretary of HHS, an 82-page document and an additional volume of 173 pages of technical appendixes.[115,116] Of the 21 recommendations, the first 16 addressed the updating factor and the remainder spoke to adjustments of DRG classifications and weights. Of major importance is the recommendation that the reimbursement update factor should be the estimated hospital market basket increase minus 1 percent for a combination of technology, productivity, and case mix improvements with an overall projected increase of 1 to 3 percent. Action was recommended on improving the labor market area definitions and on adjustments for hospitals serving a disproportionate share of low-income patients. In addition, it was suggested that newer data be used to recalibrate DRG weights and noted that ProPAC will continue to study the scheduled pace of transition to a national payment rate. All 21 recommendations are listed below.

1. Amount of the update factor to rise 1 percent; estimated 1 to 3 percent overall increase.

Hospital Market Basket

2. For FY 1986, a single market basket should be continued for hospitals under PPS.
3. Separate market baskets should be used for psychiatric, rehabilitation, and long-term care hospitals.
4. Market basket wage components should be split into three categories, each with separate weights: Managers and Administrators; Professionals and Technicians; and Other Hospital Workers.

5. There should be a study of the advantages and feasibility of developing an Employment Cost Index for the hospital industry.

6. ProPAC will study the effects of changes in the minimum wage on hospital workers.

7. Prior substantial market basket forecast errors should be corrected in the update factors.

8. If necessary, the HHS Secretary should seek statutory change to correct for market basket forecast errors.

9. Market basket weights should be rebased at least every five years.

Discretionary Adjustment Factor

10. For FY 1986, the allowance for productivity, scientific, and technological advancement, and hospital product change should be set at − 1 percentage point reduction.

11. Prospective payments to individual hospitals and in the aggregate should reflect real changes in case mix.

12. For FY 1986, exempt hospitals should receive a − 1 percentage point reduction adjustment as in number 10.

Hospital Labor Market Areas—Area Wage Index

13. The Secretary should improve definitions of hospital labor markets considering inner-city, suburban, and rural differences as soon as possible.

Disproportionate Share Hospitals

14. In FY 1986, the Secretary should develop and implement an adjustment methodology for hospitals treating a disproportionate share of indigent patients.

15. In FY 1986, the Secretary should establish a definition of disproportionate share hospitals using broader boundaries than merely the numbers of Medicaid patients.

Rebasing the Standardized Amounts

16. Standardized amounts used to determine the hospital PPS payments should be recalculated using cost data reflecting hospital behavior under PPS.

DRG Classifications and Relative Weighting Factors

17. All DRG weights should be recalibrated using the 1984 PATBILL data set.

18. DRGs involving cardiac pacemakers—DRGs 115, 116, 117, and 118— should be recalibrated in the same manner as other DRGs.

19. Cataract extraction and intraocular lens implantation, DRG 39, should be recalibrated in the same manner as other DRGs.

20. Cases in which Percutaneous Transluminal Coronary Angioplasty (PTCA) is the principal procedure should be removed from DRG 108 and temporarily assigned to DRG 112 before calibration, reducing payment in the interim.

21. No change is recommended in DRG classification or weights at this time for Bone Marrow Transplantation and Infective Endocarditis.

Notably, ProPAC did not recommend the development of a severity of illness index. According to ProPAC's executive director, the term "severity" is used as a catchall for a variety of problems.[117] Some ProPAC members were concerned that the 1 percentage point reduction for technology, productivity, and product change would be seen as an endorsement of the shift to outpatient care and a stifling of scientific advancement. According to ProPAC's chairman, the members did take "tight federal finances" into their deliberations. Therefore, the recommendations indicate that there should be no change in aggregate payments and somewhat dilute the financial changes suggested.[118] Nevertheless, hospital industry commentators see the modest ProPAC update increase as better than the no-increase payment freeze pushed by the federal administration. In addition, the hospital representatives support ProPAC's recommendations and have had good interactions with the commission.[119]

On April 1, 1986, ProPAC submitted its second annual report to the secretary of HHS. There were 33 recommendations included the following seven major areas: update factor of 2.8 percent increase for FY 1987; sharing of gains by revising the formula for inpatient deductible; phasing capital payments into PPS by FY 1987; incorporating technological change into recalibration of DRG weights; imparting information to Medicare beneficiaries about PPS and specifically about average length of stay; PROs reviewing the entire episode of care and also selected outpatient surgery cases; adjusting the payment formula to include disproportionate share for hospitals serving indigents and to adjust for labor market differences in urban and rural areas.[120]

Studies, Reports, and Demonstrations

The Secretary is required to study and report to Congress on the following:

- Capital Related Costs: due within 18 months after enactment (October 1984).

- Annual Reports on the Impact of the Prospective Payment Methodology: due annually at the end of each year for 1984 through 1987.

- Physicians' Services to Hospital Inpatients: during FY 1984, the Secretary is required to begin the collection of data necessary to compute, by DRGs, the amount of physician charges for services furnished to hospital inpatients classified in those DRGs, to include recommendations in a report to Congress by July 1, 1985.

- Urban/Rural Rates: due at the end of 1985 as part of the 1985 annual report. Two other studies of the urban/rural distinction due by January 18, 1985, including the effect on rural hospitals of the rates for DRGs with high fixed nonlabor components and the feasibility of varying by DRG the labor/ nonlabor components of the payment rates. A study is due prior to September 1, 1984 on further refinements to the payment system, including determining a percentage of the payment amount of a regional basis.

- Prospective Payments for Hospitals Not Included in the System: whether, and the method under which, hospitals not paid under the prospective system can be paid on a prospective basis for inpatient services; due at the end of 1985 as part of the 1985 annual report.

- Payments for Outliers/Intensity: due by the end of 1985 as part of the 1985 annual report.

- Payments for All Payers of Hospital Care: due by the end of 1985 as part of the 1985 annual report.

- Impact on Admissions: due by the end of 1985 as part of the 1985 annual report.

- Impact of State Systems: due by the end of 1986 as part of the 1986 annual report.

- Sole Community Hospitals, Information Transfer Between Parts A and B, Uncompensated Care, and Making Hospital Cost Information Available: due no later than April 1, 1985.

- Payments to Hospitals in the Territories, Including Puerto Rico: due before April 1, 1984.

- Skilled Nursing Facilities (SNFs): due prior to December 1, 1984.

- Nurse Anesthetists: possible Medicare hospital reimbursement methods which would not discourage the use of certified registered nurse anesthetists by hospitals; due as soon as is practicable.

- Wage Index: develop an appropriate wage index, taking into account wage differences of full-time and part-time workers, due 30 days after enactment (August 18, 1984). Also, a study of criteria for modification of a hospital's wage adjustment if such adjustment does not reflect the wage levels in the labor market serving the hospital. Federal revision of the wage index was noted in the September 3, 1985 *Federal Register*.

Legislation and Budget Proposals Affecting PPS

Deficit Reduction Act of 1984 (P.L. 98-369)

This Act includes the following changes to the Medicare prospective payment system:

Limits on payment rate increases.   This provides that the rate of increase in the prospective payment rates be equal to the market basket plus one-quarter percentage point in FY 1985. It prohibits the Secretary from establishing a percentage increase in the payment rates for FY 1986 greater than market basket plus one-quarter percentage point.

Rural hospital provisions.   This provides that a hospital classified as a rural hospital may appeal to the Secretary to be classified as a rural referral center based on criteria established by the Secretary, to be implemented by October 1, 1984. It provides that a hospital located in a Metropolitan Statistical Area that contains more than one census region be deemed to be in the region in which a majority of the hospitals in the same area are located or, at the option of the Secretary, the region which accounts for the majority of the Medicare discharges. It also provides that hospitals located in areas reclassified from urban to rural be allowed a two-year transition to the rural rates. It requires the Secretary to study the urban/rural payment differential with respect to (1) the advisability of making adjustments in the nonlabor component of DRGs with high fixed nonlabor costs and (2) varying by DRG the proportion of the labor and nonlabor components of the federal payment amount, due within six months of enactment. The provision requires the Secretary to study further refinements to the prospective payment system to address problems of differences in payment amounts to specific hospitals, including determining a percentage of the payment amount on a regional basis, due prior to September 1, 1984.

Payment for nurse anesthetists.   This removes the costs of certified registered nurse anesthetists from the prospective payment system for cost reporting periods beginning on or after October 1, 1984, and before October 1, 1987. Such costs will be paid on the basis of reasonable costs. It requires the Secretary to study methods of reimbursement for use of CRNAs in hospitals.

Prospective payment assessment commission.   This clarifies that the commission is an independent body responsible for requesting appropriations.

Wage index.   Requires the Secretary to conduct a study to develop a wage index taking into account wage differences of full-time and part-time workers, not later than 30 days after enactment, and to adjust payment amounts to reflect any changes made in the wage index. Requires the Secretary to study criteria by which an adjustment could be made in a hospital's wage index if the index did not accurately reflect the hospital wage levels in the labor market serving the hospital. As noted earlier, the wage index was adjusted in the Federal Register of September 3, 1985.

Budget Proposals in the 99th Congress

Submitted February 4, 1985, the President's FY 1985 budget included several proposals affecting the Prospective Payment System. In its press release on the FY 1986 budget, HHS indicated that these initiatives are part of an overall framework in the President's FY 1986 budget to constrain government spending in order to reduce the federal budget deficit. Proposals are described and analyzed below:

Freeze PPS Payment Rates in FY 1986 at the FY 1985 Levels. (HHS Savings Estimate: Outlays of $1.8 Billion in FY 1986 and $12.733 Billion in FY 1986-FY 1990.)   A regulatory rate freeze is consistent with the freezes placed on other programs in the federal budget, according to the Administration. This freeze will improve the solvency of the Medicare Hospital Insurance Trust Fund.

Administration arguments state that the rates in effect for FY 1985 will be sufficient in FY 1986 because: (1) productivity improvements made by hospitals (as measured by declines in hospital employees, length of hospital stays, and admission rates) are reducing their costs so that rate increases are not justified; (2) excess payments may have been made to hospitals in FY 1985 because the market basket index used to update the rates from FY 1984 to FY 1985 was overestimated; and (3) DRG coding problems—such as an overestimation of the base year costs that are built into the hospital-specific portion of the current rates and incentives for cases to be classified in more costly DRGs in order to maximize reimbursement—also may be causing overpayments to hospitals.

Final rules in the September 3, 1985 Federal Register upheld the Medicare freeze and take effect on October 1, 1985. HHS considered more than 2,000 comments after the proposed freeze was published in late June 1985. HCFA argued that the freeze was generous since their data indicated that the Medicare reimbursements should have been reduced by almost 3 percent in 1986. However, a reduction was rejected as appearing punitive. In addition, there is some Congressional action to overturn the freeze and provide a 1 percent increase in the DRG rates.

Opponents of the DRG payment rate freeze argue that (1) a freeze on DRG payment rates in the context of a budget-wide freeze cannot be justified if certain federal programs, such as defense, are not frozen; (2) although many hospitals have initiated certain cost-cutting measures, they still face increases due to inflation in the costs of goods and services they must purchase and to the continuing increase in the complexity of the cases they treat (due to the aging of the population and to the trend to treat less severely ill patients in an ambulatory setting, leaving the more seriously ill to be treated in hospitals); and (3) instead of their FY 1986 payments being frozen at FY 1985 levels, some hospitals will actually receive less in FY 1986 because the budget does not propose to freeze the phase-in of the blending of hospital-specific, regional, and national rates.

Freeze Payments for Direct Medical Education Costs Indefinitely. (HHS Savings Estimate: Outlays of $150 Million in FY 1986 and $2.71 Billion in FY 1986-FY 1990.) This is a proposal to use regulatory authority to indefinitely freeze Medicare payments to hospitals for direct medical education costs at the level received by each hospital in the hospital's cost reporting year which ended in 1984. An HHS press release indicated that, in 1984, Medicare reimbursement for direct medical education costs was about $1 billion. This proposal would be effective for hospital cost reporting years beginning July 1, 1985, which is the month in which most teaching hospitals begin their cost reporting periods. Administration indicates that the freeze is in keeping with the freezes placed on other programs in the federal budget. This will be the first step towards imposing limits on direct medical education costs. In fact, payments were frozen in actions noted in the *Federal Register* of July 5, 1985.

Questions relate to whether the Medicare program, which was designed to pay for medical services to its beneficiaries, should continue to underwrite the costs of medical education through its payments to teaching hospitals. Such support is also challenged in view of the apparently adequate supply of physicians and other health care professionals.

Opponents of the freeze argue that there appears to be no programmatic justification for this proposal except in the context of a budget-wide freeze. Teaching hospitals argue that their costs for salaries and fringe benefits for residents and teachers will rise over time, resulting in Medicare not paying its fair share of these costs. Teaching hospitals are also concerned that other payers for hospital care may follow Medicare's precedent in reducing support for the direct costs of medical education programs. Another problem mentioned is that freezing such payments locks in the current configuration of direct medical education costs among hospitals; would this proposal exclude new hospitals from receiving payments for direct medical education costs?

Eliminate the Doubling of the Indirect Medical Education Payment. (HHS Savings Estimate: Outlays of $695 Million in FY 1986 and $6.595 Billion in FY 1986-FY 1990.) This proposal seeks legislative authority to eliminate the doubling of the indirect medical education adjustment which Congress included in the original PPS authorizing legislation. The Administration argues that there is no empirical justification for the Congress to double the factor used to calculate the indirect payment from 5.795 percent to 11.59percent. HHS also argues that the indirect adjustment increases the DRG payments to all teaching hospitals, whether they need the adjustment or not. Others argue that the adjustment resulted in windfall gains to certain teaching hospitals and provides incentives for these hospitals to increase the size of their residency programs in order to maximize payments from Medicare.

Indirect adjustment is a proxy to account for a number of factors, possibly increasing costs in teaching hospitals. Some may be related to the teaching activity, such as greater use of tests by residents; some may not, such as any inability of the DRG case classification system to account fully for the more severely ill patients who are treated at teaching hospitals. Critics argue that any factors legitimately resulting in higher costs for any hospital, not just teaching hospitals, should be addressed directly by adjustments for severity of illness or uncompensated care.

Opponents of this proposal argue that the financial viability of teaching hospitals will be affected if they are not allowed an adjustment to the DRG payment rates sufficient to account for their higher costs. Some argue that the doubling be left as is until a method is developed to address problems such as severity of illness and uncompensated care. Others propose that the adjustment factor be reestimated with more recent and more accurate data.

Freeze FY 1986 Limits on Payments to PPS-Exempt Hospitals at FY 1985 Levels. (HHS Savings Estimate: Outlays of $20 Million in FY 1986 and $185 Million in FY 1986-FY 1990.) This is a proposal to use regulatory authority to freeze the FY 1986 limits on payments to PPS-exempt hospitals and hospital units at FY 1985 levels. PPS-exempt hospitals and hospital units are paid on the basis of their actual reasonable costs, subject to rate of increase limits established by P.L. 97-248, the Tax Equity and Fiscal Responsibility Act of 1982. This rate of increase limits system operates as follows: in the first year of the limits, a target rate percentage (market basket plus 1 percentage point) was applied to a hospital's allowable inpatient operating costs per discharge in the base period to yield a target amount (or limit) for that hospital in that year. In subsequent years, a new target amount is determined for each hospital by applying the applicable target rate percentage amount to the previous period's target amount. If the hospital's costs are lower than its target amount, a PPS-exempt hospital is paid its actual costs plus a bonus. If its costs exceed its target amount, it is paid its target amount. These conditions have been muted by a notice in the *Federal Register* of September 3, 1985 which freezes exempt hospitals at 1985 levels.

For hospital cost reporting periods beginning in FY 1985, the applicable target rate percentage used to update the previous period's target amount was set by law at market basket plus one-quarter of a percentage point. For FY 1986, the Secretary has the authority to set the target rate percentage which, by law, cannot exceed market basket plus one-quarter of a percentage point. This proposal means that such hospitals would be paid their actual costs in FY 1986, subject to the same target amounts which applied in FY 1985. Thus, hospitals whose actual costs were below their target amounts in FY 1985 could potentially receive greater reimbursement from Medicare in FY 1986 if their actual costs are higher than in the previous year.

Administration supports the freeze, indicating that it is consistent with the freeze on other programs in the federal budget and on payments to PPS hospitals. This freeze is opposed for many of the same reasons that the freeze on payments to PPS hospitals is opposed, including the cost increases hospitals face each year due to inflation, the increasing elderly population, and the increasing costs of technology. It has also been argued that the freeze for PPS-exempt hospitals may have a greater impact than the PPS payment freeze because such hospitals have not had the incentive in the past to institute cost-saving measures to the same degree that hospitals under PPS have done.

Future of PPS

Numerous questions have been raised about the Medicare prospective payment system. Questions range from the broader issues of whether this particular system should have been approved and implemented in the first place, or whether it should be expanded to cover all payers for hospital services, to more technical questions about the details of the system. Legislation providing for the new payment system was passed rapidly as part of the Social Security Amendments of 1983 (P.L. 98-21). There are certain critics who believe that the Medicare hospital reimbursement changes were included without sufficient examination of the potential impact of such changes. Other critics believe that the DRG payment system, although implemented in New Jersey under a demonstration project sponsored by HHS, had not been sufficiently tested to determine if it were suitable as a model for the nationwide Medicare hospital payment system.

Even supporters of the change in Medicare hospital reimbursement have raised questions about its impact. Those concerned about rising Medicare hospital costs and shortfalls in the Medicare Hospital Insurance Trust Fund question whether the system will achieve sufficient savings. Others are concerned that the DRG payment rates are not large enough to adequately pay hospitals for their services. Impacts of the system have been questioned for the elderly (e.g., will quality of care change?), for hospitals (e.g., will they be adequately or excessively reimbursed?), for health insurers (e.g., if Medicare's payment rates are not sufficient to cover hospital costs, will hospitals charge other insurers more to make up any shortfall?).

This system is very much in transition. HHS has indicated that many aspects of the system will continue to be analyzed and may be changed in the future. Congress enacted certain changes to the system in P.L. 98-369, the Deficit Reduction Act of 1984. In addition, Congress specified in P.L. 98-21 that many issues concerning the system, such as how to pay for capital-related costs, are to be studied and addressed in the future. Thus, even as some are trying to ascertain the impact of the system, the system is changing.

References

1. *A Guide for Physicians. Diagnosis-Related Groups and the Prospective Payment System* (Chicago: American Medical Association, February 1984).

2. "DRGs: The Changes Will Not Be Easy," *Journal of Indiana State Medical Society* 76, No. 9 (1983):592-593.

3. H. L. Lang, "A Physician Looks at DRGs," *Western Journal of Medicine* 141, No. 2 (1984):248-255.

4. S. Lewis, "Prospective Pricing and DRGs," *Western Journal of Medicine* 140, No. 1 (1984):123-128.

5. R. L. Mullin, "DRGs: The Doctor's Role," *Journal of Family Medicine* 3, No. 12 (1983):3-7.

6. C. M. O'Brien, "The Reality of the DRG System," *Ear, Nose and Throat Journal* 63, No. 6 (1984):255-261.

7. B. C. Vladeck, "Medicare Hospital Payment by DRG," *Annals of Internal Medicine* 100, No. 4 (1984):576-591.

8. *The Prospective Payment System* (training material for staff orientation), (Philadelphia: Albert Einstein Medical Center, undated.)

9. *A DRG Primer* (Wallingford, CT: Connecticut Hospital Association, February 1983).

10. J. T. Lynch, "DRG Primer," *Connecticut Medicine* 47, No. 9 (1983):552-558.

11. R. L. Mullin, "DRGs: A Brief Description," *Connecticut Medicine* 47, No. 5 (1983):281-282.

12. *The DRG Maze*. Unravelling the Mysteries of Hospital Reimbursement *in New Jersey* (Princeton, NJ: New Jersey Hospital Association, 1979.)

13. J. M. Gaynor, Jr., D. A. Kant, and E. M. Mills, "DRGs: Regulatory and Budgetary Adjustments," *Nursing and Health Care* 5, No. 5 (1984):275-279.

14. B. Rusynko, "DRGs. Who, What, How, Where?" *Today's OR Nurse* 6, No. 4 (1984):8-13.

15. F. Shaffer, *DRGs: Changes and Challenges* (New York: National League for Nursing, June 1984), Pub. No. 20-1959.

16. C. E. Smith, "DRGs: Making Them Work For You," Nursing 85 *15, No. 1 (1985):34-41.*

17. M. K. William, "DRGs—A Primer," *Nursing Economics* 1, No. 2 (1983):135-137.

18. R. F. Averill, "The Design and Development of the Diagnosis Related Groups," *Topics in Health Record Management* 4, No. 3 (1984):66-76.

19. R. F. Averill and M. J. Kalison, "Development and Interpretation of the Diagnosis Related Groups (DRGs)," *Healthcare Financial Management* 38, No. 2 (1984):72-74, 78-84.

20. C. L. Scanlon, *The Medicare Prospective Payment System. What It Is and How It Works,* Presentation at seminar at SUNY Health Science Center, Stony Brook, NY, June 15, 1984.

21. M. L. Vaida, "The Development of DRGs," *CHA Insight* 7, No. 8 (December 27, 1982):1-4.

22. "Prospective Payment: DRG Era Dawns," *Washington Report on Medicine and Health* 37, No. 35 (September 5, 1983):1-6.

23. C. N. Wilson, "Financial Management Issues. The DRG," *Hospital Pharmacy* 19, No. 2 (1984):109-122.

24. D. Wirtschafter, "The Impact of DRGs on Medical Management," *American Journal of Medical Sciences* 21, No. 1 (1984):86-95.

25. *Description and Analysis of Medicare Prospective Rate Setting* (Washington, DC: Healthcare Financial Management Association, 1983).

26. A. Dobson, *Prospective Payment: Current Configuration and Future Direction,* Presentation to Prospective Payment Assessment Commission, Washington, DC, February 2, 1984.

27. F. K. Goldschmidt, *The DRG System in New Jersey* (Trenton: New Jersey State Health Department, undated).

28. T. Jemison, "Medicare DRG Guide Published: Reviews, Indices, Waivers Abound," *U.S. Medicine* 19, No. 18 (September 15, 1983):4, 18, 19.

29. J. P. Lundy, *Medicare: Prospective Payments for Inpatient Hospital Services,* Congressional Research Services, Library of Congress, Washington, DC, updated March 6, 1985.

30. J. O'Sullivan, *Medicare,* Library of Congress, Congressional Research Service, Washington, DC, Issue Brief No. IB84052, updated 1985.

31. R. S. Schweiker, *Report to Congress. Hospital Payment for Medicare,* USDHHS, Washington, DC, December 1982.

32. *Diagnosis Related Groups. The Effect in New Jersey. The Potential for the Nation,* USDHHS, Health Care Financing Administration, Pub. No. 03170, March 1984.

33. Flip Chart on DRGs (press material), USDHHS, Health Care Financing Administration, August 1983.

34. *Medicare Prospective Payment, Probable Effects on Academic Health Center Hospitals, Short-Term and Long-Term Options,* (Washington, DC: Association of Academic Health Centers)/Association of American Medical Colleges, April 1983).

35. K. Casey, "Hospital Bills—Six Part Series on DRGs," *The News Tribune* (New Jersey), August 27-September 1, 1984.

36. W. Greenberg and R. M. Southby, *Health Care Institutions in Flux* (Arlington, VA: Information Resources Press, 1984).

37. P. L. Grimaldi and J. A. Micheletti, *Diagnosis Related Groups. A Practitioner's Guide* (Chicago: Pluribus Press, Inc., 1983).

38. P. L. Grimaldi and J. A. Micheletti, *DRG Update* (Chicago: Pluribus Press, 1984).

39. P. L. Grimaldi and J. A. Micheletti, *Prospective Payment, The Definitive Guide to Reimbursement* (Chicago: Pluribus Press, Inc., 1985).

40. Shaffer, DRGs: *Changes and Challenges.*

41. R. J. Shanko, *Physician's Guide to DRGs* (Chicago: Pluribus Press, Inc., 1984).

42. E. Levine and F. G. Abdellah, "DRGs: A Recent Refinement of an Old Method," *Inquiry* 21 (Summer 1984):105-112.

43. C. Asparro, *DRGs and Prospective Pricing* (New York: Arthur Anderson & Co., November 15, 1984).

44. "The Development of Diagnosis Related Groups (DRGs)," *DRG Monitor* 1, No. 1 (1983):1-8.

45. Ernst and Whinney, *The Medicare Prospective Payment System,* New York, E & W No. J58475, 1983.

46. Ernst and Whinney, *The Medicare Prospective Payment System,* Changes in the Final Regulations, New York, E & W No. J58506, 1984.

47. Ernst and Whinney, *The Revised DRGs,* New York, E & W. No. J58442, May 1983.

48. Peat Marwick Mitchell & Co., *Analysis of Regulations Implementing the Medicare Provisions of the Tax Equity and Fiscal Responsibility Act of 1982,* Chicago, IL, December 10, 1982.

49. Lundy, *Medicare: Prospective Payments.*

50. "Medicare Hospital Rate Hike About 4%," *American Medical News* 27, No. 25 (June 29/July 6, 1984):3, 7.

51. J. Fochtman, "Hospitals May See Smaller Medicare Increases," *Medical Marketing and Media* 19, No. 8 (1984):4.

52. D. L. Gibbons, "AMA Delegates Want Growing Influence of Outsiders on Medicine Curtailed," *Medical World News* 25, No. 14 (July 23, 1984):15-16.

53. J. Finn, "Medicare Prospective Pricing, Compromise," *Hospitals* 58, No. 19 (October 1, 1984):39-40.

54. J. Fochtman, "DRG Reg Fine Tuning," *Medical Marketing and Media* 19, No. 11 (1984):14.

55. "Freeze, DRG Cuts Pending in Conference, $1 Billion Cut From Medicare," *American Medical News* 27, No. 24 (June 22, 1984):124.

56. "$2.8 Billion in Cuts Sought for Medicare in 1986," *American Medical News* 27, No. 47 (December 21, 1984):1, 19.

57. S. McIlrath, "Diverse Coalition Opposes Medicare Cuts," *American Medical News* 28, No. 11 (March 15, 1985):8.

58. D. P. Wagner, T. D. Wineland, and W. A. Knaus, "The Hidden Costs of Treating Severely Ill Patients: Charges and Resource Consumption in an Intensive Care Unit," *Health Care Financing Review* 5, No. 1 (1983):81-86.

59. "$2.8 Billion in Cuts Sought," *American Medical News*.

60. "Report: Medicare Payment Inadequate for ICU Stays," *American Medical News* 28, No. 11 (March 15, 1985):42.

61. J. H. Keffer, "The Impact of TEFRA and DRGs on Laboratory Medicine," *Syva Monitor* 2, No. 2 (1984):8-10.

62. "DRGs Affect Specialists Most," *American Medical News* 27, No. 24 (June 22, 1984):24.

63. "Burn Centers Losing Money on Admissions," *Hospitals* 58, No. 10 (May 16, 1984):40.

64. C. Petty and J. H. Hopkins, "Anesthesia Drugs and Supplies," *Association of Operating Room Nurses Journal* 40, No. 4 (1984):606-613.

65. K. B. Carter, "A $1,400 Headache for Hospital Treatment," *Star Ledger*, New Jersey, February 1, 1985.

66. U.S. Government Accounting Office, *Excessive Respiratory Therapy Cost and Utilization Data Used in Setting Medicare's Prospective Payment Rates*, Washington, DC GAO/HRD-84-90, September 28, 1984.

67. R. Green, "Health Care Rationing: Can It Happen Here?" *Medical World News* 25, No. 21 (November 21, 1984):50-51, 58, 63-64, 69-70, 72, 74.

68. "$156,000 Loss Prompts Hospital to Seek Changes in DRG Payment Plan," *Medical World News* 25, No. 14 (July 23, 1984):10-11.

69. G. S. Hughes, "Diagnosis Related Groups" (letter), *Annals of Internal Medicine* 101, No. 1 (1984):138.

70. Green, "Health Care Rationing."

71. L. Kahn, "Bleak Future Seen for Nation's Hospitals," *Hospitals* 56, No. 24 (December 16, 1982):24, 28.

72. "Lloyd's of London to Sell DRG Policy," *Hospitals* 59, No. 1 (January 1, 1985):41.

73. "Northstar/BeneCorp Introducing DRG Stop-Less Policy," *Hospitals* 59, No. 8 (April 16, 1985):53.

74. "Part VII. Medicare Program: Changes to the Inpatient Hospital Prospective Payment System and Fiscal Year 1985 Rates: Final Rule," *U.S. Federal Register* 49, No. 171 (August 31, 1984):34777.

75. C. Mickel, "Congress, HHS Consider DRG Adjustments," *Hospitals* 58, No. 7 (April 1, 1984):37.

76. J. E. Wennberg, "Should the Cost of Insurance Reflect the Cost of Use in Local Hospital Markets?" *New England Journal of Medicine* 307, No. 22 (November 25, 1982):1374-1380.

77. C. Wallace, "Rural Hospitals Attack Payment System," *Modern Healthcare* 14, No. 5 (1984):48.

78. "Opposition to DRG Attestation Form Renewed," *American Medical News* 27, No. 25 (June 29/July 6, 1984):23.

79. Ibid.

80. S. Porter, "How Ohio Hospitals are Coping with DRGs," *Ohio State Medical Journal* 80, No. 4 (1984):263-265.

81. D. Lefton, "Rural Hospitals Press HHS for Overdue DRG Rate Report," *American Medical News* 28, No. 8 (February 22, 1985):1, 24.

82. Ibid.

83. "Medicare to Adjust Payments," *New York Times* (April 2, 1984).

84. "Medicare Change is Proposed," *New York Times* (April 2, 1985).

85. Lefton, "Rural Hospitals."

86. Mickel, "Congress Considers Adjustments."

87. "Eleven Ohio Hospitals Sue Over PPS," *Hospitals* 58, No. 6 (March 16, 1984):17.

88. "Eleven Ohio Hospitals to Appeal Ruling on PPS Classifications," *Hospitals* 58, No. 23 (December 1, 1984):31.

89. Ibid.

90. "DRG Horror Stories Told in Congress; Data Awaited," *Modern Healthcare* 14, No. 4 (1984):41, 44.

91. Mickel, "Congress Considers Adjustments."

92. Wallace, "Rural Hospitals."

93. S. McIlrath, "Congress Hears DRG Horror Stories," *American Medical News* 28, No. 10 (March 8, 1985):1, 33.

94. B. C. White, *Testimony Before Task Force on the Rural Elderly, Select Committee on Aging,* (February 26, 1985).

95. McIlrath, "Congress Hears Stories."

96. Ibid.

97. "New Medicare System Seen Hurting Patients," *The News Tribune* (New Jersey), March 30, 1985.

98. "An Honest Broker for Fine-Tuning Medicare," *Hospitals* 58, No. 19 (October 1, 1984):102, 104-105.

99. American Medical Association, *Diagnosis-Related Groups and the Prospective Payment System,* Chicago, IL, (February 1984):11.

100. "An Honest Broker," *Hospitals.*

101. M. Lesparre, "PPS Commission Explores Charge, Political Implications," *Hospitals* 58, No. 2 (January 16, 1984):29, 31.

102. J. K. Iglehart, "Washington News Analysis. Prospective Payment Commission," *Hospital Progress* 65, No. 2 (1984):20.

103. Lesparre, "PPS Commission."

104. J. Finn, "ProPAC Gears Up for Action on Prospective Prices," *Hospitals* 58, No. 20 (October 16, 1984):32-33.

105. "ACP Offers Help on DRGs. Testimony Before Commission Emphasizes Partnership," *American College of Physicians Observer* 4, No. 4 (1984):1, 7.

106. C. Wallace, "Congress, Business Toy with More Cost Cuts," *Modern Healthcare* 14, No. 5 (1984):38.

107. "An Honest Broker," *Hospitals.*

108. Ibid.

109. E. Friedman, "PPS Needs Overhaul to Survive: Altman," *Hospitals* 58, No. 22 (November 16, 1984):33.

110. "Donald Young, M.D.: Assessing PPS," *Hospitals* 59, No. 2 (January 16, 1985):113-114.

111. J. Finn, "ProPAC Keeping Its Options Open," *Hospitals* 58, No. 23 (December 1, 1984):37.

112. Finn, "ProPAC Gears Up."

113. Ibid.

114. C. Mickel, "Disproportionate Share Hospitals Draw Attention of AHA, Others," *Hospitals* 59, No. 2 (January 16, 1985):37.

115. *Report and Recommendations to the Secretary, U.S. Department of Health and Human Services,* Washington, DC, April 1, 1985.

116. *Technical Appendixes to the Report and Recommendations,* Prospective Payment Assessment Commission, Washington, DC, April 1, 1985.

117. "DRG Rates Should Rise Slightly in '86," *Medical World News* 26, No. 8 (April 22, 1985).

118. S. McIlrath, "Panel Suggests 1% to 3% Hike in 1986," *American Medical News* 28, No. 12 (March 22, 1985).

119. "DRG Rates Should Rise," *Medical World News.*

120. *Report and Recommendations to the Secretary, U.S. Department of Health and Human Services.* Washingtion, D.C.: Prospective Payment Assessment Commission, April 1, 1986.

CHAPTER 2
Exceptions to the Rules:
State Waivered Programs

There have been numerous attempts to develop and test hospital prospective payment mechanisms. An Office of Technology Assessment report reviewed per case and DRG payment systems in California, Idaho, Georgia, Maryland, and New Jersey.[1] Some systems have been mandatory, others have been voluntary. In 1972, Congress encouraged state prospective rate-setting demonstrations. This resulted in a variety of approaches including waivers from the Medicare and Medicaid programs. Key regulatory features and operating aspects of 17 state-legislated hospital cost containment programs were abstracted by Esposito et al. as of May 1982. Attention focused on programs requiring the disclosure, review, or legislation of hospital rates and budgets.[2] Another state-by-state survey in 1983 collected information on rate setting, financial disclosure or charge comparisons, health planning, contracting, Medicaid, freedom of choice, PPOs, and business coalition activities. Hospitals reported concerns about belt-tightening, increased state-mandated hospital rate-setting, moratoriums on capital improvements, the uncertain future of health planning, and the hospital/physician strains with a possible future exacerbation as the DRGs come into being.[3] Now, state legislatures are taking action on establishing feasible alternatives to retrospective cost-based reimbursement to contain increases in hospital expenditures. However, not all systems were applicable to a Medicare-only system. Therefore, the federal government developed criteria for a waiver from the Medicare PPS.

Guidelines for Waivers

In the Tax Equity and Fiscal Responsibility Act of 1982 (TEFRA), three conditions were listed for state rate-setting programs to meet to be considered for a waiver from the federal Medicare system.

1. State system applies to "substantially all" nonfederal acute care hospitals in the state and reviews are made of at least 75 percent of all inpatient expenses, including Medicaid.

2. State system equitably treats all payers, hospital employees, and patients and gives the Secretary of HHS "satisfactory assurances" of that.

3. State's system, over a three-year period, will not cost the federal government more than it would have cost under the Medicare system.[4]

Passage of the Social Security Amendments of 1983, which set up the federal PPS, added two more waiver criteria.

1. State's system does not exclude HMOs or CMPs from negotiating directly with hospitals concerning payment for inpatient hospital services.

2. State's system prohibits Medicare Part B payment for nonphysician services to patients except in narrowly prescribed circumstances.[5]

However, waivers are granted at the discretion of the Secretary of HHS. In 1982, Massachusetts and New York received approvals from then Secretary Schweiker for state cost control programs that do not use the DRG methodology. After that, Secretary Schweiker announced new criteria saying waivers would only be granted to states using the DRG system. That guideline caused conflict because the Secretary cannot deny a waiver simply because the state's system is not based on DRGs.[6] However, Wallace reported that the "DRGs only" rule came too late to block most waivers to states to substitute for the Medicare PPS. "All those who wanted waivers (with the exception of Washington) got them," according to FAH's Bromberg.[7]

Four states had waivers exempting them from participation in the federal Medicare PPS: Maryland, Massachusetts, New Jersey, and New York. Only New Jersey and Maryland still have waivers.

Programs in each of the four states are described. However, New Jersey's DRG effort is given special attention since the federal government patterned its national PPS on the New Jersey model.

Maryland: Guaranteed Inpatient Revenue (GIR)

Maryland's cost containment system controls revenue to hospitals using a DRG case mix adjustment process. Patient classification grouping schemes vary from hospital to hospital; base periods for cost calculations also vary and individual patient charges relate to the specific intensity of services rendered instead of per case averages.[8]

Program Description

In 1972 there were 46 acute hospitals and 12 specialty hospitals subject to the Maryland Health Services Cost Review Commission's jurisdiction. Those numbers were 52 and 12 in 1983. Rate review authority extends to all acute hospitals in the state and to private specialty hospitals. Both budget review and formula methodologies are used for rate-setting purposes. This system of rate setting was years in development and continues to undergo refinements as new methodologies are developed.

Initial rate review responsibility requires the Commission to determine the reasonable costs of providing individual hospital services. These costs and certain statistics for measuring the volume of each department are reported via the Uniform Accounting and Reporting System. According to the Commission, inefficiency should be reviewed at the department level prior to allocations to revenue-producing departments. Direct costs of the revenue-producing departments are also reviewed for reasonableness. The Commission must not only assure that the total costs of the hospital are reasonably related to the total services offered by the hospital, but is also obligated to permit a hospital to charge reasonable rates which will permit the institution to render the effective and efficient services in the public interest. Behind the reasonableness test is the theory that the same services should cost approximately the same amount at similar hospitals, and that a high cost may indicate an inefficient and wasteful operation. Hospitals have the opportunity to discuss rate increases with the Commission staff as well as to have formal rate review hearings before the Commission if they believe they need to justify costs which have been challenged. The Commission reviews any questions on a case-by-case basis and will consider special justifications for a hospital's costs. Their regulations also allow for input and cross-examinations by representatives of the major payors including Blue Cross, the Health Insurance Association of America, Medicare, Medicaid, and others. These payers are referred to as DIPS (Designated Interested Parties).

Process of Rate Review

Three underlying methodologies are used in the process of rate review: (1) full rate review, (2) the inflation adjustment system, and (3) the Guaranteed Inpatient Review System. The first is the method by which the Commission establishes the reasonableness of a hospital's rates; the second is the system by which a hospital's rates are typically adjusted on an annual basis; and the third is the per-case prospective reimbursement system employed by the Health Services Cost Review Commission. A thorough understanding of these systems and how they interrelate is essential to an understanding of hospital rate setting in Maryland.

A full rate review evaluates a hospital's costs in light of the Commission's legislated requirements. This task is accomplished by comparing the hospital's actual costs to standards of reasonableness. Separate standards are established for each of the four components of a hospital's rate base. These levels, described below, evolved from the development of the Commission's Uniform Accounting and Reporting System.

Level I   Direct Operating Costs
              Patient Care Centers
                 Routine
                 Ancillary

              General Service Centers
              Primarily Fixed
              Primarily Variable

Level II   Capital Facilities Allowance
              Building
              Equipment
                 General Allowance
                 Capital Intense Departments

Level III   Other Financial Considerations
              Miscellaneous Additional Expenses
              Auxiliary Enterprises

Level IV   Working Capital, Bad Debts, and Charity
              Care Payer Differential

A particular feature of the Maryland Rate Setting System is that all payers accept the Commission's basic definition of full financial requirements. That definition includes the cost of reasonable bad debt and charity care. In most other states, such a provision is not included and hospitals located in inner-city areas have suffered financial hardship. Recognition of these costs as part of a hospital's full financial requirements has been credited in part for the support the Commission has enjoyed from the hospital industry.

An Inflation Adjustment System (IAS) was developed as a voluntary system to annually adjust a hospital's rates to provide long-term incentives for reducing costs and predictability of future revenues, and to remove the administrative burden on both the hospitals and the Commission staff of annually conducting a full rate review on every hospital.

IAS is voluntary in the sense that hospitals which have passed a case mix adjusted per-case screening test and are in compliance with the Commission's reporting requirements may elect to automatically have their rates adjusted to account for inflation, volume changes, and price compliance. Hospitals which fail to qualify for the inflation adjustment or believe they require higher rates than provided by the IAS have the option to submit a full rate application. The case mix adjusted per-case screening test was initially established by the Commission in December 1979.

By and large, the IAS is an automated procedure which, through a series of calculations, adjusts a hospital's rates for the following factors:

1. Factor cost inflation

2. Unusual or government mandated costs

3. Price variances

4. Volume variances

5. Guaranteed inpatient revenue adjustment

In 1977, the Commission realized that the most serious deficiency in its system was reflected by the unbridled growth in patient lengths of stay and ancillary testing. In comparison to the rest of the nation, Maryland ranked near the top in both cost per admission and average length of stay. It was clear that restraining the growth in unit rates would not be sufficient to control hospital cost inflation.

As noted previously, the inflation adjustment system includes volume adjustments which act to discourage volume increases by paying only variable cost for volume increases. This constraint does nothing to actively encourage decreases in volume and there is even some debate as to whether the variable cost percentages are low enough to discourage growth.

A Guaranteed Inpatient Revenue system (GIR) was established specifically to address these problems. It was the first case mix adjusted per case prospective reimbursement system and preceded the development of the implementation of the New Jersey DRG and the Medicare national prospective payment system. While the GIR shares some characteristics with these programs, it differs in a number of fundamental ways. Similarly, the GIR establishes in advance a limit on per case (or per admission) reimbursement. All these systems permit hospitals to keep at least a portion of the savings they are able to generate by remaining below the prospective limit. Like those systems, the GIR provided an additional adjustment to account for new services and technology. Finally, all these systems provided for the special treatment for "outliers" or cases which are for one reason or another atypically high or low cost. At this point, however, the similarities end.

Currently, 37 of 54 hospitals representing 86 percent of revenue are on the traditional GIR, the modified GIR, or the Capitation Payment System.

In a 1981 evaluation of the Maryland program, the management of Bon Secours Hospital in Baltimore considered the GIR system "a substantial improvement over previous rate setting and reimbursement systems."[9] However, at the time the administration did not consider DRGs to be a valuable tool. On the other hand, the Johns Hopkins Hospital chose to use the DRG method as they participated in the GIR because of the potential for accurate reimbursement. "Our experience . . . confirmed this assumption. Since 1979, our reward for more efficient performance (GIR reward) . . . increased from $1 million to $8 million (1983)."[10] Over that same time period, deducting the hospital's large GIR rewards, Maryland still saved $16 million because the hospital charged less than it was allowed to by the rate setting commission.

A study of 20 Maryland hospitals operating under GIR concluded that "controlling for case mix has a highly significant impact on the amount of revenue hospitals receive under such a program. In addition, the manner in which case mix is defined has a significant impact, and it produces different effects for different hospitals."[11]

According to the Maryland Health Services Cost Review Commission, data from a 1983 analysis showed that 46 hospitals had a profit and seven had profits in excess of $3 million. Eight hospitals posted a loss. Total hospital profits in the state went from $3.4 million in 1982 to $57.8 in 1983. Part of the huge jump was due to the Commission's overestimating anticipated inflation adjustments by two percentage points.[12]

Interestingly, the president of the Maryland Hospital Association says that patient dumping does not occur because the payment system has no incentives to transfer high-cost patients to other facilities.[13]

An AHA study of the impact of the Maryland payment system reported that "hospitals were openly enthusiastic about the system."[14]

Currently, the Maryland system reports hospital costs averaging 3 to 4 percent below the national average. Strong support continues from the Maryland Hospital Association with a spokesman stating: "Right now, with the instability of the federal system, we have no desire to be a part of it."[15] With hospital costs staying below the national average, Maryland officials believe that they have an indefinite waiver.[16] HCFA has agreed to continue Maryland's waiver until June 1987.[17]

Massachusetts: Maximum Allowable Cost (MAC)

Blue Cross of Massachusetts initiated a prospective hospital reimbursement system for its private business on October 1, 1981. This system was extended to all payers one year later.[18] In Massachusetts, the prospective payment system was based upon establishing a maximum allowable cost (MAC) to be paid to the hospitals in a given year. That MAC fluctuated with adjustments for volume and inflation.

Program Description

Medicare utilized a reimbursement system called MAC-M, the Blue Cross MAC contract. The system was administered by Blue Cross, the Medicare intermediary.

Base year. From the base year fiscal 1981, the MAC-M system established a prospective limit on the rate of cost increase for the majority of hospital costs. After the first reimbursement year, the system functioned on a rate-to-rate basis. Reimbursement for each subsequent year was based on the rate in the previous reimbursement year, rather than on actual costs. MAC-M definitions of allowable costs and the cost-finding processes were similar to Medicare principles.

An adjustment allowed costs in a reimbursement year associated with filling nursing positions which were vacant in the base year to be added without incurring a penalty. This adjustment enabled hospitals to fill positions which were vacant due to the nursing shortage.

Certain costs not incurred for the entire base year were annualized to compute base year costs, if they were under consideration prior to May 11, 1981. Expenses falling into this category included wage and fringe benefit increases deviating from normal wage and salary policies, determination of need projects, new services, and changes in physician billing practices from nonhospital-based to hospital-based (and vice versa).

A number of costs were reimbursed on an actual cost basis (pass-through costs): depreciation; capital allowances, interest expense; renal dialysis; home health services; malpractice insurance; sick, vacation, and earned time accruals; and other costs as approved by the MAC Exception Review Board (MERB).

Trended forward. Base year costs trended forward to the reimbursement year using the Rate Setting Commission's seventy-nine cost category proxies and each hospital's cost structure to develop a hospital-specific, composite inflation index (Harbridge House Methodology). If the actual inflation for labor costs was lower than projected, no adjustment was made. But if the actual inflation for labor costs was higher than projected, the difference was adjusted in the subsequent year.

Productivity. In accordance with Section 3 of Chapter 372 of the Acts of 1982 (Massachusetts General Laws), a series of "productivity" reductions applied to Medicare's payment liability under the MAC system.

In determining reimbursable costs for fiscal year 1983, total reimbursement, including MAC costs and costs reimbursed outside the MAC, were reduced by a productivity factor of 2 percent. Fiscal years 1984 and 1985 also had a 4 and 6 percent productivity factor applied respectively.

Financial incentives.   A number of financial incentives encouraged reductions in length of stay, limited increases in ancillary service utilization, and shifted treatment from inpatient to outpatient. Incentives operated by assigning different fixed-to-variable cost ratios for changes in the volume of inpatient care, inpatient ancillary services, and outpatient ancillary services. In addition, a neutral corridor was assigned for volume decreases in those services where a decrease in utilization was desired (e.g., for decreases in the use of inpatient ancillary services up to 4 percent, there was no corresponding decrease in reimbursement).

Settlement process.   A year-end settlement process was similar to the one used by Medicare with one important exception. Aggregate hospital financial requirements were allocated to each third-party payer based upon calculations of each program's proportionate share of the hospital's total patient care activity. Medicare allocated costs by department rather than in the aggregate. In addition, routine patient care services were settled on a proportional charge basis rather than the Medicare per diem cost basis.

Other operational factors.   Under the demonstration system the hospitals and Medicare each shared one-half of the difference between the rate of increase in the aggregate Medicare payments in Massachusetts and the rate of increase in aggregate Medicare payments nationally.

MERB reviewed cost increases associated with new services and programs, volume and case mix changes, and extraordinary changes in factor costs which were reasonable and not accounted for within the MAC formulas. MERB was composed of two Blue Cross/intermediary representatives, two hospital representatives, and three independent professionals. Blue Cross, as the intermediary, represented Medicare on issues presented to the MERB.

Following are examples of the types of costs reviewed by the MERB upon the request of a hospital:

- Capital and operating costs associated with determination of needed projects.

- Disaster loss.

- Changes in the age and health status of patients treated.

- Regionalization of services.

- Health maintenance organization affiliations.

- Program, service, and health systems development costs associated with the following types of projects:

emergency medical services
medical training programs
mergers, corporate reorganizations, and hospital closures.

In sum, "Massachusetts hospitals operated on a revenue cap computed on the basis of the state's prospective payment contract with the Blues, with allowances for volume, case mix and inflation."[19]

The Massachusetts Hospital Association Board of Trustees voted unanimously not to support a new waiver proposal, and the state legislature concurred.[20] Consequently, the waiver expired and Massachusetts came under HCFA's national plan as of October 1, 1985.

New York: All-Inclusive Per Diem Rate

In a study of New York's prospective hospital rate setting program using 1974-1976 data, Ruchlin and Rosen commented that the process of rate regulation was not adequately researched. Specifically, these investigators related process factors such as rate stability and coordination of rate setting across all third party payers to the objectives of the prospective initiative such as cost containment. At the time of this study, New York's prospective plan included the statewide Medicaid program and the eight Blue Cross insurers operating in the state. Despite the limitations of the research, Ruchlin and Rosen reported that state rate regulators realized the need for review of all sources of hospital revenue to yield maximum cost containment results.[21]

New York State's Medicare waiver, effective from January 1, 1983 to December 31, 1985, follows through on the control of hospital revenue issue by creating an all-payer system. In hearings before a Congressional Committee on the PPS/DRG proposal, Robert M. Crane, director of the Office of Health System Management for the New York State Health Department described the payment mechanism:

> In New York State we reimburse hospitals on the basis of an all-inclusive per diem rate. Because of the size and complexity of New York's health care system, we use a formula-based methodology rather than a time-consuming budget review process.[22]

A spokesman for the Hospital Association of New York State, representing the 350 facilities, also pointed out that the payment rates were hospital-specific and therefore more equitable.[23]

Following joint investigations by New York State officials and hospital industry representatives of case mix studies and DRGs, the New York's Prospective Hospital Reimbursement Methodology (NYPHRM) was implemented under the Medicare waiver. A leaflet detailing the NYPHRM was widely distributed by the Hospital Association of New York State.[24]

Put another way, "Hospitals in New York are assigned to peer groups based on size, location, and case mix and have per diem allowances adjusted to meet an annual revenue cap."[25]

Program Description

Conditions leading to waiver. Since 1969, New York State has been attempting to control inpatient hospital costs by building cost containment incentives into the rate-setting methodology. After 1976, the state's efforts intensified, resulting in a more stringent reimbursement system for Medicaid and Blue Cross. This resulted in overall hospital costs in New York increasing at a rate significantly below the national average. However, in the state's view, two problems existed which had to be resolved before the state could have a truly rational system of health care financing. The first problem was the existence of numerous facilities with serious financial difficulties created by patients who could not afford to pay their hospital bills. The second problem was the conflicting cost containment incentives created by Medicare's retrospective reimbursement system. In order to resolve these problems, New York submitted three requests to HCFA to bring Medicare under the state's system to establish all-payer cost controls. As a concession for this provision, a methodology was established to reimburse hospitals for bad debt and charity care. The state's third proposal, NYPHRM, was approved by HCFA in December, 1982 and was effective January 1, 1983. The Office of Research and Demonstration established evaluation criteria for the waiver which required that the increase in total Medicare reimbursement under the waiver be at least 1 percent less than the national average.

General information. This waiver encompassed the period January 1, 1983 through December 31, 1985, and included all third-party payers, although commercial payers were treated differently than Medicare, Medicaid, and Blue Cross. NYPHRM covers inpatient hospital care at approximately 300 facilities certified under Article 28 of the New York Public Health Law. Psychiatric hospitals were not included in the demonstration project. Estimated Medicare reimbursement to these facilities for 1983 was roughly $3,138,000,000, while estimated Medicaid reimbursement for the same period was $1,693,000,000.

Basically, NYPHRM was a comprehensive revenue cap system under which rates were established prospectively using 1981 costs, apportioned-based on charges, as the base year for all three years of the project. Base year allowable costs using audited cost data were determined through the use of peer group comparisons with ceilings on ancillary costs and a combined routine cost/length of stay ceiling. Costs in excess of the ceilings, based on a percentage of average peer group costs, were disallowed in the rate-setting calculation. For Medicare reimbursement purposes, the ceiling disallowances were phased in so that in

1983, only 25 percent of the ceiling disallowances were imposed. The 1984 Medicare rates reflected 50 percent of the ceiling disallowances and the 1985 rates reflected 75 percent of the disallowances.

Once allowable costs were determined, rates were calculated by inflating the costs by a trend factor developed by an independent panel of economists and dividing those costs by inputed patient days based on minimum utilization standards. There were also a number of add-ons to the rate. The two basic ones follow:

1. Bad debt and charity care—a factor of 2 percent was added to 1983 rates and pooled regionally to pay for bad debt and charity care. This factor increased during 1984 and 1985.

2. Discretionary add-on—a factor of 1 percent was added to rates to mitigate the impact of spending above trend and to allow for technological improvements, and so on.

Adjustments to the prospective rates were limited to changes in volume, case mix, services provided, increases in labor costs, or revisions necessitated by base year audits. Commercial payers paid charges with the condition that such charges not exceed the Blue Cross rate by more than a certain percentage.

Details of the NYPHRM system are described in Part 86-1 of the NYS Department of Health's regulations. All changes to those regulations had to be approved by the New York State Hospital Review and Planning Council which is appointed by the Governor. The regulatory change process is a very public one. In addition, all proposed changes to 86-1 were submitted to the federal project officer and were also reviewed by the Regional Office. The New York State Department of Health explored the possibilities for 1986 when the waiver ended. No decisions were made to request the project be continued under Section 1886.

Key areas where NYPHRM differed from Medicare cost reimbursement principles and PPS follow:

- Bad debt and charity care—Under NYPHRM, it was partially paid for.

- Capital costs—For Medicare purposes, capital costs were treated as a pass-through in 1983, and for 1984 and 1985 followed current Medicare principles in effect regarding capital costs, except that accelerated depreciation was recognized on major moveable equipment. A moratorium was instituted by New York State after NYPHRM began for all capital costs incurred during calendar year 1983. Affordability criteria were established for reimbursement of capital cost in 1984 and 1985.

- Malpractice costs—In 1983, malpractice costs were reimbursed based on average cost. In 1984 and 1985, one-third and two-thirds, respectively, of malpractice costs were apportioned on the basis of payer experience, with the remainder being reimbursed based on average cost.

- Inflation—Under PPS, base year data is updated to FY 1984 using an update factor based largely on hospital-related costs. New York State used a trend factor based on various indices representing other than hospital cost increases. The New York trend factor was generally significantly below the national rate of increase for health care as shown below:

Hospital Inflation Rate		NY Trend Factor (approximate)
1981	15.9	10.5%
1982	15.0	8.0%

- Length of stay—PPS clearly provides incentives for hospitals to minimize length of stay. A prospective per diem system like New York's provided a different incentive. However, the volume adjustment and length of stay penalty within NYPHRM worked to make the system neutral with respect to length of stay.

Cost reports for 1981 have now been completely audited. This resulted in an adjustment of 1983 reimbursement rates which are trended forward from the 1981 base year. Substantial over-payments probably resulted on a one-time basis as an outcome of the 1981 audits.

HCFA concerns.   There were no specific HCFA concerns for the waiver project in New York. However, an ongoing monitoring of the reimbursement system was necessary to determine the efficacy of continuing that system, either as a waiver, or an all-payer methodology, or converting the state to PPS.

Review of rate setting methodology.   A statistically valid sampling was performed for hospitals for which rates had been set under the New York State waiver. This review was performed by federal regional office staff to determine if payments were made in accordance with the waiver provisions. PPS base year audits were performed by New York Blue Cross—Medicare Part A and Traveler's Insurance Company for 100 percent of the hospitals participating in the waiver project.

Monitoring of operations under the waiver.   An ongoing review was conducted by employing a sampling methodology to assure that proper payments were established, paid, adjusted, and updated for providers covered under the waiver in accordance with the terms and provisions of the waiver. In addition, a review protocol was prepared and implemented for such areas as: prospective rate setting, distribution of funds in bad debt and charity care pools, appeals and adjustment of revenue caps, and the causes and effects of overpayments.

Determining Hospital Specific Rate.   This procedure essentially involved

- Having the intermediary perform 1982 (Base Year) audits of cost report data submitted by the hospitals

- Trending cost data forward to project 1984 PPS payment rates

- Comparing the previously determined 1984 PPS projected payments with actual and projected 1984 payments under the waivers for all hospitals covered by the waiver within New York State

- Verifying the accuracy of PPS base audit and PPS rate setting.

NYPHRM offered significant improvements over previous systems. While some hospitals found revenues reduced, most received greater income, and the industry benefited financially. In effect, NYPHRM balanced the needs of all parties including the hospital industry, third-party payers, government, and the public.

As early as February 1984, it was reported the HCFA might terminate New York State's waiver from the Medicare PPS. A state legislator said that HCFA believes "New York is getting an unfair share of Medicare dollars."[26] That comment was reinforced by an executive from the state's Office of Health Systems Management who remarked, "If we don't prove the waiver is working, there is no incentive for HCFA to give us another waiver."[27]

In March 1985, the reports continued ominous for a new waiver. Despite a hospital cost reduction of three to four percent below the national average, George Allen, president of the state's hospital association, said that they may not support a new waiver request because Medicare will no long pay waivered states more than nonwaivered states. Even more threatening, the state health department commented that "New York may not seek a new waiver because savings from the system are no longer clear-cut."[28] Although average daily costs appeared good, the state's length of stay was higher than the national average. That length of stay issue was publicly aggravated in April 1984 when the state's PRO, the Empire State Medical, Scientific and Educational Foundation, disallowed almost 14 percent of Medicare payments to hospitals because care was unnecessarily prolonged. Based on a review of 24,000 patient charts, that 14 percent rate compared with a 3 percent disallowance rate prior to the new review process initiated on November 1, 1984. If the 14 percent disallowance continued, New York State hospitals could be denied an estimated $80 million in 1985. Large teaching hospitals in New York City would be the biggest losers.[29]

Both the Hospital Association of New York State and the New York State Health Department were lukewarm about a new waiver request. Finally, the New York State legislature voted not to seek an extension of the Medicare waiver.

New Jersey: DRG-Specific Rates Per Case

Dating back to the late 1960s, New Jersey has a history of activities related to controlling the high cost of hospital care. Under the state's Commissioner of Insurance, a cap was placed on Blue Cross payments to some hospitals. This was followed by a prospective budget review system initially administered by the Hospital Research and Educational Trust of New Jersey and later shifted to the state health department.[30] Next came Standard Hospital Accounting and Rate Evaluation (SHARE), a more stringent mandatory budget review program applied to Blue Cross and Medicaid patients and based on a reasonable cost per day.

In an extensive and comprehensive review of SHARE, Rosko undertakes a multidimensional analysis of the program from 1975 to 1982. He suggests that SHARE did contain hospital costs but at the same time the program threatened the viability of most inner-city facilities. Rosko suggests that suburban hospitals were able to shift costs while the inner-city hospitals were limited in their ability to do likewise.[31] Shaffer blends in the political aspects of SHARE with the election of a new governor, Brendon Byrne, and the appointment of a new health commissioner, Joanne Finley, both committed to cost containment. Logically, SHARE was abandoned because "it failed to introduce sufficiently powerful cost containment encouragement."[32]

After SHARE, in the mid-1970s, Jersey received a $3 million grant from HCFA to develop a prospective reimbursement system using DRGs. In 1978, New Jersey passed a law mandating the gradual implementation of a per case payment system covering all payers. A Hospital Rate Setting Commission was given the power to adopt an approach that ties payment rates directly to the patient's DRG. In May 1980, 26 hospitals began billing patients on a DRG-specific rate per case. By October 1982, all New Jersey hospitals had been brought into the DRG system.

Each patient is assigned to a specific DRG on discharge, and the hospital is paid a previously specified rate for that DRG. All classes of payers must pay the assigned rate to the hospital regardless of the actual amount of resources consumed in treating the patient. Exceptions include "outlier" cases where the length of stay is unusually short or long relative to the mean stay in the DRG; cases where the hospital stay ends with death; when the DRG is a low-volume category; or when discharge is against medical advice. These outlier cases are paid according to the hospital's charges which are also controlled under a preexisting rate-setting approach.

DRG rates assigned to a hospital are constructed from data on the hospital's own costs as well as those of all other similar major teaching, minor teaching, and nonteaching hospitals in the state. A hospital-specific preliminary cost base (PCB) is first established by taking the hospital's actual expenditures in a base year (two years before the rate year). This PCB includes direct patient care costs, indirect (overhead) costs, allowances for the replacement of capital facilities, bad debt and charity care, and working capital. Only the direct care component of the PCB is assumed to vary with the DRG. Direct care costs are allocated among DRGs using formulas that presumably reflect actual resource use by patients in various DRGs. For example, nursing costs are allocated among the hospital's DRGs according to the percentage of total patient days in each DRG, while ancillary department costs are allocated among DRGs on the basis of the percentage of total department charges in each DRG.

Each hospital's DRG-specific average direct patient care cost computed as above is the basis for calculation of a statewide average cost per DRG, which becomes a standard DRG rate. A hospital's rate becomes a blend of the hospital's own average direct care cost per DRG and the peer group average (or standard) DRG cost. The portion of each cost average that is used (i.e., the hospital's own or the standard) varies across DRGs, depending on the amount of statewide variance in the costs of treating patients within a given DRG. If there is substantial variation in the costs of treating a DRG, greater reliance is placed on the hospital's own cost experience. The percentage of the statewide standard cost used in setting rates ranges from a low of zero percent to a high of 100 percent, with most DRGs falling into the 40 to 75 percent ranges.

After DRG-specific direct care costs are estimated, hospital-based physician costs and overhead costs are added, and the total is inflated to the rate year. Other allowable costs (e.g., allowances for capital facilities and equipment and charity care) are calculated and allocated among DRGs on a percentage basis. Hospitals are then paid these final DRG-specific rates throughout the rate year.

Under this system, hospitals may keep any surplus achieved by reducing per-case costs, but beginning in the 1982 rate year, a part of any surplus resulting from increasing admissions is taken back in the final reconciliation. Similarly, increases in costs per case must be absorbed by the hospitals, but revenue losses due to decreases in admissions are moderated by a formula at reconciliation.

In theory, this method of DRG price construction contains built-in annual adjustments to DRG rates through changes in the base-year costs to reflect changing levels of resource use. A hospital's rate for a particular DRG could change as a result of either changes in its own costs of providing services or statewide peer group changes in the costs of treating the DRG. The rate facing a particular hospital can change even if its own and the statewide peer-group average costs do not change. For example, if the variance among patients in the cost of treating cases in a particular DRG were to decrease due to greater standardization of treatment across the state, the rate in subsequent years would be based more heavily on the statewide average cost and less on the hospital's own costs than in the previous year. In practice, staff and budget limitations have precluded timely updating of the base year.

Changes in specific DRG rates are also possible through an appeals process. Any interested party, be it a hospital, a payer, a patient, or the Commission itself, may request a review of a rate in one or more DRG category if it believes it is offering services using new, more costly technology.

In testimony before the House Select Committee on Aging in March 1983, Charles F. Pierce, Jr., Deputy Commissioner of the New Jersey State Health Department, discussed experiences with DRG reimbursement. He recounted DRG construction, data requirements, implementation, evolution, monitoring, technology, and flexibility. Pierce concluded: "We feel very strongly that DRGs have a great benefit in terms of allowing hospitals to use available resources wisely and to help contain health care costs for payers and consumers."[33]

Goldberg also reviewed the DRG system in New Jersey, but he paid attention to the differences between the federal version and system in New Jersey.[34]

New Jersey—United States Differences

A state health department executive identified unique characteristics of the New Jersey plan which are significantly different from the national system:

1. New Jersey has an all-payer system.

2. Each hospital in New Jersey has a separate and individualized set of rates for all 468 DRGs.

3. Uncompensated care, bad debts, and charity care are all fully reimbursed.

4. Outpatient services are paid at a flat rate, with no regard to DRGs.

5. Payer discounts, or percentage discounts, are awarded to insurers for economically quantifiable benefits.[35]

Other analysts added shadings and nuances with more points about New Jersey/United States differences. A hospital administrator noted the reimbursement of capital costs on a pass-through basis and the educational classification by teaching activities.[36] Chenoweth astutely observed that New Jersey traditionally had higher average lengths of stay and the hospitals could initially reduce the stays to adjust to DRGs. In addition, "New Jersey's hospital population is reasonably homogenous in terms of size, the smallest hospital having about 150 beds."[37] Another hospital manager pointed out that New Jersey's system allows for adequate outliers, about 30 percent compared to a much lower percentage—5-6 percent—

in the national program.[38] In an evaluation of the New Jersey DRG program, May and Wasserman label the requirement that all payers pay the hospitals' DRG rates the most important difference because that prohibits cost shifting among payers.[39]

New Jersey Plan Legally Invalidated

Riverside General Hospital, Secaucus, New Jersey, sued Secretary Heckler, contending that HHS did not follow procedural requirements defined in the Medicare Act prior to the initiation of the New Jersey experiment. Judge John J. Sirica of the U.S. District Court for the District of Columbia found that HHS did not comply with a statutory duty to submit written reports to the House Ways and Means Committee and the Senate Finance Committee at least 30 days before implementing the prospective pricing demonstration in New Jersey. In addition, Judge Sirica stated that the Secretary failed to comply with her own internal approval procedures before granting the waiver to New Jersey to begin the experiment. HHS argued that the demonstration was a state plan and therefore not subject to the provisions of the Medicare Act. Although the court found HHS's actions illegal, the nature of relief for Riverside General Hospital was uncertain since national legislation already implementing the PPS would be unaffected. Both parties were ordered to submit additional arguments on the matter of the injunction.[40] At this time, there has been no further action on this suit.

DRG Evaluation in New Jersey

In a comparative study of the waivered programs in Maryland and New Jersey, Frankenstein and Mintz found that "New Jersey hospitals were tolerant of the system, but less enthusiastic."[41]

A major comprehensive evaluation occurred in November 1983 as the first federally-sponsored national conference focused on "Diagnosis Related Groups: The Effect in New Jersey. The Potential for the Nation." Proceedings from that conference reported on the impact of DRGs in the following areas:

- Financial Departments
- Medical Records
- Quality Assurance
- Data Processing
- Nursing
- Payers

- Utilization Review

- Medicaid

- Teaching Hospitals

- Inner City Hospitals

- Industry's View

- Government's View

- Evaluation

- Implications[42]

Since the New Jersey system served as a model for the national PPS, the 225-page report provides a source document for the cost-effective approach espoused under the Medicare PPS.

However an editorial in the New York Times proclaimed the failure of a hospital diet. New Jersey's DRG plan caused the hospitals to gain weight (inflate costs) instead of slimming down (reducing costs). According to the editorial, "Hospitals covered by the new program in the first year received $2.3 million more, on average, than they would have received under the old system."[43] Congress was advised to heed the warning from New Jersey.

In a response to the editorial, New Jersey's health commissioner, J. Richard Goldstein, called the conclusions premature. He enumerated the benefits of New Jersey's DRG plan, such as providing care for uninsured patients, bringing inner city hospitals back from the brink of bankruptcy, eliminating cost shifting, realizing that needed start-up costs amounted to only one-half of one percent of a hospital's total budget and taking a cautious, not political, stance to maintain quality of care. In addition, Goldstein cited AHA data from 1980 to 1982 showing that New Jersey dropped from the eighteenth most expensive health care state to the thirty-second. He suggested "a suspension of the prognosis."[44]

While not exactly defending the New Jersey program, the president of the American Hospital Association called the Times editorial a disservice to the DRG concept. McMahon cited reduction in length of stay and admissions as a result of the national PPS/DRG effort as well as contained costs in comparisons from 1982 to 1983. His criticism continued that "lumping the two programs (N.J. and U.S.) together is nothing more than comparing apples to oranges."[45]

Another letter from the chairman of the N.J. Medical Society's DRG Committee agreed with the editorial's point on costs. However Primich disagreed that the hospitals are to blame due to inappropriate admissions and diagnostic gamesmanship. With a flair for alliteration, Primich called DRGs "illogical, impersonal and often inhumane." Blame for the situation was placed on state law, particularly that section allowing $250 million in uncompensated care to be factored into DRG rates to prop up inner city hospitals that had huge deficits.[46]

Five volumes, produced by researchers for the Health Research and Educational Trust of N.J. (HRET) provide a comprehensive evaluation of the state's DRG program.[47-51] May and Wasserman present selected conclusions on organizational impacts, economic and financial impacts, and an overview of the evaluation's findings. Significantly they state: "Even though some of the hospitals in New Jersey have been reimbursed by DRGs for almost 4 years, it is still not possible to state unequivocally that the system has been a complete success or a failure."[52]

Todd, a prominent New Jersey general surgeon and an AMA activist, made a similar evaluation: "After almost three years' experience with this program in New Jersey, I cannot tell you whether this is a good program, a bad program, whether or not it saves money or whether or not it has any effect on quality."[53] He also warned about overzealous emphasis on saving money. "Probably, the thing to be feared most is the merchandising of health for purely economic reasons."[54]

One of the HRET studies presented a history of the politics of the evolution of DRG rate regulation in New Jersey. Morone and Dunham pinpoint the DRG story with the precipitating events, the conflict and confusion among the participants, and the role of the state and federal governments. Although the investigators do say that the start and the finish of the DRG story is arbitrary, they raise a thoughtful question: "Does the tight state control of hospitals in New Jersey represent the future of all American hospitals?"[55]

In New Jersey's application for a continuation of its federal waiver from the PPS plan, Governor Kean estimated that $126 million would be saved from 1985 to 1987. Furthermore, he stated that the waivered states—New Jersey, New York, Massachusetts, and Maryland—saved a total of $1 billion in 1983 for Medicare services and he predicted similar savings in the future if the waivers continued. Between 1980 and 1983, the state's health commissioner claimed that New Jersey saved $299 million, reduced to $149 million because of a 13.5 percent increase to hospitals of $80 million.[56]

However, the Medicare savings in New Jersey do have their doubters. An economic and financial analysis of the DRG program by HRET did not come to a definitive answer. J. Joel May, HRET President, in commenting on saving money, said "It is still not possible at this point [February 1984] to pass final judgment."[57] In addition, New Jersey's PPS is significantly different from the federal PPS and that further dilutes implications for federal cost savings. A New Jersey Hospital Association official noted that the state is among the lowest in its dollar rate per admission.[58] Yet, Morristown Memorial Hospital anticipated a $500,000 loss in 1983 despite tightening up and cross-subsidizations. However, the medical director did expect the hospital to be back in the black for 1984.[59]

Jeffrey Wasserman, HRET Vice President for Research, was not completely pessimistic as he spoke about the 1983 losses in New Jersey hospitals.

> Not only is there no proof that the DRG system has saved money, but it is possible that the system has caused more money to be spent than would otherwise have been spent.[60]

Bringing the cost containment argument up to 1985, Medical Economics declared that the entire $3 billion hospital industry in New Jersey showed "a paltry $3 million profit in 1983—hardly more than break-even." Furthermore, the magazine said that was the "first taste of profit since DRG began five years ago." With 32 hospitals reporting losses, the other 60 or so were "just barely in the black."[61]

Another 1985 report in a local newspaper proclaimed that "Jersey Hospital Costs Rank Below Nation and Region."[62] This data was contained in a report from the New Jersey Hospital Association. From 1979 to 1983, statistics quoted that New Jersey residents spent $386 less for a hospital stay than other patients in the nation and $623 less than in other northeastern states. Officials of the Association stressed the savings accrued from the federal Medicare program that covers 40 percent of all hospital patients in the state.

To say the least, the New Jersey experience has advocates on both sides of the profit and loss column.

Battle for a New Waiver

About July 1984, a headline on the front page of American Medical News declared "N.J. to lose Medicare Waiver."[63] In a letter to the state health department, HCFA Administrator Carolyne Davis said that "HCFA had concluded that the program might cost Medicare 'significantly' more than if New Jersey hospitals were reimbursed under Medicare's national rules."[64] This HCFA action was motivated by the fact that New Jersey increased its DRG rate 13.66 percent on June 1, 1984 as compared to a 4 percent increase projected by HCFA for nonwaiver states. Speaking for the N.J. State Health Department, Seamans posited that HCFA's declaration was politically motivated. He said, "The current Administration would be inclined to have no waivers to gain centralized control of the entire Medicare system."[65]

Another article confirmed that New Jersey had been notified in the summer that HCFA intended to let the waiver lapse at the end of the year. However, the state was told that it could apply for a waiver by September 30, 1984.[66]

Political, community, and government individuals and organizations geared up to reverse the HCFA decision. Intensive work progressed on preparing the waiver application as mass media also spread the word about the potential bankruptcy of hospitals catering to the poor. Eight hospitals spending 10 percent or more of their annual budgets on charity care, ranging from $3.4 million to $10.1 million, were listed in the newspapers. Dollar savings were also featured in news stories. New Jersey claimed to have saved Medicare $229 million since 1980. However, in 1985 New Jersey will cost Medicare $28 million, but in 1986 and 1987 projected savings total $154 million, for a net gain of more than $125 million over the three-year period. This was the first time New Jersey released figures to support its cost containment statements.[67]

Keeping up the campaign, New Jersey's health commissioner told a symposium audience of health care experts that the state's DRG plan is being revamped to cut increases of $30 to $50 million projected for 1985 spending to secure another Medicare waiver.[68]

Going right to the top, Governor Thomas Kean released a letter he sent to President Reagan asking for his support. In his letter he said: "Prompt positive action on our new waiver applications will serve as an indication of your Administration's continued commitment to the role of states in finding new ways to meet the challenge of rising health care costs."[69]

Coming down to decision time in early December 1984, a chairman of a New Jersey State Assembly Committee was holding hearings on the state's cost containment program. An aide to Governor Kean prevailed upon the Chairman to delay testimony from critics until after the first of the year. It was agreed that nobody wanted to do anything to jeopardize the critical stage of the waiver negotiations.[70]

By December 30, 1984, a New York Times headline predicted "U.S. Extension of Health Plan in Jersey Seen."[71] This newspaper reported the positive action despite strong misgivings by HCFA and the Office of Management and Budget over the costs. Government financial studies projected that the New Jersey system would cost Medicare $23 to $50 million more over the next three years than if the national program was in effect. "According to federal and state health officials, political arguments prevailed over financial studies."[72]

As predicted, Governor Kean announced the new three-year waiver extension on January 2, 1985 with these words: "We are extremely pleased that New Jersey can continue its successful, pioneering method of containing hospital cost escalation. Everybody wins with this decision."[73]

Announcements also appeared in many publications, including the New York Times,[74] Medical World News,[75] and American Medical News.[76] Thanks were offered to Senators Bradley and Lautenberg and the House delegation for their bipartisan support in intensively lobbying for the waiver extension.[77] A New Jersey Hospital Association official credited Governor Kean's 11th-hour appeal with saving the waiver.[78]

On the negative side, HCFA limited the waiver to inpatient care and declined to extend the waiver to outpatient services despite a U.S. District Court order to do so. State officials are still concerned with reversing HCFA's decision. In addition, HCFA made the new waiver subject to provision that the state must:

- Consult with and provide relevant information to HCFA not less than 60 days before making any material changes in the system

- Allow HCFA to monitor actual cash payments under the state system for discharges that occur during each calendar quarter of the waiver, including the impact of lump sum reconciliation amounts that were incurred before the waiver.

- Submit within 30 days a plan to revise rates if the state's actual quarterly ratio exceeds the projected ratio by less than 2 percent.[79]

Despite the political heroics, the Medical Society of New Jersey continues to oppose the DRG system, regarding the method as an experiment. For its part, a New Jersey Hospital Association spokesman echoes the sentiments of others, saying, "It's my understanding that the Reagan Administration doesn't want waivers."[80]

Waiver Round-up

New Jersey earned its waiver extension through dint of hard political infighting. Maryland continues its waiver "on a rolling three-year period."[81] New York State lost its waiver as of December 31, 1985. In voting "no" on the waiver renewal, the New York State Hospital Association agreed with the State's Health Commissioner.[82] In addition, as early as April 1985, published reports indicated that New York was not going to extend this waiver and was going to go into the federal PPS.[83,84] Massachusetts also went the nonwaiver renewal route, with the Massachusetts Hospital Association Board of Trustees voting unanimously to oppose a waiver application in May of 1985.[85] HCFA continues to push for a national PPS/DRG cost containment mechanism. In sum, the momentum seems to be toward folding all the Medicare reimbursement methods into a single uniform system.

Waivers: Good or Bad?

In February 1984, the FAH published a study entitled, "The Potential Inequities of Medicare Waivers in DRG System Explored." This study was conducted by the FAH's director of research, Samuel A. Mitchell. Estimates projected that the waivers granted to Maryland, Massachusetts, New Jersey, and New York produced a $342 million "windfall" in 1982 for the hospitals in those states. Furthermore, the FAH study stated that the windfall reduces Medicare payments to hospitals in the other 46 states by $36 per case.[86] Adjustments for case mix and teaching costs would have lowered the windfall, but the FAH claimed data was unavailable. In any event, the total would still be significantly more than if the four waivered states were under the federal DRG plan.

The timing and the objective of the FAH study was attributed to political motivation. HCFA officials had already expressed concern about the 17 percent of Medicare expenditures going to the four waivered states and some state waivers were up for renewal at the time. FAH, representing investor-owned hospitals, finds "state rate review about as popular as the plague,"[87] and opposes continuation and/or expansion of state rate-setting efforts.

Presidents of the four state hospital associations quickly condemned the FAH report and cited the following glaring omissions:

- No adjustments for the more severe case mix index in the four states

- No provision for medical education payments to cover the 27 percent of the nation's medical and dental residencies in the four states

- Failure to mention that Massachusetts and New York were not yet waivered and couldn't be included in the 1982 database

Failure to mention that federal legislation requires that states not receive funding in excess of what federal PPS would pay without a waiver.[88]

A spokesman for the four state hospital associations summed up their angry reactions: "The conceptual flaws that maim the study are so obvious and the analysis so biased that it should be readily apparent to even the most casual observer that the motivation is questionable and the results fallacious."[89]

Following this battle between the waivered states and the FAH, an editorial in *Modern Healthcare* called for an end to state waivers from the Medicare PPS. It was noted that HCFA hinted that waivers were going to end and no new exceptions would be granted. "This is the only sensible way the federal government can go. The reason is simple: State waivers increase HCFA's administrative and claims processing costs. The federal government's staff . . . would have to be greatly expanded so individual state programs could be monitored."[90]

Hospital trustees and managers were urged to fight efforts in their own states to secure waivers from the Medicare PPS. HCFA was urged to make the Medicare PPS apply to all hospitals in the nation.

References

1. U.S. Congress, Office of Technology Assessment, *Diagnosis Related Groups (DRGs) and the Medicare Program: Implications for Medical Technology. A Technical Memorandum*. Washington, DC, OTA-TM-H-17, July 1983, pp. 70-75.

2. A. Esposito, M. Hupfer, C. Mason, and D. Rogler. "Abstracts of State Legislated Hospital Cost-Containment Programs," *Health Care Financing Review* 4, No. 2, (1982):129-158.

3. "The States and Health Care: Girding for DRGs, Budget Cuts and Rate Control Fights," *FAH Review* 16, No. 5, (1983):16-36.

4. R. V. Peterson. "Waiver Provisions Allow State Opt-Outs from Federal PPS," *Health Law Vigil* 6, No. 16, (August 5, 1983):7-9.

5. Ibid.

6. Ibid.

7. C. Wallace. "DRGs—Only Rule Too Late to Block Most Medicare Waivers to States," *Modern Healthcare* 12, No. 11, (1982):16-17.

8. H. A. Cohen. Comments on Kinzer and Warner's "The Effect of Case Mix Adjustment on Admission Based Reimbursement," *Health Services Research* 18, No. 2, (Summer, 1983):226-232.

9. A. M. Powers. "DRGs: Optional in Maryland's GIR System," *Hospital Progress* 62, No. 1, (1981):47-48.

10. G. D. Zuidema, P. E. Dans, and E. D. Dunlap. "Documentation of Care and Prospective Payment. One Hospital's Experience," *Annals of Surgery* 199, No. 5, (1984):515-521.

11. D. Kinzer and M. Warner. "The Effect of Case Mix Adjustment on Admission Based Reimbursement," *Health Services Research* 18, No. 2, (Summer, 1983):209-225.

12. "Maryland Hospitals' 1983 Profits Soar, Rate Setters Say," *Modern Healthcare* 14, No. 4, (1984):11.

13. "States and Healthcare," *FAH Review*.

14. C. Frankenstein and R. Mintz. *Some Effects of New Payment Incentives on Hospital Human Resources in Maryland and New Jersey.* Public Policy Analysis paper, The American Hospital Association, undated.

15. C. Bankhead. "States Assess Waiver Status," *Medical World News* 29, No. 5, (March 11, 1985):92.

16. Ibid.

17. A. Andersen, HCFA, Office of Demonstrations and Evaluation. Personal communication, October 15, 1985. "Maryland Gets Unexpected Waiver Approval from HCFA," *Hospitals* 59, No. 7, (April 1, 1985):17.

18. R. J. Rogen. *Testimony at Hearings on PPS before U.S. Senate Finance Committee on Health,* February 17, 1983, pp. 221-224.

19. Bankhead. "States Assess Waiver Status."

20. "Massachusetts Hospitals Oppose Application for Medicare Waiver," *Hospitals* 59, No. 11, (June 1, 1985):19.

21. H. S. Ruchlin and H. M. Rosen. "The Process of Hospital Rate Regulation: The New York Experience," *Inquiry* 18, (Spring, 1981):70-78.

22. R. M. Crane. *Testimony on PPS before U.S. Senate Finance Committee on Health,* February 2, 1983, pp. 149-156.

23. *Statement submitted to U.S. Senate Finance Committee on Hearing on PPS,* February 17, 1983, p. 430.

24. Hospital Association of New York State. *New York's Prospective Hospital Reimbursement Methodology (NYPHRM), 1983-1985.* Undated leaflet.

25. Bankhead. "States Assess Waiver Status."

26. D. E. L. Johnson. "New York, Other States Resist UB-82," *Modern Healthcare* 14, No. 3, (February 15, 1984):32.

27. Ibid.

28. Bankhead. "States Assess Waiver Status."

29. R. Sullivan. "Review Bars 13.9% of Payments By Medicare to Hospitals in City," *New York Times,* April 9, 1985.

30. Frankenstein and Mintz. "Effects of New Payment Incentives."

31. M. D. Rosko. "The Impact of Prospective Payment: A Multi-Dimensional Analysis of New Jersey's Share Program," *Journal of Health Politics, Policy, and Law* 9, No. 1, (Spring, 1984):81-101.

32. F. A. Shaffer. "DRGs: History and Overview," *Nursing & Health Care* 4, No. 7, (1983):388-396.

33. C. F. Pierce, Jr. "The New Jersey Experience with DRG Reimbursement," *Testimony Before House Select Committee on Aging,* Princeton, NJ, March 28, 1983, p. 18.

34. H. H. Goldberg. "Prospective Payment DRGs: New Jersey and the USA," *Neurology* 34, No. 8, (1984):1073-1076.

35. C. F. Pierce, Jr. "The Impact of DRGs on Payers," DRGs: *The Effect in New Jersey. The Potential for the Nation,* USDHHS, HCFA, Pub. No. 03170, March 1984, p. 135.

36. H. Holzberg. "Implications of DRGs for Hospitals," Presentation at a seminar on *The DRGs: A Prognosis for New York State,* at SUNY Health Sciences Center, Stony Brook, NY, June 15, 1984.

37. J. Chenoweth. "DRGs: What's the Future Bottom Line for Health Care?" *Topics in Health Record Management* 4, No. 3, (1984):32-45.

38. Beth Israel Hospital, Newark, NJ, *Inservice DRG Training Material.* Undated, pp. 6-7.

39. J. J. May and J. Wasserman. "Selected Results from an Evaluation of the New Jersey Diagnosis Related Group System," *Health Services Research* 19, No. 5, (1984):547-559.

40. "Court Invalidates New Jersey DRG Plan," *Hospitals* 57, No. 16, (August 16, 1983):22.

41. Frankenstein and Mintz. "Effects of New Payment Incentives."

42. DRGs: *The Effect in New Jersey. The Potential for the Nation.* USDHHS, Health Care Financing Administration. HCFA Pub. No. 03170, March 1984.

43. "Failure of a Hospital Diet" (editorial), *New York Times,* April 2, 1984.

44. J. R. Goldstein. "Health Cost Curbs: Give Jersey DRGs Time," New York Times, April 12, 1984.

45. J. A. McMahon. "National System With a Difference," *New York Times,* April 12, 1984.

46. F. J. Primich. "The Added $250 Million," *New York Times,* April 12, 1984.

47. H. Boerma. *The Organizational Impact of DRGs.* Volume IV-B. Health Research and Educational Trust, Princeton, NJ, January 1983.

48. A. B. Dunham and J. A. Morone. *The Politics of Innovation. The Evolution of DRG Rate Regulation in New Jersey. Volume IV-A.* Health Research and Educational Trust, Princeton, NJ, January 1983.

49. *Economic and Financial Analysis. Volume II.* Health Research and Educational Trust, Princeton, NJ, February 1984.

50. *Case Mix Classification, Data, and Management. Volume III.* Health Research and Educational Trust, Princeton, NJ, February 1984.

51. J. Wasserman. *Introduction and Overview. Volume I.* Health Research and Educational Trust, Princeton, NJ, June 1982.

52. May and Wasserman. "Selected Results."

53. J. M. Todd. "The DRG Experience in New Jersey," *Missouri Medicine* 81, No. 7, (1984):408-410, 412.

54. Ibid.

55. J. A. Morone and A. B. Dunham. "The Waning of Professional Dominance: DRGs and the Hospitals," *Health Affairs* 3, No. 1, (Spring, 1984):73-87.

56. R. Cohen. "Kean Stresses Saving Under Medicare Plan," *Star Ledger,* (New Jersey), October 12, 1984.

57. Health Research and Educational Trust of New Jersey, *DRG Evaluation. Economic and Financial Analysis. Volume II,* Princeton, NJ, 1984, p. xi.

58. "Report Shows Rise in New Jersey Hospital Costs," *Hospitals* 58, No. 8, (April 16, 1984):25.

59. P. C. Smith. "We Tightened Up, Still Lost a Bundle," *Hospital Tribune* 16, No. 2, (February 15, 1984):3.

60. P. C. Smith. "With DRGs, New Jersey Hospitals More in Red Than Ever," *Hospital Tribune* 16, No. 2, (February 15, 1984):3.

61. "DRG: What Do You Cut After You've Cut Out the Fat?" *Medical Economics,* March 18, 1985.

62. "Jersey Hospital Costs Rank Below Nation and Region," *Star-Ledger,* (New Jersey), May 2, 1985.

63. D. Lefton. "New Jersey to Lose Medicare Waiver," *American Medical News* 27, No. 25, (June 29/July 6, 1984):1, 13.

64. Ibid.

65. Ibid.

66. M. R. Traska. "State Programs Expect to Keep PPS Waivers," *Hospitals* 58, No. 20, (October 16, 1984):41-42.

67. J. Whitlow. "Jersey Defends Hospital Fee Curbs as More Fair, Less Costly Than U.S. Plan," *Star-Ledger* (New Jersey), September 27, 1984.

68. "New Jersey to Revamp DRG Plan in Hopes of Securing Medicare Waiver," *Hospitals* 58, No. 20, (October 16, 1984):23, 25.

69. R. Cohen. "Kean Stresses Saving Under Medicare Plan," *Star-Ledger* (New Jersey), October 12, 1984.

70. J. F. Sullivan. "Testimony Delayed for Critics of Jersey Health Cost System," *New York Times,* December 4, 1984.

71. R. Sullivan. "U.S. Extension of Health Plan in Jersey Seen," New York Times, December 20, 1984.

72. Ibid.

73. D. Kenyon. "DRG Plan Wins Extension," *The News Tribune,* January 1, 1985.

74. "System Extended for Hospital Bills," *New York Times,* January 3, 1985.

75. Bankhead. "States Assess Waiver Status."

76. C. Cancila. "New Jersey's Medicaid Waiver Renewed by HCFA," *American Medical News* 28, No. 2, (January 11, 1985):8.

77. Kenyon. "DRG Plan."

78. Bankhead. "States Assess Waiver Status."

79. Cancila. "New Jersey's Medicaid Waiver."

80. Ibid.

81. Traska. "State Programs."

82. "Draft Legislation in New York Would Terminate Waiver," *Hospitals* 59, No. 10, (May 16, 1985):20, 24.

83. R. Sullivan. "About 25% of Beds in Hospitals in City are Empty, State Reports," *New York Times,* May 2, 1985.

84. R. Sullivan. "Decline in Hospital Use Tied to New U.S. Policies," *New York Times,* May 16, 1985.

85. "Massachusetts Hospitals Oppose Application," *Hospitals.*

86. C. Wallace and D. E. L. Johnson. "FAH, Four Waivered States Tussle Over Study on Effect of Rate Setting," *Modern Healthcare* 14, No. 4, (1984):138, 141.

87. Ibid.

88. D. Lefton. "State Hospital Groups Hit FAH Report on Waivers," *America Medical News* 27, No. 6, (February 10, 1984):1, 7.

89. "Waivered States Deny Higher Costs," *Hospitals* 58, No. 5, (March 1, 1984):17.

90. "End State Waivers" (editorial), *Modern Healthcare* 14, No. 5, (1984):5.

PART II
IMPACTS ON
THE HOSPITAL

CHAPTER 3
Operational Management Variables for Inpatient Services

Arguments abound about the ethical aspects of medical care versus the business of medicine. Similarly, discussions focus on whether hospital care is an industrial venture or a community service. Prospective payment, using DRGs, emphasizes the business of hospital care. Administrators must be capable of running an institution without falling into a negative cash balance.

Managerial decisions fall into two categories: those concerning the operation of the facility and those pertaining to the facility's structural organization. Operational variables include the overall cost containment environment, the hospital's case mix, the severity of illness issue, reimbursement for capital costs, medical technology, marketing services, and procedures known as "gaming the system." Structural variables deal with items such as the type of institutional auspices, participation of trustees, legal aspects, physician/administration relations, implementation activities, and the creation of new positions to move the new reimbursement plan along.

These administrative options are influenced by a wide range of vested interests inside and outside the hospital. However, there appears to be a consensus that PPS has effectively applied a business ethic to the management variables. Executives may be forced to make unpleasant choices under the banner of effective management principles.

It is readily apparent that every hospital must place cost-containment strategies at the forefront of their operational philosophy. In the toss-up between hospitals as a community service and hospitals as a business, community service appears to be the loser. That loss could lead to a rationing of services and to judgments about the ethical nature of managerial determinations regarding hospital operations.

Using the Robin Hood technique of taking from the rich to give to the poor, administrators may be able to shift costs to cover inadequately reimbursed services. However, that management option could disappear if all-payer reimbursement systems evolved from the Medicare PPS/DRG model.

Case mix is another prime operational concern of hospital managers. Under the DRG payment mode, a direct relationship exists between the hospital's case mix and its financial viability. To achieve some control over case mix, administrators will create greatly expanded informational systems to generate the vital data for rational decision making. Of course, managers will have to significantly increase their hospitals' computerization in order to execute these responsibilities.

Directly related to case mix deliberations, the severity of illness aspects of DRG payment rates occupies extensive managerial time. A number of operational choices exist to justify the use of additional resources to care for patients with severe—and not DRG average—illness. While medical care experts debate which severity of illness technique to adopt, the government contends that the problem is already accommodated in the PPS/DRG model by outliers, exemptions, and other mechanisms for additional funding.

Even though admissions and length of stay are under the direct control of the attending physician, there are management aspects to consider. In addition, the use of medical technology is closely allied to the length of stay and the severity of illness. Operationally, nonphysician administrators may have a great deal more input into acquisition decisions under the PPS/DRG program.

Getting down to the bottom line mentality of front line managers, hospital executives have plunged into the typical industrial marketing activities of selling their products. Starting with the concept of hospital product lines, administrators have adapted commercial salesmanship techniques to attract customers to their facilities. This salesmanship mode also raised the issue of DRG manipulation or the newly coined disease of "DRG Creep." A new argot emerged to describe ways to get the most DRG reimbursement possible for the illnesses being treated in the hospital.

The operational components of hospital management are profoundly influenced by the all-encompassing blanket of cost containment ideology. In turn, that philosophy has stimulated the intensive business-like approach to running a hospital.

Cost Containment

It is quite possible that more high level management decisions will be based on cost containment principles than on any other factor dealing with the aggregate components of health care services. Concerns about the rapidly rising costs of health care took hold in Congress and resulted in a variety of legislation aimed at curbing inflation while still maintaining quality care.

In late 1982, Somers, a prominent health economist, discussed moderating the rise in health care costs. She concluded that, "there are no shortcuts to containment of health care costs."[1] In considering the same topic, Alper pointed out that doctors, patients, and hospital administrators—those most directly concerned with hospital care—"have no common rallying point for cost control."[2] Even after the federal government indicated a move toward a PPS using DRGs which would provide such a rallying point, Crosby "emphasized that it would take a lot more creative strategies than those encompassed in a DRG plan to bring costs under control."[3] Powers noted prior governmental actions to obtain "more for less" and emerged with a mathematical ratio: "History shows that the half-life of any proclaimed 'answer' to the problem of health care costs normally is about two years, which not coincidentally is roughly the usual term of office of an HEW (now HHS) Secretary."[4]

Despite the caveats, DRGs are the mechanism touted to achieve the elusive goal of containing costs. In addition, the concept appears to have gained acceptance as an effective cost containment strategy. In a 1984 survey report sponsored by the Equitable Life Assurance Society, 76 percent of the public and 71 percent of hospital administrators found the DRG system "very" and "somewhat" acceptable. Physicians did not agree: 61 percent found DRGs "not very" or "not at all" acceptable. However, even 58 percent of the physicians do concede that DRGs will be effective in controlling costs.[5] Furthermore, major American industries also endorse health care cost containment efforts and approve of actions to lower the inflationary upward trend.[6] In discussing an ideal reimbursement system, Saline described the roles for the government, providers, employers, and the insurance carriers. He opted for a "more or less free enterprise" approach with all the participants helping in the evolutionary process.[7]

Actions for Profit

Bromberg enumerated eight actions that hospitals will be encouraged to take in the name of cost containment:

1. Limit the growth in the number of hospital employees.

2. Limit wage and benefit increases.

3. Reconsider capital expenditures that increase operating costs.

4. Consider specialization in DRGs that are economical.

5. Urge physicians to order more preadmission testing to reduce length of stay and inpatient testing.

6. Urge physicians to order fewer ancillary tests per patient.

7. Make arrangements with alternative, less expensive providers for post-hospital care.

8. Seek price discounts on supplies.[8]

From a management view, these eight actions tighten costs and increase profits. Interestingly, under the retrospective payment system, these actions would have decreased revenue without adding anything to the profit margin.

In a related manner, Doremus identified five variables playing a major role in costing outpatient care. Using slightly different language with management phrases, the items include the following:

1. Physician Practices—process of selecting inputs to achieve output, skill, and so on

2. Quality of Inputs— ancillaries supplied by hospital

3. Patient—response to treatment, general physical condition, and so on

4. Illness—thousands of potential combinations of diagnostic and surgical procedure codes as well as individual codes

5. Patient's Degree of Being Healed—finished product of the hospital.[9]

Cost Accounting

To achieve cost containment objectives, hospitals will have to adopt modern cost accounting procedures. Cleverley succinctly explains the determination of true costs, the different types of costs, and the evaluation of accounting systems.[10] An entire issue of DRG Monitor relates the method to PPS, stressing the importance to the viability of the hospital.[11] A health care consultant emphasizes the development of product lines in the manager's tasks.[12] Sophistication is added with discussions about net contribution variance analysis[13] and determining the contribution margin for DRG profitability.[14]

These few examples all lead to an understanding of a competitive market approach to cost control using modern accounting mechanisms. Generally, hospitals have not had to operate like industrial firms pricing out each element of the finished product to arrive at a final selling price for the merchandise. In addition to pricing, cost accounting procedures create data that are helpful in planning for additional cost containment measures.

Health Planning Lessons

In applying the experiences of health planners to the problem of cost containment, Waters and Tierney reflect upon the hard lessons learned when the emphasis switched from access to the "bottom line." They came up with 10 guidelines.

1. Open-ended third party financing of health care is unrealistic.

2. A la carte financing of health care is inherently inflationary.

3. Separate financing systems lead to cost shifting.

4. Separate has not proved to be equal in health care.

5. Government is not well suited to deliver health care services, except in special circumstances.

6. Performance follows money; reimbursement encourages activities.

7. There is no such thing as a good monopoly in health services.

8. Quantity and costs of medical care delivered in a given community are directly related to the number of hospital beds and physicians and the pattern of medical practice, not to the level of disease.

9. External regulation of medical care is a negative, stifling approach.

10. The science of clinical medicine is not exact and needs a stronger database.

These commentators believe that the hard lessons, enumerated above, can be applied to national health programs to result in "appropriate access to high quality health care at a reasonable cost."[15]

Who Controls Costs?

Hospital administration experts are quick to point out that the upward cost trend is not solely within their control. "Hospitals do not admit, treat or discharge patients—doctors do."[16] In fact, physician specialists do even more so. About 42 percent of medical specialists' services to Medicare patients take place in hospitals, as compared to about 19 percent for general practitioners.[17] However, Hyman, a founder of Private Doctors of America, compares the $155.18 electrical contractor's bill for replacing a $3.64 circuit breaker to the physician's role in hospital costs. He concludes that the doctor does not control hospital costs and suggests referring the complaining patient to the proper bureaucrat in Washington, DC.[18] Blitzer, chief economist for Standard & Poors Corporation, commented that "health care doesn't follow the pattern of a typical market economy."[19] For that reason, he said that "Medicare's prospective payment system is a quick fix that won't put the brakes on escalating health care costs in the long term."[20] In addition, Blitzer commented that DRGs will only affect price but will not integrate the volume.

Volume and Price

In an 1980 article, Thompson dealt with volume and price considerations. He defined cost "as total expenditures per unit of population" with the end goal expressed in the equation, Total Cost = Volume × Price.[21] Prior governmental efforts to control volume took the form of a Regional Medical Program (RMP), Utilization Review (UR), Professional Standards Review Organizations (PSROs), Health Systems Agencies (HSAs) and Health Maintenance Organizations (HMOs). Price control came about through state and local hospital cost control programs and rate setting regulatory bodies. Rochester, New York's Maxicap experiment did try to control both volume and price. Thompson concludes: "What this means, then, is that any program aimed at deescalating hospital costs in this country must control both the volume and price factors, and must involve physicians, hospital boards, and administrators if there is to be any real effect on long-term or short-term costs."[22]

Three strategies are identified that could directly or indirectly influence the prices of hospital services.

1. Treating specific conditions on an outpatient basis instead of an inpatient basis, i.e., ambulatory surgery

2. Transferring services to an outpatient basis, i.e., preadmission testing

3. Reducing lengths of stay and admissions in hospitals, i.e., early discharge planning.

In conclusion, Thompson posited: "The only system now operative which can deal with the complex interrelationship between the volume and price of services is the DRG system."[23]

Writing in the *Harvard Business Review*, Egdahl disagrees with Thompson's conclusion. He notes the DRGs' limitations and is negative about cost control: "The current push to pay hospitals for the care of medical patients by diagnostic related groups does not involve 'volume' controls, and health costs will rise as the volume of services increases."[24]

Rationing Resources

In relating the issue of resource use to costs, the President of the American College of Physicians equated cutting costs with using health resources properly. Reitemeier talked about access limitations and reductions in services while stressing the appropriate use of available resources.[25] Even while applauding the inflationary slowdown, a *New York Times* editorial also raised the specter of resource curtailment. "Some 'rationing' of health care seems inevitable and remains an urgent subject for debate."[26] A feature article in *Medical World News* asked if health care rationing could happen in the United States.[27] In response, the comment was that "health care rationing is inextricably linked with cost containment."[28] In fact, the President of the Union of American Physicians and Dentists stated that "diagnosis related groups were conceived as a rationing program."[29] Schwartz, coauthor of a book on rationing health care, coldly analyzes the cost containment impact on resource use: "The idea that by getting rid of the fat we can keep the current system is a myth. The only way to cut costs will be to deny benefits to some people or deny benefits for some diseases."[30]

A number of issues and trends related to resource allocation—the euphemism for rationing—will figure in the linking of cost containment to whatever emerges. These identified issues will require equitable resolutions.

- Cost containment legislation is directly linked to reduced benefits.

- Rationing plans need to be developed.

- Nobody is rushing forward to make rationing decisions.

- A basic level of care has yet to be defined.

- American values regarding death and dying may require an overhaul.

- A lack of a solution to the economic and ethical problems could lead to a national health insurance program.[31]

Expanding a bit on the terminal care issue, Ginzberg noted that many excessive health care costs are related to the high cost of dying in America. While he agreed that medical technology saves lives, Ginzberg said that "medicine can't provide perpetual life."[32] He urged the American public to modify their attitudes and to comprehend the limitations of health care services. Others have suggested ways to avoid health care rationing.

- Resolve variations in medical practice resulting in cost reductions and saving the system without rationing.

- Reduce demands on the hospital system through insurance copayments and deductibles and better use of outpatient services and a stress on healthful living.

- Emphasize prevention and accept medicine's limitations in treating terminal illness.

- Initiate a means test for Medicare patients and allow hospitals to bill for unreimbursed costs.[33]

While it appears incongruous to talk about health care rationing in one of the richest countries in the world, the subject is not merely idle talk. Regardless of which words are used to describe the situation, the United States has to consider the appropriate effective and efficient use of its health care resources.

Cost Shifting

Hospitals that experience losses under the DRG reimbursement mechanism can attempt to shift costs to patients covered by programs other than Medicare. "Simply put, through the cost shift, private patients subsidize uninsured people and public program beneficiaries."[34] Other insurers may pay more than the DRG rate for exactly the same services. A booklet from the Health Insurance Association of America, a trade organization, estimated the charges shifted to the private sector at $7.9 billion in 1983 and $8.8 billion in 1984.[35] When the federal PPS began in 1983, a *New York Times* editorial called attention to the possibility of cost shifting.[36] Almost a year later, another Times editorial noted that the cost shifting phenomenon did not occur.[37] A trade association representing private hospitals, the Federation of American Hospitals (FAH), also challenged the cost shifting assumption. FAH felt that all economy measures affecting productivity and effectiveness would apply to all patients regardless of who picks up the tab.[38] Pointing out the basic flaw that DRG rates do not apply to more than half of all hospital care, an anecdotal impact statement appeared in a 1984 letter to the editor: "Knowledgeable hospital administrators readily concede that despite Medicare's restrictive payment system, they are not likely to have much difficulty balancing their budgets as long as they can make up the shortfall through increased charges to non-Medicare patients."[39]

When asked if they approved of cost shifting, 87 percent of the hospital administrators polled did not condone the technique. Obviously, those participating in the poll were not the "knowledgeable" ones mentioned above. Physicians and the public also disapproved by 87 and 74 percent, respectively.[40] As an aside, Cain comments that when only two parties are involved, it is called cost sharing and is applauded.[41]

Avoiding the value connotations, Ginsburg and Sloan identify three sources of payment differentials.

1. Limitations in the cost finding accounting systems that are used to allocate costs

2. Costs of hospital activities that are not directly attributable to the care of paying patients, such as charity care and unfunded research

3. Prudent purchasing policies of insurers that pay "reasonable" costs.[42]

Options suggested to resolve the problem include grants to hospitals for bad debts and charity care, all-payer hospital rate setting, and an antitrust exemption to allow commercial insurers to negotiate lower rates with hospitals.[43] Meyer adds consideration of a ceiling on the tax free status of employer contributions to employee health insurance or a redesign of Medicare benefits to include more cost sharing, catastrophic coverage, and/or a voucher arrangement.[44]

Ginsburg and Sloan conclude that the cost shifting resolution resides in broad policy decisions that rely on market forces or regulation to contain health care costs.[45]

Case Mix: The Source

"Of all the new management challenges hospitals will face, however, case mix management looms as one of the most important."[46] This statement was delivered by Jack W. Owen, executive vice president of the American Hospital Association at a conference on health care institutions in flux. Changing health care reimbursement in the 1980s was the flux that was discussed from a variety of viewpoints.[47]

Hospital Products

Underpinning the importance of the case mix concept is the fact that "a hospital will have to manage and control its case mix to keep out of the red under Medicare's new system. Case mix is synonymous with product mix."[48] This health care consultant went on to discuss the development of product families, the setting up of product families, and "dynamic" product families. In taking a business-oriented view of a hospital, a private health care insurer noted that "the unavoidable basic question is: What does the hospital produce?"[49] Dr. E. A. Codman, a prominent Massachusetts surgeon, addressed that question in 1914: "What, then, are the products of a large hospital, whether in the form of healed wounds, healthy babies, faithful nurses, promising young surgeons and physicians, or in the more abstract forms or original ideas on pathology or treatment, model methods of administration, or such intangible things as enthusiasm and ideals?"[50]

Bringing the consideration into the present, in December 1984, Berki remarked that "current discussion of hospital 'product lines' is in terms of the mix of DRGs, or the case mix."[41] Without mincing words, a group of hospital management experts developed a program matrix to "essentially represent what industrial corporations call 'product lines.' For the hospital, product lines are patient groupings."[52]

Case Mix and Hospital Cost Relation

In conducting an evaluation of economic variables related to the efficiency of health services, Feldstein argued that hospital costs were related to case mix.[53] He changed the prior emphasis on institutional factors to one centering on the characteristics of patients. "Since then it has come to be universally accepted that hospital costs and case mix are positively correlated."[54] A number of other studies confirm the direct relation between case mix measures and cost.[55-58] In assessing the AUTOGRP case mix classification system, Young and her colleagues pointed out that "programs in prospective budgeting and hospital rate setting are increasingly in need of differential case mix information in order to more accurately relate reimbursement to production costs and performance."[59] After investigating the effect of case mix adjustment on prospective admission-based reimbursement, Kinzer and Warner concluded: "The results of this analysis indicate that controlling for case mix has a highly significant impact on the amount of revenue hospitals receive under such programs."[60]

Linking case mix concepts to DRGs, Goran stated that DRGs define a hospital's product based upon a case-mix reimbursement system.[61] Interestingly, Goran called attention to the possibility of clinicians inflating the complexity of their cases to result in "case mix creep."[62] While sounding off on the related new hospital-acquired disease "DRG Creep," Simborg also echoed Goran's point about DRGs and case mix: "Today, the use of DRGs is virtually synonymous with case mix measurement, and it has become the standard method to describe hospital outputs for any use."[63]

While Reiss recognizes that case mix per se is only a valuable tool, he does attribute a major advantage to the technique. In addition to using case mix to link medical definitions of problems to finances, case mix can also relate to quality, safety, and other issues.[64]

There does not appear to be any doubt that case mix is synonymous with hospital reimbursement methods. However, the relation can depend upon what definition and purpose is assigned to the case mix measures. It is also relevant to note that an article, 12 years before the federal PPS was implemented, found that each hospital's case mix changes little from year to year.[65]

Case Mix Defined

Starting out with a managerial approach, Reiss says that "case mix provides a measure of output for the health care delivery system."[66] Ament adds more detail, defining case mix as the "distribution of a hospital's patients among different diagnostic, age, and operative groups."[67] Likewise, Hulm and Burik state that "a hospital's case mix is the number and proportions of particular case types or disease groups. These groups can be referred to as the hospital's product line or programs."[68] In its glossary of terms, the Office of Technology Assessment report combined resources with patients and noted that case mix is "the relative frequency of admissions of various types of patients, reflecting different needs for hospital resources."[69]

In an economic and financial analysis of the DRG program in New Jersey, the investigators identified the desirable elements of an acceptable case mix measure as follows:

- Case mix must be based on reliable information that is easily accessible at a reasonable cost.

- Each patient must be assigned to one and only one group.

- Case mix must be medically meaningful to physicians and understood by the hospital personnel who will work with it.

- Patients who consume resources of relatively equivalent value must be grouped together.

- Case mix must be useful for administrative and planning purposes.

- There must be sufficient versatility so that the groups can be combined in various ways for different purposes.

- Benefits of using the scheme must justify its costs.[70]

Yale University researchers, in a 1975 study of case mix and resource use, compared 34 diagnostic groupings in 18 hospitals in Connecticut. In addition to marked differences in resource use, they came to one inescapable conclusion: "There is a substantial difference in the diagnostic mix of patients treated in hospitals that are seemingly delivering the same product and fulfilling the same role in their communities."[71]

Case-Mix Complexity

To add to the vagaries of a case-mix definition, Averill explained case mix complexity as "an interrelated but distinct set of patient attributes that include severity of illness, prognosis, treatment difficulty, need for intervention and resource intensity."[72] He then proceeded to give precise meanings for each of the five patient attributes. Reiss also illustrates the complexity of case-mix applications by defining 32 data items used in measurements.[73]

Despite the varied definitions, two distinct and essential parts of case mix measurements are repeatedly identified:

1. Grouping of clinically homogeneous patient categories

2. Specification of resources required for clinically appropriate management of the patient groupings linked to resource costs.[74,75]

Case-Mix Index (CMI)

Using the essential components of case-mix measures, a case-mix index (CMI) can be developed. Lave et al. define a CMI as a "a scalar measure of the relative costliness of the inpatient cases treated in a particular hospital compared to those treated in the 'average' or 'typical' hospital."[76] Thus, for all hospitals, the CMI is 1.0; hospitals with CMIs above 1.0 spend more to treat their patients while hospitals with CMIs below 1.0 spend less. Under the PPS law, each hospital calculates its own hospital specific CMI using Medicare Provider Analysis and Review (MEDPAR) data and actual Medicare costs.[77] Grimaldi explicitly details the calculation and adjustment of Medicare CMIs and the DRG methodology.[78]

Keeping the definitions in mind, the purposes for using case mix can be considered as another part of managerial options.

Purposes of Case-Mix Measurements

Depending upon the initial purpose of gathering case-mix measurements, an optimal method is selected. Case-mix measures could be used for purposes such as reimbursement, quality assurance, management, policy decisions, and research. Regardless of the purpose, significant data requirements accompany any but the most rudimentary measures. This variation in purposes "has been a barrier because it appears that the optimal measure may be different"[79] according to the anticipated purpose.

Hornbrook applies case-mix measures in three general areas: policy, administration, and research.[80] Examples in each area follow:

Policy	Administration	Research
Reimbursement	Quality Control	Estimation of Variable
Planning	Planning and Budgeting	Cost Estimation
Program Evaluation		Production Estimation[81]

In relation to using case-mix measures for reimbursement alone, Butler and Bentley identify 10 major policy issues encountered by payers and hospitals.

1. Choosing the measure

2. Tying the measure to reimbursement

3. Determining which costs are related

4. Allocating costs to diagnostic groups

5. Identifying, collecting, and processing the data

6. Defining atypical patients

7. Examining historical trends

8. Deciding which third parties will participate

9. Meeting the needs of different types of hospitals

10. Designing an exception process.[82]

In concluding, Butler and Bentley call for the policy issues to be clearly defined and explained to all concerned parties so as alleviate fears about institutional survival. "Hospitals and third parties should understand that choices are available."[83]

While examining future directions for case-mix applications, Reiss details three general purposes that relate to Hornbrook's use of case-mix measures. However, Reiss does add the vested interests of the patient and the funding body into the purposes:

1. Payment

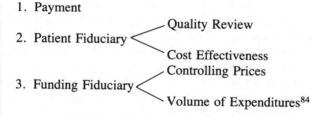

2. Patient Fiduciary ⟨ Quality Review / Cost Effectiveness

3. Funding Fiduciary ⟨ Controlling Prices / Volume of Expenditures[84]

Regulation is another purpose aligned with the use of case-mix measurements. "The state of the art in hospital regulation requires the use of case-mix data for regulatory purposes."[85] Of course, it should be pointed out that the above statement appeared in an article by the executive director of a state rate setting commission. Nevertheless, Cohen and Atkinson list five major regulatory purposes and add a sixth for exploration:

1. Budget review to determine the appropriate rate level

2. Charge setting to determine the appropriate rate structure

3. Public disclosure

4. Capital expenditure review and health planning

5. Utilization review

6. Epidemiological studies.[86]

Both Hornbrook and Cohen and Atkinson specify the use of case-mix measures for health planning. Greenberg and Kropf developed cost-effective criteria for five specific elements in coronary care units. Chart abstracts from 19 New Jersey hospitals provided the case-mix data to allow the researchers to illustrate criteria norms lower than accepted health planning standards for average length of stay, CCU beds needed per 100,000 population served and per 100 general service beds, CCU discharges per AMI (acute myocardial infarction) discharge, and AMI discharges per 1,000 population served. These investigators concluded that "the case mix method . . . is a powerful, inexpensive tool for relating the clinical, cost and utilization aspects of hospital care . . . The case mix method should also be used to evaluate the cost effectiveness of other forms of hospital care. . . ."[87]

Another purpose of case-mix measures relates to the quality of care. Gerber et al. compare case mix, costs, and outcomes between faculty and community services at Stanford University Medical Center in California. After adjustment for case mix and patient characteristics, statistically fewer patients died when cared for on the faculty service, with the difference being particularly larger for patients at greater risk.[88] With case-mix analysis showing higher costs on faculty services despite similar patient groupings, the policy issue of the relation between expenditures and quality of care raises a crucial question: Do you contain costs or do you save lives? Investigators admit the difficulty of ascertaining the contributions of aggressive faculty service care. They also note the difficulty of judging whether the reduced mortality justified the cost. Yet, they urge that hospital mortality rates be monitored as well as hospital expenditures.

Case-Mix Data

However, it is clear that any effort to move toward case-mix reimbursement . . . must be accompanied by recognition that the project cannot succeed without extensive data collection and data processing capabilities; participation by and cooperation among providers, payers and those designing the system and patience and a commitment to thoroughly explore the options available.[89]

Few, if any, disagree with the emphasis upon the collection of reliable data in any chosen case-mix system for reimbursement. In fact, current journals in the health care field carry a burgeoning number of advertisements that offer to make the data collection task manageable for institutions.

Lichtig detailed the data requirements and specifically cited examples of patient identification data, patient demographic data, patient stay data, clinical data items, physician data, and charge data—about 23 bits of information.[90] When the volume of data is high, critics contend that the problem of accuracy and errors is a considerable hurdle to overcome. Bentley typically notes advantages and disadvantages,[91] while Reiss also debates pros and cons in talking about future applications of case mix.[92] In addition, critics focus on specific problems in case-mix use, such as in public vs. nonpublic hospitals,[93] end stage renal disease patients in a hospital case mix as opposed to treatment elsewhere,[94] and differences in the care of patients in intensive care units (ICUs).[95] A Chicago hospital explained how they prepared for a case-mix system to meet DRG reimbursement requirements. Their case-mix system compared the hospital's case mix to that of the community, improved resource allocation, prepared physician practice profiles, and collected data for rate negotiation. Three types of reports were generated: physician profile reports, hospital diagnostic profile reports, and patient origin reports. Administrators at the hospital felt that the case mix data system provided information for "in-depth analysis of sophisticated issues."[96]

There is no need to belabor the point—everyone agrees that data is the critical mass in any case-mix system.

Case-Mix Limitations

Limitations of case-mix measurements, particularly when used for reimbursement, have been noted by many. Goran, for example, listed several of the special needs or problems of hospitals that would not be reflected in the case mix: research needs, compatibly narrow clinically-relevant patient groupings, inaccurate data, hospital classifications, teaching services, and financial incentives.[97] An epidemic of "DRG Creep" was predicted by Simborg. He defined the disease "as a deliberate and systematic shift in a hospital's reported case mix in order to improve reimbursement."[98] In a more expansive view of methodological limitations in case mix hospital reimbursement, Williams et al. delineated faults in hospital peer group measures as well as in patient classification measures using case-mix data. While the review focuses on reimbursement, the authors note that the limitations also apply to other uses of case-mix measures. Among the limitations detailed are those relating to subgroup combinations, sequencing explanatory variables, combining clinical and statistical criteria, trim points, practice patterns changes, implementation, payment schedules, normalcy assumptions, hospital characteristics, and linearity. To meet the case-mix limitations, Williams et al. propose a comprehensive hospital reimbursement system with a significant role for case-mix measures: "Hospitals would be assigned to peer groups using the hospital classification system instead of policy considerations alone. Patients would be assigned to case types using the patient classification system, and hospitals would be paid different rates for different patient types according to the hospital's peer group schedule of case-mix rates."[99]

Variations in case mix and hospital characteristics would be accounted for in the classification mechanisms.

Case Mix and Computer Programs

Arons describes more than 50 years of commitment to case-mix systems by Presbyterian Hospital in New York City, including one of the first medical applications of electronic data processing using punched data cards.[100] In 1984, the Milton S. Hershey Medical Center in Pennsylvania began using a computerized case-mix management system to generate more than 20 reports grouped into six major categories:

1. Physician and payer profitability

2. Financial and clinical performance reports by clinical service and physician for Medicare patients

3. Financial and clinical summary reports for PPS by MDC, DRG, and physician

4. Financial and clinical performance reports for all patients.

5. System standards reports.

6. Edit report.[101]

In evaluating the new case-mix management information system, Hulm and Burik remarked that between late 1982 and late 1983, about 26 new computerized systems were marketed.[102] These case-mix programs differed from existing information techniques because clinical and financial information was integrated for management planning and budgeting purposes. Twelve characteristics of case-mix management information systems deal with purchase or leasing, vendor aid, flexible reports, comparative standards, confidentiality, and the integration into the system of different case-mix methodologies.[103]

Case-Mix Classification Systems

Analysis of case-mix classification systems has resulted in similar groupings, although different terminology is used to distinguish the approaches. An Office

Exhibit 3-1   Case-Mix Classification Systems by Grouping

Institutional/Indirect/Index-Value/Scalar	Patient Level/Direct/Diagnostic
Ad hoc groupings[107]	Commission on Professional and Hospital Activities (CPHA), List A[112]
Information Theory[108,109]	International Classification of Diseases, Ninth Revision, Clinical Modification (ICD-9-CM)[113]
Resource Need Index (RNI)[110]	Disease Staging[114]
Single Index-Hospital and Service Area Characteristics[111]	Patient Management Categories[115]
	Severity of Illness Index[116,117]
	DRGs[118]

of Technology Assessment report separates the case-mix approaches into institutional and patient level measures.[104] Williams et al. identify direct and indirect approaches.[105] An evaluation by the Health Research and Educational Trust of New Jersey classifies one grouping as index-value or scalar measures while the other is labeled diagnostic measures.[106]

Generally, one approach to case-mix measures, called the institutional, indirect, scalar, or index-value approach, uses hospital and service area characteristics gained through such techniques as factor and cluster analysis. The other approach to case-mix measures, called the patient level, applies direct care, or diagnostic approach, clinical and statistical information based on empirical practice and medical records data. More recently, the thrust of case-mix measures stresses the direct care/diagnostic approach through DRGs with the others considered as alternative case-mix measurements.

A combined listing follows with references cited for the differing approaches (Exhibit 3-1).

CPHA List A evolved into ICD-9-CM and that classification system was folded into the DRGs. Reviews of case-mix measurements by Bentley and Butler,[119] Hornbrook,[120] and Plomann[121,122] agree that DRGs, disease staging, patient management categories, and severity of illness now occupy center stage for consideration as case-mix measurements. Other methods mentioned included the following:

- Veterans Administration Multilevel Care Groups (MLC). A refinement of progressive patient care that matches variable resource needs of patients with different levels of care to identify average resources and costs.[123]

- AS-SCORE (Age; Systems (organs); Single system involved; State of disease; COmplications; REsponse to therapy). Patients are placed into four levels of severity based on clinical data. This evolved into the severity of illness index.[124]

- MD-DADO (MD; physician; Discharge Abstract; Data Optimal). Allows for adjustment to reflect local factors such as physician preferences and type of diseases characteristic of a specific patient population.[125]

- Generic Algorithms. Develops medically logical algorithms that group patients into resource consumption by diagnosis, procedures, sex, or age.[126]

- Grade of Membership (GOM). Evaluates the heterogeneity of reimbursement categories and service groups in multivariate terms.[127]

Siemon reviewed 1970 to 1981 literature on case mix and data quality.[128] He points out that experts believe that case mix can explain about 80 percent of the differences in hospital costs. Based on the literature, Siemon comments that "it is generally agreed that the most satisfactory input for case-mix measures would be patient-oriented data."[129] However, reliable patient-oriented data is not easily available according to Siemon's overview. That situation led to the use of proxy variables such as patient days, hospital size, and services available. DRGs use length of stay as a proxy variable for cost. In any event, the use of meaningful proxy variables is not clear. A major issue that relates to patient-oriented data is the severity of illness and a number of approaches to that problem are under investigation.

Severity of Illness

One of the heated arguments relative to the management of the prospective payment plan centers on the DRGs' ability or inability to reimburse for actual resources rendered to patients. Health care providers maintain that the DRGs are not homogeneous and that there is no such thing as an "average patient." Critics claim that services rendered to hospital patients relate to the severity of that individual's ailments. Hornbrook states that the severity of illness can be related to the stages of the disease following an expected natural history. Four types of natural history are identified: self-limiting; terminal; non-self-limiting, acute; and non-self-limiting, chronic. Exhibit 3-2 illustrates disease severity classifications over time. In relating the allocation of resources to severity, Hornbrook compared three types of reimbursement: capitation, fee-per-diagnosis, and fee-for-service. He noted that in fee-per-diagnosis, the DRG method, "the same fee applies even if the patient is severely ill."[130] Furthermore, the

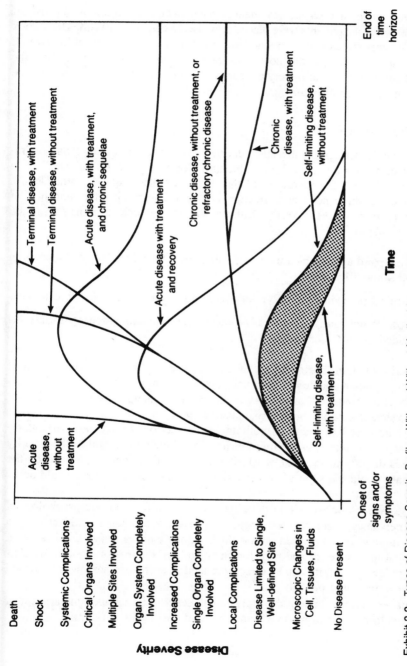

Disease Severity

Death

Shock

Systemic Complications

Critical Organs Involved

Multiple Sites Involved

Organ System Completely Involved

Increased Complications

Single Organ Completely Involved

Local Complications

Disease Limited to Single, Well-defined Site

Microscopic Changes in Cell, Tissues, Fluids

No Disease Present

Terminal disease, with treatment

Terminal disease, without treatment

Acute disease, with treatment, and chronic sequelae

Acute disease, without treatment

Acute disease with treatment and recovery

Chronic disease, without treatment, or refractory chronic disease

Chronic disease, with treatment

Self-limiting disease, without treatment

Self-limiting disease, with treatment

Onset of signs and/or symptoms

End of time horizon

Time

Exhibit 3-2   Types of Disease Severity Profiles, With and Without Medical Intervention

Source: M. C. Hornbrook, "Allocative Medicine: Efficiency, Disease Severity, and the Payment Mechanism," *Annals of the American Academy of Political and Social Science* 468 (1983): 17.

point was made that physicians made ethical decisions regarding the use of resources when the patients were placed into disease categories. While Hornbrook concluded that the capitation method was more effective for controlling overall resource use, the fee-per-diagnosis was the compromise choice. Therefore, the issue of severity does not merely concern cost containment but also involves the basic concept of appropriate care for patients.

Severity Definitions

In its report to Congress, the HHS defined severity of illness as "risk of immediate death or permanent loss of function due to a patient's disease."[131] In explaining further, the report stated that "it is a concept of risk rather than a concept of resource need or utilization that is a disease specific concept."[132] According to the report, severity of illness was accommodated in the PPS in the following ways:

- Principal diagnosis as a main variable allows for allocation of resources in DRG classifications.

- Surgical procedures in DRG definitions allows for related added resources.

- Age, complicating, or comorbid conditions affecting resource use are included in DRG derivations.

Variations within specific DRGs of resource use, according to the report, must consider physician practice patterns and other factors as well as severity of illness.

Smits et al. contend that severity of illness depends upon your vantage point as a physician, a nurse, or as a manager/payer.[133]

Physicians tend to focus on pathologic impacts on the patient, particularly complications and the possibility of death. This view may not relate the severity of illness directly to the cost of care. A severely ill patient, as defined by the physician, could die soon after admission and relatively few costs could accumulate.

Nurses view severity within the physician's definition but add psychological and dependency needs to their scope. However, a physician could classify a patient as low severity based on the illness alone while a nurse could rate that individual high severity and plan for an episode of depression or anxiety. This nursing view of severity can be directly related to cost since nursing time would be used to treat that patient.

Managers/payers concern themselves with severity based upon the amount of resources to be used in treatment and the total cost of the services.

Most of the literature on the severity of illness seems to seek a generic definition. If the above differing viewpoints are accurate, a qualifier may be required in any severity of illness classification scheme.

DRGs and Severity

DRGs were first designed as a management system for hospitals, as a utilization review instrument, and for research. In relation to severity, only the physician's and the manager's viewpoints were incorporated. "The nursing perspective was conspicuously absent from DRG construction . . ."[134] This can be explained by the fact that hospital accounting methods did not include nursing resources as a separate line item and dependency and psychological services were not measured.

Experience has already indicated that there are wide ranging variations within specific DRGs that are directly related to the severity of the individual's illness. This could mean that the facility would incur a severe financial loss, since the DRG payment remains the same regardless of the severity not compensated for by outliers, direct, or indirect education adjustments. Smits et al. identify eight possible causes for DRG instability.

1. Error in discharge or cost data

2. True outlier case

3. Physician patterns of practice

4. A small number of rare DRGs

5. Uniform Hospital Discharge Set (UHDDS) data limitations

6. ICD-9-CM limitations

7. Nursing severity data lacking

8. Medical severity descriptions vague.[135]

These investigators, including one of the original Yale University DRG researchers, concluded: "Discussions of severity issues are often confused by the inclusion of erroneous cases, by an assumption that the elimination of outliers is a desirable goal, or by a firm belief that increased sickness will of necessity correlate with increased cost. High levels of sickness and high levels of cost are not necessarily the same thing: an effective severity measure may well identify certain less costly subgroups of the severely ill."[136]

DRGs and the severity of illness concept may also have to consider the "contribution margin" included in the DRG payment. Contribution margin is the difference between the DRG payment the hospital receives and the variable actual cost of treating that patient. "Researchers contend that as much as 60 percent of a hospital's costs may be fixed costs."[137] Suppose that payment for DRG 39 is $1,500. As little as $600 may cover laundry, food, drugs, patient supplies, and direct care and is the variable marginal cost. Thus, $900 ($1,500 minus $600) becomes the contribution margin to the fixed costs of the hospital. Keegan asserts that hospitals would "see a big contribution margin for DRGs in which patients are less severely ill and a smaller contribution margin for DRGs in which the patients are more seriously ill."[138] However, it should be noted that the source of this concept is a vice president for finance at a hospital and he is obviously presenting a managerial stance. It would appear that he is advising managers that severity would not make that much of an impact providing the adminstrator knows what the true costs are for each DRG.

On the other hand, a recent study at Stanford University Hospital reaffirms the charge that "DRGs alone may be an inadequate basis for reimbursement to hospitals."[139] That conclusion was based, in part, on the increased severity of illness within DRG groups and between DRGs.

Measures of Illness Severity

A number of methods for determining the severity of specific illness have been proposed, including the following:

- Diagnosis Related Group (DRGs)
- Patient Severity of Illness Index (PSI)
- Disease Staging
- Patient Management Categories (PMCs)
- Medical Illness Severity Grouping System (MEDISGRPS)®
- Relative Intensity Measures (RIMs)

Each of these measures seeks to find objective methods to classify illness that account for the resources used to treat an individual having a specific condition. Homogeneous groupings of patients having similar ailments and consuming like amounts of resources is the goal of such measurements. Developers aimed to account for the interactions of multiple diseases and changes in the patient's condition during the hospital stay.

In an editorial in the *Journal of the American Medical Association,* Eisenberg addressed the issue of equitable reimbursement and the severity complication. He commented on PSI, PMC, and disease staging and was encouraged by the integration of "an appropriate degree of clinical judgment" in those mechanisms.

Furthermore, this AMA official noted that the "eventual acceptability of any system depends greatly on the degree and quality of clinical judgment and information incorporated into it."[140] Pointedly, Eisenberg remarked that the DRG system lacks an appropriate degree of clinical judgment. Gonnella also addressed the need to reduce inappropriate homogeneity in case-mix classifications. Furthermore, he noted the inconsistency of medical logic in the use of DRGs as the unit of measurement.[141] His comments were related to an article by Iezzoni and Moskowitz on the clinical overlap among medical diagnosis related groups.[142]

Diagnosis Related Groups (DRGs).   As indicated earlier, the DRG system makes allowances for surgical procedures, age, complications, and comorbidity; it has 470 principal diagnostic classifications, adjustment for excessive length of stay, and direct and indirect educational allowances. In the opinion of the federal government, these variables accommodate the severity of illness issue.

Patient Severity of Illness Index (PSI).   Dr. Susan D. Horn and her associates at Johns Hopkins University have been most closely associated with the severity of illness index. Early on, Horn and Schumacher applied information theory measures of case mix to clinical measures and demonstrated a statistically significant relation.[143] Five key patient attributes were used to assess severity in the AS-SCORE system: age, organ systems, disease stage, complications, and response to therapy. That approach was the precursor to the severity of illness index.[144]

Seven variables relate to the patient's illness in determining the level of severity for the index scaling:

1. Stage of the principal diagnosis

2. Complications of the principal diagnosis

3. Concurrent interacting conditions that affect the hospital course

4. Patient dependency on hospital facilities and staff

5. Extent of nonoperating room life support procedures

6. Rate of response to therapy or rate of recovery

7. Impairment remaining after therapy for the acute aspect of the hospitalization.[145]

Dimensions 1, 2, and 3 indicate the severity of illness that the patient brings to the hospital. Variables 4 and 5 reflect the burden placed on the facility and are minimally affected by the hospital staff and practice patterns. "It is believed that they are the least significant variables in predicting overall severity of illness." Items 6 and 7 measure the patient's response to the hospitalization.[146]

Using these seven dimensions, experienced raters evaluate data in the medical record, and score the patient at one of four levels of severity for each of the seven variables (Exhibit 3-3). Then an overall rating is made on a four-point scale integrating all the rankings. These four levels are on an ordinal scale; distinctions between the four levels have no significance and may not be equal. This rating is generic and patient-specific, not disease-specific. Using the PSI, the investigators found that "reductions of variance of over 75 percent are not uncommon."[147] In addition, experienced raters agreed more than 90 percent of the time on the scoring with no more than one to two minutes added to the review of data.

However, the severity of illness index uses discharge information on the entire hospital stay. Medical practice behavior could influence the severity ratings. Muller sharply notes shortcomings: "It is applied to the entire stay rather than classifying cases based on condition at admission. . . . Nevertheless, this feature makes it difficult to interpret the index, because several of the component variables . . . may reflect not only the severity of the condition, but also the inadequacies of treatment, i.e., faulty decisions or faulty execution, or both."[148]

Based on a number of studies of the use of and comparison of the severity of illness index against other reimbursement mechanisms, Horn and her associates found more homogeniety in their method.[147-149] They state: "Content validity, face validity, and predictive validity of the Severity of Illness Index have been demonstrated in various ways. We conclude that the Severity of Illness Index case mix grouping system is both reliable and valid."[152]

Disease Staging.   In 1748, John Fothergill wrote about the four stages of sore throat attended with ulcers. Illness and treatments were described at each stage.[153] However, progress to this time has still not resolved the problem of measuring the severity of illness.

Disease staging was developed with the principal involvement of Dr. Joseph S. Gonnella of Jefferson Medical College in Philadelphia[154] and Daniel Z. Louis of SysteMetrics, Inc. in California.[155-157] This concept borrows from clinical medicine, especially oncology. Diseases are generally divided into four stages of increasing severity in a progression toward death.

Stage 1. Conditions with no complications or problems of minimal severity
Stage 2. Problems limited to an organ or system; significantly increased risk of complications
Stage 3. Multiple site involvement; generalized systemic involvement; poor prognosis
Stage 4. Death.[158]

Exhibit 3-3 Patient Severity Index Characteristics by Stages

Level	Stages of Principal Diagnosis	Complications	Disease/Disability Interactions	Patient Dependency	Procedures	Response to Therapy	Impairment, Residual Effects
1	asymptomatic manifestations	no or very minor complications	no interaction	low dependency	noninvasive diagnostic procedures	prompt	no residual effects
2	moderate manifestations	moderate complications	low interaction	moderate dependency	therapeutic and invasive diagnostic procedures	moderate delay	minor residual effects
3	major manifestations	major complications	moderate interaction	major dependency	nonemergency life sustaining procedures	serious delay	moderate residual effects
4	catastrophic manifestations	catastrophic complications	major interaction	extreme dependency	emergency life sustaining procedures	no response	major residual effects

Source: Adapted from information in S. D. Horn, P. D. Sharkey, and D. A. Bertram, "Measuring Severity of Illness: Homogeneous Case Mix Groups," *Medical Care* 21, no. 1 (1983): 26–30.

Exhibit 3-4   Disease Staging—Medical and Coded Criteria

	Diagnosis: Diabetes Mellitus; Etiology: Metabolic		
Stage	Common Description or Name of Condition	Alternate Description or Synonym	IDC-9-CM Codes That Define Each Stage and Substage
1.0	Diabetes mellitus	Hyperglycemia, "sugar diabetes"	775.10, 790.20, 250.00-250.01, 250.80-250.91
2.1	Diabetes mellitus with an infection in one or more systems (e.g. skin, genital tract, urinary tract)	Diabetes mellitus with complications of infectious nature: pyoderma, impetigo, furunculosis, monilial vulvitis, monilial skin infection, cystitis, urethritis, epididymitis, prostatitis, pyelonephritis	Stage 1.0 + 320.00-342.90, 245.00-245.10, 254.10, 289.20-289.30, 420.00-422.99, 424.91, 429.89, 447.60, 480.00-488.00, 510.00-510.90, 511.10, 513.00-513.10, 526.40, 566.00-587.90, 589.50, 572.00, 577.00, 580.81, 590.00-590.30, 595.00-596.40, 595.89-596.90, 597.00-597.80, 598.00-598.01, 599.00, 601.00-801.90, 603.10, 604.00-604.99, 607.10-807.20, 590.90, 608.00, 608.40-608.81, 611.00, 614.00-618.11, 618.30-617.90, 680.00-686.90, 711.00-711.99, 728.00, 730.00-730.39, 730.80-730.99
2.2	Diabetes mellitus with septicemia	Diabetes mellitus, infection, and associated toxins of bacteria in bloodstream	Stage 1.0 + 038.00-038.90
2.3	Diabetes mellitus with acidosia	Diabetic acidosis or ketosis Diabetes with ketonemia or ketonuria	Stage 1.0 + 588.80, 791.80, 276.20-276.40; 250.10-250.11
2.4	Diabetes mellitus with retinopathy but without loss of vision, or glomerulosclerosis (without azotemia), or neuropathy (peripheral or autonomic), or gangrene (tissue breakdown)	Microangiopathy Kimmeisteil-Wilson disease Arterial insufficiency with associated tissue breakdown	Stages 1.0-2.3 + 337.10, 362.18, 443.81, 443.90, 446.60, 447.10, 581.81, 785.40, 354.00-356.90; 357.20, 362.01, 250.40-250.74

Exhibit 3-4 (contd.)

3.1	Diabetes mellitus with acidosis and coma, or retinopathy and loss of vision, or necrotizing papillitis, or azotemia	Diabetic coma with ketosis or acidosis Proliferative retinopathy Papillary necrosis, medullary necrosis	Stage 2.4 + 278.20, 369.00-369.90; Stages 1.0-2.4 + 583.70, 780.00, 790.60, 584.50-586.00, 590.80-590.81; 362.02, 250.30-250.31
3.2	Diabetes mellitus with hyperosmolar coma	Nonketotic, hyperosmolar hyperglycemic coma	250.20-250.21
3.3	Shock		Stages 1.0-3.2 + 458.00, 458.90, 785.50-785.59, 788.50, 994.00, 994.80, 995.00, 995.40, 958.40, 998.00, 999.40, 689.10-10-869.14, 639.50
4.0	Death		Stages 2.2-3.3 + Death

Source: D. Z. Louis, *Disease Staging: A Clinically Based Approach to Management of Disease Severity. Volume I: Executive Summary*, SysteMetrics, Inc., Santa Barbara, CA, August 1983, pp. 10, 15

For each stage, substages such as 1.1 and 2.2 indicate increasing severity within a stage. Exhibit 3-4 illustrates the stages, common name, alternate description, and the ICD-9-CM codes defining each stage and substage for diabetes. A panel of 23 medical experts, using most common diagnosis frequencies, developed medical staging criteria for 420 separate medical conditions that do not depend upon the treatment resources used.[159] In this approach, the emphasis is upon the medical meaningfulness of the criteria and there is no attempt to integrate all the variables contributing to hospital costs or resource needs. Criteria are numbered and grouped into 15 body systems with each of the 420 conditions described.[160] Another report gives the coding for all the staged diseases.[161]

A computer software package to stage disease was developed by SysteMetrics to classify patients into any of the 420 diagnostic categories. An ordinal stage within each category is also assigned; a capability of 1,680 options (420 diseases × 4 stages). According to Jon Conklin, a senior health care analyst for SysteMetrics, "We found that for some DRGs, staging significantly reduces variations in costs and length of stay."[162]

In a comparison study of disease staging and DRGs, there was not much difference in explaining length of stay. Bed size accounted for all payment structure differences, including teaching status, location, and type of hospital control. Researchers found that severity of illness is distributed more uniformly across hospitals than medical resources. For homogeneous groupings, the investigators felt that disease staging might function as well as DRGs and also provide better incentives.[163]

Questions remain regarding the homogeneity of the stages with respect to resource use, the incomparability of the severity of each stage of a specific disease with the same stage of a different specific disease, the nonaccountability of comorbidity and the fact that some diseases are difficult or impossible to stage.[164] Despite these drawbacks, a SysteMetrics research report expressed high hopes:

> We believe that staging now provides a clinically sound approach to the development of medically homogeneous patient clusters that can be used by physicians, hospital administrators, health services researchers, and government policy makers in their efforts toward an improved understanding of the difficult issues of quality, cost, reimbursement, management, and planning which face the health care delivery system.[165]

Patient Management Categories (PMCs).   Young and her associates at Blue Cross of Western Pennsylvania are most closely linked to the development of PMCs. Characteristics of PMCs include the following:

- Patient types are defined within disease/disorder groups by physician panels before patient discharge abstract data are used to operationalize the classification.

- Levels of severity are incorporated in the design and definition of PMCs.

- Category assignment is unaffected by the actual sequence of discharge diagnoses for a patient, i.e., principal versus secondary placement.

- Single disease patients having multiple related diagnoses are differentiated from comorbid cases.

- Computer programs assign patients to PMCs using discharge abstract data and can be used with any data base compatible with Uniform Hospital Discharge Data Set (UHDDS) information.[166]

PMCs aim to produce clinically specific groupings with distinct diagnostic and treatment procedures reflecting the total resources required for effective care of the specific patients in each grouping. A relative cost weight derives from examination of actual detailed expenses, patient-related costs, and costs of the service centers producing hospital revenue. Panels of physicians identified 800 PMCs based on actual clinical experience treating patients (See Exhibit 3-5).

Application of the PMC methodology to 797,833 discharges from western Pennsylvania hospitals in 1983 found that 96 percent could be placed into 766 PMCs. In fact, 75 percent of the discharges used 117 PMCs; 287 PMCs described 90 percent of the case load.[167] Even though PMCs allow for a patient to be placed into as many as five categories, the 1983 analysis revealed that about 66 percent of the patients fell into a single PMC, 31 percent had comorbid conditions, and about 4 percent were not able to be categorized based on the discharge abstract data.[168] However, patients covered by Medicare contributed 52 percent of the comorbidity cases. Importantly, people classified in a single PMC may have multiple ICD-9-CM diagnosis codes. Of the 66 percent in a single PMC, 58 percent used multiple diagnosis codes to define a single disease process. Nevertheless, PMCs distinguish comorbid combinations quite differently from DRGs. Of 3,117 patients having both of two clinically distinct PMCs—Chronic Bronchitis/Asthma and Stable Angina w/o operation— the DRG classification resulted in 108 categories.[169] Within DRG 121 dealing with Acute Myocardial Infarction, there are eight clinically distinct PMCs. While five of the eight PMCs are similar in resource use, three indicate medical management regimens that utilize significantly more hospital resources: namely, congestive heart failure without operation, cardiogenic shock, and congestive heart failure with operation.

Severity of illness is incorporated into the PMCs when the clinical specificity is identified. "Relative costliness of each PMC is quantified rather than the severity of the illness."[170]

There are limitations to the PMC system according to Young. Only one category assignment is permitted within a disease or disorder group to maintain computerization management. A person with multiple upper extremity fractures is placed into one PMC, whereas an individual with head injuries as well would be put into two PMCs. While the anticipated resources used for medical management within the multiple fracture PMC may be similar, this has to be tested.

Another limitation relates to the manner in which the ICD-9-CM diagnosis codes contain the specificity and accuracy of the PMC system. Hypertension as a diagnosis, for example, may be a true coding but may not really indicate the active medical management during a specific hospitalization.

Even with the constraints, Young states the case for PMCs: "By using multiple related diagnoses that represent a stage, unique manifestation, and/or complication of a single disease process, severity of illness distinctions among patient types are included in the classification and single disease patients are differentiated from patients with comorbid conditions."[171] In a later editorial, Young

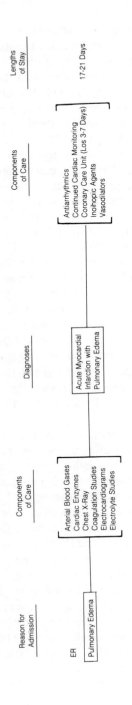

Exhibit 3-5 PMC for Acute Myocardial Infarction with Edema

Source: Blue Cross of Western Pennsylvania, Hospital Case Mix Measurement Overview, Unpublished, June 1983.

reaffirmed her belief that PMCs could substitute for DRGs and address the problem of clinical overlap more equitably.[172]

Medical Illness Severity Grouping System (MEDISGRPS)®. On admission, the MEDISGRPS system classifies hospital patients into one of five severity of illness groupings based upon clinical findings and the potential for organ failure. Brewster and Jacobs,[173,174] developers of this method, claim that MEDISGRPS is an objective technique because 67 reasons for admission and about 500 key clinical findings (KCFs) are used directly from the medical record to determine severity and not subjective ratings. On the basis of KCFs, patients are assigned to the following severity categories:

Severity Group 0   None of the MEDISGRPS key clinical findings

Severity Group 1   Minimal findings where there is a low potential for organ failure

Severity Group 2   Either acute findings connoting a short time course with an unclear potential for organ failure, or severe findings that involve a high potential for organ failure, but when such failure is probably not imminent

Severity Group 3   Both severe and acute findings, meaning there is a high potential for organ failure and a short time course is indicated

Severity Group 4   Critical findings that indicate the presence of organ failure[175]

Severity of illness on admission is reviewed at a later date during the patient's hospital stay. For example, in a 16-day length of stay, severity reviews take place on the fourth, tenth, and sixteenth days. Exhibit 3-6 shows an admission and review for a patient admitted with gastrointestinal bleeding.

Chief presenting complaints such as shortness of breath, chest pain, and abdominal pain form the basis for the 67 reasons for admission. While the reason for admission does not influence the severity categorization, it does allow for case-mix grouping. In the study groups, the following 12 reasons for admission accounted for 73 percent of all admissions:

Chest pain	Focal weakness
Shortness of breath	Fever/chills
Abdominal pain	Nausea/vomiting
Changed alertness	Dizziness
Diffuse weakness	Back pain[176]
Extremity pain	
Admission for cardiac catheterization	

Exhibit 3-6 Sample MEDISGRPS Patient Abstract

Reason for Admission—G.I. Bleeding

Admission Review Date: 12/21/83
Admission Severity: Group 2

Second Review Date: 12/30/83
R2 Severity: Group 3

Physical Exam Findings:
 ? Ascites
 Blood in Stool

Miscellaneous Procedures:
 Units of Blood Transfused: 9

Endoscopy: Duodenal Ulcer

Laboratory Findings:
 HCT: 33
 SGOT: 150
 AKP: 151

Laboratory Findings:
 HCT: 18
 SGOT: 180
 AKP: 141
 Amylase: 90

Vital Signs:
 BP: 80/50
 Pulse: 140

Source: Reprinted with permission of MediQual[SM] Systems, Inc.

In addition, reason for admission severity evaluations show an ability to predict patient health status outcomes and the use of hospital resources.

Key clinical findings emerged from observations of house officers at morning intake rounds and answer the question: How does the physician know how sick a patient is? After validation at seven hospitals and modification, about 500 key clinical findings remained to permit severity classifications for all types of patients, excluding psychiatric admissions. An example of severity of illness using KCFs is illustrated in Exhibit 3-7. Although a diagnosis is listed, this is merely for reference purposes. Severity in MEDISGRPS is not based on the diagnosis, an inaccurate severity indicator. KCFs may range from five per patient to about twenty when death is imminent. Patients are placed into the severity group with the highest KCFs. According to Dr. Brewster, "Most admissions at level two or higher are 'disease driven' and their rates are probably epidemiologically very constant around the country."[177]

In contrast with DRGs using diagnosis and discharge data, the MEDISGRPS system arrives at costs based on how sick patients are on admission and during their hospital stay. Exhibit 3-8 shows the differences for DRG 122 using the MEDISGRPS severity rankings.

MEDISGRPS is computerized and is being used in about 21 hospitals with 100 to 800 beds in different parts of the nation. Installation costs run about

Exhibit 3-7 Representative Key Clinical Findings and Their Assigned MEDISGRPS Severity Group for Principal Diagnosis of Acute Myocardial Infarction

	Severity Group 1	Severity Group 2	Severity Group 3	Severity Group 4
EKG	Ischemia Atrial Fibrillation	Myocardial Infarction (acute) (extension)	3rd Degree Heart Block	
Chest X-Ray	Cardiomegaly		Congestive Heart Failure	
Physical Exam	Rales			Coma
Cardiac Catheterization		Cardiomyopathy		
Laboratory	PO_2 60-69 CPK 121-239	PO_2 45-59 CPK 240+	PO_2 <45	
Vital Signs	Respirations 25-32	Respirations >32		

Source: Reprinted with permission of MediQual(SM) Systems, Inc.

Exhibit 3-8 Charge and Length of Stay Indicators by MEDISGRPS Admission Severity Group for DRG 122 (Circulatory disorders with acute myocardial infarction without cardiovascular complications, discharged alive)

Admission Severity Group	Patients	Avg. Charges		Avg. Length of Stay
		Total	Ancillary	
0	0			
1	9	$3,389	$1,493	7.8
2	138	5,207	2,080	12.3
3	31	6,090	2,703	12.7
4	10	8,190	3,483	19.1
Total	188	$5,424	$2,229	12.5

Excluding Morbidity, Deaths, and Transfers Hospital 11001—FY 1983 October 1984
Source: Reprinted with permission of MediQual(SM) Systems, Inc.

$10,000 to $15,000 plus an annual licensing fee of $7,000 to $35,000, depending on bed size.

Dr. Brewster feels that Medicare DRGs will be abandoned after some "fiddling around to make them more equitable" because they are neither "clinically based" nor "easily understood" by physicians.[178] This prediction is seconded by Walter

McClure of the Minneapolis Center for Policy Studies, as he stresses MED-ISGRPS' "doctor-defensible algorithms" and advises, "Scrap DRGs and replace it with this."[179]

Relative Intensity Measures (RIMs).   As a measure of illness severity, relative intensity measures (RIMs) addresses the problem of pinpointing nursing resources used to care for specific patients. This is particularly important because nursing costs can account for up to 35 percent of direct patient care costs and up to 50 percent of a typical hospital's nonphysician personnel budget.[180] Traditionally, nursing costs were included in room and board as a flat rate regardless of nursing intensity. To resolve the problem of nursing intensity, attention must be given to severity classifications as they are linked to nursing services.

Diggs reviewed a variety of patient acuity classification schemes and noted the use of weighted patient classification systems using points or hours. He stated that the nursing crisis had to be resolved with nursing productivity answers.[181] Efforts to discover methods of associating specific nursing services with units of time and then a cost factor have been reported at a number of facilities.[182-184]

Additional classification systems for nursing departments were described by Bermas and Slyck, members of a nationwide consulting firm. Four patient systems based on disease, procedure, acuity/severity, or a combination were detailed. Regardless of the patient classification system chosen, the authors suggest the following criteria:

- No need for complex calculations.

- Use columns, not rows, for easier calculations.

- Does not use zeros.

- Combines into permanent record.

- Includes other activities.

- Includes "significant others."

- Emphasizes reporting accuracy.

- Involves nurses.[185]

Early development of the RIMs method was reported upon by Caterinicchio, one the principal investigators testing the technique in New Jersey.[186-188] A rather intensive critique of RIMs by Grimaldi and Micheletti[189] was answered by Caterinicchio in a later issue of *Nursing Management*.[190] In their review, Grimaldi and Micheletti found the research design flawed. They cited statistical problems, questionable assumptions, counterintuitive results, and doubtful managerial applications because of the complexity of the RIMs method. In his counter, Caterinicchio pointed out the errors of the critics and explained the study sample, the data collection techniques, the skill mix, the empirical results, and the statistical cost allocations. These conflicting reports from health care experts familiar with the DRG system shed light on basic RIM issues for consideration in reimbursement methodology.

Studies in New Jersey from 1977 to 1979 tabulated minutes of nursing and non-nursing interventions for the following categories of services:

Nursing	Non-nursing
Assessment and planning	Transport
Health teaching and information giving	Dietary
Emotional support and counseling	Housekeeping
Medications and treatments	Miscellaneous[191]
Physical functions	

After that breakdown, the RIM process specifies RIM costs, counts the number of RIMs per case, and calculates the average RIMs used within each DRG. "Simply put, the cost per RIM is the relationship between the total actual cost of nursing in the institution and the number of minutes of nursing time used by recipients of care. One RIM equals one minute."[192]

To determine the RIMs per case, each case is classified into a nursing resource cluster (NRC) which represents a homogeneity of resource use during an average length of stay. There are a total of 13 NRCs which include all 23 Major Diagnostic Categories (MDCs) and all 467 DRGs. Then, one of the 13 predictive NRC equations is used to calculate the number of RIMs per case. Major variables affecting RIM include primary diagnosis, admission and discharge status, length of stay, and whether or not surgery was performed. It is possible that patients within the same DRG may have RIMs calculated using a different NRC equation.

Finally, the number of RIMs is multiplied by the cost per RIM and averaged for all the cases within a DRG category. This yields an average cost of nursing per DRG. Cost per RIM is calculated by dividing the hospital's total actual nursing costs by the total number of RIMs estimated for all patients.

Exhibit 3-9 illustrates the application of RIM methodology to a typical patient who is assigned to DRG 179 (Inflammatory Bowel Disease).

Importantly, RIMs will fluctuate with trends in nursing care and shifts in services provided by other members of the health care team. Joel addresses this point citing attributes of RIMs:

- RIMs are relative, not absolute. There is no increase in the dollar amount of the nursing budget. RIMs merely provide a method of equitable distribution of nursing costs over the patient population.

Exhibit 3-9   Application of RIMs Methodology for a Typical Patient

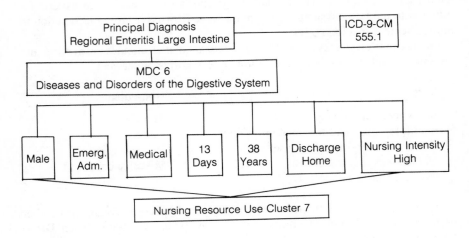

Equation for Nursing Cost Allocation:
Y (RIMs) = 927.003 + 50.761 (LOS 1.5)

Explanation of RIMs Equation Nursing Resource Cluster 7

Y = 927.003 + 50.761 (LOS 1.5)

Where Y = dependent variable; total indexed nursing units of service (RIM's) in minutes for patient in hospital:

927.003—constant (fixed) nursing units of service in minutes over the length of stay;

50.761—length of stay coefficient predicting the change in nursing units of service in minutes with each unit change in length of stay;

LOS—independent variable; length of stay in days for patient in hospital.

Total minutes of activity over length of stay is found by using the actual LOS of 13 days:

Y − 927.003 + 50.761 (13¹·⁵)   Y − 927.003 + 50.761 (46.872)
Y − 927.003 + 2379.278   Y − 3306.281 minutes or 55.105 hours

Accordingly, this patient consumed approximately 3306 minutes or 55 hours of nursing services over his 13-day period of stay.

Exhibit 3-9   (contd.)

Price per RIM is calculated as follows	Nursing Costs for DRG 179

Your hospital's total
  Actual Nursing Costs = $ 7,000,000

Total RIMs estimated
  From all your patients =   42,000,000

$$\frac{\$7,000,000}{42,000,000 \text{ RIM's}} = \$0.17 \text{ price per RIM}$$

When the price per RIM is known, the nursing cost for the example patient in Nursing Resource Use Cluster 7 in Exhibit I can be determined as follows:

Total minutes (RIMs) of Nursing Activity consumed during the 13th day LOS = 3,306,281

Price Per RIM = $0.17
3,306,281 × 0.17 = $562.07

- Patient 1 = $ 562.07
- Patient 2 = $ 600.25
- Patient 3 = $ 555.25
- Patient 4 = $ 595.75
- Patient 5 = $ 618.20
- Patient 6 = $ 538.00
- Patient 7 = $ 560.00
- Patient 8 = $ 510.00

TOTAL $4,539.52

$$\text{Number of Cases } \frac{\$4,539.52}{8} = \$567.44$$

Average Nursing Cost for DRG 179.

Source: G. P. Smith, "The RIM Development and Impact on Nursing Mangement," in *DRGs: The Effect in New Jersey. The Potential for the Nation*, HCFA Pub. No. 03170, March 1984, pp. 96, 97.

- RIMs are not a staffing tool. Resource consumption is measured, but day-to-day staffing decisions are still necessary.

- RIMs are not a measure of pure nursing. Relative resources are measured and nurses could be engaged in non-nursing activities.

- RIMs are not perfect. Yet, benefits to hospitals and the nursing profession appear to outweigh criticisms.[193]

Even with the RIMs limitations noted, Joel looks to the future of nursing with anticipation of better things to come from RIMs: "A process is set in motion; today a cost center, tomorrow a revenue-generating center; next, role clarification and purification as nurses become valued therapeutic commodities; eventually, appreciation of the need for extremely sophisticated nurse clinicians to maximize the progress of selected patients; finally, nursing as an independently contracted provider profession in hospitals."[194]

Management Aspect of Admissions and Length of Stay

While admission of a patient and hospital length of stay fall within the purview of the attending physician, there are also management aspects. Immediate reaction to this type of statement instills fear of interference with the physician/patient relationship. Pictures arise of a callous executive putting the profit and loss statement above all humane concerns. Hopefully, this is not so and the managers are only directing activities to promote effectiveness and efficiency. Therefore, the obvious impact on interactions between the hospital management team and the attending physicians is contained within formal organizational boundaries and not in treatment regimens.

Admissions

A director of admissions at a community hospital told a convention audience that admitting improves the hospital's efficiency and helps to cope with DRGs. She reported on the results of a survey by Touche Ross & Company, a consulting health management firm, as follows: "Effective admission scheduling and discharge planning can contribute significantly to operating revenues in the PPS/DRG environment. Maximized bed utilization and timely admission processing contribute to improved admission volume and reduced length of stay . . . Appropriate scheduling concepts should be applied to improve patient turnaround times and utilization levels."[195]

Changes in admissions procedures include providing social services with a daily copy of the administrative record and adding other data items helpful in discharge planning, such as estimated length of stay, emergency contacts with names of other household members, and the county of residence.[196] In addition, she stressed the public relations impact of the admissions department. Not only does the department deal with patients and their families, but it also works with the admitting physicians and with other hospital units such as medical records and finance.

In April 1983, prior to the initiation of the federal PPS/DRG plan, one expert predicted that although there would be closer and more frequent review of admitting records, there would not be much daily change in work activities. However, Allen did raise the issue of "unnecessary admissions to increase hospital profit."[197] This concern was also addressed by the Kennedy-Gephardt proposal to save Medicare. Under the bill, hospitals would be reimbursed at 40 percent of the regular Medicare rate for all Medicare admissions in excess of a base number. States having their own plans would reimburse at 50 percent for excessive admissions.[198] However, the PPS/DRG program does not appear to have stimulated unnecessary admissions.[199,200] An AHA and an Iowa Hospital Association study also confirmed a small admission variation.[201,202] It would appear that hospital managers have not produced the PPS/DRG backlash of increasing admissions to increase profits.

Length of Stay

At the same time that reports told about static or declining admissions, the length of stay data showed a definite decline of about two days in average length of stay (ALOS).[203] Again, this was confirmed in AHA and Iowa Hospital Association studies. Studies by the National Center for Health Statistics, using 1981 and 1982 hospital discharge survey data, also confirm a drop in length of stay for patients 65 and older. These studies also showed regional differences from the U.S. average of 10.1 ALOS days: Northeast, 12.3 North Central, 10.3 South, 9.4 West, 8.2. In addition, ALOS tended to increase with bed size, ranging from 8.1 to 11.5. These studies applied DRG groupings to the data.[204]

Comparative data of this nature obviously invite management probes into rationales, particularly with the projections for a national reimbursement rate scale. Can administrators modify and change behavior to contain costs, especially with regard to physicians, nursing services, and ancillary resources?

Tulane Medical Center, New Orleans, started a physician education program that brought about a 1½-day decrease in the ALOS of Medicare patients. An executive said that "the medical center is training physicians to become 'product line managers'" and includes patients' bills and costs with the chart for discussion on rounds.[205] Green commented that it may sound harsh, but hospitals have to look at the patient as a product.[206]

A nursing study concluded that length of stay was the most important predictor of nursing services regardless of age and medical complexity. These researchers believe that the ability to allocate nursing costs using their methodology gives hospital management significant leverage. "Responsible nursing administration may now take advantage of this knowledge to manage professional nursing resources more efficiently."[207] Furthermore, effective control can be exercised over the ancillary services directly related to nursing.

Ancillary services can be categorized into activities in diagnostic and therapeutic areas and those related to the "hotel" function of the hospital. Berki et al. note that the intensity and timing of those services as rendered are potentially within the control of the providing institution. Both these variables are linked to length of stay and are used to measure hospital efficiency.[208] Even though the services are ordered by the physician, they are rendered by employees of the hospital and thereby directed by management.

Case-mix, severity of illness, and length of stay are all connected with the operational use of medical technology. The appropriate way to include money for technology advancements in the DRG payment rate has evoked considerable debate. Arguments range from the accusatory—that innovation will otherwise be stifled—to the resigned— that there is no real benefit to the patient. Even before the introduction of DRGs, these technology issues engendered heat. There is no reason to expect the controversy to lessen under PPS.

Medical Technology and DRGs

Between 1977 and 1982, medical costs increased 107 percent. According to a report by the Office of Technology Assessment (OTA), approximately 28 percent of this rise was related to overuse of medical technology.[209] A basic consideration in the additional expenditures under Medicare is the impact upon morbidity and mortality. A conclusion of the OTA report addressed that issue: "There is substantial evidence to suggest that inappropriate use of medical technology is common and raises Medicare and health system costs without improving quality of care."[210]

In a review of hospital reimbursement under Medicare, Lave also suggested that expensive technologies should meet effectiveness standards "to be measured in terms of their effect on both the extension and the quality of life."[211] On the other extreme, a letter to the editor of *American Medical News* from a practicing physician expressed the pessimistic view that under DRGs "technology will wither away; the cheapest treatment must be used."[212] A similar implication appeared in a study of intensive care at a large teaching hospital, where it was calculated the hospital lost $10,567 per discharge for an annual loss of $4.7 million. This hospital "may be forced to decrease or discontinue provision of medical intensive care units and other types of high technology care to severely ill patients."[213]

Under the prospective payment system, after 1985 DRG payment rates were to be raised up by one percent allowing for technology advances. Representing 285 manufacturers of health care products, Buzzell testified for the Health Industry Manufacturers Association (HIMA) at Congressional hearings on PPS. While HIMA supported the concept of PPS, the group did express concern about potential effects on new technology. Buzzell noted that PPS could jeopardize quality health care by inhibiting the development of new technologies. Since the payment rates are based on hisorical data applying to established technology, the reimbursement would be biased. This could limit the availability of new diagnostics and therapies.[214]

A special 28-page report on technology developments appeared in a July/August 1983 issue of *FAH Review*.[215] This report covered medical technology issues such as nuclear magnetic resonance (NMR), artificial organs, the ethics of technology use, the position of industry manufacturers, technology assessment, and the transfer of technology from academia to community hospitals—all factors affecting potential technology utilization.

NMR is an example of a rapidly expanding technology where the use of such a modality may cause payment problems. In fact, it has been suggested that mobile NMR scanners and freestanding imaging centers would be the appropriate locations to bypass reimbursement difficulties.

Artificial organs in development included a wearable kidney, an electrode-controlled arm, electrodes to turn acoustic wave forms of speech into electronic forms within the ear, and a new type of polymer material for artificial blood vessels.

Industry obviously will be greatly affected by the reimbursements authorized for medical care and the use of technological advances. Sounding the theme of the industry, Olseth linked medical technology to cost containment: "Technology can play an important role in moderating health care costs. It can improve hospital productivity and generate long-term savings. In addition, technology can facilitate delivery of care at cost-effective sites."[216]

Technology Assessment

Technology assessment evaluating the advantages and disadvantages of new modalities is a major problem in the PPS. Dr. H. David Banta, of the OTA, said that the DRG payment plan will mark "really the first time that concern for medical technology assessment has become a part of the decision making process on rates of payment for health care services."[217] This viewpoint was repeated in a variety of statements in a health policy report in the *New England Journal of Medicine*.[218] Quotes from a Congressman, an assistant HHS secretary for health, an Institute of Medicine report, and an OTA report card all attest to the "serious shortcomings in the national system of health care technology assessment." Banta felt that "the hospital administrator is going to become very conservative about technology."[219]

Transfer of technology from the research laboratory to the bedside often fails. Information on new technologies is readily available since researchers need to publish the results of their work. However, practitioners often do not have time to read these articles or may not understand the jargon of academia. As a result, new technology may never really be integrated into the everyday practice of medicine.

OTA Report

With the issues raised and the potential for affecting the quantity and the quality of health care, the Subcommittee on Health and the Environment asked the OTA to examine the relation of DRGs to medical technology. This resulted in the publication of "Diagnosis Related Groups (DRGs) and the Medicare Program: Implications for Medical Technology. A Technical Memorandum" in July 1983.

In summary, the OTA report concluded that DRG payment incentives may be expected to affect technology use in the following ways:

- Overall, the number and intensity of ancillary inpatient procedures can be expected to decrease. However, procedures that can be shown to lower the cost per case will increase.

- DRG payment will encourage the movement of technologies into the home, particularly for posthospital care. Settings of technology use are likely to be influenced by DRG payment. Influential incentives work in conflicting directions and are sensitive to key features of program design.

- DRG payment is likely to influence the specialization of services, but the magnitude and direction of those effects is unknown. Incentives to reduce costs encourage concentration of capital intensive technologies in fewer institutions. Conversely, increasing competition will create incentives for widespread acquisition of some technologies.

- Greater product standardization can be expected as more expensive models and procedures are eased out of the marketplace through competition. This change in technology product mix likely results from the downward pressure of the price and quantity of supplies and on capital if that is included in the DRG rate.[220]

In general, technologies that are cost-reducing to hospitals will be encouraged; cost-raising technologies will be discouraged. Exhibit 3-10 identifies four types of technological innovation and cost effects as well as incentives for adoption.

To Buy or Not to Buy

Anderson and Steinberg asked the basic technology acquisition question: to buy or not to buy? It was their opinion that the DRG legislation aimed to "encourage a slower and more cost conscious approach to the adoption of new technologies and equipment."[221] Disincentives and counterbalancing forces to technology acquisition were identified as follows:

Disincentives.   A one percent limit on fund increases for technology despite a historical annual increase of four to five percent is a major disincentive. A smaller piece of the pie will be available as health care providers will have to use the already available resources more effectively.

Exhibit 3-10 Four Types of Technological Innovation by Effects on Capital Cost, Operating Cost, Total Cost, and Incentives for Adoption

Type of innovation	Direction of effect on:			Incentives for adoption	
	Capital cost per case	Operating cost per case	Total cost per case	With capital in rate	Without capital in rate
I. Cost-raising, quality-enhancing new technology	+	+	+	↓	↓
II. Operating cost-saving innovations					
A.	+	−	+	↓	↑
B.	+	−	−	↑	↑
III. Capital cost-saving innovations					
A.	−	+	+	↓	↓
B.	−	+	−	↑	↓
IV. Service/procedure disadoption ...	−	−	−	↑	↑

Type I   raises all components of hospital care per case.
Example—intensive care monitoring.
Adoption disincentive regardless of payment mode.

Type II   uses capital investment to save costs but may (A) or may not (B) lower the total cost per case.
Example—automated laboratory testing
Adoption incentive reversible by payment mode as in reduced operating cost with increase in total cost per case as in (A).

Type III substitutes expendable labor for capital equipment.
Example—manual lab test more effective than automated.
Adoption incentive reversible by payment mode as in increased operating cost and reduced total cost per case as in (B).

Type IV   uses new knowledge to show services/procedures to be ineffective/unsafe
Example—PPB therapy (intermittent positive pressure breathing)
Adoption incentive regardless of payment mode.

Source: U.S. Congress, Office of Technology Assessment, *Diagnosis Related Groups (DRGs) and the Medicare Program: Implications for Medical Technology. A Technical Memorandum*, OTA-TM-H-17, July 1983, pp. 40–42.

Recalibration of payment rates do not take place often enough and result in a DRG lag in accounting for technology advances. In addition, historical hospital charges resulted in technologically complex DRG procedures being systematically underpriced when compared with simple DRG procedures. Traditionally, hospitals cross-subsidized expensive procedures with less costly ones.

Counterbalancing Forces.   Physicians are motivated to seek the best quality care regardless of the cost. It is likely that physicians will pressure hospital administrators to purchase the "biggest and the best."

Hospital administrators will have to acquire the latest equipment and offer the newest services to attract and to hold their patients in the increasingly competitive marketplace.

Additional technological considerations identified by Anderson and Steinberg deal with issues concerning choices and services.

- Cost-saving diagnostic and therapeutic innovations will be selected for economic reasons. However, it may be difficult to determine accurate increases or decreases in costs. Often, new procedures and equipment are used "in addition to, rather than instead of, existing alternatives."[222]

- Short-term savings rather than long-term savings will be preferred. A hip replacement that costs more and lasts longer avoids repeat surgery for the patient. However, the DRG payment does not cover the newer longer-lasting prosthetic, while repeat surgery is covered as a new admission. Interests of patients, hospital administrators, and society may not agree on technology utilization.

- A bias against technologically intensive DRGs could emerge as hospitals choose a case mix of "DRG winners" and "DRG losers." This "could induce hospitals to stop performing technologically complicated procedures or discourage them from investing in innovations that increase the safety with which the procedures are performed."[223]

- Outpatient procedures will become more common as hospitals choose to establish their own services or contract with freestanding facilities.

State-of-the-Art Decisions

One hospital's choice between two pacemakers illustrates the problems many facilities face in choosing between state-of-the-art and less sophisticated technologies. Valley Hospital in Ridgewood, New Jersey, lost $150,000 in 1982, part of that due to a $2,000 loss on each pacemaker implant. The hospital paid $4,000 to $5,000 per device, although another model was available for $1,995.

A major drawback to the less expensive model was that it could be programmed for only one of the three pacemaker functions. According to Dr. John E. Strobeck, a cardiologist at Valley Hospital, "In practice, the number of times I had need to reprogram output can be counted on one hand."[224] The manufacturer of the new pacemaker offered cost savings, but lost out to the health care industry's continued appetite for the latest technologies. Understandably, the manufacturer questioned such logic saying that "it makes no sense to implant a Ferrari and use it like a Volkswagen."[225] This was borne out in an 1985 ProPAC study. "A Report on the Appropriateness of Medicare Hospital Payments for Pacemaker Implantation."[226] This report said that financial incentives could lead institutions to curtail pacemaker services.

Magnetic Resonance Imaging (MRI) is another piece of technology representing an economic risk under DRG payments. Charges can not be recouped under the DRG rate and there may be a choice not to use MRI for economic reasons.[227] One proprietary hospital chain emphasizes professional education as vital to cutting diagnostic imaging costs per case.[228]

Decisions on new potential cost-saving procedures and technology include the following innovations:

Laser surgery	Nutritional support
Endoscopy	Enzyme therapy
Angioplasty	X-ray film systems
Ultrasound	Computerized drug formularies
Implantable infusion pumps	Laboratory equipment
Wound closure devices and catheters	Dictation devices
Digital substraction angiography	Recombinant DNA technology
Lithotripters	Organ transplantation
Immunodiagnostic procedures	In vitro fertilization[229-231]

In addition, hospital managers are looking to move services outside of the hospital into ambulatory and home care locations. A full day conference on high technology and home health care covered topics such as respiratory care, home dialysis, and parenteral nutrition.[232] At a meeting of the National Health Lawyers Association in 1985, Schatz also covered similar issues on medical technology from the manufacturers' and providers' points of view. He cited strategies such as specialization, alternate funding, alternate reorganizational structures, engineering research actions, corporate mergers, and joint provider/manufacturer opportunities. In conclusion, Schatz also predicted a shift to ambulatory care, more patient self-care, exposure to legal liability, and a reexamination of technology incentives.[233]

Goodhart, an expert on technology policy for the AHA, pointed out four reasons why decisions are not easy to make regarding technology use:

1. Frequently, the effects of technology application are nonquantifible.

2. Comparisons of the effects of technology in different situations are difficult.

3. Resource allocations, in many hospitals, are still highly political.

4. Frequently, a new technology is obsolete before it is fully paid for, due to medical advances.[234]

The New Jersey Example

Hospital administrators in New Jersey go beyond clinical application in evaluating the acquisition of new technology or the initiation of new procedures. Criteria includes consideration of staff increases and maintenance costs, along with a productivity analysis. In addition, a marketing perspective views the potential for a profitable product line. This type of decision-making reduces the influence physicians have over incorporation of new technology into the health care system. "The DRG system has translated medical practice management into terms nonphysicians can understand," according to a health care consulting expert.[235]

Another New Jersey lesson occurred when Hackensack Medical Center (HMC) appealed to the Hospital Rate Setting Commission regarding its investment in technology— and won. HMC purchased a diagnostic Dyna Camera which obviated the need for surgery in many cases. However, the decrease in surgery resulted in lower reimbursement for the hospital unmatched by an equal reduction in costs. Patients and the system were benefiting, but not the hospital. Using DRG statistics, HMC was able to show a correlation between the use of the Dyna Camera and the loss of revenue. This appeal was won as a direct result of using DRG generated data.[236]

A Decreasing Allowance for Technology

A Congressional Budget Office (CBO) proposal to modify PPS suggested removing the 1 percent technology allowance annual increase. CBO estimated that the technology reduction would save the federal government $8.3 billion between 1985 and 1989.[237] Shortly thereafter the Senate Finance Committee voted to eliminate the 1 percent technology allowance.[238] Health care professionals contend that some patients could be denied the benefits of medical advances. Hospitals will not buy technology unless costs are saved.[239] In the Deficit Reduction Act of 1984, the Congress cut back the 1 percent technology allowance to no more than one-quarter of 1 percent for FY 1985.[240]

This Congressional action serves to "intensify the bias against technology embedded in the DRG system," according to Daniel P. Bourque of the National Committee for Quality Health Care.[241] Adding the technology allowance reduction to the DRG-lowered prices, Bourque comments on the decreased likelihood of diagnostic and treatment breakthroughs to improve health care.

In summary, the PPS, using DRGs, rewards hospitals for the use of innovations that reduce operating costs. Therefore, hospital managers will seek technology that does the following:

- Attracts admissions of profitable DRGs

- Reduces patient length of stay

- Controls the use of ancillary services

- Analyzes case and payer mixes for management decisions

- Targets services to unique markets

- Reduces operating costs while improving productivity.[242]

Marketing and Management

Carolyne Davis, HCFA Administrator, says that the federal government intends to be a "prudent buyer," paying for specific hospital services outcomes.[243] To fulfill HCFA's intent to get its money's worth, hospital executives will have to be "assertive risk-taker managers."[244] However, Schonfeld believes that most hospital plans are not creative and most top executives do not know marketing. Experts at an American Marketing Association health services seminar told the audience that "without salesmanship, even the most prestigious hospital or clinic won't survive in today's competitive marketplace."[245]

Simply and emphatically, Studnicki peels away the allure of the successful high-powered proprietary executive in explaining marketing:

> There are four ways, and only four, in which the profit of the business can be increased.
> 1. Increase production volume.
> 2. Increase selling price per unit.
> 3. Decrease variable costs per unit.
> 4. Decrease fixed costs.[246]

Two basic hospital marketing concepts are identified by Seymour, an Ernst & Whinney health care consultant, to explain what PPS means in the health care system: (1) publics and exchanges, and (2) marketing mix. A public is also called a market or a market segment and an exchange takes place between the public and the hospital. Publics served by hospitals include accreditation agencies, business groups, donors, employees, patients, payers, physicians, professional organizations, providers, regulators, suppliers, trustees, and volunteers. Examples of publics and exchanges follow:

- Patients secure improved health and hotel-like services and in exchange the hospital receives payment.

- Physicians admit patients to the hospital to produce revenue in exchange for a place to treat their patients.

- Trustees get community recognition, prestige, and a feeling of doing good, and in exchange the hospital gets their direction and expertise.

Marketing mix adds in four elements: product, price, place, and promotion. In Seymour's analysis, the term strategic program unit (SPU) is used to describe the hospital's product. After SPUs are developed, the hospital can classify them on a portfolio matrix. Considering profitability against market growth possibilities on high to low scales produces a four cell grouping of patients and/or departments into cash cows, rising stars, question marks, and dogs. These labels applied to SPUs are self-explanatory from a marketing sales approach.[244] Price includes the federal government's stimulated competition. Place refers to delivery sites such as hospital, ambulatory care, after care, and group centers. Promotion refers to mass media advertisements and other means of alerting the community to the availability of services.

An analysis of this nature by the hospital management team could profoundly affect sales and marketing planning. Community Memorial Hospital in Toms River, reacting to the DRG plan in New Jersey, sought to demystify DRGs for specific target publics. This hospital's public relations department published materials for many audiences: a quarterly, *The Inside Story*, a newsletter for important people in the community; a continuing education monthly, *DRG Briefings*, for medical/dental staff; a handbook for physicians; and a leaflet for patients.[248] Henrotin Hospital in Chicago uses radio spot announcements, Sunday newspaper ads, and magazine ads "to inspire consumers to use hospital services."[249] Psychiatric hospitals were told by a health policy expert to define their services and to sell themselves better.[250] One hospital chain even offered to absorb the Medicare deductibles for elderly patients admitted to their facility. Roerig, a pharmaceutical, likewise provided a marketing stimulus to hospital administrators. This firm announced that it would provide hospitals with certain medications at no charge to complete therapy for Medicare patients who remain hospitalized after the DRG allowance lapses.[251]

Obviously, salesmanship and marketing costs money. A communications expert urges hospitals to budget one to two percent of gross revenue for marketing and advertising. However, Strum warned that hospitals with large-volume DRG business will have trouble allocating funds to advertising. On the other hand, hospitals with opportunities to increase their market share of private paying patients will spend money to achieve that goal.[252]

DRG Manipulation

DRG Creep

In a June 25, 1981 article in the *New England Journal of Medicine,* Dr. Donald W. Simborg reported on "DRG Creep. A New Hospital-Acquired Disease."[253] Dr. Simborg predicted that DRG creep would be an epidemic in the 1980s. "DRG Creep may be defined as a deliberate and systematic shift in a hospital's reported case mix in order to improve reimbursement."[254] Lewis clarifies the situation when he notes that "DRG creep involves the subtle shift upward from lower cost categories to higher cost ones."[255] Hence, the DRG classification "creeps" in some direction to result in the hospital's receiving more money for the services rendered to patients covered by Medicare. Altman called it "DRG Gallo," projecting a 12 to 15 percent manipulation rate.[256]

Simborg realized the potential for DRG creep in an examination of data at the University of San Francisco's hospital. In the 1978 medical records, there were 159 patients who had a major surgical procedure, as well as chronic nephritis, chronic pyelonephritis, or other renal disease as a secondary diagnosis. Using the 1978 data, the 159 patients fall into 64 DRGs with a weighted average of $4,210. If the sequence of diseases were changed, these patients classify as DRG 238 (Diseases of the Kidney and Ureter with Surgery) with an average charge of $9,322. This changed sequencing of the diseases shifted the costs by more than $800,000. In some cases it would be difficult to justify renal disease as the principal diagnosis; in some cases it would be appropriate. Using a computer program to "optimize" the DRG classifications would have resulted in a 14 percent increase in reimbursement for the hospital.[257]

Considering the results of the study at UCSF's Hospital, Simborg made three sharp observations about DRG creep:

1. If the computer editing had been used on the hospital's discharge abstracts, the institution would have received "an unprecedented windfall profit."

2. Incorrectly reported principal diagnoses may have increased, but the high error rate would have probably neutralized the noticeable increase.

3. DRG creep "is a blatantly unethical method."[258]

Other forms of DRG creep besides computer optimization were cited by Simborg. Continuing physician education and the use of expensive and sensitive diagnostic studies are additional forms. Physician education could involve teaching clinicians to be aware of legitimate medical gray areas in arriving at a diagnosis. "When does 'probable transient ischemic attack' become the more costly 'possible stroke'?"[259] When does angina pectoris (DRG 123) become myocardial infarction (DRG 121) based upon more sensitive and expensive testing than the usual diagnostic studies? From the DRG creep view, it is important to know that DRG 121 calls for about three times as much reimbursement as DRG 123. Education of physicians in this area would be important since "minor diagnostic nuances and slight imprecisions of wording have little practical clinical importance, yet under DRG payment they would have major financial consequences."[260]

Physician education regarding sequencing was formalized in the "Economic Grand Rounds" of a major hospital system. While complete and accurate documentation was lauded as the goal of the medical staff, examples illustrated the financial impact of the ordering of multiple diagnoses.

Gastroenteritis with Dehydration	DRG	182	$1,465
Dehydration with Gastroenteritis	DRG	296	$3,222
Peptic Ulcer with Cirrhosis of Liver	DRG	177	$1,898
Cirrhosis of Liver with Peptic Ulcer	DRG	202	$2,435[261]

Following publication of Dr. Simborg's article, a number of commentators responded to his observations on DRG creep. Dr. Finley, New Jersey's Health Commissioner, agreed that Dr. Simborg "described a mentality that unfortunately prevails in much of the health care industry." She spoke about the refining of information to maximize revenue but also noted that "coding-up" was easily detectible. A foreign correspondent remarked that in any reimbursement scheme "misuse of the output unit is possible." However, Grimaldi took Dr. Simborg to task and stated that his comments on DRG creep's "potential to generate windfall profits are incomplete, if not misleading." Grimaldi expressed views that DRG creep would be contained through legal constraints, audits, ethical standards, and long run financial consequences. In addition, Grimaldi took the regulators to task for constructing a payment plan with data known to be incomplete and erroneous.[262]

Dr. Simborg replied to the letters saying that he agreed that the regulators and the regulated should work together for the public's benefit. Yet, he was not optimistic that "crime does not pay for the DRG creepers" and added that "both artifical and biased alterations are perpetually rewarding." Even though the profit motive may not be dominant, the choice of clinical procedures is a complex process without a single correct answer. In closing, Dr. Simborg opined that the strength of the reimbursement vector would vary among individuals and institutions but the direction "is always the same; toward the most profitable alternative."[263]

Manipulation and Quality

In testimony before the U.S. Senate Subcommittee on Health, Dr. Howard Strawcutter, President, American Medical Peer Review Association, identified inappropriate ways to take advantage of DRG loopholes:

- Allow bias to affect the selection of a principal diagnosis for a patient with multiple diagnoses in order to obtain higher payment.

- Admit patients who might be cared for on an outpatient basis.

- Favor the admission of patients within each DRG where costs are comparatively low and stays brief.

- Withhold clinical services or substitute less expensive services, or delay use of new technologies to reduce cost during a single stay but possibly induce greater overall service use and aggregate costs during subsequent stays.[264]

Even the Inspector General of the U.S. Department of Health and Human Services pointed out a DRG loophole. Kusserow conjectured that hospitals could classify as many patients as possible into DRG 468. That DRG is for patients admitted for one condition but who receive surgery for an unrelated condition. Reimbursement for DRG 468 is higher than 409 of the other 467 DRGs. This incentive could cause hospitals to "falsely assign lower cost cases to the 468 category," according to the inspector general. He suggested abolishing DRG 468.[265]

Gaming Warnings

In a sharp warning, lawyer John T. Mooresmith of the Medical Mutual Liability Insurance Society alerted physicians that fraudulently modifying a diagnosis to get more money for the hospital could result in five years in prison and a $25,000 fine. This warning appeared in *Medical Economics* and was headlined in bold typeface, "Playing Games with DRGs is Playing with Fire."[266]

Both HHS Secretary Margaret Heckler and HCFA Administrator Dr. Carolyne Davis have repeatedly warned about DRG gaming. Secretary Heckler "put the hospitals on notice" that she "will not allow manipulation to the detriment of the public."[267] In a speech at the American Hospital Association's annual meeting, Dr. Davis explained the warning: "I want to give clear notice that, to the extent we find evidence of the system being gamed, we will aggressively pursue preadmission review and other appropriate sanctions."[268] At the annual meeting of the Federation of American Hospitals about one month later, Dr. Davis said that hospitals were not gaming the DRG system. As of February 3, 1984, Medicare transfers were similar to past years, DRG 468 dumping was not noted, with that classification accounting for only one percent of all billing, and unusual admission practices were minimal. Of the 1,200 hospitals with unusual changes in admissions, about half had reasonable explanations and about a fifth required corrective actions.[269]

Government Reaction to DRG Creep

By July 1984, the hospitals' case-mix index (CMI) showed an increase of 5.8 percent. This was 2.4 percent above the expected 3.38 percent CMI use.[270] HCFA and the Office of Management and Budget claimed that the CMI increase was the result of manipulation by hospitals. Former Secretary Heckler attributed the CMI rise to DRG creep "even though she acknowledged DHHS had no hard evidence of such gaming of the system."[271] Declining identification, a HCFA official agreed that this was more DRG creep than had been anticipated. He added: "Whether this is gaming (to circumvent the system), or whether the hospitals are just doing a better job of assigning (the diagnosis), I don't know."[272]

Jack Owen of the AHA countered that hospitals were merely updating their medical records to reflect the careful reporting of principal diagnoses. Michael Bromberg of FAH argued that Medicare patients in 1984 were sicker than those treated in 1981, the base year for the CMI.[273]

These rationales were dismissed by government experts and the DRG creep was countered by a proposed reduction in the weights assigned for cost calculations by 2.4 percent. In response to intense pressure from the hospital lobbying groups, a compromise was struck, reducing DRG prices 1.05 percent but allowing inflation adjustments to vary. However, the federal officials admonished that hospital records would continue to be scrutinized for unexplained CMI increases.[274]

Readmission Gaming

Researchers at Johns Hopkins Hospital analyzed 270,266 Medicare patients treated between 1974 and 1977. Nearly 25 percent were readmitted within two months and 5 percent within a few days. Steinberg and Anderson concluded that the DRG payment plan "could cost the government more money if the physicians manipulate the program by repeatedly admitting the same ill patients."[275] Readmissions could be stimulated by premature discharge, availability of empty hospital beds, and by physicians treating each ailment during separate admissions. Investigators calculated that each year readmissions account for about 25 percent of the Medicare medical billings.[276]

As with any new program, an argot quickly develops and takes hold in the language. In the area of DRG manipulation, it started with DRG creep and rapidly surged to include the following words with subtle meanings used to shade the intent of the PPS: education; gaming; loopholes; manipulation; optimalization; refining; up-coding; winners and losers. It appears to be axiomatic in the health care business—if there are ways to beat the system, somebody will come up with them.

References

1. A. Somers, "Moderating the Rise in Health Care Costs," *New England Journal of Medicine* 307, No. 15, (October 7, 1982):944-947.

2. P. R. Alper, "Moderating Hospital Costs," *Medical World News* 25, No. 10, (May 28, 1984):76.

3. M. Korcok, "DRG Plan Not Enough to Curb Health Costs: Speaker," *Hospitals* 56, No. 24, (December 16, 1982):17-20.

4. G. Powers, "A Lawyer's Look at Legal Bases Available to Government in its Efforts to Use DRG System," *Review, Federation of American Hospitals* 13, No. 3, (1980):38-40.

5. Equitable Life Assurance Society of U.S., *Physician's Attitudes Toward Cost Containment*, New York, NY, March 1984.

6. E. N. Berg, "Major Corporations Ask Workers to Pay More of Health Cost," *New York Times, September 12, 1983*.

7. L. E. Saline, Discussant in *Health Care Institutions in Flux*, edited by W. Greenberg and R. M. Southby (Arlington, VA: Information Resources Press, 1984), pp. 90-91.

8. M. D. Bromberg, Discussant in *Health Care Institution in Flux*, edited by W. Greenberg and R. M. Southby (Arlington, VA: Information Resources Press, 1984), pp. 124-125.

9. H. D. Doremus, "An Economic Approach to DRGs. A Reimbursement System That Limits the Cost of Hospital Care," *Hospital Financial Management* 37, No. 4, (1983):88-91.

10. W. O. Cleverley, "Cost Accounting Pins a Value to DRGs," *Modern Healthcare* 14, No. 5, (1984):172-176, 178-179.

11. "Cost Accounting Under a Prospective Payment System," *DRG Monitor* 1, No. 6, (1984):1-8.

12. C. Wallace, "Managing Along Product Lines is Key to Hospital Profits Under DRG System," *Modern Healthcare* 13, No. 9, (1983):56.

13. S. Y. Soliman and W. L. Hughes, "DRG Payments and Net Contribution Variance Analysis," *Healthcare Financial Management* 37, No. 10, (1983):78-86.

14. H. A. Kohlman, "Determining A Contribution Margin for DRG Profitability,"

Healthcare Financial Management 38, No. 4, (1984):108, 110.

15. W. J. Waters and J. T. Tierney, "Hard Lessons Learned," *New England Journal of Medicine* 311, No. 19, (November 8, 1984):1251-1252.

16. J. D. Thompson, "Regulation of Hospital Costs, Volume and Prices," in G. L. Glandon and R. J. Shapiro (eds.) *Profiles of Medical Practice* (Chicago: American Medical Assn., 1980), pp. 81-89.

17. "DRGs Affect Specialists Most," *American Medical News* 27, No. 24, (June 22, 1984):24.

18. E. S. Hyman, "Who Controls A Patient's Hospital Bill?" *Private Practice* 16, No. 11, (1984):19-21.

19. M. Tatge, "Prospective Pay's Just A Quick Fix," *Modern Healthcare* 14, No. 5, (1984):156, 158.

20. Ibid.

21. Thompson, "Regulation of Hospital Costs."

22. Ibid.

23. Ibid.

24. R. H. Egdahl, "Should We Shrink the Health Care System?" *Harvard Business Review* 62, No. 1, (1984):125-132.

25. R. J. Reitemeir, "Cutting Costs—Using Health Resources Properly," *ACOP Observer* 4, No. 4, (1984):3.

26. "Uncertain Progress on Health Costs" (editorial), *New York Times,* July 17, 1984.

27. R. Green, "Health Care Rationing: Can It Happen Here?" *Medical World News* 25, No. 21, (November 12, 1984):50-51, 58, 63-64, 69-70, 72, 74.

28. Ibid.

29. Ibid.

30. Ibid.

31. Ibid.

32. L. Kahn, "Bleak Future Seen for Nation's Hospitals," *Hospitals* 56, No. 24, (December 16, 1982):24, 28.

33. Green, "Health Care Rationing."

34. J. A. Meyer, "Cost Shifting—Passing the Health Buck," *American Medical News* 27, No. 6, (February 10, 1984):28.

35. Health Insurance Association of America, *Prospective Payment. A Sound Approach to Containing Hospital Costs,* Washington, DC, undated.

36. "A New Era in Medicine" (editorial), New York Times, September 12, 1983.

37. "Uncertain Progress," *New York Times.*

38. S. Lewis, "Speculations on the Impact of Prospective Pricing and DRGs," *Western Journal of Medicine* 140, No. 4, (1984):638-644.

39. M. A. Glasser, "Reverse Side of a Curb on Hospital Costs" (letter), *New York Times,* September 11, 1984.

40. Equitable Life Assurance Society, *Physician's Attitudes.*

41. H. P. Cain, II, "The Blue Cross and Blue Shield Perspective" in *Health Care Institutions in Flux,* edited by W. Greenberg and R. M. Southby (Arlington, VA: Information Resources Press, 1984), p. 59.

42. P. B. Ginsburg and F. A. Sloan, "Hospital Cost Shifting," *New England Journal of Medicine* 310, No. 14, (April 5, 1984):893-898.

43. Ibid.

44. Meyer, "Cost Shifting—Passing the Health Buck."

45. Ginsburg and Sloan, "Hospital Cost Shifting."

46. J. W. Own, "Coping with Medicare Prospective Payment" in *Health Care Institutions in Flux,* edited by W. Greenberg and R. M. Southby (Arlington, VA: Information Resources Pub., 1984), pp. 95-106.

47. W. Greenberg and R. M. Southby, *Health Care Institutions in Flux. Changing Reimbursement Patterns in the 1980s* (Arlington, VA: Information Resources Press, 1984).

48. P. D. Benz, "Group DRGs Into Product Families for Better Management and Control," *Modern Healthcare* 14, No. 4, (1984):110, 114, 118.

49. Blue Cross of Western Pennsylvania, *Hospital Case Mix Overview.* Unpublished, June, 1983.

50. E. A. Codman, "The Product of a Hospital," *Surgery, Gynecology, and Obstetrics* 18, (1914):491-496.

51. S. E. Berki, "The Design of Case Based Hospital Payment Systems," *Medical Care* 21, No. 1, (1983):1-13.

52. M. E. Sinioris, T. H. Esmond, A. E. Glenesk, and R. S. Newman, "Program Matrix Aids Planning Process," *Hospitals* 56, No. 8, (April 16, 1982):75-77.

53. M. Feldstein, *Economic Analysis for Health Service Efficiency* (Amsterdam: North Holland Pub. Co., 1967).

54. J. E. Siemon, "Case Mix and Data Quality: A Review of the Literature," *Topics in Health Records Management* 2, No. 4, (1982):13-22.

55. R. Ament, "The Use of Case Mix Figures in Analyzing Average Charges for Inpatients," *PAS Reporter* 14, No. 3, (1976):1-7.

56. J. D. Bentley, "HCFA Case Mix Index: Implications for Hospitals," *Hospital Progress* 62, No. 1, (1981):49-55.

57. J. D. Klastorin and C. A. Watts, "On the Measurement of Hospital Case Mix," *Medical Care* 18, No. 6, (1980):675-685.

58. J. R. Lave, L. B. Lave, and L. P. Silverman, "Hospital Cost Estimation Controlling for Case Mix," *Journal of Applied Economics* 4, No. 9, (1972):165-180.

59. W. W. Young, R. B. Swinkola, and M. A. Hutton, "Assessment of the AUTOGRP Classification System," *Medical Care* 18, No. 2, (1980):228-244.

60. D. Kinzer and M. Warner, "The Effect of Case Mix Adjustment on Admission-Based Reimbursement," *Health Services Research* 18, No. 2, (Summer, 1983):209-225.

61. M. J. Goran, "DRGs: Imperfect But Useful Reimbursement Tool," *Hospital Progress* 62, No. 3, (1981):6, 8.

62. Ibid.

63. D. W. Simborg, "DRG Creep. A New Hospital-Acquired Disease," *New England Journal of Medicine* 304, No. 26, (June 25, 1981):1602-1604.

64. J. B. Reiss, "Future Directions for Case Mix Applications," *Topics in Health Care Financing* 8, No. 4, (Summer, 1982):67-83.

65. J. R. Lave and L. B. Lave, "The Extent of Role Differentiation Among Hospitals," *Health Services Research* 6, (Spring, 1971):15-38.

66. Reiss, "Future Directions."

67. R. Ament, "The Use of Case Mix Figures in Analyzing Average Changes for Inpatients." *PAS Reporter* 14, No. 3, (1976):1-7.

68. C. Hulm and D. Burik, "Evaluating the New Case Mix Systems," *Hospitals* 58, No. 2, (January 16, 1984):92, 94, 96.

69. U.S. Congress, Office of Technology Assessment. *Diagnosis Related Groups (DRGs) and the Medicare Program: Implications for Medical Technology,* A Technical Memorandum, OTA-TM-H-17, July 1983.

70. Health Research and Educational Trust of New Jersey, *DRG Evaluation*

71. J. D. Thompson, R. B. Fetter, and C. D. Mross. "Case Mix and Resource Use," *Inquiry.* 12, No. 4, (1975):300-312.

72. R. F. Averill, "The Design and Development of the Diagnoses Related Groups," *Topics in Health Record Management* 4, No. 3, (1984):66-76.

73. Reiss, "Future Directions."

74. Berki, "The Design of Case Based Hospital Payment Systems."

75. Blue Cross of Western Pennsylvania, *Hospital Case Mix Overview.*

76. J. R. Lave, J. Pettengill, and J. Vertrees, "Case Mix Index and DRGs: Should They Be Calculated at the National or Regional Level?" *Healthcare Financial Management* 37, No. 4, (1983):64-70.

77. Ernst & Whinney, *The Revised DRGs. Their Importance in Medicare Payments to Hospitals,* E&W No. J58442, revised May 1983, pp. 5-6.

78. P. L. Grimaldi, "Adjusting to Medicare DRG Indexes and Target Ceilings," *Hospital Progress* 62, No. 1, (1983):42-47.

79. U.S. Congress, OTA, *DRGs and Medicare,* p. 11.

80. M. C. Hornbrook, "Hospital Case Mix: Its Definition, Measurement and Use: Part I. The Conceptual Framework. Part II. Review of Alternative Measures," *Medical Care Review* 39, Nos. 1 and 2, (Spring and Summer (respectively), 1982).

81. Ibid.

82. P. W. Butler and J. D. Bentley, "Ten Issues to Consider When Evaluating Case Mix Reimbursement," *Hospital Financial Management* 34, No. 6, (1980):34-42.

83. Ibid.

84. Reiss, "Future Directions."

85. H. A. Cohen and J. G. Atkinson, "Case Mix and Regulation," *Topics in Health Care Financing* 8, No. 4, (Summer, 1982):21-28.

86. Ibid.

87. J. Greenberg and R. Kropf, "A Case Mix Method for Developing Health Planning Criteria for Hospital Services," *Medical Care* 19, No. 11, (1981):1083-1094.

88. A. M. Garber, V. R. Fuchs, and J. F. Silverman, "Case Mix, Costs, and Outcomes," *New England Journal of Medicine* 310, No. 19, (May 10, 1984):1231-1237.

89. Butler and Bentley, "Ten Issues to Consider."

90. L. K. Lichtig, "Data Systems for Case Mix," *Topics in Health Care Financing* 8, No. 4, (Summer, 1982):13-19.

91. J. D. Bentley and R. W. Butler. *The DRG Case Mix of a Sample of Teaching Hospitals, A Technical Report*. Washington, D.C.: Association of American Medical Colleges, December 1981, pp. A4-A7.

92. Reiss, "Future Directions."

93. M. Schwartz, J. C. Merrill, and L. K. Blake, "DRG-Based Case Mix and Public Hospitals," *Medical Care* 22, No. 4, (1984):283-299.

94. A. L. Plough, S. R. Salem, M. Schwartz, J. M. Weller, and C. W. Ferguson, "Case Mix in End-Stage Renal Disease. Differences Between Patients in Hospital-Based and Free-Standing Treatment Facilities," *New England Journal of Medicine* 310, No. 22, (May 31, 1984):1432-1436.

95. D. P. Wagner, T. D. Wineland, and W. A. Knaus, "Hidden Costs of Treating Severely Ill Patients: Charges and Resource Consumption in an Intensive Care Unit," *Health Care Financing Review* 5, No. 1, (1983):81-86.

96. D. Burik, P. Gilroy, and A. M. Mastrangelo, "Case Mix Data System Prepares Hospitals for DRG-Based Reimbursement," *Hospital Progress* 64, No. 2, (1983):47-49, 72.

97. Goran, "DRGs: Imperfect But Useful."

98. Simborg, "DRG Creep."

99. S. V. Williams, G. F. Kominski, B. E. Dowd, and K. A. Soper, "Methodological Limitations in Case Mix Hospital Reimbursement, With a Proposal for Change," *Inquiry* 21, (Spring, 1984), 17-31.

100. R. R. Arons, *The New Economics of Health Care: DRGs, Case Mix and Length of Stay* (New York: CBS Scientific-Prager Publishing, 1984).

101. A. J. Rutigiliano, "Case Mix System Plots M.D., Dept. Performance," *Health Care Systems* (April, 1984).

102. Hulm and Burik, "Evaluating Case Mix Systems."

103. Ibid.

104. U.S. Congress, OTA, *DRGs and Medicare*, p. 13.

105. Williams et al., "Methodological Limitations."

106. Health Research and Educational Trust of New Jersey, *Case-Mix Classification, Data and Management. DRG Evaluation. Volume 3*. Princeton, NJ, February 1984, pp. 8-17.

107. Lave and Lave, "Role Differentiation."

108. R. Evans and H. Walker, "Information Theory and the Analysis of Hospital Cost Structure," *Canadian Journal of Economics* 5, No. 8, (1972):398-418.

109. S. D. Horn and D. N. Schumacher, "An Analysis of Case Mix Complexity Using Information Theory and Diagnostic Related Grouping," *Medical Care* 17, No. 4, (1979):382-389.

110. W. R. Wood, R. P. Ament, and E. J. Kobrinski, "A Foundation for Hospital Case Mix Measurement," *Inquiry* 18, (Fall, 1981):247-254.

111. Klastorin and Watts, "Measurement of Case Mix."

112. Commission on Professional and Hospital Activities. *List A: Hospital Diagnosis Groups*. Ann Arbor, MI, 1974.

113. Commission on Professional and Hospital Activities. *The Internal Classification of Diseases, 9th Revision. Clinical Modifications. Volume 1, Diseases, Tabular List*. Ann Arbor, MI, 1978.

114. J. S. Gonnella and M. J. Goran, "Quality of Patient Care—A Measurement of Change: The Staging Concept," *Journal of Medical Education* 56, No. 8, (1981) 467-473.

115. W. W. Young, R. B. Swinkola, and D. M. Zorn, "The Measurement of Hospital Case Mix," *Medical Care* 20, No. 5, (1982):501-512.

116. S. D. Horn, P. D. Sharkey, and D. A. Bertram, "Measuring Severity of Illness: Homogenous Case Mix Groups," *Medical Care* 21, No. 1, (1983):14-31.

117. S. D. Horn, "Does Severity of Illness Make a Difference in Prospective Payment?" *Healthcare Financial Management* 37, No. 5, (1983):49-53.

118. R. B. Fetter, Y. Shin, J. Freeman, R. F. Averill, and J. D. Thompson, "Case Mix Definition by DRGs," *Medical Care* 18, No. 2, (Supplement 1983):1-53.

119. Butler and Bentley, "Ten Issues to Consider."

120. Hornbrook, "Hospital Case Mix."

121. M. P. Plomann and F. Shaffer, "DRGs As One of Nine Approaches to Case Mix in Transition," *Nursing and Health Care* 4, No. 8, (1983):438-443.

122. M. P. Plomann, "Understanding Case Mix Classification Systems," *Topics in Health Record Management* 4, No. 3, (1984):77-87.

123. Ibid.

124. Ibid.

125. Ibid.

126. Ibid.

127. K. G. Manton and J. C. Vertrees, "The Use of Grade of Membership Analysis to Evaluate and Modify Diagnosis Related Groups," *Medical Care* 22, No. 12, (1984):1067-1081.

128. Siemon, "Case Mix and Data Quality."

129. Ibid.

130. M. C. Hornbrook, "Allocative Medicine: Efficiency, Disease Severity and the Payment Mechanism," *Annals* AAPSS 468, No. 7, (1983):12-29.

131. R. S. Schweiker, *Report to Congress: Hospital Prospective Payment for Medicare,* Appendix C. USDHHS, December, 1982.

132. Ibid.

133. H. L. Smits, R. B. Fetter, and L. F. McMahon, Jr., "Variation in Resource Use Within Diagnosis-Related Groups: The Severity Issue," *Health Care Financing Review* 38, No. 11, (1984):71-78.

134. Ibid.

135. Ibid.

136. Ibid.

137. A. J. Keegan, "Hospitals Will Continue to Treat All DRGs to Snare 'Contribution Margin'," *Modern Healthcare* 13, No. 9, (1983):206, 208.

138. Ibid.

139. K. R. Jones, "Predicting Hospital Charge and Stay Variation," *Medical Care* 23, No. 3, (1985):220-235.

140. B. S. Eisenberg, "Diagnosis-Related Groups, Severity of Illness, and Equitable Reimbursement Under Medicare" (editorial), *Journal of the American Medical Association* 251, No. 5, (February 3, 1984):645-646.

141. J. S. Gonnella, "Case Mix Classification: The Need to Reduce Inappropriate Homogeneity" (editorial), *Journal of the American Medical Association* 255, No. 7, (February 21, 1986): 941-942.

142. L. I. Icozzoni and M. A. Moskowitz, "Clinical Overlap Among Medical Diagnosis-Related Groups," *Journal of the American Medical Association* 255, No. 7, (February 21, 1986): 927-929.

143. Horn and Schumacher, "Analysis of Case Mix Complexity."

144. S. L. Kreitzer, E. S. Loebner, and G. C. Roveti, "Severity of Illness: The DRGs' Missing Link?" *Quality Review Bulletin* 8, No. 5, (1984):21-34.

145. Horn, Sharkey, and Bertram, "Measuring Severity of Illness."

146. Horn, "Does Severity of Illness Make A Difference?"

147. S. D. Horn and R. A. Horn, "Reliability and Validity of the Severity of Illness Index," *Medical Care* 24, No. 2, (1986): 159-178.

148. C. Muller, "Paying Hospitals: How Does a Severity Measure Help?" *American Journal of Public Health* 73, No. 1, (1983):14-15.

149. S. D. Horn, "Measuring Severity of Illness: Comparisons Across Institutions."

American Journal of Public Health 73, No. 1, (1983):25-31.

150. S. D. Horn and P. D. Sharkey, "Measuring Severity of Illness to Predict Patient Resource Use Within DRGs," *Inquiry* 20, (Winter, 1983):314-321.

151. S. Horn, B. Chachich, and C. Clopton, "Measuring Severity of Illness: A Reliability Study," *Medical Care* 21, No. 7, (1983):705-714.

152. Horn, "Reliability and Validity of the Severity of Illness Index."

153. J. Fothergill, "An Account of the Sore Throat Attended With Ulcers," in L.A. May, *Classic Studies of Infectious Diseases* (New York: Dabor Scientific Publications, 1977). Original work published 1748.

154. J. S. Gonnella, M. C. Hornbrook, and D. Z. Louis, "Staging of Disease. A Case-Mix Measurement," *Journal of the American Medical Association* 251, No. 5, (February 3, 1984):637-644.

155. D. Z. Louis, *Disease Staging: A Clinically Based Approach to Measurement of Disease Severity. Volume 1: Executive Summary* (Santa Barbara, CA: Systemetrics, Inc., August, 1983).

156. D. Z. Louis, *Disease Staging: Medical Staging Criteria. Volume 2* (Santa Barbara, CA: Systemetrics, Inc., August, 1983).

157. D. Z. Louis, *Disease Staging: Coded Staging Criteria. Volume 3.* (Santa Barbara, CA: Systemetrics, Inc., August, 1983).

158. Louis, *Disease Staging, Volume 1.*

159. Gonnella, Hornbrook, and Louis, "Staging of Disease."

160. Louis, *Disease Staging, Volume 2.*

161. Louis, *Disease Staging, Volume 3.*

162. B. Christensen, "Staging Software Measures Severity of Patient's Illness," *Hospitals* 58, No. 9, (May 1, 1984):45-46.

163. R. M. Coffey and M. G. Goldfarb, "DRGs and Disease Staging for Reimbursing Medicare Patients," May 18, 1984, unpublished.

164. Health Research and Educational Trust of New Jersey, *Volume 3,* p. 15.

165. Louis, *Disease Staging, Volume 1,* p. 22.

166. W. W. Young, "Incorporating Severity of Illness and Comorbidity in Case Mix Measurement," *Health Care Financing Review* 38, No. 12, (Supplement) (1984):23-31.

167. W. W. Young, *Patient Management Categories.* Data presented at Annual Meeting of the American Public Health Association, November 14, 1984.

168. Young, "Incorporating Severity of Illness."

169. Young, *Patient Management Categories.*

170. Young, "Incorporating Severity of Illness."

171. Ibid.

172. W. W. Young, "Substitution Permissible," *Journal of the American Medical Association* 255, No. 7, (February 21, 1986): 942-943.

173. A. C. Brewster, R. C. Bradbury, L. A. Hyde, B. G. Karlin, and C. M. Jacobs, "A Computerized Clinical Information System for Hospital Quality Control," November 11, 1984, unpublished.

174. A. C. Brewster, B. G. Karlin, L. A. Hyde, C. M. Jacobs, R. C. Bradbury, and Y. M. Chae, "Medical Illness Severity Grouping System (MEDISGRPS): A Clinically-Based Approach to Classifying Hospital Patients at Admission," November 26, 1984, MediQual Systems, Inc. Westborough, MA, unpublished.

175. S. McIlrath, "Review Systems Based on Illness Severity," *American Medical News* 28, No. 2, (January 11, 1985):2, 17, 18.

176. Brewster et al., "Medical Illness Severity."

177. McIlrath, "Review Systems."

178. Ibid.

179. Ibid.

180. R. P. Caterinicchio, "Relative Intensity Measures: Developing a Ratio of Costs to Charges Methodology for the Pricing of Inpatient Nursing Services Under DRG Prospective Hospital Payment," in *DRGs: The Effect in N.J. The Potential for the Nation,* USDHHS, HCFA Pub. No. 03170, March 1984, pp. 88-94.

181. W. W. Diggs, "Patient Acuity Classifications," abstractedc in *Hospitals* 57, No. 10, (May 16, 1983):30.

182. H. Vanderzee and G. Glusko, "DRGs, Variable Pricing, and Budgeting for Nursing Services," *Journal of Nursing Administration* 14, No. 5, (1984):11-14.

183. M. Mitchell, J. Miller, L. Welches, and D. D. Walker, "Determining Cost of Direct Nursing Care by DRGs," *Nursing Management* 15, No. 4, (1984):29-32.

184. J. Nyberg and N. Wolff, "DRG Panic," *Journal of Nursing Administration* 14, No. 4, (1984):17-21.

185. N. F. Bermas and A. V. Slyck, "Patient Classification Systems and the Nursing Department," *Hospitals* 58, No. 22, (November 16, 1984):99-100.

186. R. P. Caterinicchio and G. P. Smith, "The Relationship Between Nursing Activity and Age," *Hospital Topics* 58, No. 4, (1980):46-50.

187. R. P. Caterinicchio, "A Debate: RIMs and The Cost of Nursing Care," *Nursing Management* 14, No. 5, (1983):36-39.

188. R. P. Caterinicchio and R. H. Davies, "Developing a Client-Focused Allocation Statistic of Inpatient Nursing Resource Use: An Alternative to the Patient Day," *Social Science and Medicine* 17, No. 5, (1983):259-272.

189. P. L. Grimaldi and J. A. Micheletti, "RIMs and the Cost of Nursing Care," *Nursing Management* 13, No. 12, (1982):12-22.

190. Caterinicchio, "A Debate."

191. G. P. Smith, "The 'RIM': Development and Impact of Nursing Management," in *DRGs: The Effect in N.J. The Potential for the Nation,* USDHHS, HCFA Pub. No. 03170, March 1984, pp. 95-100.

192. L. A. Joel, "Relative Intensity Measures and the State of the Art of Reimbursement for Nursing Services," in *DRGs: Changes and Challenges,* edited by F. A. Shaffer. National League for Nursing, Pub. No. 20-1959, June 20, 1984, pp. 57-64.

193. Ibid.

194. L. A. Joel, "DRGs and RIMs: Implications for Nursing," *Nursing Outlook* 32, No. 1, (1984):42-49.

195. N. Farrington, *Admitting Improves Hospital Efficiency: Coping With DRGs,*

Presentation at Middle Atlantic Health Congress, Atlantic City, NJ, May 22, 1984.

196. Ibid.

197. "Expert Says New DRG Bill Will Not Change Admitting Procedures," *Hospital Admitting Monthly* 2, No. 4, (1983):51-52.

198. "One Democratic Proposal to Save Medicare," *Medical World News* 25, No. 5, (March 12, 1984):95.

199. J. K. Inglehart, "Legislators Seek to Slow Phase-In of Medicare National Rates," *Hospital Progress* 65, No. 5, (1984):17, 28.

200. "Government Says DRGs Are Meeting Expectations," *American Medical News* 27, No. 19, (May 18, 1984):20.

201. "Business Declines for Nation's Hospitals," *American Medical News* 27, No. 27, (July 20, 1984):7.

202. "PPS Reduces Iowa Admissions: Study," *Hospitals* 58, No. 14, (July 16, 1984):28.

203. "Government Says DRGs Meet Expectations," *American Medical News.*

204. R. Pokras and K. K. Kublishke, "Diagnosis Related Groups Using Data From the National Hospital Discharge Survey: United States, 1982," *NCHS Advancedata,* No. 105, DHHS Pub. No. (PHS) 85-1250, January 18, 1985.

205. "Tulane Physician Education Program Reduces Lengths of Stay by 1.5," *Hospitals* 58, No. 2, (January 16, 1984):38.

206. Ibid.

207. R. P. Caterinicchio and R. H. Davies, "Developing a Client-Focused Allocation Statistic."

208. S. E. Berki, M. L. F. Ashcraft, and W. C. Newbrander, "Length of Stay Variations Within ICDA-8 Diagnostic Related Groups," *Medical Care* 22, No. 2, (1984):126-142.

209. "'High Tech' Medicine Cited in Medicare Hike," *American Medical News* 27, No. 30, (August 10, 1984):2, 15.

210. Ibid.

211. J. R. Lave, "Hospital Reimbursement Under Medicare," *MMFQ Health and Society* 62, No. 2, (Spring, 1984):251-268.

212. H. C. Moss, "Planners Haven't Learned from Mistakes, M.D. Says," *American Medical News* 27, No. 19, (May 18, 1984):6.

213. P. W. Butler, R. C. Bone, and J. Field, "Technology Under DRGs Prospective Payment. Implications for Medical Intensive Care," *Chest* 87, No. 2, (1985):229-234.

214. H. O. Buzzell, *Testimony on PPS, U.S. Senate Subcommittee on Health Hearings,* February 17, 1983, pp. 93-99.

215. "Technology '83: Looking at NMR and Other Developments as the DRG System Approaches," *FAH Review* 16, No. 4, (1983):20-34, 39-48.

216. Ibid.

217. Ibid.

218. J. K. Iglehart, "Another Chance for Technology Assessment," *New England Journal of Medicine* 309, No. 8, (August 25, 1983):509-512.

219. U.S. Congress, OTA, "DRGs and Medicare," p. 11.

220. U.S. Congress, OTA, "DRGs and Medicare," p. 5.

221. G. Anderson and E. Steinberg, "To Buy or Not to Buy. Technology Acquisition Under Prospective Payment," *New England Journal of Medicine* 311, No. 3, (July 19, 1984):182-185.

222. Ibid.

223. Ibid.

224. M. Nathanson, "New Breed of Pacemaker Vendors Helps Hospitals Cut Implant Costs," *Modern Healthcare* 14, No. 3, (February 15, 1984):158, 160.

225. Ibid.

226. S. McIlrath, "ProPAC: Heart Device DRG Rates are Fine," *American Medical News* 28, No. 12, (March 22, 1985):14.

227. B. J. Hillman, J. D. Winkler, C. E. Phelps, J. Aroesty, and A. P. Williams, "The Business Community Looks at DRG Based Hospital Reimbursement," *Health Affairs* 2, No. 1, (Spring, 1983):38-49.

228. E. F. Kuntz, "Cost-Cutting Drive Tags Imaging," *Modern Healthcare* 14, No. 3, (February 15, 1984):150, 152.

229. Ibid.

230. M. D. Goodhart, "Technology Acquisition Poses Thorny Dilemma to Hospitals," *Hospitals* 58, No. 14, (July 16, 1984):34, 38, 42.

231. W. I. Roe, "Medical Technology Under PPS: An Uncertain Future," *Hospitals* 59, No. 2, (January 16, 1985):88-90, 92.

232. "High Technology and Home Health Care," *Pride Institute Journal of Long Term Home Health Care* 3, No. 2, (Spring, 1984):1-58.

233. G. B. Schatz and S. M. Schuster, Jr., *Medical Technology: Current Issues from the Manufacturer and Provider Viewpoints,* Presentation at National Health Lawyers Association Meeting, Washington, DC, May 7, 1985.

234. Goodhart, "Technology Acquisition."

235. J. Wasserman, "Lessons from N.J. Hospitals Acquiring Equipment Under Prospective Pricing Can Learn from Others Experienced with the System," *Hospitals* 57, No. 23, (December 1, 1983):76, 78.

236. M. J. Kalison, "Technology Appeals: A Case Study," in *Physician's Guide to DRGs,* edited by R. J. Shanko (Chicago: Pluribus Press, 1984).

237. "Changes in Medicare System Could Save Billions, CBO Says," *Modern Healthcare* 14, No. 4, (1984):41.

238. J. K. Iglehart, "Compromise Proposal Eliminates Technology Adjustment in DRG Rates," *Hospital Progress* 65, No. 4, (1984):22-24.

239. C. Wallace, "Congress, Business Toy with More Cost Cuts," *Modern Healthcare* 14, No. 5, (1984):38.

240. C. Mickel, "Disproportionate Share Hospitals Draw Attention of AHA, Others," *Hospitals* 59, No. 2, (January 16, 1985):37.

241. D. P. Borque, "Technology Acquisition Under Prospective Payment" (letter), *New England Journal of Medicine* 311, No. 18, (November 1, 1984):1189-1190.

242. Roe, "Medical Technology Under PPS."

243. G. Richards, "The Next Step: The Feds and Hospitals Recognize That Payment Incentives Need Change," *Hospitals* 57, No. 6, (March 16, 1983):65-67, 71-72.

244. "Management Strategy Shift Seen with DRGs," *Hospitals* 57, No. 16, (August 16, 1983):30.

245. "Hospital's Marketing Efforts Reviewed," *American Medical News* 27, No. 17, (May 4, 1984):92.

246. J. Studnicki, "Regulation by DRGs: Policy or Diversion," *Hospital and Health Services Administration* 28, No. 1, (1983):96-110.

247. D. W. Seymour, "What PPS Means for Hospital Marketing," *Hospitals* 58, No. 12, (June 16, 1984):70-72.

248. "Demystifying DRGs," *Profiles in Hospital Marketing* 13, (First Quarter, 1984):44-47.

249. "Hospital's Marketing Efforts," *American Medical News.*

250. L. Punch, "Psychiatric Hospitals Told to Define Services and Sell Themselves Better," *Modern Healthcare* 14, No. 4, (1984):60.

251. "Pharmaceutical Firm to Share DRG Costs," *Medical World News* 27, No. 2, (January 27, 1986): 44

252. "Marketing Budgets Tied to Medicare Admission Numbers," *Hospitals* 58, No. 8, (April 16, 1984):44.

253. Simborg, "DRG Creep."

254. Ibid.

255. Lewis, "Speculations on Impact of PPS."

256. E. Friedman, "PPS Needs Overhaul to Survive: Altman," *Hospitals* 58, No. 22, (November 16, 1984):33.

257. Simborg, "DRG Creep."

258. Ibid.

259. Ibid.

260. Ibid.

261. *Physician Participation in the Management of DRG Reimbursement,* New York City Health and Hospitals Corporation, December 15, 1983.

262. "Correspondence," *New England Journal of Medicine* 305, No. 16, (October 15, 1981):961-962.

263. Ibid.

264. H. Strawcutter, Testimony on PPS. U.S. Senate Subcommittee on Health Hearings. Washington, DC, February 17, 1983, pp. 361-366.

265. "Coping with Prospective Payment for Healthcare: Loopholes, Anxiety, and Sudden Change," *Hospital and Community Psychiatry* 35, No. 3, (1984):291-292.

266. "Playing Games with DRGs is Playing with Fire," *Medical Economics,* May 28, 1984.

267. R. Sorian, "Is DRG Creep Spoiling the System?" *Washington Report on Medicine and Health,* September 3, 1984.

268. "Hospitals Warned Against PPS 'Gaming' by HCFA," *Hospitals* 58, No. 5, (March 1, 1984):22.

269. K. Guncheon, "Hospitals Not Found 'Gaming' PPS: Davis," *Hospitals* 58, No. 7, (April 1, 1984):26.

270. Sorian, "Is DRG Creep Spoiling System?"

271. "Hospitals Warned Against PPS 'Gaming'," *Hospitals.*

272. "Medicare Hospital Rate Hike About 4%," *American Medical News* 27, No. 25, (June 29/July 6, 1984):3, 7.

273. Sorian, "Is DRG Creep Spoiling System?"

274. Finn, "Medicare PPS Compromise."

275. "DRGs Could Cost Government More Money," *American Medical News* 28, No. 3, (January 18, 1985):23.

276. Ibid.

CHAPTER 4
Structural Management Variables for Inpatient Services

Structural variables deal with matters such as the physical plant, the governance style, the staffing patterns, the legal aspects, and the financial management of an organization.

Hospital executives are no different from other industry managers in that they operate within their own environment, using the resources available to them.

Within the PPS, the major managerial issues concern product line analysis, physician profit and loss, DRG profit and loss, and service contraction.[1] All of these concerns reflect the cost containment theme. On behalf of the American College of Hospital Administrators (ACHA), Lachner stressed the function of the hospital manager: "The role of the CEO (chief executive officer) is going to increase in importance as the economics of healthcare become much more visible."[2]

The impact of that statement is evident when one considers the traditionally separate hospital managerial functions. In the past, medical care was managed by medical staff while hospital administration tended to the rest of the operation. There was little crossover of administration. Under PPS, all that is changed. "The system can no longer be dominated by the demands and needs of physicians," according to Dr. Paul Ellwood, Jr., a physician and president of InterStudy, in Excelsior, Minnesota.[3] In addition, Ellwood listed four characteristics of hospitals that will continue under PPS:

1. They will have integrated risk management.

2. They will be vertically integrated.

3. They will be based on group practice.

4. They will include primary care satellites.[4]

Bassett also adds that "hospitals will have to reorient their thinking and their behavior," to survive.[5] Finally, integrating the business ethic, ACHA's Lachner comes directly to the heart of the managerial dilemma: "I think those hospital administrators who have entrepreneurial instincts are going to be survivors in the '80s and '90s."[6]

Legal Aspects

An important part of administration relates to the legal liability of members of the management team: executives, trustees, and employees—along with the attending physicians.

Starting with the basic right of the federal government to impose constraints on reimbursement, Powers contends that the legal foundation "lies in one word—jurisdiction." He claimed, in his 1980 article, that the premise "has never been thoroughly litigated."[7] Courts have ruled that "all administrative remedies" have to be pursued first. Since that route may take considerable time, the financial pressure on the hospital mounts unbearably. During those years of contention, the government's cost containment procedures remain in effect, with the funds under federal control. According to Powers, "It will—at least—take creative lawyering to show (the government's) confidence to be misplaced."[8]

Assuming the legality of the PPS, another issue relates to the hospital's ability to curtail or even revoke a physician's staff privileges for economic reasons, such as not conforming to DRG norms. Palmisano, both a physician and a lawyer, argues that most medical staff bylaws would not be clear enough on that problem. Legal due process principles mandate that there be substantive grounds for the actions. Further, the challenged physician must have reasonable notice of the charges and have a hearing before an impartial decision maker. Palmisano concluded: "The observation here is that a hospital inclined to remove a physician from staff on economic grounds may well find its action thwarted by the absence of procedural capacity to do so or by the failure of the staff bylaws to provide adequate grounds and procedures for removal consistent with due process."[9]

There have been predictions that PPS will increase the number of malpractice suits related to a lower quality of care level. Attacking the DRG plan in a letter to the editor of *American Medical News*, attorney Sambol cautioned physicians that lowering their professional standards accelerated the professional practice of lawyers.[10] While Ludlam agreed that DRGs could have serious implications, he also said that "the new payment system may actually decrease malpractice losses."[11] This decrease is to come about through a combined risk management and utilization review program. However, the pivotal role of the physician is the key to success with those malpractice-reducing activities.

Trustees

Historically, hospital trustees spent their time planning for services and developing physical settings for the delivery of such services. Additionally, the trustees used their integrative skills to resolve conflicts arising from the managerial/clinical dichotomy that divided providers and administrators in many hospital situations. With the advent of PPS, O'Gara suggests that trustees should be involved in the following activities:

- Education for themselves and others about PPS
- Review of institutional prerogatives
- Development of comparative information
- Development of performance standards
- Community and employee relations activities to maintain the hospital's image and reputation.[12]

Nevertheless, the trustees will still contend with considerable pressures from within and without under the PPS. A president of a statewide hospital association indicates where the trustees must stand: "A difficult, but necessary responsibility of trustees is to support management in carrying through organizational goals in the face of mounting medical staff pressures to serve individual physician interests."[13]

Ewell examined changes in the roles of trustees as they governed under New Jersey's DRG system. He identified five general areas for review: (1) management, (2) medical care, (3) community responsibilities, (4) strategic planning, and (5) fiduciary responsibilities.[14]

- Management changes showed a movement from a rather liberal review of the requests of the hospital administrator by the trustees to a governing group's asking tough questions of management about clinical need and financial feasibility.

- Medically, the trustees appointed physicians to every board committee to assure input. Physicians became involved in educational efforts using comparison data. This led to the establishment of a "Quality Assurance Center" to review physician practice behavior.

- Community responsibility resulted in "more aggressive questioning by the trustees about whether hospital programs should be cut."[15] At one hospital, trustees approved the closing of 10 individual clinics after this type of critical analysis.

- Strategic planning dealt with market share analysis, advertising, and competition. One hospital purchased an advertising package in *Time* magazine and *Sports Illustrated* to go to residents in their service area defined by zip codes.

- Fiduciary changes led trustees to increase the emphasis on cost control and productivity using detailed data on each unit producing services and revenues. To achieve this objective, the trustees allocated expenditures for new computer resources.

Trustees had been described as "incompetent groups of competent individuals," based on their ineffective hospital policy-making endeavors despite strong credentials in their own business or profession.[16] Now, under the PPS, the trustees are beginning to act like they do in their own businesses. New management principles in marketing, strategic planning, and competition engendered by PPS fit the trustees most comfortably. After all, they have been successful with those principles in their own business or profession.

Management Style

Now that the trustees are bringing their own managerial expertise to bear on the hospital, various management styles are emerging. Fetter remarks that the cost containment pressures induced hospitals to adopt efficient management techniques akin to "those commonly employed by manufacturing firms."[17] This, then, leads to the concept of the "product" of the hospital. A product includes outputs and inputs. Hospital inputs include labor, materials, and equipment. Outputs include items such as X-rays, medications, lab tests, nursing care, operating room facilities, hotel services, and social services. In total, outputs are the goods and services supplied to patients using resource inputs to result in a product of the hospital. "The hospital is thus a multiproduct firm with each product consisting of multiple outputs."[18]

Keeping the manufacturing model in mind, a 1983 study of 650 hospital executives by the American College of Hospital Administrators came up with 10 recommendations to help chief executive officers "survive and thrive" in the competitive environment of the mid-1980[19]:

1. Engage in more long-range strategic planning. Put less emphasis on achieving short-range objectives.

2. Develop more linkages and joint ventures with other providers. This benefits in economics of scale and a stable base of financial, manpower, and other resources.

3. Use quantifiable data on the costs and effectiveness of care in managing clinical and financial systems.

4. Be willing to take risks.

5. Get involved in the political arena.

6. Interact with leaders in other business and philanthropic organizations.

7. Initiate more team-building efforts.

8. Streamline decision making.

9. Mobilize resources to enhance productivity.

10. Uphold high ethical standards and maintain a high level of competence.[20]

Management Related Groups (MRGs)

Early on, Linder and Wagner proposed that DRGs fostered MRGs—management related groups. They defined an MRG as a group "consisting of hospital managers, medical staff and players in the healthcare scenario that analyze performance data generated by a DRG system."[21] In essence, the MRG exercises control over productivity, efficiency, and quality. These authors stress that the "R" in both DRG and MRG hinges on how closely all the hospital players are willing to *relate* to achieve success.

Several levels of MRGs can exist within the hospital to tackle specific problems. Management winners will "organize, educate and communicate with the hospital team" using MRGs.[22] Physicians are included on the management team as part of the MRG mode. A true MRG allows the hospital, as a whole, to benefit from participation in resolving business aspects of health care through an educational process. MRGs help decide what a hospital "can, should or want to do."[23]

Matrix Organization

A growing multihospital system trend in conjunction with DRGs spurred St. Luke's Hospital (Phoenix, Arizona) to adopt the matrix concept of management. "In addition to the traditional vertical chain of command for departmental management" the matrix mode "utilizes program unit managers with horizontal responsibility to coordinate efforts across divisions to meet project requirements."[24] This raises the criticism that unity-of-command is violated and can cause conflicts. However, most hospitals already have that problem in the dual authority of the attending physician and the hospital managers. To alleviate the potential administrative friction, St. Luke's employs program administrators for each specialty service or "clinical center of excellence" such as digestive diseases, heart-lung center, ophthalmology, and nursing. Program administrators exercise responsibility for a variety of complex tasks as follows:

- Serving as primary liaison between physicians and the hospital

- Analyzing marketing surveys, checking physician and patient satisfaction, and developing the program's marketing plan

- Developing, implementing, and evaluating the program's strategic, operational, and financial plan

- Recruiting physicians for St. Luke's and cultivating referrals from outside physicians

- Participating in selecting members for all board and medical staff committees in the specific specialty area

- Determining the need for new programs in the specialty area.[25]

Program administrators have both clinical and management backgrounds on a level with assistant administrators in more traditional hospital structures. Since the matrix concept does not formally appear in the organization chart, the authority of the program administrator depends upon acceptance of their leadership.

In an evaluation of the matrix system, medical staff felt that the system improved communication with hospital administration, allowed for effective responses to medical requests and problems, and enhanced the quality of patient care. In the acid test, 82 percent said that they would recommend the matrix system to other hospitals.[26]

Vertical and Horizontal Organization

Both vertical and horizontal management modes are being stimulated by PPS/DRG. Both management styles have existed within the business community for many years.

Vertical integration takes place when a hospital expands to provide a comprehensive array of goods and services to meet a variety of health care needs under the auspices of a single organization. Institutions may establish a home health agency to provide aftercare; may build or buy a skilled nursing facility to render lower cost care for patients not needing intensive acute care hospital services; may open up satellite primary care offices in shopping centers or ambulatory surgicenters; or develop hospice care units either in the facility or as part of the home health care activity. In all these situations, hospitals are adding on to existing services to offer a broad vertical spectrum of health care to a variety of populations.

Horizontal integration leads to consolidation of similar groupings of hospitals and services into multifacility systems. Voluntary hospitals may become part of for-profit chains or even form their own nonprofit chain. In any event, horizontal management aims to increase service volume, to benefit from consolidated purchasing power, and to reduce administrative overhead.

It is also possible that there could be a combination of vertical and horizontal integration with accompanying management modalities.

Contracting Services

PPS has also stimulated the growth of management of specific hospital departments under contracts with outside firms. Interestingly, few hospitals would have considered contracts for many of these services in past years.

Mental Health Management, Inc., McLean, Virginia, increased the number of psychiatric hospital units they managed by 100 percent in 1983 and expects to double or triple that number for 1984. According to the president of the company, hospitals want to gain an exception from the PPS/DRG plan for their distinct psychiatric units. Pinkert says, "We're a company with a product whose time has come, thanks to DRG."[27]

Contract management of nursing management services is offered by Janna Medical Systems, St. Louis. This company, which sells a nursing management software package, reported a large increase in inquiries about their contract management services. Company executives believe that many nursing supervisors are not prepared to cope with PPS educationally or emotionally. "There is going to be a tremendous shortage of qualified nursing administrators who are prepared to look at nursing as a business," says Lenkman, a company executive.[28]

Servicemaster Industries, Inc., Downers Grove, Illinois, provides housekeeping, laundry, and plant operation and maintenance contracts to institutions. Plant operation and maintenance contracts have surged under PPS because there is anticipation that costs can be controlled more readily by outside expertise and resources.[29] However, Mullennix argues that housekeeping contract management is not a remedy for DRG fever. He contends that an in-house operation should always cost less than contracted services, since the contractor makes a profit on the fee. Movement to contract for services is attributed to the hospital's inability to employ and retain a good executive housekeeper.[30]

Management Styles in Specific Departments

Management modes that are adopted for the larger organization obviously filter down into the individual departments. Illustrative examples deal with nutrition and purchasing.

At Holy Name Hospital in Teaneck, New Jersey, Scelzi reacted to DRGs by shortening his food service menu cycle. This resulted in reduced storage and preparation time, combining several jobs, and producing extra savings. Lighter weight foil, smaller napkins, lighter tray place mats, and smaller straws also accrued savings without detriment. In addition, Scelzi replaced an outside vending operation with his own in-house activity, increasing profits from $1,200 to $30,000 per year. His food services cut costs and built profits under DRGs.[31]

A nutrition support team concept claims to trim a patient's length of stay. Sheridan claims that nutritional support contributes to a "hospital's ability to discharge patients under DRG expense limits."[32] Nutritional support includes increased frequency of meals, enriched supplements, enteral or parenteral feeding or any type of specialized feeding. About 10 percent of hospital patients should get these services to make recovery less costly and less complicated.[33]

Stating that DRGs kicked off a whole new game, Porcelli related the changing role of the materials manager. Major functions under DRGs include reduction of overall prices paid for products and services, reduction of a costly inventory supply, paperwork simplification, avoidance of emergency deliveries, and improvement of communications among related departments. Since a wide variety of inpatient and outpatient services are affected by materials management directors, the style of administration should reflect overall cost containment objectives.[34]

Hospital Financial Management

In June 1983, Kelly and O'Brien reported that "between one-quarter and one-third of the nation's voluntary hospitals cannot generate sufficient revenue to pay expenses."[35] Urban hospitals were more seriously affected than rural facilities. Noting that nearly 25 percent of all patient discharges were covered by Medicare, the authors predicted significant financial crises for those hospitals already operating at a loss when the PPS was implemented nationwide. Lawson also added to the crisis by pinpointing the financial squeeze exerted on tertiary care centers and other hospitals trying to balance decreased revenue against the need for physical plant improvements.[36] A major burden of the management of this crisis falls within the realm of the hospital's finance department.

Major functional areas of a hospital finance department that are almost or sometimes administered include the following:

- Accounting—accounts payable, cashiering, general accounting, payroll
- Budgeting—operating, capital, cash

- Cash management and investments
- Data processing
- Grants and contracts
- Internal audit
- Management engineering
- Materials management—purchasing, central materials supply
- Medical records
- Patient accounts—billing, collection, admitting, registration
- Reimbursement[37]

As we review this inclusive listing, we can understand why a publisher's panel for Hospital Financial Management made the following statement: "Historically, administrative teams have been facilitators, coordinators, and communicators. The ball-game has changed and administrators must become managers who actively seek financial information. . . . This type of information is required if hospital managers are to maintain needed flexibility to react quickly to environmental changes."[38]

On top of the usual money problems, contradictory opinions in two respected hospital-oriented journals published one day apart add additional fuel. On February 15, 1984, an article in *Modern Healthcare* makes a case that hospital revenue bonds are a solid investment and are the single most important source of capital for hospitals. It states that Standard & Poors and Moody's both anticipate "only moderately negative effects from DRG reimbursement"[39] on hospitals issuing bonds. One day later, *Hospitals* published an article whose headline read: "Bond Ratings May Fall With Prospective Pricing System." Florida's Tampa General Hospital was the example described as "just the tip of the iceberg" relative to the impact of PPS on a hospital's ability to raise money. It was predicted that some hospitals would not be able to get into the bond market.[40]

Doody credited the Medicare PPS with three characteristics impacting upon hospital financial management: (1) prospective payment, (2) a case as a unit of payment, and (3) prices determined by DRG classification. These three characteristics put the hospital at risk for actual cost experiences, changes the relations with the medical staff, and hinges the financial manager's success on the ability to identify costs for groups of DRGs.[41]

Basically, though, Murray believes that the duties of the hospital's financial manager are unchanged from the pre-DRG period. Simply said, but implying a great expanse, the financial manager secures the assets of the institution and maintains, promotes, and assures continued financial solvency.[42]

Westfall isolated specific financial management techniques required under a PPS to measure a hospital's performance. Four general management categories emerged:

1. Initiation of product line management

2. Investigation of unit costs

3. Management of input units

4. Development of competitive pricing strategies.[43]

PPS/DRGs require hospital financial officers "to generate information which is new to them but basic to most other industries."[44]

Implementation of the PPS

According to the chairman of the New Jersey State Medical Society's DRG Committee, a 400- to 500-bed hospital may spend up to $300,000 for personnel, computer capabilities, and related office supplies.[45] Hospitals take varied approaches in planning for and actually implementing whatever is required to activate the PPS in their institution:

> An entire issue of *DRG Monitor* explained the new "ballgame" and detailed the preparations for implementation, including the identification of the players, the goals, the task assignments, and the postimplementation activities.[46]
>
> Neubauer-Rice outlined a seven step preparation for the Piqua (Ohio) Memorial Medical Center, a 150-bed acute care hospital using a PERT (Program Evaluation and Review Technique) methodology.[47]
>
> In Chicago, the Columbus-Cuneo-Cabrini Medical Center utilized a task force consisting of eight in-house PPS experts to rapidly set the PPS program into action. Each member's primary and secondary tasks are listed for an overview of the implementation process.[48]
>
> In 1981, Conner developed a management strategy for prospective case-based payment that contained seven major steps.[49]
>
> A Philadelphia consulting firm devised a five-phase system for a smooth transition into the PPS. Their approach "depends upon a logical progression: from the development of complete data, correct data by the institution, placement of the computer programs necessary to analyze that data, along with meaningful management reports, and perfection

of financial and management strategies for operating in the DRG environment.''[50]

An HCFA representative stated that ''basic management principles are applicable to all manner of business and government endeavors.''[41] He went on to enumerate the following six areas for immediate adjustments to hospital behavior: database collection, administration, organization, hospital/physician relations, volume, and quality of care. Longer-run adjustments dealt with setting objectives for long-term behavior, movement toward competition, capital investment strategies, technological adjustments, specialization, discussion of all-payer systems, supply effects, and consideration of ethical and legal questions.[52]

Based on interviews with members of the Healthcare Financial Management Association, Kovener and Palmer prepared an article on implementing PPS. Members told about their plans for ''increasing productivity, evaluating arrangements for providing ancillary and general services, marketing hospital services to other organizations, developing alternatives to acute care, and specializing in 'profitable' patient care programs.''[53]

In his book providing a guide to DRGs for physicians, Shanko includes a comprehensive implementation road map listing 27 suggestions for a smooth transition, 13 dangers to avoid, and 14 ways to improve efficiency.[54] Almost every item has been incorporated in one of the earlier methods mentioned. After regrouping and condensing the suggestions, the implementation steps are itemized in Exhibits 4-1, 4-2, and 4-3. Surely, these recommendations can be gleaned for adaptation in specific institutional situations.

DRG implementation also stimulated a host of seminars, workshops, and the like for management people throughout the nation. From a participant's perspective, Rzasa felt that the seminar planners ''tried to cram too many topics into a one-day or two-day session.'' Commenting on the uneven approach to the topic and the scare tactics, Rzasa advised managers to shop around before spending their money.[55]

Exhibit 4-1   Suggestions for a Smooth Transition to a PPS/DRG Plan

Education
1. Thoroughly educate everyone on the DRG system.
2. Key people should form an inservice education team to explain DRGs in each department, particularly physicians in each department.
3. Nursing staff should also be offered educational programs.
4. Patients and the community should be educated about the system and public information should be prepared early.
5. Making DRGs work requires the total commitment of all throughout the hospital.

Exhibit 4-1   (contd.)

Physicians
6. Plan to educate, indoctrinate, and prepare the medical staff leadership for DRGs.
7. Set up a DRG hotline in medical records and provide wallet-size cards with relevant terminology for physicians to assure access to pertinent information.
8. Encourage physicians to cooperate with medical records staff.
9. If necessary, assign administrative/clerical personnel to assist physicians with the DRG requirements.
10. Bring physicians into the management team and let them know that the hospital is depending upon them.
11. Medical staff leadership must serve as a buffer between administration and the individual practitioners.
12. Review activities should be created in each clinical department by its director to monitor physician behavior under DRGs.
13. Include the house staff physicians within the operating DRG system.
14. Physicians should be involved in overall hospital planning for the future.
15. If necessary, hire physician(s) to direct and monitor the DRG system when private practitioners are too busy.

Data
16. As soon as possible, set up an operating data processing system.
17. Acquire computer systems through purchase, rental, or lease to provide hardware and software necessary for management decision making.

Monitoring the System
18. Establish accountability in the chain of command to monitor the DRG system.
19. Create a DRG Committee representing medical records, finance, utilization review, administration, data processing, admitting, social services, and medical staff to meet regularly to review the program.
20. Include DRGs as an agenda item for continual reevaluation by the board, medical staff, and administration.
21. Set internal deadlines for a final diagnosis on the chart, for the discharge summary, for medical records to forward material to billing and for billing to mail out bills. Keep to the deadlines.

Medical Records
22. Assure that medical records staff are geared up and fully trained for DRGs.
23. Prohibit medical records from being signed out until they are processed.
24. Concurrent medical record review should take place while the patient is still in the hospital.

Business Office
25. Prepare business office to cooperate with medical records and then to issue bills accurately and quickly.
26. Train finance staff to accommodate DRGs with any necessary accounting changes.

Outside Consultants
27. Employ consultants as needed but only until the tasks can be performed in-house. Don't become overly dependent.

Source: R. J. Shanko. *"Physician's Guide to DRGs"*, (Chicago, IL: Pluribus Press, 1984), pp. 212–217.

Exhibit 4-2 Implementation Dangers to Avoid

1. Avoid adversarial situations by having medical staff responsible for implementing and monitoring the DRG system.
2. Physicians must cooperate with the DRG classification experts in medical records without being defensive or inflexible.
3. Physicians should participate and not leave DRG assignment wholly to medical records.
4. Medical staff should learn about the computer systems and not be threatened by them.
5. Physicians should continue to participate after implementation.
6. Medical staff should establish disciplinary procedures for dealing with physicians who fail to cooperate.
7. There should be open communication between physicians and administration regarding implementation and monitoring of the system.
8. Physicians must understand that there is more than one way to provide quality care. That may require changes in practice patterns.
9. Don't think DRGs aren't your problem or that they will simply go away if you ignore them.
10. Don't think the hospital's problems can all be solved by the other guy.
11. Don't deny that health care has a price tag by taking refuge in the myth that a hospital is not a business.
12. Length of stay is critical and don't assume that the hospital's record can't be improved.
13. Carefully review patient services for greater efficiency in seeking a better way to deliver health care services.

Source: R. J. Shanko, *Physician's Guide to DRGs* (Chicago, IL: Pluribus Press, 1984), pp. 218–221.

Exhibit 4-3 Suggestions to Improve Efficiency

1. Consider operating a full seven day schedule to spread fixed costs and to increase volume with only marginal additional costs.
2. Use alternative settings for self-care, hospice care, home care, and other ambulatory or outpatient care reserving the hospital for patients truly needing acute care.
3. Ancillary services such as laboratory, pharmacy, physical therapy, respiratory therapy, and other diagnostic services should be continually monitored for appropriateness.
4. Review all clinical services to measure demand and evaluate the profit and loss accounting for each.
5. Use preadmission screening to avoid unnecessary bed days.
6. Split shifts and flex time can minimize overtime and maximize hospital use in response to patient demands.
7. With nursing staff the largest group of employees, nursing costs should be reviewed to assure that the professional nursing staff is fully utilized allowing nonnursing tasks to be performed by others.
8. Consider establishing a single day surgery unit for appropriate procedures.
9. Outpatient services can probably be expanded.

Exhibit 4-3   (contd.)

10. To avoid complaints, assure patients that they are receiving all services required for their condition and are not being rushed out of the hospital.
11. Computer systems are an absolutely essential tool for hospitals in dealing with DRGs.
12. Weigh carefully the benefits of expansion versus remodeling to meet plant limitations.
13. Set up discharge planning coordinators to prepare patients to meet shorter lengths of stay with community aftercare services.
14. In evaluating different units, efficiency must be an important criterion; consider productivity pay, capital purchases, scheduling, and delays in delivering patient services.

Source: R. J. Shanko, *Physician's Guide to DRGs* (Chicago, IL: Pluribus Press, 1984), pp. 221–227.

Organizational Impact of DRGs in New Jersey

In January 1983, Boerma reported on a study of a group of matched New Jersey hospitals that evaluated the managerial and organizational impact of the DRG system in that state.[56] Hypotheses tested in the study sponsored by the Health Research and Educational Trust of New Jersey were related to the workings of the medical records department, the medical staff role in management, changes in hospital organizational modes, and the effects of available new information systems. Boerma found that the DRG system affected mainly the departmental and vice presidential levels at that time in its evolution. Chief executive officers were affected on a limited basis. Overall, the following effects on the organization were noted:

- Decentralization increased with department heads assuming more decision-making authority.

- Medical records departments changed dramatically; they added personnel and assumed more complex responsibilities as the unit integrated more with other hospital operations.

- Medical staff became involved in hospital operations and coordinating mechanisms with management increased.

- Information collection expanded in quantity and type, allowing for more sophisticated management databases for decision making.

- DRG hospitals were more "output"-oriented, while non-DRG facilities were "process or management"-oriented.[57]

A review of the literature appearing in professional journals—judging by content alone with no scientific statistical measurements—overwhelmingly buttresses Boerma's findings.

In view of management's desire to reduce the hospital's financial risk for physician behavior, it may be useful to list the medical staff control methods encountered in Boerma's study:

- A joint management/medical staff committee, usually chaired by the medical director, to review the revenue/charge statement and to determine which physicians should be audited.

- A highly respected DRG physician intermediary to act as "trouble-shooter" to discuss performance improvement with physicians identified as being "costly" to the hospital.

- A director of quality assurance in a role similar to the physician intermediary but focused on a review of medical practice.

- A director of medical education to integrate, for example, seminars on "nonprofitable DRGs" into the usual educational activities.[58]

Tied in with medical staff control is a shift in orientation by chiefs of medicine from management and governance to hospital operations. Rankings by chiefs of medicine of five hospital units in their importance to medicine are shown below comparing DRG and non-DRG hospitals:[59]

Hospital Units	Non-DRG	DRG
Administration	1	4
Board	2	5
Nursing	2 Tied	1
Laboratory	3	2
Medical Records	4	3

Investigators also divided the impacts into immediate, intermediate, and long-range effects. Immediate and intermediate effects relate to many of the findings already covered. However, in the long range area, Boerma speculates that DRGs will spur vertical integration in the future as hospitals transfer patients to newly acquired "step-down" care units such as nursing homes or home care.[60],[61] In a cautionary tone, Boerma noted that in 1983, DRGs had not really been operating long enough in New Jersey to truly forecast future events. Nevertheless, later events proved his projections about vertical integration to be reasonably accurate.

Hospital Missions and Management

Organizational impact is closely allied to the mission of the hospital and the managerial constraints imposed by that mission. For the most part, Boerma's points related to voluntary nonprofit hospitals in New Jersey. While it is true that most of the hospitals in the United States are classified as voluntary nonprofit, there are also local, state, and federal government facilities and a growing number of proprietary hospitals. Additionally, any of the facilities could also be a teaching hospital and conduct research activities.

Thus, it is not uncommon for a hospital administrator to be the chief executive for a voluntary nonprofit teaching hospital engaging in research investigations. In that situation, the managerial decisions are obviously affected by the conflicting vested interests in the facility, creating tension throughout the hospital every time a decision is made. Enveloping all that, environment is the added overlay of the business ethic imposed by the demands of the PPS/DRG regulations.

Therefore, it is important to understand how the structural mission of the hospital fits into the PPS/DRG cost containment principles and impacts on the administration of the institution.

Voluntary Nonprofit Hospitals

As the classification indicates, voluntary nonprofit hospitals do not aim to enrich their owners through their operations. In fact, these hospitals usually have a Board of Trustees as their governing body, as well as the sponsorship of religious organizations, fraternal groups, charitable agencies, and philanthropic foundations. These sponsoring groups espouse idealistic approaches to the delivery of health care. To qualify as a nonprofit organization for tax benefits, the hospitals must meet governmental legal requirements and receive a charter which states their mission, usually in terms of helping individuals and improving the condition of mankind.

An overwhelming majority of the references in the literature about PPS deal with the impact on voluntary nonprofit hospitals. Therefore, to avoid redundancy, this section looks into the managerial effects related to teaching hospitals, research implications, public hospitals, Veterans Administration and military facilities, and multihospital chains. It is also appropriate to remember that the pronounced business ethic stimulated by the PPS/DRG cost containment push makes all the hospitals more similar than dissimilar. Thus, management directives could easily apply across the board, regardless of the structural mission or auspices of the hospital.

Teaching Hospitals

Basic problem. There seems to be agreement that the basic problem of the teaching hospital is that too much of the care given is not reimbursed; in addition, it costs more because the patients are sicker. "Although they constitute less than six percent of all acute care hospitals, the hospitals belonging to the Council of Teaching Hospitals (COTH) provide almost half of the charity care in the country."[62] Furthermore, a 1981 review showed that the average cost of care in the 300-plus COTHs for each admission was about twice the cost in nonteaching hospitals. Even when case mix is held constant, teaching hospitals have higher costs.[63-66] However, a 1984 report at the annual meeting of the COTH found contrary evidence. Berman, Executive Vice President, New York University Medical Center, reported: "A study of NYU patients, using two different severity measuring systems, did not produce convincing evidence that DRGs and prospective pricing discriminated against teaching hospitals because of their treating sicker patients."[67]

Nevertheless, the prevailing sentiment still holds that teaching hospitals will be hard put upon by the DRG payment mechanism. To bolster that contention, five nonprofit hospitals filed a law suit in Washington, DC against the federal Health Care Financing Administration in early 1985. These hospitals claimed that the legislation required HCFA to grant them readjustments in reimbursements for serving "disproportionately large numbers of low-income and Medicare patients."[68] Detroit's Samaritan Health Center and Mount Carmel Mercy Hospital, Chicago's Mercy Hospital and Medical Center, Washington, DC's Greater Southeast Community Hospital, and Mercy Hospital in Toledo, Ohio joined in the suit filed in U.S. District Court in Washington. HCFA maintains that the costs do not vary significantly and the hospitals do not merit special treatment. HCFA lost the court battle and responded to the court-ordered December 31, 1985 deadline by publishing "disproportionate share" definitions and a list of hospitals in the *Federal Register* of that date. Under the HCFA definition, 89 hospitals met the criteria; only two of them are urban public hospitals. Furthermore, the definitions are of little relevance, since HCFA also stated that "we believe there is not currently sufficient evidence to demonstrate that an adjustment is warranted." Larry Gage, President of the National Association of Public Hospitals, called the HCFA decision a "travesty of congressional intent."[69]

Difference between teaching and nonteaching hospital care costs are usually attributed to the historical tripod of patient care, clinical education, and clincial research in academic centers. All three elements are an integral part of a teaching hospital's mission. As long as generous grants and third-party payers covered expenses, the teaching hospitals flourished and were able to care for the sicker and nonpaying patients.

Council of Teaching Hospitals.   These rationales were detailed at the Congressional hearings on the Medicare PPS in February 1983 by Dr. Mitchell Rabkin speaking on behalf of the Council of Teaching Hospitals (COTH). COTH represents 329 state, municipal, and private nonprofit hospitals with Medicare patients accounting for 18 percent of admissions and 28 percent of total hospital revenue in COTH hospitals.[70] Rabkin cited five broad concerns of teaching hospitals with federal policies about PPS.

1. Crucial details to evaluate PPS are lacking.

2. Methodology cannot overcome inadequate funding.

3. Statistical averages mask appropriate individual differences.

4. Teaching hospitals do more and cost more.

5. PPS threatens hospital/physician relationships.[71]

In closing, Rabkin stated that the Association approved of a prospective payment system. However, they advocated a PPS "that determines payment on a discharge basis, by type-of-case using an individual hospital's actual cost-per-case adjusted for inflation."[72]

Association of American Medical Colleges.   Along with testimony from COTH, the Association of American Medical Colleges (AAMC) also spoke at the U.S. Senate hearings on the PPS proposal. Dr. John A. D. Cooper, President of AAMC, added nine prospective payment principles advocated by the medical colleges organization. AAMC feels that PPS should:

1. Fully recognize the impact on operating costs arising from differences in hospital size and scope of services.

2. Recognize regional differences in the costs of goods and services purchased by hospitals.

3. Calculate operating costs on a "going concern" basis with full recognition of hospital capital requirements.

4. Recognize physician costs for personal medical services and for medical program supervision and administration.

5. Recognize costs resulting from manpower training programs which are accredited by an appropriate organization. Costs recognized should include those for educational instruction and supervision, student stipends where provided, program support and institutional overhead, and the decreased productivity accompanying training in the hospital setting.

6. Recognize the patient care costs associated with clinical research to bring advances in biomedical knowledge to the improvement of medical care.

7. Recognize increased costs accompanying the use of new diagnostic and treatment technologies.

8. Permit hospitals to charge patients for the differences between the program's payment and the posted charges for the services actually used.

9. Provide hospitals with statutory right to obtain administrative and judicial review of program policies and payment computations.[73]

Dr. Cooper concluded that "the defects and weaknesses of the HHS proposal are serious, raise substantial questions of equity, and assume hospitals have essentially homogeneous products."[74]

Some of the inequities espoused by the COTH and AAMC representatives were addressed in final regulations but major problems still exist. Recent experiences of teaching hospital administrators highlight the continuing difficulties.

Teaching hospital experiences. Dr. Stanley Bergen, president of a university medical center in New Jersey, commented that the Medicare PPS posed a "danger for complex care and biomedical research."[75] As an example, Foley illustrated the cost differentials in 1984 for treating a patient having a myocardial infarction at a major teaching hospital, a minor teaching hospital, and a nonteaching hospital. Respectively, the charges were $4,153, $3,484, and $3,341. Major and minor teaching hospital designation relates to the number of and specialties of approved residencies and the minimum number of residents in the programs.[76]

A former medical school dean reviewed the situation and concluded: "Obviously, the fate of academic health centers will depend on federal policy, particularly that which is related to reimbursement for care in primary teaching hospitals. . . . Nevertheless, academic health centers can no longer afford to plan on the basis of the assumption that ultimately the federal government will bail them out if they are in difficulty."[77]

Relman, the editor of the *New England Journal of Medicine,* titled his comment, "Are Teaching Hospitals Worth the Extra Cost?" His reaction to the impact of DRGs on teaching hospitals is clearly pessimistic: "But the handwriting is on the wall, and the message is plain: The special needs of teaching hospitals will no longer be automatically accommodated by a passive reimbursement system."[78]

Impact of DRGs. In a 1978 study, the Yale University group that developed the DRGs discussed a strategy for controlling costs in university teaching hospitals. They concluded that DRGs do "consider the effect of differing case mix on the three parameters of utilization, cost and quality."[79]

An exploratory 1980 study sponsored by AAMC examined the DRG case mix of 33 teaching hospitals. Taking each of the then 383 DRGs, a comparison was made for Medicare patients and all patients by number of discharges, average length of stay, average charge, and average cost. Results clearly showed that case mix does make a difference. In addition, this initial investigation indicated that teaching hospitals combined "expensive 'tertiary care' patients and relatively frequent 'routine care' patients."[80]

In 1983, a joint workshop of the Association of Academic Health Centers (AAHC) and the AAMC considered the use of case-mix classification in managing and paying hospitals. Four short-term effects of DRGs were identified:

1. Teaching hospitals would lose money caring for Medicare patients. In a study on estimated 1984 data, DRG payments at 7 to 8 percent below costs was projected. Another study noted that 10 percent of Medicare patients have very long hospital stays and $798 was to be lost on each patient treated.

2. Severity of illness averages do not work for teaching hospitals, since the patients are sicker.

3. Physician practice patterns would be difficult to change from higher severe utilization levels to customary intensity levels.

4. Technology and intensive care previously subsidized in other diagnoses would be reduced if not eliminated.[81]

Yet, despite these effects, the AAMC generally supported the PPS. Three major concerns related to the above points were detailed:

1. A lack of sensitivity of the DRGs in measuring differences in the complexity of disease in patients

2. Inaccuracies resulting from the use of average costs and average prices to make cost comparisons

3. A need for appropriate recognition of, and payment for, the many products produced by teaching hospitals.[82]

Some recognition of the teaching hospital difference is included in PPS. DRG features that accommodate teaching hospitals include the following:

- Outliers compensate hospitals for the atypical patient who uses more resources with additional payments.

- Educational programs for health professions students will be reimbursed on a cost basis to the teaching hospitals.

- Teaching hospitals will receive additional monies based on the ratio of house staff to patient beds.[83]

Rural teaching hospitals.   Hughes pointed out that university teaching hospitals in rural areas were on the short end of DRG payments. In addition to getting lower labor wage rates, the rural teaching hospital also received lower payments which do not account for the intensity of care. In the two examples cited by Hughes, the rural teaching hospital was in debt for $96,353.18—for only the care of two patients![84]

Continuing medical education.   A director of medical education questioned the impact of PPS on CME (continuing medical education). He urged hospitals to review their activities, especially the nonteaching hospitals. A possible benefit was noted in that CME may be forced to become cost-beneficial.[85]

Proxy Payment.   While the impact of DRGs does seem to be detrimental to teaching hospitals, adjustments are supposed to make up for the differences. Senator Robert J. Dole, speaking as Chairman of the Senate Finance Committee, explained his rationale for the teaching hospital's extra educational payments:

> A teaching adjustment was provided in light of doubts about the ability of DRG case system to account fully for factors, such as severity of illness, which may require the specialized, and often costly, services of teaching institutions. This adjustment is only a proxy to account for those factors which legitimately increase costs. We are hoping to find some better, more accurate method of addressing both the direct and indirect teaching costs in the future.[86]

Labeling of the educational payments as a "proxy" has engendered negative reactions to the use of that word. Critics feel that "a necessary and appropriate adjustment has been mislabeled as an educational cost."[87] It is possible that future legislators may do away with the "proxy" payment rather than consider the additional monies as an integral part of teaching center expenses.

Uninsured patients.   For years, teaching hospitals contended that case mix had to be considered in any reimbursement system,[88] because "major teaching hospitals are likely to treat a disproportionate share of patients with atypically intense manifestations of particular illnesses."[89] Of course, many of those patients may be uninsured. In some urban areas many of the patients may also be illegal immigrants in addition to being unable to pay for care. In a review of hospital reimbursement under Medicare, Lave considered the teaching hospital and uncompensated care. She stated that 30.3 percent of the patients cared for in large teaching hospitals are uninsured, as are 9.8 percent in small teaching hospitals and 8.2 percent in nonteaching hospitals.[90] Noting the limitations of Medicare, Lave recommended that the DRG payment share the cost of charity care and bad debts.

A 1985 feature article in the *Wall Street Journal* was headlined, "Hospitals in Cost Squeeze 'Dump' More Patients Who Can't Pay Bills." This article called attention to the rising numbers of uninsured patients. With examples, the writer illustrated efforts by hospitals to transfer nonpaying patients. In 1984, Cook County Hospital, a teaching affiliate in Chicago, admitted 6,000 emergency patients transferred from private hospitals.[91] Since teaching hospitals continue to accept "dumped" patients, this impact of the uninsured may increase in volume.

Clinical culture.   Teaching hospitals breed a "clinical culture" among the residents and the students. This clinical culture translates into the intensive use of resources and specialized bed units. House staff are encouraged to use the newest and the best of technology and drugs. As a result, teaching hospitals "provide patient and educational services not found in community hospitals generally."[92] Differences between care rendered by teaching faculty and community physicians were compared in a recent study at Stanford University Hospital. Based on 1,007 faculty admissions and 1,018 community admissions in 1981, the researchers concluded that costs were 11 percent higher on the faculty service, after adjustment for DRGs. However, the patients treated on the community service were 34 percent more likely to be dead at discharge. "Even if the extra costs on the faculty service are attributable to the education of the house staff and students, without corresponding patient benefits, these activities may be worthwhile."[93] It appears that teaching hospital physicians who follow an academic clinical culture may incur financial penalties for their respective institutions if hospital mortality rates are not considered along with the costs.

Fundamentally, house staff and students engage in major roles in caring for patients of faculty physicians. In that role, the house staff orders more diagnostic services for learning purposes, orders more services generally, and are unwilling to let patients die even when there is little or no improvement.

On the other hand, house staff has little to do with the patients of the community physicians. These physicians rely more on the clinical examination and their experience rather than on intensive diagnostic testing. Attending doctors know their patients better and are aware of the individual's attitudes toward heroic lifesaving measures and death. Care may be supportive rather than intensive. Thus, the clinical culture may add to the cost of care. Pointedly, the question is: Was the effort worthwhile?[94]

A number of letters to the editor followed the publication of this faculty/ community physician study. DRG inaccuracies, differing results in another study, and the truth of higher costs on a teaching service were among the issue raised.[95] Nevertheless, another recent study at Stanford University Hospital confirmed higher costs for teaching hospital patients even after extensive control measures were used to make the comparisons equitable.[96]

Atypical capital expenditures.   Another part of the clinical culture syndrome focuses on the fact that teaching hospitals have atypical capital expenditures. This may reflect their role in the development of new technology, new diagnostic procedures, and new treatment services. Although 1981 Medicare data stated that teaching hospitals averaged 5 percent capital costs compared to 7 percent for nonteaching institutions, the AAMC felt that the data did not accurately reflect the current situation.[97]

Teaching hospital management.   Garza and Evans reiterate the vulnerable areas faced by academic health centers including the charity care, the house staff expenses, the extra space for teaching, and the DRG ceilings on reimbursement. However, their article in the *Journal of School Health* looks at the future of a variety of health profession education programs.[98] These vulnerable areas could be reflected in the management of teaching hospitals.

To make it in the DRG situation, teaching hospitals must manage the facility effectively. Administrators must upgrade medical records, stress cost consciousness contrary to clinical culture, review high-cost low-volume services, contain capital costs, and emphasize medical staff relations.[99] Managers will no longer be able to excuse problems away with a reasoning that such is allowable in a teaching hospital.

In fact, Gurtner and Ruffner attack the problem head on by detailing strategies for hospitals committed to teaching and serving the poor. Their approach comes from experience developing marketing techniques for the Mt. Zion Hospital and Medical Center in San Francisco, California. Marketing segmentation is the method used to discover services which have the most potential for return on the investment. To develop survival strategies, teaching hospitals must consider the following difficult questions:

- How will your teaching programs survive with less revenue?

- What are your management information system needs?

- What is the significance of participation in your state Medicaid program?

- What is the optimal service of product mix for your hospital?

"One of the most likely options for the urban teaching hospital is a return to a former role as the referral center for a larger network." In Mt. Zion's case, the hospital reaffirmed its focus on geriatrics.[100]

Another management mode is alignment with for-profit hospital corporations to administer teaching hospitals. Relman predicts that the "medical-industrial-complex" will fail even though there have been a number of such ventures.[101]

McFadden, a university hospital administrator, also looked at the for-profit aspect. He commented: "My general view is to say that the 'price-based marketplace' is not compatible with medical education and that alternative methods to finance must be sought."[102]

A joint AAHC/AAMC workship recommended management changes to help teaching hospitals function under a DRG payment system. This report called for accounting systems adaptations and for behavior changes by physicians and house staffs. However, the report also suggested a realignment of management responsibilities including concepts of a "product line team" and/or a DRG Committee. These realignments strive to keep costs down on a floor or by specialty.[103] In concluding the report, it was suggested that the AAHC and AAMC help academic health centers improve their management by DRG, undertake studies to upgrade Medicare payments, and investigate future roles for teaching centers in the changing health care marketplace.[104]

Research in teaching hospitals. "Will the DRG Decimate Clinical Research?" was the question in the title of this article by Rabkin. His answer was in the affirmative.[105] Yarbo and Mortenson posited a cheap and simple solution; create DRG 471 for research.[106] These authors felt that the money crunch caused by the DRG reimbursement plan may cause administrators to consider "research that costs more than conventional care as an unnecessary 'frill'."[107] Presenting preliminary, but highly consistent clinical data from Oklahoma City, Long Branch, California, and New Jersey, the authors demonstrated that patients treated in clinical trials generate a majority of the costs. In addition, support for DRG 471 came from physicians treating the 8,000 patients on clinical trials in community hospitals.[108] Medical education pass-through monies are not awarded to non-teaching community hospitals. Looking to the future, researchers predicted that the additional DRG monies for medical education may disappear.[109] These concerns about payment for clinical research, much of it at teaching hospitals, are spearheaded by the Association of Community Cancer Centers (ACCC) and the National Cancer Advisory Board (NCAB).

Dr. Carolyne K. Davis, HCFA Administrator, responded to the DRG 471 suggestion in an editorial in the *Journal of the American Medical Association*. First, she noted that "it was never intended that Medicare would cover research costs"[110] whether bench or clinical. Statutory restrictions existed in Medicare prior to the initiation of the DRG system. "Consequently, there can be no establishment of a separate DRG for research.'' Later, she emphasized that ''this agency (HCFA) cannot simply establish a research DRG under the auspices of Medicare.''[111]

Dr. Davis also called attention to the fact that the PPS allows exceptions for cancer hospitals. In addition, many cancer hospitals are also teaching hospitals and receive additional direct and indirect teaching allocations.

Citing the example of the first artificial heart transplant to Dr. Barney Clark in 1982, Dr. Davis said that Medicare reimbursed the University of Utah Medical Center for all but five days of the bill for $254,068 covering 114 days. Five days were disallowed for the experimental clinical research procedure related solely to the implantation.[112]

In concluding, Dr. Davis stated that neither she nor the Secretary of HHS believes that research will suffer. Further, she closed on a strong management note: ''We trust that a well-managed hospital operating under the prospective payment system would be able to order its priorities to enable continuance of its clinical cancer research program. . . . Hospitals will likely trim away only those programs that they cannot manage efficiently or in which they have no overwhelming interest.''[113]

Looking for solutions to the lack of funding for clinical research, Rabkin suggested the following approaches:

- Educate the Congress and the nation on these issues.

- Investigate philanthropy as a resource.

- Consider industry as a resource (though it seems unrealistic.)

- Profit-making companies are an alternative, although it requires a lot of venture for a little profit.

- Stress economy in hospital expenditures.[114]

At a recent meeting of the ACCC, research specialists blasted Medicare's ''below cost'' reimbursement policies. Specifically, DRGs 401, 403, and 410 were attacked: lymphoma or leukemia in patients over 69, with or without minor surgery and/or complications and malignancies requiring chemotherapy. Yarbo, a board member of the ACCC and a university oncology director, compared cancer care to a ''loss leader'' in a supermarket sale to bring customers into the store. In strident tones, he complained: ''Hospitals are not grocery stores. We don't entice patients into a hospital for a low cost hernia operation and then persuade them to undergo a higher cost spinal fusion.''[115]

Impact summary. In an early study of a hospital behavioral model, Hornbrook and Goldfarb noted that teaching hospitals tended to have higher protection levels with beds available on any given day for emergencies. In addition, these hospitals had shorter diagnosis specific length of stays and greater diagnosis specific ancillary service utilization. Part of the behavior was explained by the resident's inexperience and uncertainty resulting in more tests and services.[116]

Even while Foley marked the contributions of teaching hospitals to improved health care, he raised questions regarding the future of teaching hospitals:

- Can we afford to subsidize medical education?

- Should patients pick up the medical education tab?

- How will the teaching hospital fare in the competitive health care marketplace?

- Will teaching hospitals be penalized for having other educational services such as extensive medical libraries, and nursing, patient, and community education activities?[117]

These questions could be compounded if third-party payers follow the lead of the federal government in adopting a PPS/DRG plan. Rabkin felt that the DRG was only the first step in a reimbursement revolution.[118]

To counter that inequitable revolution, the AAMC and the AAHC suggested changes in federal regulations to adjust for severity of illness, intensity of services, excessive numbers of low income patients, and wage level differentials. State level rate setting was also an alternative along with a variety of studies on technology, house staff payments, and education costs.[119]

New Jersey experiences.   While the differences between the New Jersey version and the federal PPS are substantial for teaching hospitals, medical centers in that state are still concerned about the future. New Jersey's PPS covers uncompensated care, more outliers are allowed, individual hospital specific rates are used, and there is less of an emphasis exclusively on cost containment. Currently, New Jersey teaching hospitals have an easier time financially. Nevertheless, Bergen calls for a study of a surtax on health insurance to create a fund to support medical education and approved research.[120] He points out the dilemma that academic centers may become too expensive for consumers and lose their support. Sources other than patient care revenue must be found to help teaching hospitals fulfill their special mission.[121]

Future guidelines.   Relman describes the phases that teaching hospitals have gone through, including generous research support, open-ended insurance coverage, and profit-making company business ventures. For the future phase, Relman posits the following recommendations for teaching hospitals:

- Garner public support for biomedical research and explain the work of teaching hospitals and the relation to research.

- Justify special treatment by showing teaching hospitals to be efficiently managed.

- Give more attention to teaching and research and less to clinical programs.

- Insist on adequate care for the poor.

- Establish that teaching hospitals are public resources and dependent upon public support.[122]

In summary, Bentley cogently observes that "many of the changes teaching hospitals must make are changes that all hospitals must make."[123]

Public Hospitals

Administrators and supporters of public hospitals generally claim that their institutions serve as a substitute for the family physician providing primary care. Furthermore, people receiving inpatient care are reported to be sicker, to need more complex services, to stay longer, and to have interrelated social and economic problems. In addition, public hospital officials also state that their physical plants are older, their wage costs higher, and their percentage of charitable, uncompensated care much higher. Based on 1981 data, New Jersey hospitals rendered close to $200 million worth of uncompensated care.[124]

Organizational association concerns.   Dr. Ron Anderson represented the National Association of Public Hospitals (NAPH) at the February 1983 U.S. Senate hearings on the PPS. He told the legislators that the public hospitals were the "safety net" for people unable to pay for health care. Twelve key facts about the nation's urban public hospitals were enumerated:

1. Public hospitals continue to take all patients regardless of ability to pay.

2. Wholesale reductions in Medicaid eligibility, benefits, and provider payments levels in many states have caused serious additional strain on the resources of public hospitals.

3. The non-Medicaid uninsured caseload of public hospitals has also substantially increased.

4. Public hospital budgets have inflated far less rapidly in recent years than the rest of the hospital industry.

5. Public hospitals have managed their resources more efficiently.

6. Public hospitals are important providers of primary and ambulatory care to poor persons who often have little or no access to private physicians.

7. There is a growing body of data which indicates poor patients are sicker, often have multiple diagnoses, and require more expensive care.

8. Public hospitals often provide special public health and other unique services to their entire community, not just to the poor.

9. Despite number 8 above, many of these special community-wide services are also in jeopardy due to substantial budget reductions in categorical health programs as well.

10. Despite the persistent Washington, DC, myth that cities and counties are not paying their way, a substantial portion of the public hospital budget comes from state and local tax revenues.

11. Public hospitals and other high volume providers of care to the poor have fewer private paying patients than most community hospitals.

12. Urban public hospitals remain the backbone of our medical education system. Yet that role may be threatened by reduced governmental support.[125]

While supporting the movement toward a PPS, the NAPH representative did comment on deficiencies in the proposal. In effect, the inequities related to the greater resources used to care for sicker and poorer patients, the longer lengths of stay, the transfer of patients from private hospitals to public centers and the exclusion of other than Medicare patients from the PPS. "In short, the prospective payment plan based on DRGs fails, in many respects, to take into account the uniqueness of the nation's public teaching hospitals."[126]

National patient comparisons.   In an effort to compare patients, Coffey examined caseloads in 67 public hospitals with patients in 247 voluntary nonprofit facilities as part of the federal government's Hospital Cost and Utilization Project (HCUP).[127] According to the author, little national data were available to confirm or refute the anecdotal evidence commonly believed to be fact. In the study, demographic, economic, and medical characteristics were compared with the medical variables, also including diagnostic patterns of treatment and severity of illness.

Important differences emerged from comparisons of public and voluntary hospital admissions in urban areas. "Urban public hospitals have larger percentages of ethnic minorities, younger patients, uninsured patients, Medicaid patients, obstetrical patients, psychiatric patients, patients with pneumonia, and patients with injuries from accidents or violence."[128] In rural counties, both types of hospitals had similar proportions of most age and diagnostic categories.

Coffey compared the seven most frequent conditions: vaginal delivery, atherosclerosis of coronary arteries, external hernia, diabetes mellitus, hypertrophy of tonsils and adenoids, cholecystitis, and diarrhea/gastroenteritis. Obviously, not all seven conditions would affect a Medicare population. However, patients with diabetes in an urban public hospital were more seriously ill. Patients with hypertrophic tonsils or adenoids and diarrhea/gastroenteritis were less ill. Patients with the other four conditions had similar degrees of severity in both types of hospitals.

This investigation concluded that "in SMSA counties public hospitals serve poorer patients than voluntary hospitals, but generally do not treat more seriously ill patients."[129]

A study from the AHA's Office of Public Policy Analysis investigated the impact of variables on Medicare cost per case. Primary variables included DRG case mix index, area wage index, and interns/residents per bed. Other variables included low income patients, Medicare patient services, bed size, and urban population base. Researchers concluded: "Contrary to expectations associated with a flawless system, virtually all of the other variables tested were statistically significant at the 95 percent confidence level."[130]

These relations held even after adjustments for the primary variables which also had positive correlations with Medicare cost per case. Reasons for the situation included delay in seeking care, lack of alternatives to hospital care, illness complications, and more required social and support services. This report recommended that the federal government consider DRG-specific price blending as an alternative toward a single national DRG rate. On an individual DRG basis, the payment could be 100 percent of the institution-specific rate, 100 percent of the national rate, or a blending of the two rates. AHA staff members shared the report with the Prospective Payment Assessment Commission as that group pondered the "disproportionate share" issue with regard to providing services to low income patients.[131]

New York City patient comparisons. Stanley Brezenoff, President of the New York City Health and Hospitals Corporation (NYCHHC), testified in 1983 before the U.S. House of Representatives' Committee on the Medicare PPS proposal. He stated that the NYCHHC operated the largest municipal hospital system in the nation:12 hospitals and 36 community care centers. Citing two studies on case mix and length of stay, Brezenoff noted that the DRG method would result in under-reimbursement and accelerated shifting of high cost patients from private to public institutions. Factors not taken into account in the DRG plan included the following, which are expected to impact on public hospitals.

- Multiple diagnoses—Fully 55 percent of NYCHHC Medicare patients have three or more diagnoses.

- Emergency admissions—NYCHHC facilities record that 75 percent of Medicare patients are admitted on an emergency basis.

- Alternate care—Medicare patients account for 57 percent of the need for alternate care follow-up such as a nursing home.

- Severity—Medicare patients with DRG 5 (septicemia) also had tuberculosis more often; 47 percent in NYCHHC facilities as compared to 19 percent in voluntary hospitals.

Modifications suggested by Brezenoff addressed the need for adjustments to account for the public hospital's charity care and the complex case load. These modifications were backed up by reports from Bellevue Hospital and comparison studies of city and private hospitals.[132]

Another study compared 12 acute care public hospitals in New York City with a matched group of nonpublic hospitals using discharge data from late 1979. This investigation sought to show "that the complexity of illnesses and lack of social support their patients have provide medically justifiable reasons for possibly higher-than-average costs that might not be recognized in DRG-based reimbursement systems for public hospitals."[133] Questions researched dealt with the case mix, the average length of stay, and variables affecting stay. Twenty of the most common discharges were compared along with major surgery and secondary diagnoses. This analysis used the original 383 DRGs, since those were the only classifications available then.

Clear differences were found between the public and voluntary hospitals. Case loads in the public hospitals were concentrated in fewer DRGs, with a higher percentage of abortion, psychiatric, and chemical dependency discharges. About one half of the 20 most common discharges were similar in both types of hospitals. Public hospitals had considerably fewer discharges where a DRG involved surgery. However, the public hospitals did have a somewhat higher rate in DRGs with a secondary diagnosis. Public hospitals had a short average length of stay. However, patients with the same DRGs did have longer average stays in public hospitals, particularly those having major surgery. Importantly, the rationale for the longer stay was linked to the higher percentage of outliers in public hospitals.

Variables such as payer status, admission status, discharge status, and principal diagnosis each explained a bit of the length-of-stay differences.

This conclusion differs from Coffey but the authors still believed that the DRG system should be implemented. Pointedly, they stated that "patients in a DRG are not a homogeneous group" as a justification for differential reimbursements.[134]

California comparisons.   A study by the California Medical Association stated that inner city and rural hospitals will bear the brunt of increased financial pressure from the Medicare PPS. "As the last resort of care, county hospitals carry a heavy Medicare, Medicaid and medically indigent caseload at less than full cost payment."[135] Location and competition inhibit public facilities from attracting insured and self-pay patients to counter their deficits. This report contended that inner city public hospitals had higher operating costs, while their rural counterparts suffered from low volume.[136]

District of Columbia comparisons.   A report from the District of Columbia Hospital Association found that an average stay in a city hospital cost $1,029 more than a stay in a suburban hospital. More than 250 hospitals were surveyed in five metropolitan areas: Washington, DC; Minneapolis-St. Paul; Chicago; Cleveland; and Philadelphia-Camden, NJ.[137] Patient care in inner city hospitals cost 33 percent more and the Medicare DRG reimbursement system tended to discriminate unfairly against the inner city facilities. Factors adding to the higher inner city costs included the following items:

- Higher wage levels for employees

- Intensity of the patients' illnesses with more comorbidities and longer lengths of stay

- Difficulty in arranging for post-acute care discharge placements

- Additional patient assistance costs such as drug abuse and alcoholism counseling, psychiatric and family counseling, and patient education services in self-care and nutrition

- Increased property-related costs, such as maintenance of the physical plant, parking facilities, security expenditures, and insurance premiums

- Higher administrative costs in trying to collect payments from underinsured and uninsured patients.[138]

In its conclusion, this report suggested separate wage indexes and added DRG compensation to account for the charity care.[139]

A public hospital's experience.   District of Columbia General Hospital is the only public hospital in Washington and is also a major teaching facility. An analysis of the hospital's data projected that DC General "would lose several million dollars over the next three years if no changes were made" in the Medicare PPS.[140] Following are the steps that DC General put forward aimed at increasing efficiency and utilization:

1. Increase admissions from an average of 1,009 per month (FY 1982) to 1,200 per month (FY 1984).

2. Decrease the average length of stay from 10.9 days (1982) to 8.6 (1984).

3. Provide services on an outpatient basis.

4. Review the establishment of an HMO type arrangement at the hospital.

5. Improve preadmission testing.

6. Intensify efforts to place patients in nursing homes if such care is required.[141]

These steps may work in the short run but public hospitals will face future problems as the DRG shifts to a single national reimbursement allowance. Partly, this is related to the general inability of a public hospital to be as flexible as its nonpublic counterparts. Another hindrance, according to this report, is that public facilities have to do more with less resources in older physical plants to treat more severely ill patients.[142]

Inner-city hospital commandments.   An administrator of an inner-city hospital in New Jersey acknowledged the burden of charity care, the teaching costs, the higher wages, and the other aspects related to additional expenditures. Yet, he said, "I am not convinced that the inner-city hospitals are faced with unique problems under DRG."[143] Out of the analysis at his hospital, the 12 commandments for DRG implementation were developed:

1. Understand your profits and losses.

2. Improve your efficiency.

3. Manage your length of stay.

4. Physicians are your partners.

5. Educate your organization.

6. Restructure senior management.

7. Adjust your financial systems.

8. Develop a case-mix reporting system.

9. Manage from your case-mix reports.

10. Volume isn't everything; it's the only thing.

11. No hospital is an island.

12. Who will pay for the poor?[144]

These commandments evolved from first finding ways to outperform other hospitals to introducing sophisticated marketing techniques, and finally to encouraging urban renewal with the intention of attracting population back into the inner city.

Stances of the federal government. At a meeting of the National Association of Public Hospitals on November 5, 1983, Dr. Robert J. Rubin, then an Assistant Secretary for Planning and Evaluation for HHS, delivered the government's view on the arguments raised by the public hospitals.[145] Dr. Rubin acknowledged the difficulties in managing a public hospital but did not promise speedy relief. He cited four frequently proposed options for easing the financial plight of public hospitals:

1. Increase DRG payments to public hospitals because of the more complicated cases treated there.

2. Increase DRG payments because of the charitable care provided.

3. Increase the capital expenditure reimbursement.

4. Establish health insurance for the unemployed.

HCFA analysis showed no relationship between the cost per Medicare patient and the proportion of public beneficiaries and did not affirm the theory that public hospitals have a more complicated case mix. Dr. Rubin stated that public hospitals already receive more money for outliers and for direct and indirect educational activities. For these reasons, the federal government decided not to exercise option 1, but they will continue to study the data.

Dr. Rubin said that the Administration opposes the use of Medicare money to pay for the care of people not eligible for Medicare. To initiate option 2 would hasten the insolvency of the Medicare Trust Fund and also change the nature of Medicare into a quasinational health insurance program.

Reviewing the complex issues related to capital costs, Dr. Rubin stated that the public hospital will continue to be reimbursed in the same manner as previously—on a reasonable cost basis. While he touched upon the problem of the hospitals with older plants receiving less, this option was also declined.

Finally, Dr. Rubin commented that the Administration had not taken an unyielding stand against health insurance for the unemployed. He posed requirements for government support of the measure.

In a strong conclusion, Dr. Rubin summed up the Administration's position on financial aid for public hospitals:

- We do *not* support arbitrary increases in Medicare reimbursement for public hospitals.

- We also *oppose* Medicare payments to cover the care of people who are not elderly or disabled.

- We *will* support, however, a *fiscally prudent* program of health benefits for the unemployed (author's emphasis).[146]

As if in response to Rubin's strong government position, an article in *Hospitals* told how to survive under PPS by cutting the length of stay. According to the administrator of quality assurance for Jackson Memorial Hospital in Miami, Florida, innovative cost cutting is the answer. Rifkin's hospital set up a PPS/DRG implementation committee and educated their physicians about managing patients in more cost-effective ways. Physicians are encouraged to do the following:

- Schedule patients for surgery as soon as possible to reduce preoperative length of stay.

- Consider the costs of antibiotics on the ordering form which now lists the expense of antibiotics directly on the form.

- Work with social service and nursing to affect timely discharges.

- Eliminate requests for portable X-rays when the patient is ambulatory.

- Monitor routine diagnostic testing.

- Inform hospital administration of PPS problems that increase length of stay.

Jackson Memorial Hospital reported that length of stay for Medicare patients was cut by one day between 1983 and 1984 and monies were also saved on other cost-cutting measures.[147]

Multi-institutional Hospital Chains

If the PPS/DRG plan aims to encourage a businesslike approach to the health care delivery system, then the trend towards multi-institutional hospital chains should not come as a surprise. In fact, the movement had started before the initiation of PPS. Furthermore, the emergence and rapid growth of multihospital organizations has not been limited to proprietary companies. Both nonprofits and for-profits have entered into this type of management style with vigor. "Overall, multihospital systems have financial advantages over freestanding hospitals, whether the chains are for-profit or not-for-profit."[148]

Fox, an academic expert on hospital management, opined that managerial control for a multihospital group "necessitates that standards and norms be developed and comparisons among hospitals be made."[149] He stated that the biggest control task was the allocation of resources and lauded DRGs as a valuable management information tool for multihospital systems.[150] In conjunction with DRGs as a tool to evaluate the hospital's product, enhanced combined resources to establish comprehensive cost accounting systems give the chains an edge in the competitive market. Using this type of cost accounting, hospitals can associate the true cost of every input with the DRG payment and get a "bottom-up" or "roll-up" cost. In addition, fixed costs can be distinguished from variable costs when making decisions on resource allocations. Finally, comprehensive cost accounting can be used for productivity considerations.[151]

Multihospital directives. In interviews with executives from nonprofit and proprietary multihospital chains, Punch presented an overview of management opinions relative to DRGs and administration trends. She collected comments from hospital administrators at the following multihospital chains:

Adventist Health Systems/US Washington, DC	76 hospitals
Baptist Memorial Hospital Memphis, TN	2 hospitals
Catholic Health Corporation Omaha, NE	24 hospitals
Evangelical Health Systems Oak Brook, IL	5 hospitals
Fairview Community Hospital Minneapolis, MN	57 hospitals
Humana, Inc. Louisville, KY	89 hospitals
Intermountain Health Care, Inc. Salt Lake City, UT	23 hospitals
National Medical Enterprises, Inc. Los Angeles, CA[152]	61 hospitals

Interestingly, a number of the nonprofits have also set up separate management subsidiary entities and enter into varying combinations of for-profit and nonprofit units offering services. One small two-hospital nonprofit psychiatric chain was purchased and converted into a proprietary enterprise with expansive plans for the future.[153]

Some typical managerial directives are listed below as examples of executive approaches in multihospital settings. These administrative tenets are valuable, regardless of the for-profit or nonprofit hospital status, if sound management techniques are to prevail under DRGs:

- Streamline and systematize hospital operations.

- Revamp cost accounting and medical records systems.

- Consolidate services system-wide for savings.

- Standardize cost efficient departmental procedures system-wide.

- Develop treatment protocols for each DRG.

- Give physicians a choice of products but ask for justification for the use of the most expensive products.

- Provide physician feedback on their performance under DRGs.

- Accelerate outpatient surgery.

- Promote local creativity in each hospital.

- Put major emphasis on changing physician's practice patterns.[154]

If the health care implications were removed from the above listing, these executive directives would sound similar to any other industrial manager turning out a product to be sold at a supermarket or a department store. Yet these managers, both nonprofit and for-profit, say they wish to avoid the "bad doc syndrome," where physicians are faulted for not meeting performance and/or productivity standards. Also, the efforts to "streamline and systemize" hospital services should not "short-circuit the patient," according to the executives.[155]

Paul M. Frison, chief executive for Lifemark Corporation in Houston, Texas— a concern that operates or provides services to 80 hospitals with a 40 percent Medicare population—regards the DRG procedures as a stimulating challenge. Frison plans to try to lower the average length of stay by about two days. He says DRGs provide "a positive shot in the arm for creatively inclined management."[156] In addition to outreach marketing and ambulatory care whenever possible, Frison says he intends to go out of his way to make his facilities the hospital of choice. He summarizes his managerial directive by stating: "We'll have to get leaner, smarter, more creative. We'll have to be better than anyone else."[157]

At a Standard & Poor's Corporation seminar on hospital credit ratings, stock analysts predicted that the proprietary hospital chains will do well in the future. This supposition relies upon corporate readiness to use market research and information processing to gain a competitive advantage. In addition, chains can experiment with a new program in one hospital to see if it works. If successful, the activity can be spread throughout the entire multihospital system.[158] There is no reason to believe that the same readiness should not prevail in the nonprofit multihospital chains.

Certificate plan for Medicare. Dr. Merlin DuVal, chief executive officer of Associated Hospital Systems (AHS), testified at the 1983 Congressional hearings on PPS. AHS is an association of 11 of the nation's largest nonprofit multiinstitutional health care systems, operating, managing, or providing contract services to more than 475 hospitals. Speaking for AHS, DuVal proposed a certificate plan for Medicare which would finance health plan choices for its beneficiaries to make in the private market. Similar to the HMO/CMP concept, three advantages were cited for the AHS' certificate plan:

1. Competitive forces of the market would produce economical health plans for the elderly.

2. There would be no need to construct and operate a nationwide hospital payment system for Medicare.

3. Government would retain the important responsibilities of assuring fair competition, maintaining consumer protection, and determining the level of health care coverage to be funded.[159]

Impact on multihospital chains. As early as May 1984, about seven months after PPS/DRG came into being nationally, a dramatic effect was noted on a multihospital chain's utilization rates. At an investors' conference, Campbell compared the 200 Hospital Corporation of America (HCA) hospitals paid by Medicare DRGs with the 200 still reimbursed on a cost basis. He said that occupancy rates, days of care, lengths of stay, and admissions all declined faster in the hospitals under PPS. Consistent with management approaches elsewhere, outpatient care increased. During the first quarter of 1984, HCA's outpatient revenue grew to $80 million, as compared to $60 million for the same period in 1982.[160]

Low, a Standard & Poor's credit rating analyst, feels that the growth of multihospital systems will increase. Small, financially-distressed hospitals will be purchased by chains. She offered a rationale for the continued growth: "Systems are not a panacea, but they do offer financial flexibility and economies of scale that are becoming more important with the advent of prospective payment."[161]

An integral part of any system is the physical plant and the fixed equipment assets located in the buildings. There has been a great deal of discussion about how to assure funding for capital costs under the PPS/DRG reimbursement mode. No resolution is immediately in sight and a number of alternative approaches have been suggested to reimburse hospitals for capital costs.

Reimbursement for Capital Costs

PPS regulations allow the following capital-related costs to be reimbursed on a reasonable cost basis as a pass-through expense:

- Net depreciation expense
- Leases and rentals
- Betterments and improvements extending use of assets
- Minor equipment cost that is capitalized
- Interest expense
- Insurance on depreciable assets
- Taxes on land or depreciable assets used for patient care
- A return on equity for proprietary providers
- Capital-related costs of related supplying organizations.[162]

In addition, six items were excluded from capital-related costs and included in operating costs.

1. Repair of maintenance of equipment and facilities
2. Lease or rental payments for repair and maintenance
3. Interest on borrowed working capital for operating costs
4. General liability insurance to provide protection other than replacement or to pay capital-related costs in case of business interruption
5. Taxes other than on assessed evaluation
6. Minor equipment costs charged off to expenses.[163]

This capital cost reasonable reimbursement approach will be in effect until a mechanism for including those costs in the DRG system is adopted. However, the historical development of paying for hospitals' capital costs via revenue bonds raises relevant concerns for the future. Keefe put it succinctly in the title of his article, "Capital Costs and DRGs—Caveat Emptor!"[164]

Revenue Bonds for Hospital Expansion

In the early 1930s and 1940s, the federal Children's Bureau and the Emergency Maternity and Infant Care Program allowed hospital capital costs to be included for patient care reimbursement.[165,166] This was soon followed by similar policies in other federal agencies, in Blue Cross plans, in AHA statements, and in the reasonable costs of capital included in the Medicare and Medicaid programs. With capital reasonable costs included in insurance payments, hospitals turned to revenue bonds to fund capital expenditures. After receiving a review and a certificate of need or other planning approval where required, the hospital also has to meet the requirements of the Securities and Exchange Commission. "Clearly, once revenue bonds are issued, the first obligation of the hospital becomes the generation of enough cash to pay off the bonds."[167] Raising money this way is much like a home mortgage, the hospital incurs a huge debt in interest over a long time period. In 1982, it was noted that some hospitals had debt services as high as $100 per patient day.[168] Between 1968 and 1981, debt-financed construction increased from 40 percent to 80 percent of total construction in voluntary hospitals.[169] Now, adding cost containment measures compounds the problem: "Any public policy to constrain hospital use and patient care costs runs counter to the legal obligations of the hospitals financed by revenue bonds. Even a small decrease in use, if coupled with rate controls, could create serious financial difficulties for most of the institutions."[170]

Bond investors, banks, and investment firms now have a financial interest in promoting the use of hospitals and increasing their revenues to pay off the bonds. From the hospital's management viewpoint, this could mean cutting unprofitable services such as Medicare and Medicaid patients, to assure funding to meet bond repayment schedules. "Those who attempt to restrain costs or reduce use are certain to face a powerful new force that is invisible to the public—bondholders and their financial spokesmen."[171] This new force was explained in several studies about facility mergers.

Merger Studies

A General Accounting Office (GAO) study of the acquisition of 54 hospitals by the Hospital Corporation of America (HCA) fueled the debate about reimbursement for capital costs. As a result of the merger acquisition, the GAO concluded that HCA's capital costs increased by $55.2 million in the first year after the deal. Those costs are reimbursed under Medicare and Medicaid regulations.[172] HCA rebutted the report, saying the increase to Medicare was $8 million and that was offset by capital gains taxes/liabilities of more than $135 million. Commmercial investors also defended HCA, commenting that the company abided by the law in allowing Medicare to reimburse for interest and depreciation. However, the GAO report was bolstered by a similar study of 30 newly acquired nursing homes and hospitals conducted by the Kansas City Regional Office of HHS.[173] On top of that, the Congressional Budget Office (CBO) proposed that

"Medicare no longer recognize the stepped-up depreciation costs of an acquired hospital."[174]

With these studies in mind, the federal govenment expressed views on the capital reimbursement issue.

HHS Capital Payment Principles

At a February 1984 annual meeting of the Federation of American Hospitals, Dr. Robert Rubin, Assistant Secretary for Planning and Evaluation, outlined three principles regarding the federal government's decisions on capital reimbursement:

1. We want to get away from government planning, not making decisions for or guaranteeing a return of investment to individual hospitals.

2. We intend to give preference to methods that reduce administrative and reporting burdens for hospitals.

3. We recognize that hospitals need both a predictable capital payment and an adequate transition period.[175]

Sensing the need to respond, a number of organizations and researchers came forth with alternate suggestions for capital cost reimbursement under the PPS. However, a number of common denominators should be kept in mind as the different recommendations are evaluated.

Alternate Generics

Capital costs of a typical hospital are only a small part of the overall budget—about 7 percent.[176] Estimates for capital expenditures in the 1980s range from $80 to $193 billion, with an acceptable Medicare target of around $100 billion.[177] One analyst pointed out that a dollar of hospital capital investment generates $1.84 in additional operating costs.[178] Another observer comments that cost reimbursement promotes capital spending by hospitals.[179]

As PPS regulations stand, there is a distinction between operating costs and capital costs. Secretary Heckler of HHS stated the government's position: "We prefer reviewing capital as a payment issue, as opposed to a government planning issue. In other words, we want to establish appropriate economic incentives for hospitals, and then permit hospital administrators to decide how those funds should be spent. This Administration favors minimizing the authority that government planners or regulators have over capital investment."[180]

PPS legislation implies that pass-through expenses increase health care expenditures without an incentive to contain costs. Therefore, the law requires a change in capital investment; the HHS Secretary is expected to review alternative ways to fold capital costs into the payment mode. If that is not done, capital costs would be approved by a state planning body.

This situation led to heated debate and divisiveness among health care providers. Special interest groups promoted their own views, creating splits between proprietary and nonprofit institutions, between those facilities able to attract funding and those that can not, and between health planners and operating executives.[181,182] Proprietary hospitals pointed out that they payed taxes, while the nonprofits rebutted with the fact that the for-profits get a return on equity. Hospitals unable to attract investors complained about the rich getting richer. Health planners tried to continue to maintain their leverage by calling for controlling capital cost expenditures through the rational design of health care systems, as opposed to individual uncoordinated expansion. Added into this tangle, the teaching hospitals pushed their need for increased capital payment because of their prominent role in scientific advances.[183]

Within the debate, conversation centers on pass-through payments or some type of consolidated price that would be industry-wide and hospital-specific.[184] When questioned, most hospital executives favored a pass-through system.[185,186]

Making distinctions between community service and business components of a hospital's goals, a Congressional Budget Office analyst countered that capital reimbursement depends upon what the United States can afford versus what is needed.[187]

Six capital reimbursement options are identified by the Health Industry Manufacturers Association:

1. Retrospective cost reimbursement without regulatory controls

2. Retrospective cost reimbursement with planning controls

3. Medicare outlays for capital subject to prearranged limits, probably via regional capital reimbursement-payment pools

4. A combination/blending approach with prospective payment for equipment costs, and retrospective cost reimbursement of plant, with some planning review or controls

5. A combination/blending approach with prospective payment for plant costs, and retrospective cost reimbursement of equipment, with some planning review or controls

6. A quasimarket approach whereby a hospital's capital costs are paid for prospectively, with the need for a planning mechanism.[188]

Capital cost issues involve conceptions about growth, scientific breakthroughs, and aggressive marketing of services. These concepts are near and dear to the hearts of trustees, physicians, and hospital administrators and lead to the diversified conflicting agendas represented in the following capital reimbursement options endorsed by different organizations.

American Hospital Association.   In August 1983, the AHA proposed a 7 percent add-on to DRG payments to cover the capital costs of hospitals. However, this AHA recommendation drew intense opposition from health care executives, particularly the for-profit managers. In addition, professional hospital associations vigorously opposed a percentage add-on.[189] This intense reaction moved the AHA to change its mind. At the February 1984 annual meeting, the AHA House of Delegates simply suggested that capital reimbursement be included in the DRG rate without being specific about how it should be done.[190] At the same meeting, the Board of Trustees declined to support pass-through payments because of the inevitability of a federal cap in the future.[191] Association officials contend that Congress and HHS will ask for the AHA's opinion. "By removing the specifics, AHA avoids sending Congress a signal that it has a solution on how to pay for capital."[192] Dr. Stuart Altman, ProPAC chairman, also supported including capital costs in DRG rates to allow for managerial tradeoffs between labor and capital.[193] This formula proposal represents a consensus, since all hospitals would be treated equally.

Federation of American Hospitals.   FAH represents proprietary hospitals and takes the position that no answer is required immediately. Michael D. Bromberg, executive director, stresses that for-profit hospitals pay taxes and that fact should be considered in any capital payment method. This stance could split the united front of non-profit and proprietary hospitals.

Rather than coming forward with their own proposal, the FAH works with other groups. One proposal called viable by the FAH adjusts capital payments based on the age of the facility with newer facilities getting higher payments. Generally, FAH members have newer facilities and would benefit from the age factor methodology.[194]

Healthcare Financial Management Association.   HFMA proposes that fixed plant and equipment costs continue to be reimbursed on an institution's reasonable cost pass-through basis. Movable equipment costs are to be added into the DRG rate. This proposal allows investors and lenders to be assured that a hospital will be able to meet its financial obligations.

Health Industry Manufacturing Association.   HIMA represents manufacturers of medical devices. They propose that capital payments be specific for each DRG. A proposal of this nature would allow for the integration of equipment costs into the clinical procedures defined within the DRG.[195,196]

Washington Business Group on Health. "The integration of capital into an all-inclusive DRG price is appropriate," according to WBGH. Furthermore, WBGH supports continued health planning after the payment decision.[197] Since WBGH, like other industry-dominated groups, is concerned with cost reductions, the concept of prospective inclusion lends itself to budgeting and resource allocation techniques.

National Committee for Quality Health Care. NCQHC is a coalition representing profit and nonprofit hospitals, hospital chains, health maintenance organizations, and suppliers of medical products and services. Assuming that a facility's age is the "single most significant variable," NCQHC suggests a uniform percentage add-on to reimburse hospitals' capital costs.[198] An index would be used to calculate the add-on; the newer the facility, the higher the index to reflect higher interest, depreciation, and leasing costs. Annually, the index would change as the hospital aged. In addition, the NCQHC proposal asks HHS to include capital in the market basket adjustments. Several issues are unresolved in the proposal, such as the return on equity for proprietary hospitals, recognition of tax payments by for-profits, and the lack of access to capital of hospitals serving low-income populations. While health care executives thought an age index was a positive move, they questioned whether the index could be developed easily.[199]

American Health Planning Association. AHPA, an association of planners and regulators, recommended a percentage add-on to DRG payments for movable equipment and a cost-based reimbursement for fixed assets. However, the health planners also "want to place a state limit on the amount of capital available for fixed assets."[200] This proposal tends to maintain a place in the health care system for the AHPA's membership in the face of the government's actions to eliminate or severely curtail health planning activities.

Case-Mix Allocation. Kalison and Averill suggest that capital be allocated based on case mix. This technique treats capital in an input manner similar to nursing and ancillary services. An end result would be a capital factor for each DRG, with the national factor determined in the same way that the DRG cost weights are calculated under PPS. Thus, the coronary bypass surgery DRG would probably have more capital factors included than an uncomplicated appendectomy. "In the aggregate, different kinds of case mixes have meaningful different overall capital requirements."[201]

Two exceptions to this proposal dealt with payment-neutral accelerated depreciation and with new technology. Since Averill was a part of the Yale University group that developed DRGs, this suggestion has a familiar approach.

Prospective Capital Reimbursement System.   Researchers compared the advantages and disadvantages of a DRG approach, a planning technique, and a PCRS method for prospective reimbursement for hospital capital costs. They concluded that the DRG method was efficient, the planning technqiue provided access, and the PCRS was both efficient and accessible.

PCRS blends three components into the proposal.

1. Physical capital allowances, maybe 4 percent of total DRG revenue

2. Financial capital allowances, maybe 6 percent of money invested in existing net fixed assets

3. Transitional capital fund, maybe three to five years to meet special needs as the pass-through system is phased out.[202]

This blended proposal distinguishes between the different incentives linked to physical and financial elements of capital costs. PCRS is thought to be superior in meeting the cost containment goals of PPS. While this investigation was funded by the federal government, the authors note that the conclusions are their own.[203]

Reactions to the Alternatives

Reacting to a variety of capital payment alternatives, Dr. Robert Rubin of HHS commented on the categories of proposals.

- *Formula Proposals*. As with the AHA suggestion, these add a flat percentage on to Medicare's payments to hospitals. This could be a very expensive option as Dr. Rubin estimated a 12 percent add-on would increase Medicare payments by $1.8 billion. In addition, this system is the only one that would have to be phased in instead of being implemented all at once.

- *Hospital Specific Proposals*. Dr. Rubin called these "do nothing" proposals. Current incentives and uncertainties would remain in place. Age indexing for specific hospitals, as proposed by NCQHC, creates "youth creep" as hospitals strive to make their assets ever younger.

- *Combination Proposals*. HFMA suggested mixtures of payment for fixed costs and movable equipment costs and Dr. Rubin said that was "naive." There would be no chance that Congress would continue the cost-based system. A pass-through system for fixed equipment and plant costs would account for the majority of a hospital's capital expenditures.

• *Allocation Proposals.* As AHPA recommended, states would limit total capital payments to hospitals within the state. Dr. Rubin pointed out that none of the waivered states allocated capital funds that way. If the idea had merit, he believed that the states with waivers would have experimented with the method.[204]

On the positive side, Dr. Rubin did say that there should be a phase-in of the capital payment policy so older hospitals don't get locked into low rates. He also stated that the hospital's age was the prime factor impacting on capital spending.

At a speech before the Illinois Hospital Association, Dr. Carolyne Davis, former HCFA administator said: "The fact is, there are no ultimate truths in projecting hospital capital spending."[205] She estimated the range from $49 to $231 billion between 1981 and 1990, with HCFA projecting $112 billion for that period. However, those numbers could change drastically, depending upon inflation and renovation cycles. Davis added: "Regardless, the chances of a capital crisis for hospitals are close to nil."[206]

HHS Report Delay

Speakers at a FAH seminar in New Orleans in 1985 felt that the federal government had moved capital reimbursement to the back burner. In conjunction with the federal government's actions, the hospitals were also not pushing because Medicare capital reimbursement is a relatively small share of outlays— $2 to $3 billion. Therefore, Congress has until October 1, 1986 to take mandated legislative action if no report is forthcoming from HHS. At the same seminar, Randy Teach, HHS Deputy Assistant Secretary, did hint about the Department's leanings on specific points. He raised questions about continuing the return on equity, about paying for previously reevaluated assets, about paying twice for Hill-Burton funded assets, and about paying for unused hospital beds. In addition, there was a consensus that health care providers ran a risk in the postponement of the capital reimbursement decision. With the federal government continually looking to cut costs, capital could be a promising candidate.[207]

Structural Variables Impact Summary

As with the operational variables, the overriding impact of the structural variables on hospital administration resides in the overlay of accepted American business practices upon the health care delivery system. Corporate management styles are moving to the forefront for hospital trustees, on the executive level, and for lower management employees. Attending physicians, in actuality a volunteer part of the hospital's organization, are now recognized as a vital cog in management to maintain the hospital's viability.

Declared mission objectives and sponsorship of the hospitals do bring specific considerations to bear in management decisions. However, the PSS/DRG requirements tend to push governmental, voluntary nonprofit, and proprietary hospitals into closer proximity on management approaches to the resolution of problems. Hospitals with teaching responsibilities and with ongoing research activities claim to be treated unfairly within the PPS, but the government responds that the regulations already contain remedies, such as additional funds for outliers, direct and indirect education awards, and exemptions.

In like fashion, public hospitals stake a claim to increased DRG payment rates on their above-average amount of unreimbursed and charity medical care rendered. Furthermore, the claim is made that patients are sicker and stay longer in public hospitals. Again, the government disagrees and points to the extra monies for direct and indirect education and outliers.

In line with the thinking of corporate America, the health care industry moved into the multihospital concept in a big way. Multihospital entities exist on a for-profit as well as a nonprofit basis. Under either auspices, management methods and techniques are borrowing from the guidebooks of the American Management Association, rather than from the American Medical Assocation—both AMAs.

These structural variables play a vital role in the decisions of hospital managers. Combining these variables with the operational components, it is evident that hospital executives will have to reorient their thinking to keep their institutions running smoothly under PPS/DRG, financially and otherwise.

References

1. J. C. Bassett, "Cost-per-Case Reimbursement: A Challenge to Hospital Management," *Topics in Health Record Management* 4, No. 3, (1984):1-9.

2. L. Punch, "How Will CEOs Fit into Healthcare Puzzle? ACHA Studies Future Roles," *Modern Healthcare* 14, No. 3, (February 15, 1984):48-52.

3. "Doctor Cooperation Needed Under PPS," *Hospitals* 58, No. 5, (March 1, 1984):26.

4. Ibid.

5. Bassett, "Cost-per-Case."

6. Punch, "Healthcare Puzzle."

7. G. Powers, "A Lawyer's Look at Legal Bases Available to Government in Its Efforts to Use the DRG System," *Review, Federation*

of American Hospitals 13, No. 3, (1980):38-40.

8. Ibid.

9. D. J. Palmisano and R. J. Conrad, "DRGs, Bylaws, and Staff Privileges: Is Confrontation Inevitable?," *The Hospital Medical Staff* 12, No. 12, (1983):9-15.

10. M. G. Sambol, "Attorney Hits DRG Pay Plan," *American Medical News* 27, No. 23, (June 15, 1984):6.

11. J. E. Ludlam, "Payment Systems, Cost Management, and Malpractice," *Hospitals* 58, No. 21, (November 1, 1984):102-104.

12. N. O'Gara, "Prospective Payment Encourages a Board's Integrative Skills," *Hospitals* 57, No. 6, (March 16, 1983):88-90.

13. Ibid.

14. C. M. Ewell, "A Look at How New Jersey's DRG System is Changing Board Roles," *Trustee* 37, No. 1, (1984):24, 28-29.

15. Ibid.

16. Ibid.

17. R. B. Fetter, "Diagnosis Related Groups: The Product of the Hospital," *Clinical Research* 322, No. 3, (1984):336-340.

18. Ibid.

19. Punch, "Healthcare Puzzle."

20. Ibid.

21. J. Lindner, Jr., and D. A. Wagner, "DRGs Spur Management Related Groups," *Modern Healthcare* 13, No. 5, (May 1983):160-161.

22. Ibid.

23. Ibid.

24. R. Boissoneau, F. G. Williams, and J. L. Cowley, "Matrix Organizaton Increases Physician, Management Cooperation," *Hospital Progress* 65, No. 4, (1984):54-57.

25. Ibid.

26. Ibid.

27. L. Kahn, "PPS Spawns New Contract Management Growth Areas," *Hospitals* 58, No. 3, (February 1, 1984):67-68.

28. Ibid.

29. Ibid.

30. G. Mullennix, "Housekeeping Contract Management Not a Rx for DRG Fever," *Executive Housekeeping TODAY* 5, No. 3, (1984):20-23.

31. G. J. Scelzi, "Cut Costs and Build Profits Under DRGs," *Food Management* 18, No. 8, (1983):27-28.

32. L. Punch, "Nutrition Support Can Trim Stays," *Modern Healthcare* 14, No. 3, (February 15, 1984):164.

33. Ibid.

34. V. Porcelli, "The Changing Role of the Material Manager Under DRGs." Presentation at Mid-Atlantic Health Congress, Atlantic City, NJ May 22, 1984.

35. J. V. Kelly and J. J. O'Brien. *Characteristics of Financially Distressed Hospitals,* Hospital Cost and Utilization Project Research Note 3. USDHHS Pub. No. (PHS) 83-3352, June 1983.

36. C. E. Lawson, "Pervasive Health Implications of Medicare's Financial Crisis," *New York Times,* September 15, 1983.

37. A. J. Sperazzo, "Financial Management of Hospitals," *American Journal of Hospital Pharmacy* 41, No. 6, (1984):935-941.

38. M. Mannisto, "Managers Wanted," *Hospitals* 57, No. 6, (March 16, 1983):91-93.

39. J. Illyes, "Hospital Bonds' Track Record Trips Up Critics Who Contend Bonds Are Risky," *Modern Healthcare* 14, No. 3, (February 15, 1984):180, 182, 184.

40. P. Gapen, "Bond Ratings May Fall with Prospective Pricing System," *Hospitals* 58, No. 4, (February 16, 1984):43, 46.

41. M. F. Doody, "Impact of DRGs on Hospital Financial Management," In *DRGs: The Effect in New Jersey. The Potential for the Nation.* USDHHS, HCFA Pub. No. 03170, March 1984, p. 51.

42. R. E. Murray, "Hospital Financial Management Under the New DRG System," In *DRGs: The Effect in New Jersey. The Potential for the Nation.* USDHHS, HCFA Pub. No. 03170, March, 1984, pp. 52-53.

43. G. Westfall, "Financial Management Techniques Under a Prospective Payment System," In *DRGs: The Effect in New Jersey. The Potential for the Nation.* USDHHS, HCFA Pub. No. 03170, March, 1984, pp. 54-58.

44. Ibid.

45. C. Keenan, "Hospitals' PPS Start-Up Costs May Be Hefty," *Hospitals* 58, No. 1, (January 1, 1984):25.

46. "Preparing for the Implementation of PPS and DRGs, It's a New Ballgame" *DRG Monitor* 1 No. 8, (1984):1-8.

47. R. Neubauer-Rice, "Preparing for the DRG-based Prospective Rate System," *Quality Review Bulletin* 9, No. 8, (1983):236-9.

48. R. J. Annis, "Task Force, Staff Education Ease Transition to Prospective Payment," *Hospital Progress* 65, No. 2, (1984):50-52, 74.

49. R. A. Conner, "A Management Strategy for Prospective Case Based Payment," *Health Care Management Review* 6, No. 4, (1981):57-63.

50. "Moving into DRG," *Cost Containment Newsletter* 5, No. 10, (March 24, 1983):3-6.

51. A. Dobson, "The PPS Incentive Structure—How Will the Nation's Hospitals React?" in *DRGs: The Effect in New Jersey, The Potential for the Nation*. USDHHS, HCFA No. 03170, March 1984. pp. 117-121.

52. Ibid.

53. R. R. Kovener and M. C. Palmer, "Implementing the Medicare Prospective Pricing System," *Healthcare Financial Management* 37, No. 9, (1983):74-78.

54. R. J. Shanko, Physicians Guide to DRGs Chicago, IL: Pluribus Press, 1984, pp. 212-226.

55. C. B. Rzasa, "DRG Seminars from a Participant's Perspective," *Quality Review Bulletin* 9, No. 10, (1983):286-288.

56. H. Boerma, *Organizational Impact of DRGs. DRG Evaluation Volume IV-B*. Health Research and Educational Trust of New Jersey, Princeton, New Jersey, January 1983.

57. Ibid., pp. IX-X.

58. Ibid., pp. 47-48.

59. Ibid., P. 49.

60. Ibid., P. 70.

61. M. Snyder, "Study Looks at How DRGs Change Hospital Organization, Management," *The Internist* 24, No. 6, (1983):16.

62. A. S. Relman, "Who Will Pay for Medical Education in Our Teaching Hospitals?," *Science* 226, No. 4670, (October 5, 1984):20-23.

63. E. R. Becker and B. Steinwald, "Determinants of Hospital Casemix Complexity," *Health Services Research* 16, (Winter, 1981):439-458.

64. A. P. Frick, S. G. Martin and M. Shwartz, "Case Mix and Cost Differences Between Teaching and Nonteaching Hospitals," *Medical Care* 23, No. 4, (1985):283-295.

65. J. D. Thompson, R. B. Fetter, and Y. Shin, "One Strategy for Controlling Cost in University Teaching Hospitals," *Journal of Medical Education* 55, No. 3, (1978):167-175.

66. C. A. Watts and T. D. Klastorin, "The Impact of Case Mix on Hospital Cost: A Comparative Analysis," *Inquiry* 17, No. 4, (1980):357-367.

67. E. Friedman, "Case-mix Severity Found Not to Affect Hospital Revenues," *Hospitals* 58, No. 23, (December 1, 1984):32.

68. "Hospitals Sue for Price Adjustments," *Medical World News* 26, No. 6, (March 25, 1985):34.

69. "Definitions of Needy Hospitals Attacked," *Medical World News* 27, No. 4, (February 24, 1986):25.

70. M. T. Rabkin, Testimony at Hearings on PPS. U. S. Senate Subcommittee on Health, February 2, 1983. Washington, DC, pp. 103-108.

71. Ibid.

72. Ibid.

73. J. A. D. Cooper, Testimony at Hearings on PPS. U. S. Senate Subcommittee on Health, February 2, 1983, Washington, DC, pp. 115-124.

74. Ibid.

75. S. S. Bergen, Jr. and A. C. Roth, "Prospective Payment and the University Hospital," *New England Journal of Medicine* 310, No. 5, (February 2, 1984):316-318.

76. T. J. Foley, "Impact of DRGs on Teaching Hospitals," In *Diagnosis Related Groups: The Effect in New Jersey. The Potential for the Nation*. USDHHS, HCFA Pub. No. 03170, March 1984, pp. 183-184.

77. R. H. Ebert and S. S. Brown, "Academic Health Centers," *New England Journal of Medicine* 308, No. 21, (May 27, 1983):1200-1208.

78. A. S. Relman, "Are Teaching Hospitals Worth the Extra Cost?" *New England Journal of Medicine* 310, No. 19, (May 10, 1984):1256-1257.

79. Thompson, "One Strategy."

80. J. D. Bentley and P. W. Butler, *The DRG Case Mix of a Sample of Teaching Hospitals: A Technical Report*. Washington, DC: Association of American Medical Colleges, December, 1981, p. 26.

81. *Medicare Prospective Payment. Probable Effects on Academic Health Center Hospitals. Short-Term and Long-Term Options*, Association of Academic Health Centers and Association of American Medical Colleges. Washington, DC, April, 1983, pp. 4-6.

82. J. A. D. Cooper, "Medicare's Prospective Payment System and the Teaching Hospital," *Journal of Medical Education* 58, No. 11, (1983):906-907.

83. J. D. Bentley, "Changing Hospital Payments: Implications for Teaching Hospitals," *The Hospital Medical Staff* 12, No. 9, (1983):2-3, 6-8.

84. G. S. Hughes, "Diagnosis Related Groups" (letter), *Annals of Internal Medicine* 101, No. 1, (1984):138.

85. J. H. Thorpe, "DRGs, PPS and CME," *AMA Continuing Medical Education Newsletter* 13, No. 3, (1984):5-6.

86. Cooper, "Medicare's PPS."

87. Ibid.

88. S. LaViolette, "Hospitals Split Between Praise, Distrust of DRGs," *Modern Healthcare* 10, No. 7, (1980):100-101.

89. B. C. Vladeck, "Medicare Hospital Payment by Diagnosis Related Groups," *Annals of Internal Medicine* 100, No. 4, (1984):576-591.

90. J. R. Lave, "Hospital Reimbursement Under Medicare," *MMFQ Health and Society* 62, No. 2, (Spring 1984):251-268.

91. "Hospitals on Cost Squeeze 'Dump' More Patients Who Can't Pay Bill," *Wall Street Journal*, March 8, 1985.

92. Bentley, "Changing Hospital Payments."

93. A. M. Garber, V. R. Fuchs and J. F. Silverman, "Case Mix, Costs, and Outcomes. Differences Between Faculty and Community Services in a University Hospital," *New England Journal of Medicine* 310, No. 19, (May 10, 1984):1231-1237.

94. Ibid.

95. "Letters to the Editor from J. E. Van Gilder, L. F. Eichenfield and A. B. Bindman, R. B. Saizow, et al., M. S. Blumberg, and response by A. M. Garber, et al.," *New England Journal of Medicine* 311, No. 11, (September 13, 1984):737-739.

96. K. R. Jones, "Predicting Hospital Charge and Stay Variation," *Medical Care* 22, No. 3, (1985):220-235.

97. "Prospective Payment," *Hospitals*.

98. D. Garza and D. W. Evans, "Boom or Bust: Future of Health Profession Education," *Journal of School Health* 53, No. 8, (1983):494-498.

99. Bentley, "Changing Hospital Payments."

100. W. H. Gurtner and J. K. Ruffner, "Strategies for Hospitals Committed to Teaching and Service to the Poor," *Hospital Forum* 27, No. 1, (1984):57-59.

101. Relman, "Teaching Hospitals."

102. G. B. McFadden, "Impact of DRGs on Teaching Hospitals," In *Diagnosis Related Groups: The Effect in New Jersey. The Potential for the Nation*. USDHHS, HCFA Pub. No. 03170, March 1984, pp. 185-186.

103. *Medicare PPS*, "AAHC/AAMC," p. 9.

104. Ibid., p. 15.

105. M. T. Rabkin, "Will the DRGs Decimate Clinical Research?" *Clinical Research* 32, No. 3, (1984):345-347.

106. J. W. Yarbo and L. E. Mortenson, "The Need for Diagnosis Related Group 471," *Journal of the American Medical Association* 235, No. 5, (February 1, 1985):684-685.

107. Ibid.

108. J. G. Katterhagen and L. E. Mortenson, "Clinical Research Patients Generate Significant Losses Under Diagnosis Related Groups (DRGs)," *Seminars in Oncology* 11, No. 3, (1984):xxxv-xxxvi.

109. Ibid.

110. C. K. Davis, "The Impact of Prospective Payment on Clinical Research," *Journal of the American Medical Association* 253, No. 5, (February 1, 1985):686-687.

111. Ibid.

112. Ibid.

113. "New Medicare Payment System Seen Threatening Clinical Research Projects," *American Medical News* 28, No. 6, (February 8, 1985):39.

114. Rabkin, "Will DRGs Decimate Research?"

115. "DRGs: Cancer Patients' New Malignancy?" *Medical World News* 26, No. 8, (April 22, 1985):6, 7, 9.

116. M. C. Hornbrook and M. G. Goldfarb, "A Partial Test of a Hospital Behavioral Model," *Social Science in Medicine* 17, No. 10, (1983):667-680.

117. Foley, "Impact of DRGs."

118. Rabkin, "Will DRGs Decimate Research?"

119. *Medicare PPS*, AAHC/AAMC.

120. Bergen and Roth, "PPS and the University Hospital."

121. S. S. Bergen, Jr., "The Effect of DRG Based Per Case Payments on Academic Medical Centers," In *Diagnosis Related Groups: The Effect in New Jersey, The Potential for the Nation.* USDHHS, HCFA Pub. No. 03170, March 1984, pp. 187-188.

122. Relman, "Teaching Hospitals."

123. Bentley, "Changing Hospital Payments."

124. H. A. Murray, "Impact of DRGs on Inner City Hospitals," In *DRGs: The Effect in New Jersey, The Impact for the Nation.* USDHHS, HCFA Pub. No. 03170, March 1984, p. 188.

125. R. Anderson, *Testimony on PPS.* U. S. Senate Subcommittee on Health Hearing, February 2, 1983, Washington, DC, pp. 221-241.

126. Ibid.

127. R. M. Coffey, *Patients in Public General Hospitals: Who Pays, How Sick?* USDHHS Pub. No. (PHS) 83-3344, September, 1983.

128. Ibid., p. 19.

129. Ibid., p. 20.

130. American Hospital Association, Office of Public Policy Analysis. *An Analysis of Medicare/Low-Income Patient Involvement and Other Hospital Factors.* Chicago, IL: November 28, 1984, p. 3.

131. Ibid.

132. S. Brezenoff, *Testimony on PPS.* U. S. Senate Subcommittee on Health Hearings, February 17, 1983, Washington, DC, pp. 477-498.

133. M. Shwartz, J. C. Merrill, and L. K. Blake, "DRG-Based Case Mix and Public Hospitals," *Medical Care* 22, No. 4, (1984):283-294.

134. Ibid.

135. "New Pressures Seen on Public Institutions," *American Medical News* 27, No. 6 (February 10, 1984):22.

136. Ibid.

137. "Study Cites High Costs for Hospitals in Inner Cities," *American Medical News* 27, No. 39, (October 19, 1984):30.

138. "Study Suggests Large City Hospitals Most Affected by DRG Payment Rule," *U. S. Medicine* 20, No. 23, (December 1, 1984):20.

139. "Study Cites Costs," *American Medical News.*

140. V. R. Iglehart and K. S. Taneja, "Prospective Payment System: Experience of a Public Hospital," *Journal of the National Medical Association* 76, No. 8, (1984):765-767.

141. Ibid.

142. Ibid.

143. K. G. Halpern, "Impact of DRGs on Inner City Hospitals," In *DRGs: The Effect in New Jersey. The Impact for the Nation.* USDHHS, HCFA Pub. No. 03170, March 1984, pp. 189-193.

144. Ibid., pp. 190-191.

145. R. J. Rubin, "Speech before the National Association of Public Hospitals," Sonoma, California, November 5, 1983.

146. Ibid.

147. "Public Hospitals Can Survive PPS, Cut LOS," *Hospitals* 59, No. 2, (January 16, 1985):75-76.

148. M. Tatge, "Chains Will Do Well Under Prospective Pay: Analysts," *Modern Healthcare* 14, No. 5, (1984):158, 162.

149. R. T. Fox, "DRGs: A Management Control Tool in Hospitals and Multiinstitutional Systems," *Hospital Progress* 62, No. 1, (1981):52-53.

150. Ibid.

151. M. Nathanson, "Comprehensive Cost Accounting Systems Give Chains an Edge," *Modern Healthcare* 14, No. 3, (February 15, 1984):122, 124, 128.

152. L. Punch, "Physicians Must Alter Practice Patterns Under DRGs: Chains," *Modern Healthcare* 14, No. 3, (February 15, 1984):114, 116, 118.

153. C. Wallace, "For Profit Psychiatric Hospital Firm Will Seek Niche in Small Urban, Rural Areas," *Modern Healthcare* 14, No. 3, (February 15, 1984):64, 66.

154. Punch, "Physicians Must Alter Practice Patterns."

155. Ibid.

156. C. Holmes, "Will DRGs Change The Way Multis Do Business?," *Texas Hospitals* 39, No. 4, (1983):39-41.

157. Ibid.

158. Tatge, "Chains Will Do Well."

159. M. K. DuVal, *Testimony on PPS*. U. S. Senate Subcommittee on Health Hearings, February 17, 1983, Washington, DC pp. 350-360.

160. G. Richards, "PPS Has Dramatic Effect on Use of HCA Hospitals," *Hospitals* 58, No. 12, (June 16, 1984):21.

161. Tatge, "Chains Will Do Well."

162. M. J. Kalison and R. Averill, "The Response to PPS: Inside, Outside, Over Time," *Healthcare Financial Management* 38, No. 1, (1984):78-88.

163. J. Keefe, "Capital Costs and DRGs—Caveat Emptor!" *Radiology Management* 6, No. 2, (1984):35-38.

164. Ibid.

165. J. Feder, Medicare: *The Politics of Federal Hospital Insurance* (Lexington, MA: D. C. Heath, 1977), p. 53.

166. I. Wolkstein, "The Legislative History of Hospital Cost Reimbursement: A Position Paper For The Secretary's Advisory Committee on Hospital Effectiveness," USDHEW, 1967, pp. 3-4.

167. G. Wilson, C. G. Sheps and T. R. Oliver, "Effects of Hospital Bonds on Hospital Planning and Operations," *New England Journal of Medicine* 307, No. 23, (December 2, 1982):1426-1430.

168. Ibid.

169. K. Guncheon, "HHS Has Broad Principles for Capital Pay Under PPS," *Hospitals* 58, No. 2, (April 1, 1984):26, 31.

170. Wilson, Sheps and Oliver, "Effects of Bonds."

171. Ibid.

172. C. Wallace, "GAO Report Triggers Payment Debate," *Modern Healthcare* 14, No. 3, (February 15, 1985):30, 32.

173. J. E. Mistarz, "Two Reports May Expedite Capital's Inclusion in PPS," *Hospitals* 58, No. 4, (February 16, 1984):26.

174. Wallace, "GAO Report."

175. "For-Profits' Meeting Examines DRG System, Capital Payment Options," *Hospital Progress* 65, No. 4, (1984):20-21.

176. P. L. Grimaldi, "Reimbursement of Capital Costs," *Nursing Management* 14, No. 12, (1983):61-64.

177. Keefe, "Capital Costs and DRGs."

178. S. Lewis, "Speculations on the Impact of Prospective Pricing and DRGs," *Western Journal of Medicine* 140, No. 4, (1984):638-644.

179. Grimaldi, "Reimbursement."

180. W. J. Unger, "DRGs and the New Medicare Prospective Rate-Setting System: Business Implications and Strategies for Success," *Syva Monitor* 2, No. 2, (1984):2-5.

181. C. Wallace, "New Proposals Complicate Debate," *Modern Healthcare* 14, No. 4, (1984):28-30.

182. Lewis, "Speculations."

183. "Teaching Hospitals' Capital Cost Debated," *Hospitals* 58, No. 10, (May 16, 1984):20.

184. G. Warner, "Exploring the Options of Medicare Payment for Capital," *Hospitals* 58, No. 6, (March 16, 1984):66-67.

185. Ibid.

186. M. Tatge, "Industry Execs Unhappy with Capital Proposals," *Modern Healthcare* 14, No. 4, (1984):28-29.

187. J. Finn, "Debate Heats Up Over Capital Plan," *Hospitals* 58, No. 7, (April 1, 1984):37-38.

188. HIMA Issues Paper on Medicare Payment for Capital, Health Industry Manufacturers Association: Washington, DC, June 15, 1984.

189. C. Wallace, "Hospital Execs Divided on Political Strategies," *Modern Healthcare* 14, No. 3, (February 15, 1984):28.

190. Ibid.

191. "DRG Rate Setting, Capital Payments Examined," *Hospital Progress* 65, No. 3, (1984):20.

192. Wallace, "Hospital Execs."

193. E. Friedman, "PPS Needs Overhaul to Survive: Altman," *Hospitals* 58, No. 22, (November 16, 1984):33.

194. Wallace, "Hospital Execs."

195. Ibid.

196. "PPS Should Include Capital Equipment Cost, HFMA Says," *Hospitals* 58, No. 1, (January 1, 1984):28.

197. Wallace, "Hospital Execs."

198. Ibid.

199. Tatge, "Industry Execs."

200. Finn, "Debate Heats Up."

201. Kalison and Averill, "Response to PPS."

202. B. R. Neumann and J. V. Kelly, "Prospective Reimbursement for Hospital Capital Costs," USDHHS, National Center for Health Services Research, November, 1983.

203. C. Mickel, "Capital Cost Study Recommends Blended Approach," *Hospitals* 58, No. 5, (March 1, 1984):31.

204. "Old Hospitals Need Capital Payment Phase-in: Rubin," *Modern Healthcare* 14, No. 5, (1984):34.

205. "PPS Capital Report Due in Early 1985: Davis," *Hospitals* 59, No. 2, (January 16, 1985):26.

206. Ibid.

207. "Capital Reimbursement On The Back Burner?" *Medical World News* 26, No. 8, (April 22, 1985):36-37.

CHAPTER 5
Medical Records:
Front and Center

Revolutionary Changes

Within the DRG system, where so much depends upon comprehensive data and the accurate coding of illnesses, medical records departments will be a key component of any health care management process. "Medical records is the cash register operator for the hospital. Therefore, the administrator had best watch this operation very carefully."[1] This conclusion was affirmed by some of the leading accounting firms in the United States as the DRG system was implemented on October 1, 1983. Comments from these firms appeared in an article in *Hospitals* entitled, "Medical Records Hold Key to PPS." These accounting experts agreed that the medical records department is now "the basis for the financing of the hospital."[2]

Along with the financial importance, the medical records department has also moved out of dark, basement quarters into the executive suite. In fact, "RRAs (Registered Records Administrators) may be more important in hospital management than executives who hold master's degrees in business administration," according to a college professor in the field.[3]

This combination of responsibility for data and income is changing medical records people from librarians into data managers, from cost generators to revenue enhancers. "Helping their hospitals collect billions of dollars in federal reimbursement will become the top priority of medical records departments."[4] About 7,000 RRAs and 13,000 ARTs (Accredited Record Technicians) will be interpreting the patient's medical stay into proper DRGs and saving and making money for their employers.

Even prior to the actual federal implementation of the DRG system, Bruce Vladeck, an official familiar with the experiences in New Jersey, predicted "a revolution in medical records."[4] Not only will medical records departments find themselves reeducating physicians in chart completion, they will be training competent coders and learning to integrate computers into the operation. There will also be revolutionary changes as financial information is linked together with medical record clinical data.

Medical records experts had also recognized the impact of the prospective payment plan early on. In April 1982, a guest editorial in the *Journal of the American Medical Record Association* pointed out: "There has never been a greater opportunity than now."[6] This editorial served as a primer, reviewing the federal government's DRG system and commented on the technical complexities. Jackson summed up, "Clearly no hospital professional is in a better position to understand and be able to interpret DRGs than medical record practitioners, who should take advantage of the opportunity to add this knowledge to other skills and thus materially contribute to the management of the hospital."[7]

Appropriately, the increased importance of medical records departments and personnel should lead to a jump in status and salary increases for medical records staff members. An assistant vice president of one of the large for-profit hospital chains, herself an RRA, compared the situation to a profit and loss statement: "Coded inpatient discharge data—once used primarily for research, quality assurance studies, or simple statistical output—in recent months has become a primary focus in medical record departments and perhaps the essence of a hospital's bottom line and survival for the 1980s."[8]

Drawing on his experiences working for the New Jersey Hospital Association, Grimaldi addressed the impact of the DRG system for medical records departments. He detailed the informational requirements, the DRG assignment process, the responsibility for coding accuracy and completeness, quality control measures, and the maximizing of reimbursement. "For the first time," he concluded, "the coding of medical information will determine hospital reimbursement."[9]

Role of American Medical Record Association

Located in Chicago, the American Medical Record Association (AMRA) is the professional organization that speaks for the practitioners of their art. Two documents present consensus AMRA views about DRGs. One lists procedural guidelines for using health care data for reimbursement (See Exhibit 5-1). Another discusses the AMRA's role in prospective payment. Both of these documents endorse the concept of using qualified medical record personnel to perform the tasks described in the guidelines and other material. In all cases, the material clearly points out the pivotal role of the physician in recording the information on the patient's chart. Even while the guidelines state that a qualified medical record person should select and code the DRGs, there is obviously no intent to bypass or supersede the attending physician. In the conclusion of the guidelines, the point is strongly made:

Exhibit 5-1 Procedural Guidelines for Using Health Care Data for Reimbursement

1. Hospital medical record must be primary data source. Qualified medical record personnel should code and sequence diagnoses and procedures based on definitions in the Uniform Hospital Discharge Data Set (UHDDS).
2. Principal diagnosis should be selected and coded by qualified medical record personnel based on review of the physician's documentation in the medical record. Educational programs should be conducted by medical record personnel to familiarize medical staff with UHDDS definitions, DRGs, and the need for correct ordering of diagnoses.
3. "Qualified medical record personnel may exercise discretion in sequencing the listed codes in the absence of a clear principal diagnosis."
4. Medical records should be searched to identify other diagnoses related to the patient's stay.
5. Hospital documentation policies must ensure that complications and comorbid conditions impacting on DRG assignment are reported on the billing form.
6. Principal procedure should be selected and coded by qualified medical record personnel based upon the complete record.
7. Medical record personnel should become familiar with procedures used in the determination of DRG assignment.
8. In conjunction with the business office staff, medical record personnel should make sure that correct age and discharge status are recorded on the patient's record as well as the billing form.
9. Length of stay should be accurately recorded noting the time of admission and discharge.
10. "Ethical medical record practitioners must ensure that each medical record contains appropriate documentation to support the principal diagnosis, principal procedure, qualifying complications and comorbid conditions used for the DRG assignment of a patient."

Source: Summarized from American Medical Record Association, Revised May 1983.

Although neither the UHDDS (Uniform Hospital Discharge Data Set) definitions nor the ICD-9-CM classification system was developed for reimbursement purposes, AMRA believes qualified medical record personnel can conform to the high ethical standards of AMRA while collecting uniform hospital data to fulfill the requirements of the prospective system, and enhance hospital reimbursement.[10]

While the leaflet explaining the role of the AMRA in PPS covers the health record, health care data, DRG coordination, and DRG validation, there is a statement that will appeal to hospital administrators everywhere. ". . . medical record personnel may assign, as the principal diagnosis, the diagnosis using the most resources when the documentation reveals two or more diagnoses, any of which could be the principal diagnosis. This assists the hospital in remaining financially viable."[11]

Again, this document also talks about each member of the health care team contributing to high quality records, accurate data collection and efficient record-keeping systems.

In 1982, HCFA studied the quality of data submitted by hospitals and others to them. A review of the coding data indicated numerous errors in the selection of the correct diagnosis and codes. Recommendations by HCFA included the following:

1. More trained personnel are needed to identify the correct principal diagnosis and principal procedure.

2. Medical record personnel should perform all coding on claims to address the problem of quality coding.

3. Medical record department should be responsible for submitting all diagnoses and procedures to the business office.

4. Periodically, the quality of the work must be checked.[12]

Since HCFA is the federal agency most directly concerned with DRGs, these recommendations lend solid support to the similar recommendations made by the professional association.

Medical Record Data Needs

With the evident direct relation between the information contained in the medical record and the financial stability of the institution, it is obvious that the data to be collected should be clearly specified. For complete health care documentation, the American Medical Record Association recommends that a medical care facility do the following:

- Clearly delineate the required contents of medical records.

- Ensure that all clinical information pertaining to a patient's care is centralized in the patient's record and accessible when needed.

- Offer an inpatient analysis program to assist physicians and other health care team members in recording their findings and observations concurrently with events, rather than after patient discharge.

- Develop policies, rules, and regulations to ensure that every record is completed within a time period which assures completeness and accuracy of discharge data and reduces health information processing costs.[13]

These guidelines deal with the establishment of the proper environment for the collection of medical record data. A management approach to the situation describes the required standard operating procedures that the health care institution should develop and maintain.

Specific Medical Record Data

Proceeding from the overall guidelines to the specific—what are the actual bits of information that need to be entered in the record? For DRG assignment, six bits of information are required:principal diagnosis, secondary diagnoses, principal and other procedures, age, sex, and discharge status. However, most administrators will be analyzing additional data as listed in Exhibit 5-2. Data listed in Exhibit 5-2 goes far beyond the routine collection of information for the assignment of DRGs.These bits of data are considered part of a management information system that allows decision makers to arrive at conclusions based upon reliable evidence. However, it may cost more to secure all the data and

Exhibit 5-2 Suggested Data for Collection and Medical Records

For DRG Assignment
- Principal diagnosis
- Secondary diagnoses
- Principal and other procedures
- Age using birth date
- Sex of patient
- Discharge status including admission and discharge dates

Patient Stay Data
- Admission class; emergency/elective
- Referral source; transfers
- Special care units; ICU, CCU
- Days in special care units
- Transfer designations
- Payor code
- Certified days
- Department attending patient
- Readmission

Charge Data
- Total charges
- Charges by cost center

Patient Identification Data
- Hospital ID number
- Medical record number
- Billing number

Patient Demographic Data
- Zip code
- County-municipality code

Clinical Data
- Procedure dates
- Admitting diagnosis
- Major diagnoses and major procedures
- Consultations by speciality

Physician Data
- Attending physician code
- Principal surgeon code
- Other physician code

Sources: L. K. Lichtig, "Data Systems for Case Mix," *Topics in Health Care Financing* 8, no. 4 (Summer 1982): 13–19. "Building a DRG Management Information System, Part I," *DRG Monitor* 1, no. 3 (1983): 1–4.

outweigh the utility to the administrators. "Therefore, the goal is not to achieve perfection, but is to maximize data quality and usefulness."[14] It should be evident that this type of DRG management data collection system portends great potential for getting the most value for health dollar expenditures. Integrating the financial and clinical information for analysis before decision making can only be beneficial to those required to make choices. On the other hand, making the decision purely on a financial basis must fall short in comparison and could be detrimental to the population being served.

In addition, the information relates directly to areas that the federal government will be monitoring. This monitoring relates to the investigation of facilities that may be "gaming" the DRG system to secure the most reimbursement possible. Specific review will look into admissions, length of stay, outliers, transfers, and DRG assignment. Therefore, hospitals would be judicious to review that data themselves to avoid future problems affecting payments.

Based on experiences in New Jersey, Bennett, a director of medical records at a local hospital, emphasizes the need for complete diagnoses from the attending physician, the timeliness of recording data, the alliance with the billing department, and the use of an ongoing review while the patient is still in the hospital.[15] At that hospital, a flow sheet is appended to the chart to allow medical records personnel to document all data required for DRG assignment before the patient is discharged.

Data and Management

Data listed in Exhibit 5-2 will be used by hospital administrators for a variety of purposes.

To assign patients to the proper ICD-9-CM and the DRG group, the bits of information are obvious.

Likewise, the patient identification information allows for easy referral back or for tracking when the patient receives services at more than one facility.

Patient demographic data can be used for planning and marketing as well as patient origin studies. In addition, these data could be used for epidemiologic investigations.

Patient stay data allows the facility to distinguish between emergency or urgent admissions and elective admissions. Referral sources detail where patients are transferred from, such as a skilled nursing home or through the ER. Special care unit data tells if the patient was treated in intensive care, coronary care, or isolation. This relates to the severity of illness and the resource consumption issue. Days in special care unit information logically relates to length of stay and resource use. Transfer data allows for the flow of patients to another facility and also reviews the discharge practices. Payer coding identifies third-party payers as well as individual payers and case-mix comparisons can be made.

Certified days relates to the length of stay for specific conditions as set forth by utilization review groups. Attending department comparisons can be made with this type of data collected for each attending service. Readmission information reveals practice patterns and can identify possible problems regarding the quality of care.

Clinical data can be used by management to pinpoint the practice patterns of their physicians regarding procedures, diagnoses, and consultations.

Physician data can be used to identify the behavior patterns of the physicians in the facility. This is similar to routine identification codes required for the patient.

Charge information allows the facility to relate the individual services to the various centers providing the services. Furthermore, this data could be linked to individual physicians and patients. Analysis here merges the billing and clinical data for management scrutiny.

Impact of Medical Record Data

At a national conference on the effect of DRGs in New Jersey and the potential for the United States, an official of the Health Care Financing Administration enumerated the lessons to be learned about medical records departments.Savitt spoke about timeliness, principal diagnosis identification, completeness, accuracy, and the changing role of medical records departments.These comments were based upon experiences in New Jersey where the DRG system had been in effect for about three years.

Quality and Timeliness of Data in Medical Records

Quality and timeliness are closely linked because the longer the delay between recording the information and the patient's discharge, the more likely that the data will be incomplete. Documentation in the medical record is vital. "If the record has only garbage in it, that is all that can be abstracted and coded."[16] Therefore each diagnosis must be fully described, including all modifiers. Following that, all procedures must be fully described and identified; entries must be made in a timely manner in the record. To achieve the quality and the timeliness, physicians can be guided and encouraged to improve their medical record entries. Some hospitals include boxes on the record forms to stress the information needed. Almost all hospitals initiate educational programs for all team members regarding the data required for the medical record. In a follow-up, the medical records department should monitor the quality of the entries and report back to the staff regarding any necessary changes in reporting.

Abstracting and Coding: Principal Diagnosis

Obviously, a complete medical record filled out comprehensively will make abstracting and coding easier. Nevertheless, special attention has to be given to the selection of the principal diagnosis, the selection of procedures, and then the accurate coding. "In New Jersey the hospital assigns the DRG and the accuracy of DRG assignment is monitored by the State."[17] Errors in coding can be detrimental to the institution and cost dollars and time in reviewing records. At this point, there will be issues relating to who makes the DRG assignment and the cooperation of the health care team in the total activity.

Billing Department Coordination

"There will be great concern by hospital management that the reported data maximize reimbursement."[18] As a bottom line comment, this indicates that medical records bears a large part of the responsibility for the financial stability of the hospital. Bills that are returned for errors or corrections merely mean a delay in payment. Thus, the medical record department and the billing department must coordinate their activities to produce a smooth flow of reimbursement monies. In the past, many hospitals did not have a solid line of communications between those two departments.

To effect this merger, the Hospital Research and Educational Trust of New Jersey has developed a computer software program to merge clinical and financial data. This program, called PBCS (Planning, Budgeting, and Control System) has been licensed to the Commission on Professional Hospital Activities (CPHA) by HRET. CPHA plans to market the program with prices ranging from $12,000 for a small hospital to $30,000 for larger facilities. As an extra, hospitals using PBCS will be able to compare their data with information from other institutions using the system.[19]

Coulton used a social work department to illustrate the integration of the cost data with the professional activities. Even though the content is social work, the extensively detailed explanation could also be used for a model in health and medical care. She divides the model into inputs, processing, and outputs.[20]

Inputs included social work procedures, with each procedure having its own form. Procedure forms will have data such as patient identification information, a worker code, problem status, type of problem, type of service, and time required for the procedure. Standard units of service defined by the average time it takes to carry out the task should be explicitly defined. For example, a community referral takes .05 hours; counseling takes 0.4 discharge planning takes 0.8 and family treatment takes 1.9. In addition to the standard units of time, productivity standards are also indicated.

Processing requires computer hardware and software sufficient to handle the workload. Tasks to be undertaken include the updating of the procedure file, analysis of utilization patterns, calculation of patient care productivity, cost calculations, matching records from social work with patient records, analysis profiles, and compilation of services other than patient care.

Outputs determine the bottom line in the merging of clinical and financial data. These are the so-called products of the hospital. Reports will emphasize productivity, costs, utilization, and effectiveness. Social work departments estimate that 65 to 75 percent of their services are in patient care. This should be reflected in the cost reports and productivity.

To carry out the merger of clinical and financial data, Coulton noted that several prerequisites are vital:

- Each department has to prepare a list of all specific patient care services defined exactly and detailing what constitutes each unit of service.

- Data collection forms have to be devised along with written instructions and whatever numerical codes are required for identification.

- Each department has to conduct time studies to establish average times for each unit of patient care service and productivity standards.

- High-risk criteria should be established for individuals who do not fall into the average service unit designations.

- Data processing procedures need to be spelled out in detail.

- Staff needs to be trained on how to use the system.[21]

Lichtig also talked about the merging of clinical and financial data and enumerated the options for information processing as follows:

1. Data can be entered in each department on a single form.

2. Data can be sent to a central office for entry on a single form.

3. Data can be entered into a single computer in each department.

4. Data can be entered on separate computers and merged by the system.

In all cases, however, caution should be taken to assure that the data entered is for the same patient by checking the name, the ID number, and admission and discharge data.[22]

Payer Feedback and Monitoring

This is closely aligned with prior impacts in that the payer may be calling upon the hospital to verify the princial diagnosis and procedures. When data are late, the payer will accept corrections. When data are in error, the payer will expect reassignment and withhold payment. In either case, the facility will be required to ensure that the flow of information is accurate and coordinated to the payer.

Hospital Internal Response

At first, institutions will be spending large sums of money for automated equipment and computer programs to enhance the ability of staff to meet the data needs. Anything that the vital medical record department wants it is likely to get in the first blush of this enormous task. However, as real life sets in, the "department will be expected to do more and more, and do it better and better, with less and less."[23]

In summary, Savitt concludes that the tasks can be accomplished, that the physicians do respond, and that the medical records departments will gain much from the DRG reimbursement system.

Errors and Medical Record Data

Patterns

Errors contained in medical records material have to be of concern to administrators within a DRG system. There is a direct link between the medical record data and reimbursement that cannot be ignored as previously, when the payment mechanism was based solely upon the per diem retrospective method. Burick and Nackel observed that discharge abstracts often contained classification and coding errors, did not include all diagnoses, and varied according to the individual physician's documentation and the individual coder's interpretations.[24] In a 15-year review of the literature on data quality, Simeon concluded that common errors of medical records included inaccurate record data, inaccurate classification, and incomplete coding.[25]

Patterns in medical record data were delineated by Appleton and Schneider as they used a focused review technique to discover if the errors adversely affected reimbursement. Four error modes emerged:

1. Incorrect sequencing of the principal diagnosis

2. Omission of significant secondary diagnosis

3. Omission of codable procedures

4. Wrong assignment of ICD-9-CM codes.[26]

In going back to the process of editing the record data to arrive at DRG coding, a number of specifics were identified as probable causes, including the following:

- A usual principal diagnosis code appearing in a secondary diagnosis position.

- No secondary diagnoses, even though patient's age, length of stay, or principal diagnosis anticipates such entries.

- Underlying causes coded in secondary positions, with nonspecific and symptom codes in principal diagnosis.

- Noncorresponding surgical and principal diagnosis codes.

- No surgery codes where diagnoses and length of stay indicate such expectations.

- Use of two codes where ICD-9-CM calls for a combination code.[27]

Institute of Medicine Studies

When discussing data errors, most investigators usually cite the studies of the Institute of Medicine. In each study, a sample of patient records was reabstracted by a trained team of registered record administrators and compared with the original data. Findings from these studies indicated that the hospital data on admission date, discharge date, and sex were highly reliable. However, this was not so when diagnosis and procedure data were examined. Medicare data was reliable in only 59.5 to 64.1 percent of the cases.[28] A major possible limitation with the data resides in the fact that the information was based on 1974 and 1977 patient information and the data was not used for payment purposes.[29] All three IOM studies 30-32 concluded that there is a "substantial level of imprecision and error" in hospital discharge data.[33] In fact, the 1974 study even referred to payment: "Diagnosis-specific discrepancies are of sufficient magnitude to preclude such data for detailed research and evaluation, or to measure diagnostic case mix as an indication of intensity of services that could then form the basis for determining reimbursement rates."[34]

Furthermore, the IOM studies did not show any significant improvement in data accuracy between 1974 and 1977.[35]

Obviously, errors contained in medical record information are not a new problem.[36] Research in the past has consistently illustrated the tendency to encode incorrect information. Now when coding takes on such major importance, these errors can cause serious harm to an institution's financial stability.

Coding Errors

A study of 15 hospitals in New York revealed factors responsible for coding errors. In order of importance, these factors were:

1. Coding from incomplete medical records, particularly those with incomplete discharge summaries and face sheets

2. Hospital policies requiring the coder to do so in conformity with the information provided by the physician on the face sheet and summary alone

3. Assuming the information was complete, lack of expertise in coding and sequencing.[37]

This study stated that the data errors had severe financial impact upon the hospitals. "Losses ranged from $50,000 to several million dollars in one fiscal year."[38] Another study, confined to surgical practice, came to a similar conclusion about the relation between coding and pricing of services.[39]

In another review of the quality control of diagnosis and procedure coding, investigators identified a different typology of coding errors. First, it was noted that "coding is a relatively subjective, independent task."[40] Errors then fell into three classifications:

1. Clerical errors involving careless mistakes

2. Judgmental errors when an individual makes a subjective mistake

3. Systematic errors due to incorrect procedures in carrying out tasks.[41]

Clerical errors occur about 2 percent of the time. This could involve transposed numbers, 245 for 254, or misread words, *peroneal* for *perineal*. Estimates for judgmental errors range as high as 10 percent although there is no accurate occurrence. Systematic error rates are the most important and some estimate that 70 percent of the errors can be attributed to this factor.[42]

Problems in the systematic classification can be traced to four potential sources:

1. Terminology selection inaccurate or incomplete

2. Wrong code selected for the terminology

3. Additional code required but missing

4. Sequencing error.[43]

In addition, systematic errors are signficant because there is the potential to affect every record in the institution. Yet, it is possible, once detected, to design a method to catch these systematic errors. Once the method becomes standard operating procedure, the facility can eliminate the largest source of errors through systematic correction of systematic errors. A management difficulty with the detection and correction of systematic errors lies in the fact that physicians, who may be providing inadequate data, do not fall under the purview of the medical record administrator responsible for the coding system.

Impact of Medical Record Errors

It is evident that without the tie to reimbursement, the impact of medical record errors would not be considered as serious a problem as it is now that the DRG system has arrived. A number of studies have investigated impacts such as errors on case mix patterns, financial loss or gain, and comparative recording.

In an early study at the University Hospitals of Cleveland, Doremus and Michenzi reviewed a 20 percent sample of Medicare patients discharged in 1978; 262 patients were selected from the 959 records for the study. Data from the records was reabstracted by registered record administrators and placed into DRG classifications. Results showed "widely divergent diagnostic and surgical data that results in a significant variation in DRG classification and reimbursement ceilings."[44] Two major reasons for this conclusion lay in the problem of data transmitted to Medicare and inaccurate and incomplete recording of diagnostic and surgical information in the record.

Corn assigned DRG numbers to each of 2,774 discharges from 56 New Jersey hospitals using 1977 data. He concluded that 18.5 percent of the principal diagnosis codes were not in agreement with the reabstracted codes. Errors regarding age, principal diagnosis, secondary diagnosis, and the procedures for both of those caused 475 of the 2,774 patient records (17 percent) to be placed into the wrong DRG. While there was an absolute mean error of $74.59 per discharge, the canceling out of overpayment and underpayment resulted in a net underpayment of $8.25 per discharge. This interaction led Corn to conclude that "prospective reimbursement appears to be relatively insensitive to errors in patient data, because errors resulting in underpayments are largely compensated by errors resulting in overpayments, yielding a small net error."[45] At the time that Corn did this study, 1981, he suggested that there might be little to gain by investing time and effort into reducing the error level in patient data. However, he did comment that the situation could change because of the shift to the ICD-9-CM coding system and the fact that data would be directly linked to reimbursement in the future. He also suggested that the principal diagnosis and major diagnosis be defined on the face sheet. This would allow the attending physician to look at the medical record and make a determination. Also, attention should be paid to reducing sequencing errors, since that is a major source of errors in reimbursement.

Investigators in the state of Washington took a statewide stratified random sample of discharges during 1978 and 1979. Abstracts were chosen of people having diabetes as the principal or other diagnosis. A total of 4,466 records were discovered; 3,691 with a principal diagnosis of diabetes. "After reabstracting, only 60 percent of the sample were found to be unequivocally correct. In another 23 percent, the correct principal diagnosis could not be determined with certainty. Furthermore, 10 percent of the cases where diabetes mellitus was coded as another diagnosis were ambiguous as to whether diabetes actually was the principal diagnosis."[46] Effects of these errors on admission rates, length of stay and hospital payment are also considered in this study. However, this study found that "despite substantial errors and ambiguities in coding, there is little variability in diagnosis or DRG specific average length of stay,"[47]

Using Medicare data from 26 community hospitals in Minneapolis-St. Paul, Johnson and Appell compared the HCFA data with medical record information. Three questions were posited for investigation:

1. What is the degree of correspondence between HCFA claims data and hospital medical record data?

2. Does bias exist in the data?

3. What are the financial implications of the data?[48]

For 1980, the agreement level ranged from 31 to 74 percent, with an average concordance about 50 percent of the time. A trend emerged that showed that the larger tertiary care hospitals were in agreement less often and the smaller suburban hospitals had the higher agreement percentages. In 1981, the range remained similar but the agreement rate rose to 53 percent with the same trend exhibited by type of hospital. Potential data errors identified included the diagnosis or procedure code in error, omission of secondary diagnosis or procedure data, and age and/or sex code missing, wrong, or invalid.

Bias was measured by comparing hospital case mix indexes. When hospital medical record data are contrasted with HCFA claims data, the medical record index is statistically higher—about 4 percent in absolute terms. Thus, the HCFA claims data understated the hospital case mix and missed accurately representing the complexity of the hospital's patient load.

Financial impacts were substantial for the hospitals in this study. "Bias in the Medicare claim data has a dramatic effect on hospital reimbursement. Although the average hospital will be underpaid by 4.1 percent, some hospitals may gain as much as 89 percent in Medicare reimbursement while others may lose as much as 26 percent."[49] As with the agreement on diagnosis, the larger tertiary care facilities are most likely to lose funding, while the smaller hospitals are most likely to gain revenue.

Bindman et al. did a retrospective review at Mount Sinai Hospital in New York of the charts of 43 patients with a 1982 discharge diagnosis of chronic obstructive pulmonary disease (COPD)—DRG 88. Charts were examined to evaluate the physicians' documentation, the completeness of the abstract, and the validity of the discharge diagnosis. Discrepancies were sorted into abstractor error, physician error, disease overlap categories, and incomplete chart information. More than half of the primary diagnoses were correct, 25 of the 43. Yet, 42 percent, 18 out of 43, were considered to have justifiable grounds for a different diagnosis. Researchers judged that physician errors were the cause in nine instances, abstractor error in one, and disease overlap in nine (one case with more than one error). Translating this into financial impact, reviewer assigned DRGs increased revenue by 4.4 percent, $6,012. If the reviewer coded to maximize the DRG classification, revenue went up 8.9 percent, to $12,170. Furthermore, the reviewers considered the increased reimbursement appropriate for the resources used for the assigned DRG classification as medically justifiable.Markedly, even though six months had passed before the reviewers examined the 43 charts, there were still 12 charts that were incomplete. Missing information could have been used by abstractors to properly classify the patients into the appropriate DRG category. These investigators called attention to the importance of educating physicians as to the vital role that the face sheet and chart play in hospital reimbursement. In this study, medical record abstractors made additions to the face sheets in 56 percent of the cases.[50]

Improving Medical Record Data

To resolve some of the difficulties revealed by the various studies on the quality of data in medical records, the federal government's Health Care Financing Administration is distributing a computer program to fiscal intermediaries. Designed by Health Systems International (HSI) of New Haven, Connecticut, the software package is called "Medicare Code Editor." This program runs on IBM mainframe computers and it screens claims before DRG classification and payment for the following errors:

- Invalid DRG codes
- Obvious inconsistencies
- Questionable coverage, such as liver transplants.

Using this computer program, the fiscal intermediary can return rejected Medicare claims to the hospital for recording and resubmission.[51]

A statement by researchers who reaccessed earlier record data and found errors presents an overview comment on improvement: "Further, the quality of the diagnostic and surgical data found in the medical record should be improved to the extent that it can be considered reliable for use, not only for case mix determination, but also for management reporting, quality assurance, utilization review, diagnosis costing, program planning, and research."[42]

Homogeneity of DRGs

A basic premise of the DRG classification scheme is that similar patients will use similar resources. This point was examined early in a number of articles in the *Journal of the American Medical Record Association*. Several investigators commented on homogeneity; some were affiliated with the New Jersey Hospital Association, another was a DRG coordinator for a New Jersey area hospital. These authors related their experiences from a state in which DRGs were already being used for payment.

In an 1980 article, the authors concluded that their review of statistical and medical data "strongly supports the conclusion that the majority of DRGs are not homogeneous."[43] At that time, 26 New Jersey hospitals were classifying patients into 383 DRGs. Their conclusion related to the huge variances in the resources required for specific DRGs. Other factors mentioned as responsible for the differences were age, race, sex, and socioeconomic factors.

After the DRGs were revised into 470 classifications, the same investigators published another article in the same medical record journal on "Homogeneity Revisited" in April 1982.[54]

After explaining the revised DRG classification system, the authors defined statistical and economic homogeneity. This definition raised the possibility that the DRGs could be statistically homogeneous but not economically so. In practical terms, the new DRGs seemed to be medically meaningful, but the patients still required a variable amount of resources. These researchers commented that "considerable economic heterogeneity still exists and will continue to exist as long as the number of groups cannot exceed 500."[45] In fact, they said that the economic disparity presented a strong case against the use of a uniform payment based on specific diagnoses.

Homogeneity arguments of a similar nature continue to be raised. Critics talk about integrating relative concepts such as the staging of disease, the severity of illness, resources intensity measures, and others to accurately indicate the resources consumed in the case of specific patients. This all boils down to the assumption by many health care professionals that there is no such thing as an average patient.

Staff Cooperation

Basically, a critical situation arises because medical, nursing, and other staff members—especially in hospitals reimbursed via DRGs—have become increasingly involved in hospital management operations. Physicians and nurses become administration managers responsible for the products of the hospital and integral cogs in the machinery of efficiency and effectiveness.[56] "An unprecedented responsibility has suddenly been thrust into physician's hands for the financial viability of the hospital in which they practice medicine."[57]

Physician Resistance

A physician consultant to the Commission of Professional and Hospital Activities (CPHA) was asked about the impact of DRGs. Dr. John A. Lowe responded that physicians and medical record personnel will bear the brunt of the impact. While he didn't believe that a good medical record department would have too much trouble, he did raise a relevant issue: "But the primary problem with DRGs is in getting closer cooperation between physicians and medical records personnel so that it's possible to get the correct information into the system."[48]

According to Ertel and Harrison, physicians consider entries such as principal and primary diagnosis and procedures as "reporting artifacts" having little "to do with the real business of providing care."[49] By custom and training, physicians report data in terms of clinical management relative to the phrasing and sequencing of information.

Physician Guidelines

Obviously, medical records staff and physicians should communicate freely to arrive at the appropriate classification. Serlucco and Johnson, an accountant and a DRG coordinator, respectively, detailed guidelines for a physician to use to assure comprehensive medical record documentation (Exhibit 5-3). Since physicians play a major role in the four key areas of admissions, inpatient services, discharges, and medical records, their relation to the DRG plan has apparent impact.

It is important for medical records staff to stress to physicians the need for timely completion of the medical record, the need to document all relevant diagnosis and procedures, and the relationship between the principal diagnoses and complicating and comorbid conditions.

Exhibit 5-3 Physician Guidelines for Medical Record Documentation

Guidelines for Medical Record Documentation

1. Enter all final diagnoses in one place on the medical record, ideally on the face sheet, discharge summary, or final progress note.
2. Document all conditions treated or observed during the patient's hospitalization.
3. Finalize all impressions made by consulting physicians; enter a diagnosis on the face sheet.
4. Use exactly the same medical term in all references to condition or diagnosis. (Slight word changes could alter the ICD-9-CM code selection).
5. Clarify disease interactions. Is admission a by-product of an underlying condition, such as cateracts due to diabetes or fracture due to bone metastasis? Is this condition a metastatic process rather than a primary malignancy?
6. Identify the principal diagnosis even if more serious conditions are subsequently noted.
7. Document each major or minor procedure on the face sheet at the time it is performed. In this way, it will be easily identifiable for coding and chronological sequencing.
8. Standardize departmental definitions of conditions, such as premature newborn.
9. Avoid recording only symptoms if clinical judgment indicates a definitive diagnosis.

Source: R. J. Serculo, and K. Johnson, "Importance of The Medical Record Process in a DRG Based System," *Quality Review Bulletin* 9, no. 9 (1983), 269.

All this information is intended strictly for records and not to imply interferences in medical judgement. Rationalization for physician cooperation with medical records personnel include the following:

- Hospitals will secure appropriate payments.
- Payer appeals will be lessened.
- Management analysis and comparative cost performance will be accurate.
- Certificate-of-need applications will be substantiated.
- A reliable database will be established.[60]

In a book devised as a physicians' guide to DRGs, Shanko devoted about 30 pages to questions doctors ask about medical records. More than 30 specific questions were detailed and eight exhibits were also used to explain the relationship between medical records personnel and physicians. The doctors inquired about timeliness, complete reporting, professional responsibilities, length of stay, and the decision-making obligations of physicians and medical records staff. Clearly, the physicians indicated that they needed some education about the DRG system and that they didn't understand the role of medical record personnel in the process of DRG classification. On the other hand, the physicians clearly understood the financial implications of entering data on the medical record to allow the hospital to garner the appropriate reimbursement.[61]

DRG Coordination

Some hospitals set up a DRG coordinating committee that includes representation from quality assurance, utilization review, financial management, medical records, discharge planning, and medical staff liaison.[62] This group deals with information-gathering groups within the hospital to better use the data and to avoid duplication. Another output of this committee is the policy of sending medical record staff onto the nursing floors to review diagnosis while the patient is still in the hospital. This would allow discussions with the attending physicians before the information is entered into the patient's record.[63]

In advocating this type of DRG coordination, the American Medical Record Association recommends the following coordination activities:

- Providing an information resource person to keep hospital employees up-to-date on regulations and information

- Assuring that medical and financial data are merged to reflect accurate coding, abstracting, and DRG assignments

- Evaluating the information to pinpoint causes of variance in physician practice patterns, in support from departments, or other causes

- Providing liaison to individual physicians and to medical committees to resolve differences

- Supplying support to DRG coordination via timeliness policies, qualified coders, record reviewers, and computer system.[64]

There have been suggestions that a new position of DRG Coordinator be created to assume the critical responsibilities.[65] In this vein, Flanagan and Sourpas prepared a job description listing qualifications, major responsibilities, and a job summary (Exhibit 5-4). Medical records personnel are among the most likely choices to fill a newly created DRG Coordinator position.[66] A pivotal issue with such a coordinating position revolves around the authority of that individual to make the decisions and have the clout to carry them out.

Observations from New Jersey

Boerma evaluated the DRG program in New Jersey and examined the relations between medical records personnel and the medical and nursing staffs. His

Exhibit 5-4 Job Description—DRG Coordinator

Title: DRG Coordinator

Job Summary: Directs implementation of and compliance with prospective payment system requirements. Participates in design and implementation of DRG management system to ensure the provision of high quality care in a cost-effective manner.

Qualifications: Baccalaureate degree required; master's degree preferred. Background should include courses in statistics, economics, financial management, health care organization and delivery, and management. Knowledge of medical record management, utilization review and reimbursement regulations required. Must have experience in needs assessment, planning, organizing, implementing and evaluating systems and procedures.

Major Responsibilities

1. Coordinates interdepartmental systems and information flow related to prospective payment.

2. Develops, institutes and maintains systems to analyze case mix data.

3. Coordinates the development of DRG appeals.

4. Develops methods to ensure minimal coding error rates.

5. Conducts concurrent and retrospective case mix review.

6. Identifies possible problems in utilization or quality of care, refers problems to appropriate individual or area for correction.

7. Identifies cost center problem areas and suggests or develops methods for more efficient functioning.

8. Chairs institutional DRG task force.

9. Maintains accurate case mix records and develops appropriate management reports for use by administration, medical staff and department heads.

10. Serves as resource person for hospital and medical staff on questions related to prospective payment system.

Source: J. B. Flanagan, and K. J. Sourapas, "Organizational Issues and Ideas, Part IV," *Journal of the American Medical Record Association* 55, no. 2 (1984): 16.

conclusions indicated that interactions were closer in DRG hospitals due to higher interdependency levels, increased awareness, formalization, and information flow. Specifically, he observed the following:

- Information flow increases significantly

- Relationships are more formalized and the units have significantly more knowledge about each other's work

- Relationship is significantly improved between nursing and medical records departments.

- All three units perceive a higher degree of interdependence.

- More communication takes place.

- Task differentiation is similar.[67]

Physician Education

Medical schools should include material in the curriculum on record keeping. In addition, the team approach to data handling should be stressed with physicians as a integral member of the group.[68] Physician education should incorporate the following principles:

1. Teaching definitions of principal diagnosis and principal procedures in accordance with the DRG system

2. Instructing how notes entered on a patient's chart relate to the DRG system, particularly with respect to accuracy and comprehensiveness

3. Stressing the timeliness of the completion of the patient record

4. Emphasizing the cautious use of the resources necessary for the patient and the associated costs.[69]

Exhibit 5-5 illustrates the practical application of the four points on medical education. Admission complaints and discharge diagnosis were listed on the chart by the attending physician in the order stated. In reviewing the reason for the patient's admission to the hospital, the tests, and the treatment regimen, the correct principal diagnosis should be chronic obstructive pulmonary disease, which also classifies the patient into a higher payment DRG category. As Ertel and Harrison stated: "The most effective legitimate method to increase payments without an actual change in case mix is to increase the accuracy with which patient diagnoses and procedures are reported."[70]

An official of HCFA reported on the impact of DRGs on medical record departments based upon experience in New Jersey. He believes that New Jersey showed that medical records can be timely, can identify the principal diagnoses, can be complete, and can be coded accurately, and that medical staff can work cooperatively with medical records personnel. In addition, Savitt said that "the most satisfying lesson from New Jersey has been the response by physicians to the need for providing better and more complete information in a timely manner."[71]

EXAMPLE: Selection of Principal Diagnosis Using UHDDS Definition

PATIENT: Age 66

ADMISSION COMPLAINTS: Shortness of breath on exertion
Cold Lower Extremities
Intermittent Claudication

DISCHARGE DIAGNOSES:	DRG CATEGORY	WEIGHT*
Peripheral Vascular Disorder	130	.9886
Chronic Obstructive Pulmonary Disease	88	1.8713
Hypertension	134	.7185

PRINCIPAL DIAGNOSIS: Chronic Obstructive Pulmonary Disease

BASIS: Reason for admission
X-ray findings
Treatment

Reference*: Health Care Finance Administration, List of DRGs and Weights, October 1, 1982.

Exhibit 5-5 Principal Diagnosis Selection Options
Source: E. MacDonald, "Accurate Medical Records to Have Key Impact on Hospitals in a DRG Case Mix System," *FAH Review* 16, no. 2 (1983): 58.

Therefore, medical records personnel should pursue cooperation from physicians, nurses, and others. Based on prior experience, there is no reason not to anticipate success.

Physician Attestation

In the final rules on the prospective payment system, published in the *Federal Register* issue of January 3, 1984, Section 405.472(d)(2)(i) (now revised and redesignated as 412.46 (a) and (b), was an item regarding DRG validation:

(i) The attending physician must, shortly before, at, or shortly after discharge (but before a claim is submitted), attest to in writing the principal diagnosis, secondary diagnoses, and names of procedures performed. The following statement must immediately precede the physician's signature: "I certify that the identification of the principal and secondary diagnoses and the procedures performed is accurate and complete to the best of my knowledge. (Notice: Intentional misrepresentation, concealment, or falsification of this information may, in the case of a Medicare beneficiary, be punishable by imprisonment, fine, or civil penalty.)"

Reactions from Medicine

Organized medicine reacted to the requirement published in the *Federal Register* with vocal and intense opposition. One journal noted that this violated Section 1801 of the Medicare law that stated that the federal government would not exercise control or supervision over the practice of medicine.[72] There was also an objection to the fact that the notice about the failure to comply and punishments were printed in capital letters.[73] A physician from Bartlesville, Oklahoma, writing to his U.S. Senator, put it strongly: "This is not only absurd and unnecessary, but it also presumes that I am dishonest and a cheater and will dictate erroneous and incorrect discharge summaries. . . . Not only does this make extra work for the hospital administration and record department, but it also is a gross insult to my integrity and will not save one dollar of Medicare money."[74]

This attitude was reinforced by Dr. John D. Abrums, president of the American Society of Internal Medicine, who said: "Our members (18,000 physicians) find this statement patently offensive, since it implies that physicians may willfully provide inaccurate information concerning a patient's condition."[75]

In a letter to the editor of the *New England Journal of Medicine,* Dr. Dennis L. Angellis's comment appeared under the title, "Government Insults Physicians." Dr. Angellis made the following three points:

1. Physicians are aware of the government-mandated consequences.

2. There was no need to remind physicians with every Medicare chart.

3. He took offense at the implication that the medical profession contains "a considerable collection of thieves, cheats, and criminals."

He also advised all physicians in the United States to have the capitalized portion regarding punishments stricken from the form.[76]

At a July 1984 meeting of the American Medical Association's House of Delegates in Chicago, the representatives were "most adamant" about the attestation requirement of the DRG program. Dr. William S. Weil said: "They've allowed Congress to insult the physician by implying he's dishonest."[77] A resolution was passed asking the AMA to work toward the elimination of the attestation statement. An editorial in the official newspaper of the AMA, *American Medical News,* also asked that attestation be rescinded. Two reasons were cited; the statement was unnecessary and there was an implication that HCFA felt that physicians would falsify the data.[78]

HCFA Counterreactions

Reacting to the "storm of protest," HCFA revised the attestation statement required on the discharge summary as follows:

> I certify that the narrative descriptions of the principal and secondary diagnoses and the major procedures performed are accurate and complete to the best of my knowledge.[79]

Furthermore, the hospital is to certify that the physician has signed a statement indicating knowledge of the following cautionary notice:

> Medicare payment is based in part on each patient's principal and secondary diagnoses and the major procedures performed on the patient, as attested to by the patient's attending physician by virtue of his or her signature on the discharge summary sheet. Anyone who misrepresents, falsifies, or conceals essential information required for payment of federal funds may be subject to fine, imprisonment, or civil penalty under applicable federal laws.[80]

Medicine's Continuing Objections

Even with the revised language, the AMA still called upon HCFA to rescind the attestation rule. Pointedly, the AMA noted that the revised language omitted the "intentional" aspect of any effort to falsify the data. Under the new wording, the AMA noted the broader requirement and the possibility that physicians could be accused in cases of mere error or unintentional fault.Several objections were detailed:

- Physicians are aware of the obligation to report accurate and complete information. Customarily, physicians have done so in the medical records. In addition, the Joint Commission on Accreditation of Hospitals (JCAH) already requires that type of data.

- Physicians are aware that intentional concealment, misrepresentation, and falsification of information is ethically, morally, and legally wrong and subject to civil and criminal penalties.

- Existing law already contains applicable penalties and the attestation is not needed to prosecute a physician for violations of the Medicare law.[81]

In a letter to the administrator of HCFA, Dr. James H. Sammons, AMA Executive Vice-President, commented that the modifications were an improvement but the AMA still felt the physician attestation was simply unnecessary. Nine specific objections were cited and the AMA membership was urged to contact their legislators to protest.[82]

Hospital Management and Medical Records

As already noted, medical records personnel may be more vital to hospital administrators than business administration graduates.[83] Data emanating from the medical records department will be used for market analysis and strategic planning. In the pro-competitive health care system, that information will be the life blood of the facility. Medical records departments are involved in management functions such as data processing, quality assurance, utilization review, physician peer review, corporation counsel work, hospital certification, market analysis, and strategic planning. This change is all part of a move for medical records personnel to become "assertive data managers."[84] In that role, the reliance of hospital administrators on medical records departments is apparent. Lichtig observed that "the management reporting aspect of a DRG data system is the key to its success."[85] He also added that data quality is a critical consideration and this has been amply noted elsewhere.

Hospital Administration Guidelines

Management personnel realize the value of the data capabilities of the medical records department under the DRG system. In view of their intended uses of the information, administrators are being advised to insure the quality of the data by following suggestions for medical records departments:

1. Hire qualified coders with experience and training in medical terminology, basic anatomy, and physiology.

2. Evaluate procedures between medical records and billing departments for the submission of DRGs.

3. Determine if approved UHDDS definitions of principal diagnosis and principal procedure are used.

4. Check to see if medical records staff routinely examine the chart for reporting all pertinent diagnoses, procedures, complications, and comorbidities.

5. Check on timeliness and accuracy of abstracting and coding functions and monitor costs associated with DRGs.

6. Check on medical records department's procedures for assuring accuracy and data quality control.[86]

This list was compiled by a registered records administrator and shows the benefit of her experience and training in the field. In addition, this RRA is also a vice president of a proprietary hospital chain firm and brings that focus into play with the guidelines.

Supervision of Medical Records Department

Considering the critical link of medical records to management, the question of administrative reporting becomes a relevant issue. Flanagan and Sourapas identify three possible alternatives for reporting: to the chief financial officer, to administration, or to an information processing director.[87]

Chief financial officer.   There is a trend for hospitals to combine clinical and financial data for case mix analysis. This trend flows from the direct use of medical record information for billing purposes. Therefore, it is logical to consolidate the admitting department, medical record department, and business office under the chief financial officer. However, critics are concerned that any services unrelated to reimbursements will be slighted or eliminated.

Administration.   In theory, the administrator has an overview of all departments and will not focus solely on payment-related services. An added benefit for medical records could be the opportunity to be involved in planning and policy activities.

Information processing director.   Using this alternative, one division would cut across all units and interact with medical, nursing, and ancillary staff and administration on patient care and resource use. A wide range of data-related tasks would be performed. Furthermore, under this reporting choice, communication with external review agencies such as professional review organizations would be enhanced.

All of the three alternatives are possible options. A choice will relate to the unique characteristics and needs of the specific facility's structure.

Management Reports from Medical Record Data

A prime concern of the administrator is the high variance DRG with extremes in the use of resources. Other areas of managerial attention will focus upon high volume DRGs, high cost DRGs, costs by cost center, and individual physician performance. Examples of management reports generated to meet those concerns were illustrated in the *DRG Monitor*, a newsletter on DRGs. Seven different types of administrative reports and possible actions were detailed:

Case mix and length of stay by DRG. Data in this report dealt with changes in case mix and in number of patient days. For example, the information showed that DRG 10, Neoplasm of Nerves, increased by 82 percent over two years; length of stay for that DRG increased by 135 percent. Therefore, a review for changes in treatment patterns and the presence of new physicians was indicated.

Case mix and length of stay by DRG by payer. In this report, local hospital data are compared to federal LOS standards. Total patient days, the number of patients, and the average LOS for each payer class are also compared. In analysis, DRG 140, Angina Pectoris, showed that these patients were discharged earlier than the federal LOS norm. Medicare patients in this group comprised more than half of the load. If the LOS rate stays favorable and the actual cost is also lower than the DRG allowance, DRG 140 would be favorable financially for the hospital.

Patient distribution by payer. Distribution here concerns the number of patients by the different payers in the 23 major diagnostic categories within the DRG scheme. Examination revealed that 38 percent of the hospital's population was covered by the Medicare program with payment on the basis of DRGs. Neurology and Respiratory major diagnostic categories had 62 and 73 percent Medicare case loads. Therefore, management should review those DRGs falling within MDC 1 (Neurology) and MDC 4 (Respiratory) first to track the use of resources.

DRG cost and reimbursement by payer. This report contains data about the cost per case, the reimbursement by payer, and the income. Two DRGs stand out in the report; DRG 12 (Degenerative Nervous System Disorders) and DRG 14 (Specific Cerebrovascular Disorders). DRG 12 costs $2,211 per patient, while the payment is $1,718 for a net loss of $493 per case.

There should be a review of resource use and LOS. DRG 14 has a net income across all payers, but the 106 Medicare patients each show a loss of $57. Management should investigate to see if any savings can be gained relative to the Medicare patients.

Cost and reimbursement by medical specialty.   Data collected here deal with the medical specialty, cost and reimbursement, and net income. Reports indicate that the hospital has a positive net income in internal medicine, neurology, and psychiatry. Dermatology shows a negative balance, but general surgery does the worst regarding Medicare patients and reimbursement. Each Medicare surgical case is costing the hospital $200. This information should lead to a review of the entire Medicare population undergoing surgery at the hospital. Negative findings could be due to high risk patients in surgery, poor postsurgical care, scheduling, preadmission testing, or other generalized problems.

Cost and reimbursement by individual physicians.   Information gathered for this report includes the physician cost per case, comparative cost data, reimbursement per case, and net income. Analysis reveals that a certain physician treats patients in DRG 128 (Deep Vein Thrombophlebitis) at a cost of $3,082 as compared to a DRG allowance of $3,350 for an average net gain to the hospital of $1,876. However, compared to the other six physicians in the unit, this physician is above their average cost of $2,566 for DRG 128 patients at that hospital. There may be a need to change the physician's practice behavior and certainly to review the treatment differences among the physicians involved.

Cost and reimbursement by hospital department.   Data would be compiled over time for routine and ancillary hospital cost centers such as intensive care, pediatrics, laboratory, and radiology diagnostic. Reviews should be concerned with changes in case mix, volume, or excessive cost. Each DRG within the unit should be considered and the positive or negative reimbursement examined for rationales. Adjustments in any of the variables should be managerial considerations.

Since the seven illustrative management reports could be viewed as threatening by the hospital staff, there needs to be an educational effort to alert staff as to the type of data being collected and the use of that information.[88]

Computers, Medical Records, and DRGs

Regardless of which mode of management is chosen for medical records, you can be sure that computers will be the building blocks of the unit's work. In an article entitled, "Hot Times for Hospital Software," *Fortune* magazine reported that "companies that provide computer software programs to hospitals are busier than an emergency room on New Year's Eve."[89] Despite the business upsurge, the article also noted that in late 1984 only 25 percent of all hospitals were able to keep track with computers of care delivered to patients. Tracking of patient care is critical because management does not wish to exceed the cost payment for specific DRG allocations. Companies in the business of selling software computer programs have been increasing their annual earnings by at least 25 percent for a number of years. Companies mentioned in the article include SMS in Philadelphia; HBO and Co. in Atlanta; Comucare in McLean, Virginia; Mediflex Systems in Evanston, Illinois; Amherst Associates in Chicago; Systems Associates in Charlotte, North Carolina; and Continental Healthcare Systems in Kansas City. In addition, the Hospital Research and Educational Trust of New Jersey markets PBCS (Planning, Budgeting, and Control System), a case-mix planning and financial reporting system for computers.[90]

Basically, the popularity of the software computer program activity has a direct relation to profitability. Averill, one of the Yale group that developed the DRG system, and also vice-chairman and chief of product development for Health Systems International in New Haven, Connecticut, said that the DRG-related software packages will be designed "to get at opportunities for making more money."[91]

One software company provides the ability to do ICD-9-M coding and DRG assignment, along with abstracting and management reporting, chart management, master patient index, and word processing thrown in for good measure.[92]

Staging Software

A program developed by SysteMetrics, Inc. of California even integrates the concept of staging disease into the calculations intended to track the use of resources. Diseases are staged, in ordinal fashion, from one (no complications) to four (death) with severity of illness as the major variable. About 420 diagnostic conditions are included in the program's capabilities. This firm makes the software available on a licensing basis for around $3,000.00 a year for a single hospital user. However, the software will also be available from federal government agencies at a lower rate but without the intensive technical support supplied by the producer.[93] Importantly, this staging of disease concept tends to reduce the variations in the length of stay and the financial losses to hospitals claiming to have patients sicker than usual, such as municipal, teaching, and referral facilities.[94]

Characteristics of Computer Systems

Before consideration of the characteristics of a sound computer system, there must be a method of collecting concurrent information, as well as an understanding that a system is only as good as the data collected. Thus, a computer system has to weed out inferior data and secure information from a variety of units at the same time.

Using those premises as the base, a computer system that works, especially for case mix analysis, should abide by the following concepts, according to Jaggar and Pugliese:

- Information should be integrated into the system simultaneously.
- Database should be retained in a flexible (disaggregated) format.
- Ad hoc analytical capability should be available.
- Multiple grouping systems (groupers) should be available.
- There should be comprehensive support for billing departments.
- Documentation and continuing education material should be on tap.
- Prompt system-wide changes should be easy.
- Case-mix modeling and forecasting should be included.
- There should be a link to cost accounting systems.[95]

Typically, a computer system could generate reports for management that would assist decision making. Among the information routinely delivered to administrators would be the following:

- DRG frequency ranking
- Services and charges by DRG
- Charges by physician by DRG
- Length of stay by DRG
- Threshold LOS warning
- DRGs by clinical division
- DRG by zip codes
- DRG analysis by payment status
- Comparative DRGs by area, state, nation
- DRGs by positive or negative variance.[96]

Computer Clarifications

With the boom in the use of computers and software programs, information managers are in a state of confusion. Dorenfest states that a hospital "may have to use as many as five computer systems just to meet its immediate prospective payment information needs."[97] In consideration of immediate needs, the computer must generate accurate records data, adapt that data to billing and reporting mandates of the payment system, and simulate economic outputs of varied case mix situations. Longer term needs require the computer to present information on resources use patterns, to analyze physician practice patterns, and to have a cost accounting system.

Early on, Fedorowicz and Veazie discussed the unanswered questions about automated DRG systems. They talked about shared systems, in-house systems, flexibility, and implementation alternatives. Hulm and Burik also evaluated the in-house turnkey, off-site processors, and shared systems. Their conclusions are displayed in Exhibit 5-6. Furthermore, it was pointed out that all costs should be specified, including investment, installation, and operating fees. These authors also suggested securing references from users of the services and a specific listing of the support services from the vendor.[98] Essentially the choice came down to buying or renting an existing computer system or designing one geared to the unique needs of a particular facility.

In 1980, the average New Jersey hospital was asking for $86,000 for start-up costs for their information system. One rental plan cost between 55 and 65 cents per DRG discharge in New Jersey.[99]

A later study by Federowicz looked into medical record requirements and the available hardware and software. She reviewed the existing literature on the use of electronic data processing by hospitals and found that 74 percent used the

Exhibit 5-6   Computer Systems Alternatives by Strengths, Weaknesses, and Examples

Alternative	Strengths	Weaknesses	Examples—Vendor (name of system)
In-house	Well suited to institution with significant in-house data processing resources Can be customized into any desired application area Utilizes in-house files Generally suitable for use as off-site processor for other hospitals	Requires in-house resources System maintenance may be difficult Generally requires interface programs Difficult to obtain comparative statistics	Arthur Andersen & Company (CMS) Rush-Presbyterian-St. Luke's Medical Center (MCFIS) Ernst & Whinney (Case Mix Manager) Mediflex Systems (Mediflex)

Exhibit 5-6 Continued

Alternative	Strengths	Weaknesses	Examples—Vendor (name of system)
In-house, turnkey	Utilizes all data in system without interface programs No additional data processing expertise required User-friendly query Flexible	To be efficient, hospital must utilize all system applications Locked into one vendor Patient classification system alternative typically not available Difficult to obtain comparative data Generally reimbursement oriented Not as flexible in accepting data from other vendors Regular reporting capabilities may be limited	Dynamic Control Corp. (Hospital Patient Management Corp.) HBO (IFAS) Systems Associates (Saint Hospital Financial System) Pacific Health Resources (DRG Promise)
Offsite	Well suited to institution without significant in-house data processing resources Utilizes existing data files Hospital requires no additional data processing expertise Capability to provide comparative data Well suited for providing multiple patient classification systems	May require interface programs Too much time may elapse between period end and reports reaching user Confidentiality may be an issue Hospital may not be able to provide required data Ad hoc reporting capabilities may be limited and/or expensive	Commons Management (Case Plex Systems) Commission on Prof. and Hosp. Activities (several products) CDC (Control Data Business Information Services) Hospital Research and Educational Trust (PBCS) Jones-Hosplex (Hosplex Case Mix Analysis) Planmetrics (Profile MPM) Rush-Presbyterian St. Luke's Medical Center (MCFIS) Systemetrics/Peat Marwick (Hospital Data Book) Amherst Associates (Case Mix Management System) Mediflex Systems Ernst & Whinney (Case Mix Manager)

Exhibit 5-6 Continued

Alternative	Strengths	Weaknesses	Examples—Vendor (name of system)
Shared systems	Same strengths as turnkey systems	Generally expensive to use Same weaknesses as turnkey systems	McAuto (Data Demand) Shared Medical Systems (Command) Amherst Associates (Case Mix Management System)

Note: This list is not intended to be all-inclusive in terms of vendors, strengths, or weaknesses. It is intended to assist management in differentiating between alternative approaches. It is not an endorsement of alternative products or vendors by either the authors or the American Hospital Association.
Source: C. Holm, and D. Borik, "Evaluating the New Case Mix Systems," *Hospitals* 58, no. 2 (January 16, 1984): 94.

equipment for financial analysis, 13 percent for clinical use, 11 percent for administrative purposes, and 2 percent for other uses. Articles illustrated that data systems can be used for reimbursement, quality control, utilization review, clinical research, and management decision support. In addition, there were several plans that classified data systems by the sophistication of the purposes and the integration capability of financial and administrative information.[100]

By 1984, more than 58 percent of hospitals installed an automated DRG analysis system. Almost 54 percent opted for a shared service while 36 percent chose an in-house system. Shared service vendors offer a generic product useful to large numbers of hospitals at a lower cost than in-house systems. Some specific features can be integrated, but that is limited. This increase in computer DRG analysis is linked directly to the fact that "today, the medical record is, in essence, the patient's bill."[101]

Computer Security

Whenever data are put into machines, the visions of tampering and invasion of confidentiality arise as issues. Recommendations were released by the American College of Hospital Administrators (ACHA) for computer security. Stuart Westbury, President of ACHA, suggested:

- Limiting staff access to computer data.
- Establishing access codes and ID cards for use.
- Mask data when recorded to protect patients.
- Set up central department responsible for data.[102]

Another recommendation included requiring the computer company, if there is a contractual arrangement, to stipulate security in the agreement. Periodically printing the master file and cross-checking with the original data should also prevent tampering.

Medical Records Impact Summary

Administrators like to look at the bottom line of the profit and loss statement when they evaluate the contributions of any particular part of their enterprise. A single typical example should suffice: "A 65-year-old patient was admitted for abdominal pain, did not have surgery, and was discharged as having pancreatitis. This patient was classified into DRG 327 (Abdominal Pain) rather than DRG 226 (Pancreatitis). This resulted in a loss of $1,102 for the hospital."[103]

Accuracy and precision of the medical records department will have a direct effect on the finances of the hospital. As this trend continues, the impact of that department's work activities will become increasingly visible in the health care provider arena.

Hospital Trends and Medical Records

Hospitals are increasing the intensity of services rendered to patients as new technology and drugs are introduced. This immediately results in an increase in the number of documents to be filed, the number of admissions, and the complexity of coding and abstracting.

Pricing differentials in cost containment systems means that medical records will have to generate more information regarding pricing. In addition, there will be more interaction with external auditors evaluating hospital claims and the need for special analyses to be used by hospital administration in their negotiations.

Corporate restructuring, especially into proprietary ownership, may result in the use of more group discharge abstract services, with a view toward comparative analysis among the facilities in the chain.

To meet the complexity of the tasks, the American Medical Records Association developed a publication, *Data Quality and DRGs*. It was written by Rita Finnegan, executive director of the AMRA; it sells for $35.00. The main sections cover patient care data, case mix, management reporting, and self-assessment exercises.

In selected issues of the *Journal of the American Medical Record Assocation*, a librarian presents an update on prospective payment issues. Bibliographic subheadings include ambulatory care, case mix, classification systems, DRGs, illness severity, and uniform billing.

With the increase in the sheer volume of activity coupled with the complexity, medical records departments must try to achieve maximum productivity. Flanagan and Sourapas suggest that there are three major steps to improve productivity.

1. Audit and review operations to find ways to make things work better.

2. Devise methods and systems improvements and be sure to work to implement the changes.

3. Create performance standards and productivity reporting mechanisms that review employee as well as environmental factors affecting output.[104]

No matter how you view the contribution of the medical records department, they are clearly destined to move further into the limelight.

References

1. R. R. Kovener and M. C. Palmer, "Implementing the Medicare Prospective Pricing System," *Healthcare Financial Management* 37, No. 8 (1983):44-46.

2. "Medical Records Hold Key to PPS," *Hospitals* 57, No. 19 (October 1, 1983):20-21.

3. M. Nathanson, "Medical Records' New Financial Role Dramatically Shifts Hospital Priorities," *Modern Healthcare* 13, No. 4 (1983):50-52.

4. Ibid.

5. E. Friedman, "Getting to Know Us. Hospitals May Finally Learn About True Cost and Pricing," *Hospitals* 57, No. 6 (March 16, 1983):74, 78-82.

6. G. G. Jackson, "The New DRGs—ICD-9-CM," *Journal of AMRA* 53, No. 2 (1982):52-55.

7. Ibid.

8. E. MacDonald, "Accurate Medical Records to Have Key Impact on Hospitals in a DRG Case Mix System," *FAH Review* 16, No. 2 (1983):55-58, 61-64.

9. P. L. Grimaldi and M. M. Zipkas, "The Use of DRGs—Selected Implications for Medical Record Departments," *Journal of AMRA* 54, No. 2 (1983):24-30.

10. *Procedural Guidelines for Using Health Care Data for Reimbursement (rev.)* (Chicago: American Medical Records Association, May 1983).

11. *Role in Prospective Payment* (Chicago: American Medical Records Association, undated). Pamphlet.

12. Macdonald, "Accurate Medical Records."

13. Role in Prospective Payment, American Medical Records Association.

14. "Building a DRG Management Information System. Part 1," *DRG Monitor* 1, No. 3 (1983):1-8.

15. S. P. Bennett, "DRGs: A Medical Records Perspective," *Nursing and Health Care* 5, No. 6 (1984):337-339.

16. H. L. Savitt, "Impact of DRGs on Medical Record Departments," in *Diagnosis-Related Groups: The New Effect in New Jersey. The Potential for the Nation,* USDHHS, HCFA Pub. No. 01370, March 1984, pp. 60-64.

17. Ibid.

18. Ibid.

19. "Software Aids with Planning and Budgeting," *Hospitals* 58, No. 2 (January 16, 1984):35.

20. C. J. Coulton, "Confronting Prospective Payment: Requirements for an Information System," *Health and Social Work* 9, No. 2 (Spring, 1984):13-24.

21. Ibid.

22. L. K. Lichtig, "Data Systems for Case Mix," *Topics in Health Care Financing* 8, No. 4 (1982):13-19.

23. Savitt, "Impact of DRGs."

24. D. Burik, "Case Mix Studies. Statement of Qualifications," (Chicago: Price Waterhouse, undated mimeo).

25. J. E. Siemon, "Case Mix and Data Quality," *Topics in Health Records Management* 2, No. 4 (1982):13-22.

26. L. Appleton and D. Schneider, "A Methodology for Assessing Data Quality's Effect on Reimbursement," *Topics in Health Record Management* 4, No. 3 (1984):56-65.

27. Ibid.

28. *Reliability of Hospital Discharge Abstracts* (Washington, DC: National Academy of Sciences, Institute of Medicine, 1977).

29. U.S. Congress, Office of Technology Assessment, *Diagnosis Related Groups (DRGs) and the Medicare Program: Implications for Medical Technology,* Washington, DC, OTA-TM-H-17, July 1983, pp. 6, 51-52.

30. *Reliability of Hospital Discharge Abstracts,* Institute of Medicine.

31. *Reliability of Hospital Discharge Records* (Washington, DC: National Academy of Sciences, Institute of Medicine, 1980).

32. Jackson, "The New DRGs."

33. H. D. Doremus and E. M. Michenzi, "Data Quality. An Illustration of It's Potential Impact Upon a Diagnosis-Related Group's Case-Mix Index and Reimbursement," *Medical Care* 21, No. 10 (1983):1001-1011.

34. L. K. Demlo, P. M. Campbell, and S. S. Brown, "Reliability of Information Abstracted from Patient's Medical Records," *Medical Care* 16, No. 12 (1978):995-1005.

35. L. K. Demlo and P. M. Campbell, "Improving Hospital Discharge Data: Lessons from the National Hospital Discharge Survey," *Medical Care* 19, No. 1 (1981):1030-1040.

36. C. Bernard and T. Esmond, "DRG-Based Reimbursement: The Use of Concurrent and Retrospective Clinical Data," *Medical Care* 19, No. 11 (1981):1071-1082.

37. Appleton and Schneider, "A Methodology."

38. Ibid.

39. H. L. Smits and R. E. Watson, "DRG and the Future of Surgical Practice," *New England Journal of Medicine* 311, No. 25 (December 20, 1984):1612-1615.

40. B. J. Thomas and R. L. Loup, "Quality Control of Diagnosis and Procedure Coding," *Topics in Health Records Management* 4, No. 3 (1984):46-55.

41. Ibid.

42. *Reliability of Hospital Discharge Abstracts,* Institute of Medicine.

43. Thompson and Loup, "Quality Control."

44. Doremus and Michenzi, "Data Quality. An Illustration."

45. R. F. Corn, "The Sensitivity of Prospective Hospital Reimbursement to Errors in Patient Data," *Inquiry* 18, No. 4 (Winter, 1981):351-360.

46. F. A. Connell, L. A. Blide, and M. A. Hanken, "Ambiguities in the Selection of the Principal Diagnosis: Impact on Data Quality, Hospital Statistics and DRGs," *Journal of AMRA* 55, No. 2 (1984):18-23.

47. Ibid.

48. A. N. Johnson and G. L. Appel, "DRGs and Hospital Case Records: Implications for Medicare Case Mix Accuracy," *Inquiry* 21 (Summer, 1984):128-134.

49. Ibid.

50. A. B. Bindman, L. F. Eichenfield, and S. A. Geller, "Diagnosis-Related Groups: Physician and Abstractor Reliability and Financial Significance of Errors," *Mt. Sinai Journal of Medicine* 51, No. 3 (1984):237-245.

51. "Medicare Claim Analysis Software Distributed to Fiscal Intermediaries," *Hospitals* 58, No. 9 (May 1, 1984):21.

52. Doremus and Michenzi, "Data Quality: An Illustration."

53. P. L. Grimaldi and J. A. Micheletti, "On the Homogeneity of Diagnostic Related Group

(DRGs)," *Journal of AMRA* 51, No. 10 (1980):43-49.

54. P. L. Grimaldi and J. A. Micheletti, "Homogeneity Revisited," *Journal of AMRA* 55, No. 4 (1982):56-70.

55. Ibid.

56. H. Boerma, "Hospital Organization Improves," *Hospitals* 57, No. 2 (January 16, 1983):50, 59.

57. P. Y. Ertel and R. V. Harrison, "Ethical and Operational Issues Concerning DRGs and the Prospective Payment System," *Topics in Health Record Management* 4, No. 3 (1984):10-31.

58. "DRGs Impact Would Hit MDs and Medical Records Personnel," *Hospital Peer Review* 8, No. 1 (1983):1-3.

59. Ertel and Harrison, "Ethical and Operational Issues."

60. R. J. Serculo and K. Johnson, "Importance of Medical Record Process in a DRG Based System," *Quality Review Bulletin* 9, No. 9 (1983):268-272.

61. R. J. Shakno, *Physician's Guide to DRGs* (Chicago: Pluribus Press, Inc., 1984).

62. D. Burik, *Case Mix Studies. Statement of Qualifications* (Chicago: Price Waterhouse, undated mimeo).

63. "Experts Offer Computer Security Tips," *Hospitals* 58, No. 4 (February 16, 1984):19-20.

64. *Role in Prospective Payment,* American Medical Records Association.

65. "Veterans of New Jersey's System Assess DRG Based Reimbursement," *Hospitals* 56, No. 23 (December 1, 1982):35, 37.

66. J. B. Flanagan and K. J. Sourapas, "Preparing for Prospective Payment. Organizational Issues and Ideas. Part IV," *Journal of AMRA* 55, No. 2 (1984):15-17.

67. H. Boerma, *The Organizational Impact of DRGs. Volume IV-B* (Princeton: Health Research and Educational Trust of New Jersey, January, 1983), pp. 28-29, 32-35.

68. P. L. Grimaldi and J. A. Micheletti, *Diagnosis Related Groups. A Practitioner's Guide* (Chicago:Pluribus Press, 1983).

69. MacDonald, "Accurate Medical Records."

70. Ertel and Harrison, "Ethical and Operational Issues."

71. Savitt, "Impact of DRGs."

72. "Another Violation of Section 1801," *Private Practice* 16, No. 7 (1984):20.

73. D. L. Angellis, "Government Insults Physicians (letter)," *New England Journal of Medicine* 311, No. 2 (July 12, 1984):131.

74. "Another Violation of Section 1801," *Private Practice.*

75. Ibid.

76. Angellis, "Government Insults Physicians."

77. D. L. Gibbons, "AMA Delegates Want Growing Influence of 'Outsiders' on Medicine Curtailed," *Medical World News* 25, No. 14 (July 23, 1983):74, 78-82.

78. "AMA Hits Modified Attestation Statement," *American Medical News* 27, No. 29 (August 3, 1984):7.

79. "Rule on MD Attestation Should be Rescinded" (editorial), *American Medical News* 27, No. 29 (August 3, 1984:4.

80. Ibid.

81. Ibid.

82. "AMA Hits Modified Attestation Statement," *American Medical News.*

83. Nathanson, "Medical Records' New Financial Role."

84. Ibid.

85. L. K. Lichtig, "Impact of DRGs on Data Processing" in *Diagnosis-Related Groups: The Effect in New Jersey. The Potential for the Nation.* HCFA Pub. No. 03170 (March, 1984):86.

86. MacDonald, "Accurate Medical Records."

87. Flanagan and Sourapas, "Preparing for Prospective Payment."

88. "The DRG Management Information System. Making Your Management Reports Perform. Part II," *DRG Monitor* 1, No. 4 (1983):1-8.

89. "Hot Times for Hospital Software," *Fortune,* August 6, 1984.

90. J. Alsofrom, "Playing the Numbers Game," *Medical World News* 24, No. 20 (October 24, 1983):38-40, 45-46, 51-55.

91. J. Riffer, "PPS Prompts Development of Software to Monitor Costs," *Hospitals* 58, No. 7 (April 1, 1984):39-40.

92. "PPS May Boost Data Base Usage," *Hospitals* 58, No. 7 (April 1, 1984):49.

93. B. Christensen, "'Staging' Software Measures Severity of Patient's Illness," *Hospitals* 58, No. 9 (May 1, 1984):45-46.

94. J. S. Gonnella, M. C. Hornbrook, and D. Z. Louis, "Staging of Disease. A Case-Mix Measurement," *Journal of American Medical Assocation* 251, No. 5 (February 3, 1984):637-644.

95. F. M. Jaggar and D. F. Pugliese, "A PPS Essential: Case-Mix Management Systems," *Hospitals* 58, No. 9 (May 1, 1984):71, 73-74, 76.

96. Ibid.

97. S. I. Dorenfest, "Computers Can Figure Out DRGs, If You Can Figure Out Computer Market," *Modern Healthcare* 14, No. 3 (February 15, 1984):130, 134, 136.

98. C. Hulm and D. Burik, "Evaluating the New Case-Mix Systems," *Hospitals* 58, No. 2 (January 16, 1984):92-96.

99. J. Fedorowicz and S. Veazie, "Automated DRG Systems: Unanswered Questions," *Hospital Progress* 62, No. 1 (1981):54-55, 71.

100. J. Fedorowicz, "Hospital Information Systems: Are We Ready for Case Mix Applications?" *Health Care Management Review* 8.

101. C. L. Packer, "Automation in the Medical Records Department," *Hospitals* 59, No. 5 (March 1, 1985):100, 102, 104.

102. "DRGs Demand Medical Record Software," *Hospitals* 58, No. 7 (April 1, 1984):75.

103. G. D. Zuidema, P. E. Dans, and E. D. Dunlap, "Documentation of Care and Prospective Payment," *Annals of Surgery* 199, No. 5 (1984):515-521.

104. J. B. Flanagan and K. J. Sourapas, "Productivity in the Medical Records Department. Part V," *Journal of AMRA* 55, No. 3 (1984):23-25.

CHAPTER 6
Effect on Health Professionals

Physicians

"Physicians control patient-care costs; they are the purchasing agents of patient-care services. Physicians are key determinants of hospital revenue, patient-care costs and the quality of care."[1] Physicians react strongly when their unique role is questioned, constrained, or limited, and when their judgments are challenged or put to the test. DRGs have been imposed without their participation in planning, testing, or implementation; rules and regulations have been promulgated despite physicians' formal objections and against their protestations and lobbying efforts.

Physicians believe that the DRG system, in practice, interferes with their patient care decisions on admissions, process of care, and length of stay; from their point of view, their value to the hospital is being questioned and their activities controlled and limited. They fear that the quality of care has been reduced and that they are potentially liable for more malpractice suits under practice constraints.

Various specialists have unique problems with the DRG system as applied to their limited codes, and are concerned about the favored status of surgical and procedure-oriented colleagues, as compared to those with cognitive specialties and skills. Physician fee DRGs have been proposed and are expected to be finalized shortly in some form. There will be prospective payments for physician care in private offices bundled with hospital inpatient care; these payments may be adjusted for severity of illness, or time spent with each patient, or on diagnosis, or on other alternatives. As a cost containment effort, the Medicare freeze is in place; it is a reality for elderly patients.

Blasting the DRG system as a "destructive" regulatory solution to the Medicare cost problems, an internist at St. Joseph Hospital in Chicago took action. With the support of his colleagues, Dr. John B. Watson placed a $3,640 full-page advertisement in the *Chicago Tribune* that vented his anger in an open letter to President Reagan.[2]

233

Distrust mounts. Although physicians may find that a good relationship with hospitals must be maintained for mutual financial solvency, they may also feel threatened by many hospital programs: utilization review, barriers to admitting privileges, inservice education, and the credentialling and reappointment process for sanctions against physicians. The AMA has joined forces with the AHA to add strength to both lawsuits and attempts to modify federal autocracy.

Patients and families confronted with the fallout of DRG turn to physicians as negotiators with, or allies against, the system; they, however, turn on physicians when they find that the doctors' reaction is incompatible with their own perceived needs and ability to cope with the system or with life-threatening illness or disability.

Impinging on Physician Prerogatives

Physicians will be encouraged not to admit patients with complex medical problems, and will be pressured to admit people who could be taken care of on an outpatient basis.[3]

There likely will be subtle and overt pressures on physicians to shorten the length of stay and reduce services to Medicare patients.[4]

Physician reward systems at the hospital under DRG are related to admitting the least sick, and keeping them for short stays. Those that are most sick are to be managed with minimal use of high technology, lab tests, X-rays, and so on, and shunted to alternative care facilities as quickly as possible.

Outpatient surgery will not be encouraged: the overnight hernia patient will be more profitable for hospitals than the outpatient case.[5]

Instead, the spurt in growth of surgicenters and hospital-based outpatient services is founded on new medical care techniques, patient interest, insurance reimbursements, and hospitals' concern in a new revenue-producing area. This explosive growth has not really affected the quantity of inpatient surgery (only a 7 percent reduction), despite the availability.[6] More surgery is being performed, in total, in multiple settings.

With office practice not under the current PPS/DRG system, physicians may have an incentive "to perform more procedures in physicians' offices . . . the system puts the physicians in a position of conflict between the interests of their patients and financial considerations of the hospital."[7]

There, services are not monitored and are dependent solely on the individual physician and the patient satisfaction with outcome—a very, very private affair. "There will be pressures to tailor the delivery of services to the DRG allowance and a consequent stimulus to undertreatment."[8]

Limiting hospital-based availability of certain options for diagnosis and treatment in the name of economy and efficiency constrains the patients' workup and may have an impact on subsequent outcome of care. Physicians will be brought into the process of developing criteria and standardizing the process of care for certain diagnostic categories or DRGs. Rationing specialized services will stimulate discussions of the ethics of certain issues, including DNR (do not resuscitate) orders, living wills, hemodialysis for the elderly, coma care, feeding the elderly, terminal care, and so on. Each of these areas interposes the hospital's fiscal-driven needs between the physician and the patient/family needs, judgments, expectations, and process of care; each changes the nature of the doctor-patient relationship.[9-11]

Homogeneous Medical Care and Homogenized Physicians

Computers storing huge amounts of inpatient data for fiscal and administrative purposes provide opportunities for assimilation of medical information by diagnosis, by physician, and by resource utilization. Physicians view this "big brother" approach with alarm when hospital administrators, colleagues, or possibly patients have access to practice pattern information.

> The medical staff will have a very real stimulus to evaluate its members' therapeutic customs and rituals, and eventually to achieve suitable measurements of the effectiveness of care and the appropriate use of resources.[12]

> It is likely that hospitals will attempt to influence physician behavior to achieve more favorable reimbursement.[13]

> Computer monitoring of doctors that DRGs seem to necessitate can be used either as a weapon in the fighting, or as a tool to resolve it.[14]

> We are now organizing groups of three to five doctors . . . in their specialty and providing them with data on the diagnostic and treatment charges for each big-volume DRG. . . . that information, along with their own clinical judgment and medical literature searches, [is] to set standards for patient care by diagnosis consistent with DRG payments levels.[15]

Some of the software computer packages were originally developed for the hospitals in New Jersey and are based on "accounting rules designed to reveal physicians with high-cost practice patterns,"[16] but need adjustment for any particular physician or group in a specific hospital or locale. Questions are raised as to the validity of cost and clinical comparisons made at specific institutions with computer norms developed elsewhere.[17] "Certainly there will be many cases where doctors repudiate norms, focusing instead on individual patient needs. Furthermore, patients are not likely to want their physicians functioning as efficiency experts in matters pertaining to their health."[18]

Adequacy of documentation in the medical record may provide another source of contention. Richard S. Wilbur, M.D., executive vice president of the Council of Medical Specialty Societies, indicates that "physicians may be pressured to put down the most remunerative diagnosis for each patient . . . this [is] a particular problem with Medicare patients, who often have multiple ailments, such as arthritis, diabetes, and hypertension."[19]

Physicians and hospitals are concerned that medical record data might be unreliable and that discharge abstracts are faulty, causing unnecessary confrontations between physicians and hospitals, and resulting in dire fiscal consequences.[20] In addition, "problems relating to the timeliness and accuracy of the charts may strain relationships between physicians and administrators."[21]

> This system obliges hospital management . . . to review performance
> of physicians in the hospital based on productivity and profitability as
> defined by third-party payers.[22]

Joseph Boyle, M.D., Chairman of the AMA Board of Trustees, says: "Physicians don't get upset having their practices monitored—it's what's done with the results that's of concern."[23]

Physicians will be considered "losers" or "winners" for the hospital and their value will be measured accordingly. Deviations from norms will need to be reduced and practice brought into line to reduce cost outliers. This system's dependence on uniformity and standardization of practice reduces independence and results in bland, lackluster, homogenized medicine. The art of medicine is expected to decline as more algorithms of care are adopted. "If the hospital cannot survive financially without controlling the physician's activities, it will restrict privileges to physicians who cooperate."[24] Strategies to change physician behavior for inpatient care include:

- Raising their "cost consciousness"

- Educating them about DRGs

- Providing financial incentives and disincentives related to hospital finances

- Providing feedback on individual results of clinical decisions and providing comparisons to other colleagues

- Participatory management of hospital policy and decisions which might have an impact on quality of care.[25]

Sanctions against physicians may be used to curb aberrant practices and may impinge on continuing clinical privileges and reappointment to the medical staff. When renewing applications, hospital boards and trustees find the need "to ask hard questions about data and to evaluate the physicians past performance."[26]

John E. Affeldt, M.D., President of the Joint Commission on Accreditation of Hospitals, says, "Being qualified may no longer be enough . . . a hospital may well consider whether the doctor can contribute to its overall marketing plan."[27]

A recent court case in New Jersey upheld the right of a hospital board to deny reappointment to the medical staff of a physician who refused to cooperate on utilization standards and cost the hospital about a quarter of a million dollars in reimbursement.[28]

At Mount Sinai Hospital in New York City, the board approved an amendment to the medical staff bylaws stating that the hospital director may temporarily suspend admitting and clinical privileges of staff members who fail to comply with the requirements of TEFRA.[29] The hospital director also notified the medical staff of the proposed sanctions for noncompliance with PRO program requirements.

Physician and Hospital Tensions

Perhaps the most significant new development arising out of the PPS/DRG plan has to do with the financial aspects of medicine. Previously, most physicians did not bother to consider the cost of any procedure as long as the patient would benefit. In fact, surveys have repeatedly shown that physicians did not know the costs of various tests and procedures. While discussing "surgonomics," Muñoz summed up the current situation: "Physicians must now begin to examine the incremental costs and incremental benefits of their actions. This will become the challenge for the future. The days of 'costs are no object' are over!"[30]

This cost crisis has existed for a considerable amount of time. At a 1976 American Medical Association meeting, then Secretary of Health, Education and Welfare Joseph Califano squarely placed the physician in the hot seat: "The U.S. can no longer afford doctors' insensitivity to costs. . . . A profound structural, long-term reform of health care is imminent, and doctors will be in the middle."[31]

After years of practicing "defensive medicine" to assure that everything possible was done to benefit the patient and incidentally reduce the risk of a malpractice suit, physicians now are being urged to change their outlook on medical care. Hospital managers are doing the urging and thereby the physician/ hospital relationships are reoriented into conflicting interest zones. "In the hospital/physician relationship, each side must balance conflicting incentives," comments Lewis.[32]

Hospitals have to remain competitive, attract admissions, and constrain utilization of services to remain within DRG allowances. Underutilization of services could possibly lead to liability risks. Putting off technology purchases could lead to patients going elsewhere. Internal conflicts and hostility between medical staff and hospital executives could make the hospital an unpleasant place to recover from an illness.

Physicians are motivated to do everything possible for their patients by their ethical code and by prior habits of using hospital services intensely. It is possible that admitting privileges may be revoked or other sanctions taken to change the medical practice patterns of the staff.

A current headline in *Medical World News* proclaimed: "Pressures Set Hospitals, Medical Staff at Odds."[33] In a nationwide teleconference, the economic and bureaucratic pressures were blamed for creating a deep and growing chasm between physicians and hospital administrators. "DRG-itis" was the specific organism credited with the inflammation. Management monitoring of the cost effectiveness of care was and is a major bone of contention. Other sources of friction revolve around legal liability for inefficient, overcostly care, new hospital ventures infringing on traditional private practice territory, and the resolution of disputes. Describing the battlefield during the teleconference, Cannon remarked that "the spirit of cooperation is being overcome by activities, practices, and policies generating distrust and even animosity," when physicians and administrators should be working together to keep their hospital afloat.[34]

Physicians fit well into the traditional hospital managerial structure that is organized around cost and revenue centers. Most physicians associate with the unit of their concern and the manager in charge of that department. "This fragmented administrative authority is the antithesis of the patient care related integrative approach of the DRG reimbursement system."[35] In fact, Shortell calls the voluntary medical staff structure an "anachronism" that is on its way out. He suggests that medical staff privileges may be replaced by wholly independent physician groups, with their own bylaws and structure, contracting with hospitals to supply services.[36]

Spivey comments that physicians control an estimated 60 to 70 percent of health care expenditures. Under PPS, hospital managers will gain some control over the introduction of new and sophisticated equipment, because they will want to be assured that the innovations improve efficiency and lower costs. After reviewing the vantage points of both the physician and the managers, Spivey concludes that the two sides have to work together as partners. Even though the points of view may differ, cooperation will be essential. He concludes his article by stating: "Without this spirit of cooperation, all concerned will suffer—and not least, the patient."[37]

In discussing the challenge of DRG payment to hospital management, Bassett describes how a hospital can cope with the situation. He suggests that physicians be educated as to what is required of them under the DRG procedures, with emphasis upon diagnoses and the relation to reimbursement. In addition, the hospital should develop a historical database for each of its physicians and provide feedback to the individual physicians about their activities.[38] However, Young and Saltman find two limitations on the maneuverability of the hospital's managers. First, the autonomy of the physician is well grounded in a fee-for-service system of payment that creates little incentive to control costs. This traditional financial freedom of physicians also hinders the hospital's efforts to integrate physicians into the institution's control system. Secondly, the historical "power equilibrium" rested with the medical staff and a collegial decision-making apparatus evolved rather than "a hierarchical supervisory arrangement."

Young and Saltman, both academic management experts, propose the "development of a semiautonomous managerial control module for physicians, in which the emphasis is on their self-regulation as a collectively responsible group. Such a module . . . could be built around inputs per case as the cost influencing variable directly under physician control. . . ."[39] This technique incorporates the doctors into the management control system, an essential cog in any successful cost containment effort. Since the hospitals are at risk for the practice behavior of the physicians, it is vital to achieve management understandings with the physicians.

Despite the obvious need for cooperation, Shortell predicts even more turmoil when PPS expands to include physician reimbursement also. Notice that Shortell said "when," not if—since he expects that expansion to be inevitable. His prognosis for the future is bleak: "If you think there's competition and hysteria out there now between hospital administrators and doctors, it's going to increase all the more as doctors realize they'll need to increase their own market share and volume."[40]

In testimony before a Congressional committee that considered the PPS before adoption in 1983, Rabkin spoke for the Association of American Medical Colleges and told the senators that the PPS "threatens hospital-physician relationships." Bromberg, representing the Federation of American Hospitals, agreed that the delicate relationship could be abruptly changed. Headline writers for the *American Medical News*, the official American Medical Association newspaper, also agreed and proclaimed: "Congress Told DRG Plan May Hurt Hospital-MD Ties."[41] *Hospitals* collected opinions and comments from medical staff leaders about management/physician relations under PPS. Sandrick reported about the adversarial stances, the bottom line mentality of the managers, the emphasis on quality care by physicians, the impact on access to care by patients, and the joint concerns of both parties. Interestingly, she quotes John J. Coury, Jr., chairman of the AMA's Board of Trustees, responding to the situation of an overutilizing physician who refuses to change his or her practice pattern: "If a physician is grossly inefficient, grossly overutilizing, he is going to have to change his way of practice or he'll lose his staff privileges, and rightfully so."[42]

In 1984, a conference on "Physicians and Hospitals: The Great Partnership at the Crossroads" invited 36 leaders in the health care field to discuss their problems. Areas covered included the role of feedback, the evolving relationship, different organizational forms, and the multihospital systems. Iglehart reported on the conference and included numerous quotes and comments on the uneasy alliance. Thompson, a participant who helped develop the DRG system, addressed the problem: "The gauze curtain between the medical records room and the financial office must disappear, allowing both the trustees and the physicians to relate the cost of treatment to the quality of care. Armed with this information, both parties in the uneasy alliance will be managing patient care with a common set of standards, both professional and fiscal."[43]

A contradictory message arose from the varied view of these leaders in the health care industry. On one hand, the call is out to contain costs and reduce the burden. On the other hand, that is to be achieved without affecting the quality of care and without rationing the quantity of care.

Physicians as Management

While the contradiction may not be immediately resolved, forces are pressing to move physicians into the management team. McMahon posits that physicians are expected to have an expanded role in hospital management under the DRGs. He states that currently "the medical staff structure is more feudal than managerial in nature." Therefore, McMahon argues that the doctor must not only manage patient care, but also must manage the instruments of that care.[44] Even while Ellwood remarked that physician cooperation is needed under PPS, he also pointed out that doctors are not part of the PPS system at this time.[45] Speaking to an AHA National Council of Hospital Governing Boards, a partner in a national health care consulting firm told the audience that DRGs demand physician involvement in management. Ertel went even further and urged physicians to master DRGs and help the administrators rescue the hospitals. He said: "In the final analysis, only physicians can identify the inequities in the DRG payment system and sort through the gray areas."[46]

Also anticipating the enlargement of the physician's hospital management role, Smits told attendees at a 1984 annual meeting of the American College of Physicians that a hospital can't be run "in a way opaque to doctors."[47] Relating to costs, Smits, a physician, continued: "We have an obligation to practice realistic, careful, parsimonious medicine. We need to know the relative value of things. . . . This is a clinical system; it's far too important a piece of economics to be left to the economists."[48,49]

At that same meeting, a political scientist noted that administrators would gain in authority relative to physicians if DRGs worked as advertised. In addition, Sapolsky said that decision-making power would shift and managers would "direct rather than respond to physician behavior." To seize the initiative, Young and Saltman recommend a semiautonomous managerial control module run by physicians.[50] In a similar approach, Ellwood suggested the development of MeSH (Medical Staff and Hospital) to be "a newly formed corporation as a discrete business entity owned equally by the hospital and the members of the medical staff who choose to participate."[51] MeSH evenly balances rights, responsibilities, and control. However, MeSH has not been enthusiastically accepted. Ellwood believes that physicians are reluctant to change the traditional management patterns.

Thus, there appears to be agreement that physicians must cooperate with management to ensure a hospital's viability under DRGs. However, exactly how the doctors will operate as part of the management team is not clear. Some doctors—pathologists, for example—even have a fear of being fired as hospital administrators trim laboratory costs.[52] Some call for physicians to be "product line managers" in an industrial chain of command, while others lean toward doctors developing innovative managerial models to maintain controls over their own activities.

DRG coordinator as intermediary. A possible alleviation of physician/hospital tensions may occur through the employment of a new professional—the DRG Coordinator. A recent want ad for such a position described the tasks as follows: "As DRG Coordinator, you will monitor Medicare patients on admission to determine DRG and coordinate proper treatment programs. Ability to interact with all levels of management is necessary."[53]

DRG coordinators need "to be able to speak the language of physicians one minute, medical records people the next, and administration the next."[54] Therefore, it has been suggested that DRG coordinators need a solid clinical background, a strong medical records comprehension, and an understanding of finances. It may be difficult to find a person with this combination of education and experience. Coordinators have come from the ranks of nurses, utilization and/or quality assurance reviewers, medical records administrators, management, and even retired physicians. In any event, "the key to being a successful DRG coordinator is to carry information to the right people, such as chiefs of staff, physician utilization review committee heads, or administrators," according to a director of health care finances at a large urban teaching hospital and a former DRG coordinator.[55] Perhaps that is why DRG coordinators describe themselves as translators, troubleshooters, watchdogs, liaisons, and go-betweens. Hidden in this list of descriptive task analysis words is the supposition that DRG co-ordinators do not report directly to physicians. Despite the indirect line of communication, nonphysician DRG coordinators may be, in effect, telling a doctor how to practice medicine. Obviously, the possibility for conflict and confrontation is quite high. In one example, a family practitioner's medical practice patterns cost the 240-bed hospital $22,000 each quarter for the patients he treated. After reviewing the DRG coordinator's report, the hospital's utilization review committee suggested to that physician that he change his habits. He replied that he could not and left the area.[56]

Advice to physicians.   Based on their on-the-job experiences, several DRG coordinators offer the following practical advice to physicians on making PPS a smooth operation:

- Listen, keep an open mind, and try not to be insulted by what finance people do. Remember that they are following the rules and regulations that mean dollars and cents to the hospital.

- Know the financial impact of your practice patterns on your hospital. Review your standing orders, your use of pharmaceuticals, and your performance as compared to your peers.

- Educate yourself about the information systems your hospital has available to you. Get copies of printouts relating to your practice patterns and work with your administrator.

- Make sure that you have an awareness of the ground rules under which hospitals must function under PPS. This includes timely chart completion and proper diagnostic documentation.[57]

Growth and organizational mode.   Keeping up with professional inclinations, DRG coordinators formed a DRG Management Association in New Jersey, as more and more of these new professionals were appointed. Currently, the Association is expanding nationwide. An informal 1985 poll by *Hospitals* found "that they [DRG Coordinators] are popping up in all types of facilities—from small or rural hospitals to large metropolitan hospitals to multihospital systems."[58] No exact count could be given on the number employed throughout the country. Within this rapid growth pattern, a wide variation exists in job responsibilities and also in the management styles for DRG coordinators.

In the chain of command, the DRG coordinator can be an independent member of the management team, can report to the finance director, can report to the medical staff director, or can report to the hospital administrator.

Some DRG coordinators function as a one-person department while others are responsible for a number of units, such as medical records, quality assurance, and utilization review. However, most of the coordinators were already employed at the hospital as director of one of the other departments when he or she was appointed to the new position, according to the *Hospitals* poll.[59] One multihospital system has a DRG coordinator to supervise activities in all 10 member hospitals. However, another large proprietary hospital chain leaves it up to each individual facility. Still other hospitals incorporate DRG coordination responsibilities into already existing positions, such as quality assurance or utilization review management. Regardless of the management style, the *Hospitals* survey found that the DRG coordinator's responsibilities consistently included supervision of utilization review and quality assurance departments.[60]

From the administrator's point of view, the main job of someone in this new position is quite clear: "DRG coordinators analyze their hospital's DRG-related information and identify departments that are causing their facilities to lose money. Once they find them, their job is to bring the information to the appropriate groups, such as chiefs of staffs, department heads, or administrators, and help analyze the information, learn the reasons for the financial loss, and recommend ways to resolve it."[61]

Specialty Concerns

Hospital-based physicians. Services of hospital-based radiologists, as well as hospital-based radiology departments, are changing to meet the demands of efficiency and cost containment of DRG planning and implementation. These departments, which were once revenue generating on the inpatient side, are now cost centers, with the price of their services rolled into each DRG.

Managing radiology departments requires data related to utilization patterns for all types of imaging services per DRG. Services should be organized to be responsive to the emerging trends in altered use of X-rays, diagnostic procedures, and therapeutic modalities.

> DRG 14—cerebrovascular disorders, expect transient ischemic attacks. At one hospital, radiology utilization and charges had dropped significantly over a one year internal study. The manager of diagnostic radiology services and the case mix data-base coordinator then were able to focus their further studies on specific alternate procedures used in diagnosis, in order to put the cost implications into perspective.[62]

To be as cost-effective as possible, the hospital must analyze staffing, equipment, supplies, space use, and resource allocations so it can respond to the demand to expedite discharges, reduce LOS, and coordinate services with other disciplines. Functionally disjointed departments and inefficient filing, retrieval, and reporting systems are no longer tolerable. Expansion of outpatient services to aid preadmission routines and to satisfy new demands for community-based services are attractive marketing strategies that require reorganization and re-alignment of traditional services.[63,64]

Ordering radiologic tests has increased as physicians become more dependent on imaging, rather than clinical observation; incentives for reimbursement are increasingly tied to tests, and defensive practices are becoming more routine. Some tests are ordered by habit, or because of institutional demands; some are ordered to minimize clinical error. "This unfettered response has led to real and identifiable waste in the current system."[65]

Radiologists are urged to expand their role as consultant to other physicians so that the most appropriate imaging tests are ordered for diagnostic purposes. Guides and protocols for sequencing examinations and lists of indications for certain procedures, costs of exams, and other techniques can enable the primary physicians to be more cost-efficient in their diagnostic approaches. Some pread-mission testing could be performed in outpatient settings to further reduce LOS.

William P. Shuman, M.D. and his colleagues at the University of Washington School of Medicine contend, "If we physicians cannot alter expensive and sometimes irrational patterns of practice, changes will be imposed by a bureau-cracy much less interested in the quality of patient care, the morale of physicians, or the future of diagnostic imaging."[66]

As hospital-based physicians, pathologists are seeking new contractual rela-tionships with administration. Their traditional domain, laboratory testing, makes them important contributors in clinical diagnosis and case management. Given the hospital's concerns for reducing costs and reducing the number of tests per patient, the pathology department will play a significant role in cost containment. A greater emphasis on outpatient and preadmission testing will cause adminis-trators to consider moving laboratories outside the hospital. "Pathologists will seek methods to do this, either on their own or with neighboring pathologists, or laboratory companies."[67] However, if the hospitals consider doing this, "such a step is considered illegal and is part of the 'unbundling' that is forbidden."[68]

While independent laboratories might grow across the country, hospitals are not likely to expand in this area. Instead, administrators will explore shared services among institutions or with outside laboratories, so that some consoli-dation is achieved and costs are reduced.

Pathologists are urged to manage their departments efficiently by reviewing staffing, instrumentation, purchasing of supplies, inventory controls, reference laboratory services, and use of shared services. Their expertise is necessary for medical staff policy developments on preadmission testing and automatic stop orders on daily laboratory tests. They may also help to educate other physicians on appropriate testing and costs for certain procedures.

Trying to gain reimbursement for pathologist services under Part B of Med-icare, the College of American Pathologists (CAP) lost a court suit against HHS

Secretary Margaret Heckler. This "unbundling" was not permitted, and the decision was reaffirmed in a ruling issued May 11, 1984 by the U.S. Court of Appeals for the District of Columbia. That ruling upheld a 1982 federal regulation that pathologist services do not constitute consultant services and should therefore be considered under Part A of Medicare as general hospital expenses. One report of the case stated that "anatomic pathology, some consultation and the personal administration of test devices and materials are excluded from the government's cost saving measure."[69]

The attorney for the pathologists responded to the Court's decision: "The regulations go beyond what Congress intended."[70]

Stress on clinical laboratories which are directed by pathologists is widespread. The new hospital stand on lab tests is becoming, "Don't let a late lab test be the reason for keeping a patient in this hospital. Get the results faster, get the reference work back faster."[71] At the Newark Beth Israel Medical Center, a 550-bed inner-city hospital, schedule changes helped speed results to patients' charts. "We try to offer more procedures on weekends and evenings in order to have the data sooner, and the patient treated and out the door faster."[72]

Staffing is aided at other institutions which have adopted 10-hour overlapping workdays, flexible scheduling, downstaffing with technicians, and the introduction of new technology.[73]

William V. Harrer, M.D., President of the New Jersey Society of Pathologists, laments, "You keep hearing about cutting costs. . . . DRG regulation aims to offer adequate care—not quality care as I was trained to provide it."[74]

Interactions between pathologists and primary physicians can result in changing patterns of test ordering. However, caution and diplomacy are necessary in this highly sensitive area. "Certain people on the medical staff are unapproachable. At our community hospital, each physician is a little private enterprise, and nobody is going to tell some of them what to do."[75]

Physician education is a critical element for the promotion of change—by increasing knowledge of newer diagnostic tests, appropriate sequencing, and higher level of consciousness of test costs of each test and the frequency of repeated testing. Utilization review and patterns of testing for DRGs with the highest laboratory costs helps to identify specific physicians, as well as the potential for pathologists' input into protocols for testing.

In attempting to make the best of DRGs, pathologists at the West Virginia University Hospital Medical Center presented this opinion: "We firmly believe that those of us in laboratory medicine, working with enlightened clinicians, can ultimately do a better job at a lower cost . . . and . . . can develop test strategies that will prove to be more cost-effective than present methods."[76]

Other specialists. Compression of diagnoses into the 467 DRGs provides areas of concern to certain specialists. Otolaryngologists point out that some inequities are apparent:

- DRG 50, sialoadenectomy. Total parotidectomy is more complex procedure in terms of time, blood loss and hospital stay than is excision of the submandibular gland, yet the hospital will be reimbursed at the same amount.[77]

- DRG 57, tonsil biopsy reimbursement, is higher than DRG 59, tonsillectomy. While the best way to do a biopsy of a tonsil is to remove it entirely in some situations, the "hospital administrator may direct (me) to do otherwise."[78]

- DRG 49 contains all the procedures for head and neck cancer. The incentive is for physicians and hospitals to elect to care only for patients with less advanced cases of head and neck cancer.

Clinicians in obstetrics and gynecology are concerned that they will wind up in the middle. "Hospitals will be pressuring them to send patients home, while patients—aware that staying longer costs no more—will be urging their doctors to permit longer stays."[79] In addition, they are concerned that fewer tests will be allowed and that they will need "to select the most remunerative diagnosis."

Ophthalmologists provide care to many patients in the Medicare age group. They have concern about the coding system and the weights that will be assigned in their specialty:

- DRG 39 lens procedures. Does discission of an after-cataract have the same relative weight as a cataract extraction? Both are listed in this DRG.

- DRG 37 orbital procedures. Does correction of trichiasis carry the same relative weight as resection of an orbital tumor? Both are listed in this DRG.

They are aware that, as in other surgical specialties, the selection of the anesthetic used, the time in the operating room, the number of lab tests done, and the LOS affect the hospital cost and contend that "to balance these factors and still provide superior medical and surgical care will require superhuman effort."[80]

In a study of patients with rheumatoid arthritis (RA) and systemic lupus erythematosus (SLE) at the University Hospital at Indiana University School of Medicine, the implications of potential coding under DRG 240 and DRG 241 (Connective Tissue Disorders) were explored.[81] Not all patients were elderly (only 15.6%) and, unless all payers adopt the DRG payment methodology, rheumatologists may not be too concerned. However, as a specialty which is heavily dependent on OT, PT, and rehabilitation, devices and prosthetics, and one-to-one therapies, the hospital strategy to reduce ancillary services or staffing and push for outpatient services and premature discharge puts these patients at particular risk. Also under attack is the pharmacological dependence on the newer nonsteroidal anti-inflammatory drugs (NSAIDs), which are more expensive than the widely used and inexpensive aspirin, known for its propensity for toxicity, "At least 18 States have already deleted, or considered deleting NSAIDs from their Medicaid formularies."[82]

Anesthesiologists—who are currently being reimbursed under Medicare Part B for their services and for the services of the nurse anesthetists whom they employ—will need to change their arrangements with each other and with the hospitals. Under the current guidelines and regulations, effective October 1, 1986, after a three-year transitional period, nurse anesthetists will be considered hospital-based, and included in the DRGs for surgical and other procedures as appropriate. Unless other changes are made, physicians will no longer be able to be reimbursed for services by anesthetists. In the interim, no new groups of anesthesiologists and nurse anesthetists may start to use Part B in this "unbundled" manner. The American Association of Nurse Anesthetists restated the federal policy in a memo to its members: "The right to bill under Medicare Part B for the services of the nurse anesthetists whom physicians employ is strictly limited to those physicians and physician groups which have customarily employed and billed on a reasonable charge basis for their nurse anesthetists."[83] For those hospitals that currently employ or contract with nurse anesthetists for their services, payments will be made by Medicare to the hospital, which will cover these services as part of the prospective payment to the hospital.

Impacts on surgeons and surgical practice are expected to be linked to the survival of hospitals, the reduction in total beds available, and the proposed greater usage of outpatient ambulatory surgical centers. Incentives in surgery have always been to get the patient admitted, operate, and discharge early, so as to admit others. The nonsurgical practitioner who is reimbursed on the basis of each hospital visit, rather than for the total surgical procedure, has a negative incentive to discharge the patient. It is anticipated that surgeons will be favored to nonsurgeons by hospital administrators.[84]

Cognitive services vs. procedural services. Reimbursement for procedural services of a diagnostic or therapeutic nature has been more rewarding to physicians than the cognitive services, such as history-taking, physical examination, visits to nursing homes or hospitals, and consultations. "Because third parties reimburse more generously for procedural services, they create financial incentives for more surgical procedures and diagnostic evaluation."[85]

These are considered "perverse incentives" by the ASIM. That association is trying to eliminate the perpetually disproportionate compensation for certain new procedures and to obtain more appropriate compensation for cognitive services. Some examples are cited:

- A surgeon receives three to seven times more money for an hour in the operating room than for an hour in the office or at the patient's bedside.

- A gynecologist's net income from surgery is five to ten times greater than the income from counseling.

- Payment for open heart surgery may be 10 times more than the payment for the overall treatment of a child with Reye's syndrome.[86]

Under the DRG system, the same differentials favoring surgical interventions seem to pervade the payment incentives. Several common disorders for which further medical management or surgery can be justified have severe financial implications:[87]

- Valve replacement (DRG 104) brings a payment 6.8 times higher than the medically-managed case (DRG 135).

- Insertion of a pacemaker (DRG 116) payment is 3 times higher than the medical treatment of the arrhythmias (DRG 139).

- Surgery (DRG 155) triples the payment for upper gastrointestinal bleeding (DRG 175) or peptic ulcer disease (DRG 178) when drug treatments to control acid secretion and endoscopic control of bleeding have greatly enhanced medical management.

With the known variability of physician practice and geographic differences in patterns of utilization of services and procedures, the question is rightly asked, "with such differentials in payment and in the expected profit margins, how will the decisions be made between surgical and medical care of individual patients?"[88]

In response to these issues, the Kansas Blue Cross/Blue Shield plan recently adjusted its fee schedules to favor cognitive services by restructuring some of the fees (some as much as 25 percent) for procedures and for smaller changes in fees for cognitive services. Dwight Wicker, Director of Professional Relations, indicates that this new reimbursement policy in Kansas, "has not changed all that much; we're still procedurally driven, and I wouldn't say that we brought about equity, but we are at least trying to move in that direction."[89]

In addition, Mountain Affiliates—a PPO in Denver—and Massachusetts Blue Shield have altered their reimbursement scales to recognize cognitive services to a greater degree.[90]

Physician Reimbursements

Control of physician reimbursement for services to Medicare beneficiaries is considered the next step in slowing the inflationary costs of health care. Jack

Hadley of the Urban Institute classifies the following approaches to alternative physician payment schemes:

- Proposals to change physician practice arrangements
- Proposals to change how Medicare sets fee levels
- Proposals to change the unit of service for which Medicare will pay.[91]

Alternative practice arrangements. Changing practice arrangements includes multiple strategies, such as health maintenance organizations (HMOs) and social HMOs, independent practice associations (IPAs), competitive bidding, the preferred provider organization (PPO), case management, health care brokers, and the primary care broker. "HMOs and IPAs are the most prevalent alternatives actually in existence, though they cover barely more than five percent of the nonelderly and an even smaller proportion of Medicare beneficiaries."[92]

These plans change fee-for-service practice to organizational arrangements which provide incentives for physicians to monitor each others' activities. In the HMOs and the IPAs, economies can be used as incentive bonuses for the physicians. In the PPO, patients enrolled receive services at discounted fees from the referred physicians. Participating physicians anticipate an increase in the number of patients directed to them by the PPO.

Blue Cross of Massachusetts was the first insurer to contract with HCFA for provision of Medicare benefits to elderly patients through an HMO network. Their Senior Plan Network will involve 15,000 elderly, with an expectation of 25,000 enrollees by 1986, with comprehensive health benefits provided by HMOs in Worcester, Braintree, Brockton, and Chicopee. Blue Cross will receive 95 percent of the average cost of services provided to elderly enrollees in each HMO service area. This technique is being used by the federal government to encourage this type of practice arrangement.[93]

In these capitation payment systems with per capita enrollments of beneficiaries, cautions are directed toward the issues of quality of care, undertreatment because of incentives to cut services and costs, reducing access to sicker elderly patients, and the loss of free choice of physician. In addition, nationwide expansion of these systems from isolated demonstrations or experiments in local communities may not be easy for rate or premium determinations, or even yield the expected aggregate cost savings.

Physicians do not generally like capitation arrangements as a method of practice. In January 1985, the Private Practice Medical Association, disenchanted with the national medical societies, was formed to promote the benefits of fee-for-service medicine by lobbying Congress and through a public educational campaign. A similar organization in Florida requires that all members be board certified, even subspecialists.[94]

C. Burns Roehrig, M.D., ASIM president, recently said, "Doctors fear capitation would disrupt the lives of the frail elderly. These fragile people are the most dependent of all patients on a stable relationship with their doctor. The fee-for-service system works best for them—always has, and always will"[95]

In contrast to the view of organized medicine's antipathy toward capitation, David J. Ottensmeyer, president of the Lovelace Medical Foundation in New Mexico, commented, "with a growing number of physicians and a falling demand for their services, doctors can no longer rule the marketplace. In many places they'll take anything they can get."[96]

Physicians are also entering into financial contracts with hospitals in record numbers, as a means of achieving some security from the pressures and uncertainty of the competitive dynamic health care market. "Approximately 155,000 patient care physicians now have financial contracts with hospitals. More than 60 percent of these contracts are salary arrangements."[97]

In addition to the hospital-based physicians such as radiologists and pathologists and the patient care physicians, other doctors are hired by hospitals as "fulltime paid medical directors to administer clinical and medical staff activities."[98] Hospitals are directly competing with private practitioners in their new quest for revenue from ambulatory care services.

In the hospital setting, physicians are salaried and patient care is either reimbursed to the facility or to the physician, depending upon the contractual terms. Physicians may be allowed a percentage of income after generating an agreed-upon dollar amount or may be able to practice privately while actually located on the hospital premises, with ancillary support provided according to the contract.

Changing the fee system—Medicare freeze.   Proposals for mandatory fixed-fee systems by the House Ways and Means Committee, as part of the tax reform legislation, brought sharp criticism from the leadership of the AMA:

- If it happens they'll have a war on their hands. . . .

- Unwarranted intrusion into the practice of medicine. . . .

- This will bring about a form of enslavement in medicine. . . .

- We're tired of this foolishness. We have allowed Congress to insult the American doctor.[99]

Lobbying efforts successfully set aside the fixed fee schedule system which physicians regard as the beginning of national fee schedules for all services. However, the AMA was unable to block inclusion of a 15-month mandatory physician fee freeze effective October 1, 1984. That freeze is expected to save Medicare $2.9 billion over a three-year period.

House members Andy Jacobs (D-IN), Henson Moore (R-LA), and Henry Waxman (D-CA), in consultation with David Stockman, former OMB Director, designed the Medicare freeze. Their plan was included in the provisions of the Deficit Reduction Act of 1984 (P.L. 98-369), which was passed on July 18, 1984. Injunctions and hearings in Indianapolis in response to the AMA court challenges were to no avail. A lawyer for the AMA said the freeze tended to create "a two tier system of medical care, in which Medicare patients will be regarded as second class citizens. It doesn't seem consistent with President Reagan's philosophy of reducing the role of the federal government. It causes a far greater government intrusion into the relationship between the physicians and patients."[100]

John J. Coury, M.D., chairman of the AMA Board of Trustees, contends that "this singles out physicians alone among all segments of our society by forbidding them from freely entering into contractual agreements with patients."[101]

Organizations representing consumers and Medicare beneficiaries hailed the provisions of the freeze. Cyril F. Brickfield, executive director of the 17-million member AARP, remarked, "This new law has the potential for slowing down the rapid increase in out-of-pocket health care costs for older Americans."[102]

Details of the Medicare freeze were outlined in letters to all physicians and each one was requested to sign a Medicare "participating physicians or supplier agreement" (Exhibit 6-1). The participating physician accepts Medicare patients on assignment and accepts the "allowable" charge set by Medicare as full payment with 80 percent of the "allowable" paid by the program and 20 percent paid by the patient. "Allowable" charges are set by a complex formula involving concepts such as customary prevailing reasonable (CPR) charges and geographical averages for the field of practice. More than a third of practicing physicians had signed the participating physician agreements for Medicare patients by the deadline of October 1, 1984.[103]

About 50 percent of the nonparticipating physicians frequently accept assignment from Medicare on a case-by-case determination. Those physicians who had tended previously to accept assignment under Medicare were more likely to become participating physicians. This trend indicates that more Medicare patients will be treated on an assigned basis in the future and may reduce the out-of-pocket expenditures.[104]

While the freeze on fees may have been the compromise near-term solution to doing something quickly about physician fees, it is clear that greater emphasis on this arena is planned. Modification of the way physicians are reimbursed has proponents in HCFA, in Blue Shield associations, among Congressional members, and constituent organizations. Research into various techniques to slow inflation through alteration in physician reimbursement has been initiated by HCFA and several private funding groups, such as the Robert Wood Johnson Foundation.

August 24, 1984

Dear Doctor:

On July 18, 1984, the Deficit Reduction Act of 1984 became law. This law establishes a freeze on Medicare reimbursement for physician services, creates a participating physician and supplier program, and prohibits certain physicians from raising their charges to Medicare beneficiaries after June 30, 1984. The purpose of this letter is to inform you of these major changes in Medicare reimbursement and to offer you the opportunity to enter into an agreement as a Medicare participating physician.

For the period July 1, 1984 to September 30, 1985, Medicare customary and prevailing charges will be frozen at the level in effect June 30, 1984. (The amount that Medicare reimburses is the lowest of a physician's customary charge for the service, the prevailing charge for the service in the area, or the physician's actual charge.) Future updates of customary and prevailing charges will take effect October 1st of each year beginning in 1985. The data to be used for those updates will be charges for services in the period April 1 to March 31st preceding the update. (Until now, customary and prevailing charges were updated each July 1 based on charges for the prior calendar year.) Also, when prevailing charges are increased by the economic index adjustment at the end of the current 15-month freeze, there will be no "catch-up" for the economic index adjustments that are not made during the period of the freeze. In addition, in accordance with existing Medicare policy, the customary charges of newly licensed physicians will be based on the 50th percentile of the weighted customary charges used to establish the prevailing charges in effect June 30, 1984.

To be a Medicare participating physician for the year beginning October 1, 1984, you will need to file the agreement by October 1, 1984. New physicians will have additional time in which to enter into agreements. The following will apply to a participating physician, participating medical group, or other participating entities authorized to bill for physician's services.

— You agree to accept assignment for all Medicare claims during the 12-month period beginning October 1, 1984. This means that you agree to bill Medicare directly and that Medicare will pay you an amount equal to Medicare's approved charge less any deductible and coinsurance. You may not charge the beneficiary (nor collect from another party such as a private insurer) more than the applicable deductible and coinsurance amounts.

— A directory of participating physicians (and entities) will be available for Medicare beneficiaries to review at Social Security and carrier offices and at senior citizens organizations. The directory will also be available for purchase by the public. As required by law, we will be informing Medi-

Exhibit 6-1   Letter to Physicians in New York City, from Medicare Intermediary

care beneficiaries of the publication of this directory. In addition, toll free telephone lines will be maintained to disseminate the name of participating physicians. We also will be developing enhancements in our electronic billing processes for participating physicians.

— During the 15-month period beginning July 1, 1984, you may raise your charges to Medicare beneficiaries. Since participating physicians agree to accept assignment for all Medicare claims for the 12 months beginning October 1st any such increases would not affect actual reimbursement to you during this period. However, the higher charges would be recognized in the calculation of your customary charges effective with the October 1, 1985, and October 1, 1986 updates.

If you decide *not* to become a participating physician, the following will apply:

— You may continue to accept assignment on a case-by-case basis.

— You may not increase your charges to Medicare beneficiaries during the period July 1, 1984, through September 30, 1985, over what you charged for the same services during the period April 1, 1984, through June 30, 1984. (Where you had a general fee increase during the April 1, 1984–June 30, 1984 period, you may continue to charge the increased fee.) Medicare will enforce this requirement by comparing your pattern of charges for each service during the 15-month freeze period to your pattern of charges during the quarter beginning April 1, 1984. To comply with this provision, you may simply continue the actual charging practices you followed in the April–June quarter.

Example 1: Dr. A charged Medicare beneficiaries $20 ninety percent of the time and $25 ten percent of the time for a brief office visit (CPT-4 code #90040) during the April 1–June 30 period. Dr. A may not charge more than $20 in ninety percent of this billing for this service during the freeze period. He may charge up to $25 during the freeze period ten percent of the time.

Example 2: Dr. B charged Medicare beneficiaries $20 for a brief office visit during April 1984 and May and June 1984. Dr. B may not charge more than $25 during the freeze period. Occasional higher fees would have to meet the criteria stated in Example 1.

In the event we find an indication of increases in charges in apparent violation of the freeze on fees, we will provide a physician with details on the claims in question and with an opportunity to furnish an appropriate explanation.

Under the law, a physician who knowingly and willfully increases his

Exhibit 6-1, cont.

charges in violation of this prohibition is subject to assessments of up to double the amount of the violative charges, civil money penalties (up to $2,000 per violation), as well as exclusion from the Medicare program for up to five years. We will not, however, bar a physician from participation in the Medicare program who is a community's sole physician or only source of essential specialized services.

— Where a charge to a Medicare beneficiary was not made in the April 1, 1984–June 30, 1984, period, the prohibition on increases in charges does not apply. Thus, newly licensed physicians going into practice after June 30, 1984, are not legally prohibited from raising their charges in the July 1, 1984–September 30, 1985 period. Similarly, established physicians who did not provide a particular service to a Medicare beneficiary in the April 1, 1984–June 30, 1984, period are not prohibited from raising their charge for that service in the freeze period.

— Any increased charges by a nonparticipating physician during this period will not be recognized in the calculation of customary charges in the October 1, 1985, and October 1, 1986, updates. This is true even if a penalty as described above is not imposed.

— Upon request, Medicare carriers will provide you with available information about your pattern of charges during the April–June quarter. Generally, we presume this will be required where you have varying charges for the same service and your records do not readily permit you to determine the pattern of charges billed to Medicare beneficiaries.

The enclosed *Fact Sheet* describes in more detail the incentives which the legislation provides for physicians to participate and discusses other aspects of the Medicare participating physician or supplier program.

If you decide to participate, please complete and return the enclosed *Medicare Participating Physician or Supplier Agreement* to the following address below by October 1, 1984.

> Medicare Participation Agreements
> Blue Cross and Blue Shield of Greater New York
> 622 Third Avenue
> New York, New York 10017

MEDICARE
PARTICIPATING PHYSICIAN OR SUPPLIER AGREEMENT

Name(s) and Address of Participant   Physician or
                                                        Identification Code(s)

The above named person or organization, called "the participant", hereby en-

Exhibit 6-1, cont.

ters into an agreement with the Medicare program to accept assignment of the Medicare Part B payment for all services for which the participant is eligible to accept assignment under the Medicare law and regulations, and which are furnished while this agreement is in effect.

1. *Meaning of Assignment*—For purposes of this agreement, the participant accepts assignment of the Medicare Part B payment when the participant requests direct Part B payment from the Medicare program. Under an assignment, the approved charge, determined by the Medicare carrier, shall be the full charge for the service covered under Part B. The participant shall not collect from the beneficiary or other person or organization for covered services more than the applicable deductible and coinsurance.

2. *Effective Date*—If the participant files the agreement with any Medicare carrier during the 3-month period July through September of any calendar year, the agreement becomes effective on October 1 of that year.

3. *Term and Termination of Agreement*—This agreement shall continue in effect through September 30 following the date the agreement becomes effective and shall be renewed automatically for each 12-month period October 1 through September 30 thereafter unless one of the following occurs:

a. Before October 1 of any year the participant notifies in writing every Medicare carrier with whom the participant has filed the agreement or a copy of the agreement that the participant wishes to terminate the agreement at the end of the current term. In the event such notification is mailed or delivered on or before September 30 of any year, the agreement shall end on September 30 of that year.

b. The Health Care Financing Administration may find, after notice to and opportunity for a hearing for the participant, that the participant has substantially failed to comply with the agreement. In the event such a finding is made, the Health Care Financing Administration will notify the participant in writing that the agreement will be terminated at a time designated in the notice. Civil and criminal penalties may also be imposed for violation of the agreement.

Signature of participant (or authorized representative of participating organization)	Title Date (if signer is authorized representative of organization)

Exhibit 6-1, cont.
Source: Personal Communication with Florence Kavaler, M.D.

Changing the units of service medicare pays for.　Janet B. Mitchell, president of the nonprofit Center for Health Economics in suburban Boston, analyzed data for 1981 Medicare Part B claims from Michigan and South Carolina and reported on the "Alternative Methods for Describing Physician Services Performed and Billed."[105] Two systems emerged as having potential for further study by HCFA: the inpatient condition package (also known as physician DRGs) and the special procedure package.

There is a tremendous amount of "anti-physician DRG" literature emerging from the AMA and in reactions from private practitioners. These reactions relate to the impact on physician acceptance of Medicare eligible patients and to the possible detriment in the quality of care. Nothing that the government does to control physicians will please physicians. Yet, the train keeps on the track and efforts are secondarily directed at derailing and stalling.

Physician DRGs.　Feasibility of rolling physician fees into the DRG payment to hospitals is under serious consideration by HCFA.Studies of a 5 percent sampling of Medicare hospital claims and the accompanying physician service bills are being meshed to gather payment ideas.[106] For the surgical procedures, for example, the hospital data plus preadmission services, surgeon fees, assistant surgeon fees, anesthesiology fees, pathologist and radiologist fees, and post-operative out-of-hospital care are all included in the analysis.

Senator Edward M. Kennedy (D-MA) and Representative Richard A. Gephardt (D-MO) introduced legislation on February 9, 1984 to extend the DRG payment mechanism to include physician services. Under their proposal, there would be a lump sum payment for all hospital services to a Medicare patient, with the hospital and the physicians then deciding how to split up the reimbursement among themselves.[107]

However, Senator Robert Dole (R-KN) and Senator John Heinz (R-PA) are not as enthusiastic about the Kennedy/Gephardt plan because of the poor data available upon which to base new reimbursement methodologies. Senator Heinz urges caution: "Extending DRGs to physicians would mark a longer step in health care policy than our present knowledge can justify."[108]

To encourage the development of state cost control plans applied to all payers as an alternative, Senator Heinz introduced the Medicare Incentive Reform Act (MIRA). A Medicare fee schedule is suggested as substitute for physician DRGs and is based on a relative value scale (RVS) that "reemphasizes primary and preventive care and deemphasizes hospitalization and high technology."[109]

Arguments are accumulating on all sides, the AMA is applying pressure on Congress against the proposals, and the results of research studies have been inconclusive. Since the bill was introduced, support has waned for the suggested changes: Senator David Durenberger (R-MN), Senate Finance Health Subcommittee chairman, reportedly is having doubts about the physician DRG scheme.

His aide, Chip Kahn, notes: "Rushing into a DRG for physicians was a little frightening . . . research on a physician DRG had mixed results . . . and physician DRG could change the physician/patient relationship."[110]

President Reagan's Private Sector Survey on Cost Control changed its mind about physician DRGs. In their news report of January 16, 1984, concern was expressed "about bureaucrats making life and death decisions under DRGs and determined that DRGs should not be extended to physician services."[111]

Studies are being funded by HCFA[112] addressing issues on the desirability and feasibility of such payment schemes, on who should receive the payments (hospitals or physicians), and on how multiple physicians should be paid (all to the primary practitioner who in turn pays the others, or to each physician separately). Should the fees cover each patient for a week prior to hospitalization and one week after discharge? Both the Office of Technology Assessment and the Institute of Medicine are studying these issues. Congress has been urged to "wait until all the cards are on the table before we start dealing a hand which can't be played."[113]

Illustrations of the physician DRG for cholecystectomy surgical case (Exhibit 6-2) shows the variations in costs for patients with complications and with common bile duct explorations. Note the following:

- Large coefficient of variation for each DRG and all cases.

- One fifth of the sample had additional surgical procedures for an average charge of $177.00.

- A high number of patients had concurrent care visits from internists and surgeons, ICU visits, or consultations. Almost half of these patients received additional physician visits.

- Nonsurgeons, anesthesiologists, and radiologists account for one-third to almost half of the visit price.

- The surgeon's share of the total bill is smaller than might be expected.[114]

For another surgical procedure studied, transurethral resection of the prostate (TURP), variability was less in DRG 336 and DRG 337.

In medical condition packages such as pneumonia (Exhibit 6-3), it is obvious that age is an important factor—DRG 89, over age 70 as compared to DRG 90, age under 70.

Specialty characteristics of the physician performing the service is also vital in determining prices, as can be seen in Exhibit 6-4 on left-heart catheterization. Other studies showed geographical differences in prices in claims made in South Carolina when compared to Michigan claims for the same procedure.

Exhibit 6-2   Physician DRG Inpatient Condition Packages for Cholecystectomy: By DRG and All Cases[a]

	With Common Bile Duct Exploration		Without Common Bile Duct Exploration		
	DRG#195 With C.C.[b] (15.7%)	DRG#196 No C.C. (8.3%)	DRG#197 With C.C. (50.3%)	DRG#198 No C.C. (25.7%)	All Cases (n = 1,160)
Surgeon	$703 (1.00)	$672 (1.00)	$592 (1.00)	$582 (1.00)	$614 (1.00)
Assistant Surgeon	142 (0.34)	140 (0.26)	118 (0.28)	116 (0.24)	124 (0.28)
Anesthesiologist	176 (1.00)	185 (1.00)	138 (1.00)	150 (1.00)	151 (1.00)
Other Surgery[c]	250 (0.25)	145 (0.11)	171 (0.22)	135 (0.13)	177 (0.19)
Routine Hospital Visits	228 (0.62)	177 (0.40)	173 (0.55)	123 (0.31)	176 (0.48)
Concurrent Care Visits	139 (0.09)	123 (0.01)	114 (0.09)	68 (0.01)	118 (0.06)
ICU Visits	105 (0.12)	89 (0.06)	119 (0.08)	95 (0.03)	111 (0.07)
Consultations	62 (0.37)	47 (0.18)	58 (0.33)	64 (0.13)	59 (0.27)
X-Rays	115 (0.88)	98 (0.70)	83 (0.82)	73 (0.60)	88 (0.76)
ECGs	13 (0.74)	10 (0.58)	12 (0.78)	9 (0.65)	12 (0.73)
Lab Tests	55 (0.18)	62 (0.20)	41 (0.05)	44 (0.11)	48 (0.08)
Other Services	64 (0.18)	64 (0.06)	73 (0.10)	92 (0.03)	73 (0.07)
Total Package Price	$1,297	$1,087	$1,020	$885	$1,034
Coefficient of Variation	27.6%	22.2%	27.0%	25.6%	29.5%

[a]All dollars are Medicare reasonable charges. Relative frequency of each physician service is in parentheses. Excludes 142 cases who had a second major operation. This lowered the total package price from $1,122 to $1,034 and reduced the C.V. from 41% to 30%.
[b]C.C.—complicating condition.
[c]Includes all physicians' fees.
Data Base: South Carolina 1981 Medicare Part B Claims Data.
Source: J. B. Mitchell, K. A. Calore, J. Cromwell, H. T. Hewes, W. B. Stason, and H. West, *Alternative Methods for Describing Physicians Services Performed and Billed* (Health Economics Research, Inc., Chestnut Hill, MA, November 1983), p. 195.

An assessment was made of the relative values of the physician DRGs to the hospital DRGs using DRG 39, lens procedure, as the standard unit (Exhibit 6-5). Note the following:

- While lens procedure is by far the least costly to the hospital, it is the second most expensive physician DRG.

- For pneumonia, DRG 89, the hospital uses 220 percent more resources than in caring for the patient undergoing a lens procedure. For the physician DRG, only one fifth as much effort is used.

Exhibit 6-3 Physician DRG Inpatient Condition Packages for Pneumonia DRGs[a]

	DRG 89	DRG 90	
	C.C. or Age 70+ (81%)	No C.C., Age <70 (19%)	All Cases (n = 5,335)
Medical Emergency	$ 33 (0.14)	$ 30 (0.08)	$ 33 (0.13)
Other Surgery[b]	293 (0.13)	326 (0.09)	298 (0.12)
Routine Hospital Visits	206 (0.98)	163 (0.97)	198 (0.98)
ICU Visits	191 (0.09)	175 (0.05)	189 (0.08)
Consultations	89 (0.27)	85 (0.16)	88 (0.25)
Chest X-ray	28 (0.53)	23 (0.48)	27 (0.52)
Other Dig. X-rays	47 (0.19)	39 (0.14)	46 (0.18)
Body Scan	27 (0.02)	27 (0.02)	27 (0.02)
Lung Scan	70 (0.02)	49 (0.02)	67 (0.02)
Lung Perfusion Study	79 (0.01)	60 (0.01)	75 (0.01)
Other Nuclear Med. Tests	134 (0.06)	116 (0.04)	132 (0.06)
ECGs	29 (0.48)	22 (0.38)	28 (0.46)
Other Tests	63 (0.09)	56 (0.06)	62 (0.08)
Total Package Price	$339	$247	$322
Coefficient of Variation	120%	133%	122%

[a]All dollars are Medicare reasonable charges. Relative frequency of each physician service is in parentheses.
[b]Includes minor and diagnostic surgery only, e.g., bronchoscopy, thoracentesis, etc.
Database: Michigan 1981 Medicare Part B Claims Data.
Source: J. B. Mitchell, K. A. Calore, J. Cromwell, H. T. Hewes, W. B. Stason, and H. West, *Alternative Methods for Describing Physicians Services Performed and Billed* (Health Economics Research, Inc., Chestnut Hill, MA, November 1983), p. 199.

- Within related groups of DRGs, the hospital and physician weights are similar.

- Older patients and patients with complicating conditions use up more hospital and more physician resources.

Dr. Mitchell has expressed concern that physicians see too few patients to be able to balance cases on which they lose money with cases on which they make more than average. "The potential per case losses could be quite large, and per-practice losses could be devastating."[115]

There are some specialties which might gain under physician DRGs, such as family practitioners, obstetrician-gynecologists, and psychiatrists. Others may lose, such as cardiologists, cardiac and thoracic surgeons, neurosurgeons, and pulmonologists. Internists can either gain or lose with equal chance. In general, physicians who treat sicker patients fare worse in expected payment.[116] Because of the large coefficients of variation within each DRG and the complexities of variations in clinical practice approach to patients with the same medical DRG, "DRGs for surgeons appear to be most feasible and should be tried first."[117]

Exhibit 6-4   Physician DRG Inpatient Condition Packages for Left Heart Catheterization[a]

Physician Component	Cardiologist (65.1%)	Internist (19.3%)	Multi-Specialty Group (14.6%)	All Physicians
	Specialty of Physician Performing Catheterization[b] (percent of claims)			
Cardiac Catherization #1	$516 (1.00)	$422 (1.00)	$527 (1.00)	$500 (1.00)
Cardiac Catheterization #2	380 (0.02)	475 (0.01)	272 (0.03)	369 (0.02)
Right Heart Catheterization	172 (0.03)	200 (0.01)	35 (0.01)	162 (0.02)
Injection Procedures for Catheterization	85 (0.03)	112 (0.04)	75 (0.01)	88 (0.03)
Routine Hospital Visits	153 (0.92)	121 (0.80)	159 (0.70)	148 (0.86)
Concurrent Care Visits	93 (0.07)	—	131 (0.05)	99 (0.05)
ICU Visits	143 (0.24)	85 (0.16)	196 (0.22)	146 (0.22)
Consultations	63 (0.27)	64 (0.23)	58 (0.33)	62 (0.27)
Catheterization X-Rays	75 (0.12)	58 (0.20)	77 (0.07)	70 (0.13)
Cardiac Nuclear Imaging	49 (0.07)	30 (0.01)	34 (0.09)	45 (0.06)
Other X-Rays	41 (0.84)	37 (0.84)	36 (0.88)	40 (0.84)
ECGs	14 (0.85)	15 (0.81)	20 (0.86)	15 (0.84)
Stress Tests	34 (0.08)	34 (0.24)	33 (0.13)	34 (0.11)
Echocardiography	50 (0.09)	33 (0.05)	52 (0.32)	49 (0.12)
Other Services	303 (0.18)	240 (0.14)	288 (0.39)	297 (0.21)
Total Package Price	$851	$677	$910	$825
Coefficient of Variation	58.3%	41.7%	73.5%	60.4%

[a]All dollars are Medicare reasonable charges. Relative frequency of each physician service is in parentheses.
[b]Specialties shown represent 99% of all left heart catheterization claims (N = 522)
Database: South Carolina 1981 Medicare Part B Claims Data.
Source: J. B. Mitchell, K. A. Calore, J. Cromwell, H. T. Hewes, W. B. Stason, and H. West, *Alternative Methods for Describing Physician Services Performed and Billed*, (Health Economics Research, Inc., Chestnut Hill, MA, November 1983), p. 204.

This view was further reinforced from studies in Boston of Medicare data for New Jersey and South Carolina. Investigators found that "diagnosis alone is a poor indicator of physician costs, primarily because of the variability in clinical practice and the severity of illness not reflected in the DRG."[118]

Relative Value Scale (RVS).   An AMA lobbyist said, "We need an ace in the hole." Both the AMA and the ASIM are supporting relative value scales (RVS) for determining reimbursement of physician services under Medicare.

RVS is a method of quantitative analysis of weights and ranks to enable comparison of individual medical and surgical services and procedures. It is not

Exhibit 6-5   Relative Cost Weights: Hospital vs. Physician DRGs[a]

	Medicare DRGs	Hospital Wts.	MD Wts. So. Carolina	MD Wts. Michigan
No.	Description			
14	Specific cerebrovascular disorders, except TIA	2.7000	—	0.3585
15	Transient ischemic attacks	1.3319	—	0.2963
16	Non-specific cerebrovascular disorders with C.C.	1.7150	—	0.4484
17	Non-specific cerebrovascular disorders without C.C.	1.6750	—	0.2643
39	Lens procedures	1.0000	1.0000	1.0000
89	Pneumonia with C.C.	2.2014	—	0.2046
90	Pneumonia without C.C.	1.9659	—	0.1491
195	Cholecystectomy with common duct exploration and C.C.	4.3293	1.1278	—
196	Cholecystectomy with common duct exploration and without C.C.	4.1106	0.9452	—
197	Cholecystectomy without common duct exploration and with C.C.	2.9677	0.8870	—
198	Cholecystectomy without common duct exploration and without C.C.	2.5453	0.7696	—
336	Transurethral resection of the prostate with C.C.	2.0118	0.8687	—
337	Transurethral resection of the prostate without C.C.	1.6948	0.8365	—

[a]All weights have been standardized by DRG 39, lens procedures.
Analysis: Hospital weights have been calculated based on the relative weights for Medicare prospective payment, published in the Federal Register, 9/1/83. The physician weights for the two states were calculated from 1981 Medicare Part B Claims Data.
Source: J. B. Mitchell, K. A. Calore, J. Cromwell, H. T. Hewes, W. B. Stason, and H. West, *Alternative Methods for Describing Physician Services Performed and Billed* (Health Economics Research, Inc., Chestnut Hill, MA, November 1983), p. 213.

a fee schedule, but when a conversion factor is applied, RVS can be used as such. For example, if the RVS for a service is 2.5 and the conversion factor is 30, then the fee would be $75.

In a study by Hsiao and Stason concerning the development of RVSs for a limited number of medical and surgical services, the results indicated important differences between existing reimbursement levels and those which integrate resource cost values. Comparisons were made between the California Relative Value Study and prevailing Medicare charges, and the model using resource cost values.

After standardizing the variations in complexity among different procedures, the prevailing Medicare charges, expressed in terms of hourly rates of reimbursement, range from $40 per hour for the general practitioner to more than $180 per hour for an ophthalmologist performing a lens extraction.

By comparison, general surgeons tend to average between $150 and $200 per operating room hour for the surgical procedures analyzed.

The question has been raised as to whether these differences are justified and, if so, on what basis.[119]

Recently the Massachusetts Rate Setting Commission began using an RVS for physician reimbursement under its Medicaid and Workers' Compensation programs,[120] as do some insurance companies and other Workers' Compensation programs elsewhere. "In the middle 1970s, 35 state medical societies and eight medical and surgical specialty organizations used relative value studies or guides.Today, only the Florida Medical Association and the American Society of Anesthesiologists use an RVS."[121]

However, in 1979, the Federal Trade Commission (FTC) issued a consent order to the California Medical Association prohibiting the development of an RVS for physician fees. Petitions were filed recently with the FTC requesting the agency to remove its restrictions in consideration of the changed conditions and new laws. In August 1984, the FTC altered its position in response to a similar petition from the American College of Obstetricians and Gynecologists and is still deliberating its position regarding the American College of Radiology.[122]

In the *Washington Report on Medicine and Health,* a reliable FTC official indicated that there are no antitrust impediments to HCFA designing a Medicare PPS for physicians based on RVSs. However, FTC cautioned that "physician associations not be involved in determining the 'conversion factor' that translates the RVS into prices."[123]

There is reported speculation that "HCFA may be using the antitrust issue to force the involvement of nonphysician groups in the work on the RVS system."[124]

"The AMA and the ASIM favor a RVS based on resource costs. The AMA would include physician time, complexity of skill, training, overhead and professional liability. Internists and surgeons would be on the same scale."[125] As internists, the ASIM wants greater weight to be given to cognitive services and preventive care and less to the procedural, technical, or surgical services. ASIM is planning its own in-house study to come up with recommendations.[126] Generally, the AMA notes that, although the RVS may be like a fee-for-service schedule, it is preferable to the physician DRG and would be less constraining and disruptive to the way physicians practice.[127]

On January 16, 1985, in response to the HCFA request, the AMA submitted a proposal to seek a grant to develop an RVS for physician services. All services contained in the AMA's *Current Procedural Terminology, Fourth Edition* (CPT-4) would be covered and the study would take about two years to complete. This RVS would then be used by third-party payers to establish the conversion factor. Plans include utilization of a 30-member consortium of medical specialty societies as a steering committee and a 10-member technical advisory panel of academics, nonphysicians, health consultant firms, and representatives of the health insurance industry and the federal government.[128]

In discussions of the AMA's interest in developing the RVS model, several physicians indicated their opposition to national RVS scales which would not take into consideration geographic variations. Others opposed the principle of using a fee schedule for government reimbursement. AMA President Boyle pointed out that fee schedules, although they may not be so labeled, were already used by third parties for Medicare, "although we usually don't know what the schedule is."[129]

HCFA did not accept the AMA's proposal and awarded a 30-month contract to Hsiao at Harvard School of Public Health to expand on his previous RVS research and to draw up a resource-based RVS for physician services. More than 160 AMA-nonminated physicians and 1,200–1,600 other physicians will be asked to participate and to represent every major medical and surgical specialty, with the results to be brought forth to a 25-member consensus panel.[130]

Congress is not generally impressed with the RVS system. One House staff member revealed that "there's no sentiment on this side of the Hill for RVS. It's just another form of fee schedule."[131]

Alternative reimbursement proposals. Several alternative methods for reimbursement of physicians are described in the Mitchell study. A special procedure package has more favor and seems more feasible than others described.

Special Procedure Packages (SPPs). Some precedent exists for this methodology in the current Medicare payments for surgeons' inpatient services which include pre- and postoperative visits in the hospital. This methodology could be extended so that the physician performing the procedure would submit a bill which includes other related physician services—anesthesiologist, radiologist, assistant surgeon services—in a single bill. For diagnostic procedures, this would be similarly structured as in the therapeutic procedures. There would be no redundant bills for office and hospital visits, currently usual, as in endoscopies or cardiac workups.

Office Visit Packages (OVPs).   An office visit would be the unique payment unit with some case mix modifiers such as

- Visit type—new or established patient
- Diagnosis—Ambulatory Visit Group (AVG), an analog to DRGs
- Reason for visit—initial, return, return with new symptoms
- Patient demographics—age

Multiple providers of lab tests and ancillary services would be combined into the primary physician billing. Inpatient activity would be excluded.

Ambulatory Condition Packages (ACPs).   This is distinguished from OVPs because the extended time interval for the diagnosis is taken into consideration. For chronic conditions treated in ambulatory centers or private offices, a fixed time period would be established for treating the patient's diagnosis. For example, hypertension or diabetes management for three months, with the physician being responsible for all ambulatory care rendered for the condition during that period (Exhibit 6-6). Given the multiple chronic illnesses of the elderly, defining care in only one package provides logistic problems and may increase out-of-package care costs.

Collapsed or Recombined Procedure Packages (CPPs).   Use of the CPT-4 system involves 6,132 separate procedure codes for medicine, surgery, anesthesia, radiology, and pathology. Physicians have wide latitude in choosing billing codes for the same service. Collapsing or recombining some of these codes would help reduce the "gaming" possibilities of upgrading codes for higher billing purposes. If brief versus intermediate office codes exist, the incentive may be to "upgrade" the nominal (name only) terms to the more lucrative code. In addition, laboratory tests have been listed separately under current Medicare billing rules. This "unbundling" does not serve as a constraint on the frequency or rate of lab testing, thereby increasing charges. Claims reviewers currently monitor physicians' services and lab tests as if they were medically unrelated.

Indemnity Proposals.   Indemnity insurance[132] reimburses the insured beneficiary—the Medicare-eligible patient—a fixed amount for a covered service. This method is seen as an attractive alternative to the customary prevailing reasonable (CPR) method of fee determinations currently being made by the third-party carriers for Medicare.

Patients have an incentive to seek care from lower-priced physicians and to keep the savings from the indemnity payment. For physicians, the fee-for-service system is undisturbed and fees can be changed based on practice costs, market forces, and technology. However, physicians may be motivated to be competitive in price to attract Medicare patients.

Exhibit 6-6 Ambulatory Condition Package (ACP): Specialty Differences in Three-Month Condition Packages for Hypertension[a]

	Specialty of Package Physician[b]				
	GP-DO (10.4%)	GP-MD (24.1%)	Internist (35.5%)	General Surgeon (6.4%)	Multi-Spec. Group (16.6%)
No. of Visits to Package Physician	2.8	2.6	2.2	2.6	2.2
Percent of Cases:					
Second Physician Involved	28.9%	27.3%	29.8%	32.9%	25.9%
X-Rays	25.8	23.9	27.8	20.0	29.1
ECGs	17.6	18.3	24.9	11.9	16.7
Injections	23.0	21.8	7.2	17.6	8.3
Office Surgery	15.4	12.5	14.9	13.8	17.6
Lab Tests	55.2	48.7	46.6	36.4	23.9
No. of Lab Tests[c]	8.7	8.9	8.8	6.6	11.0
Total Ambulatory Package Price	$151.55	$133.95	$137.02	$109.07	$121.58
Coefficient of Variation	139%	134%	135%	136%	140%
Percent of Patients Hospitalized	14.1%	14.9%	16.2%	16.1%	11.9%
Total Condition Package Price	$279.95	$258.78	$280.00	$249.20	$248.07
Coefficient of Variation	191%	181%	181%	200%	213%
% of Total Price Attributed to Package Physician	63.8%	64.7%	61.9%	66.1%	67.8%

[a]All dollars are Medicare reasonable charges.
[b]Specialties shown represent 58.5 percent of total physician sample.
[c]For patients with any lab tests.
Database: Michigan 1981 Medicare Part B Claims Data.
Source: J. B. Mitchell, K. A. Calore, J. Cromwell, H. T. Hewes, W. B. Stason, and H. West, *Alternative Methods for Describing Physician Services Performed and Billed* (Health Economics Research, Inc., Chestnut Hill, MA, November 1983), p. 179.

Indemnity schedules could be developed with sensitivity to geographic variations and could be coupled with assignment options.

Physician Reimbursement Generalizations. Each of these alternative physician reimbursement packages is linked to examples from historical billing claims reviews; the pros and cons of each have been expertly debated. However, the ability to move from the narrow research base to the political arena of acceptable practical implementation is quite difficult. Pressure to do something, even if imperfect, is upon the policy makers. Senator Robert Dole (R-KN), Finance Committee chairman, pinpointed the situation: "Physicians are among the highest paid professionals in this country. Their average income is about two and a half times that of the average family's. We can't expect Medicare beneficiaries to put up with higher out-of-pocket expenses if doctors aren't willing to moderate their fees at the same time."[133]

Representative Henry Waxman (D-CA) recognizes that Congress will be taking action before they are completely informed. "We are about to make budgetary decisions. I'm very worried about what impact those decisions will have on the quality of care. We don't have their evaluations of what is taking place."[134]

However, James S. Todd, M.D., the AMA's senior deputy vice president, recently argued that excessive physician services cannot be controlled through reimbursement policies, but only with tough utilization review. He said, "Doctors are getting mixed signals. On the one hand, society wants more and more high tech, new tech, life extending innovations like artificial organs, organ transplants and machines that can see inside the body, but on the other hand, doctors are told to bring down medical costs. You can't have it both ways."[135]

As John Iglehart, a health policy analyst for Project Hope and a frequent contributor to professional journals, astutely observed, "There's a growing concern about the volume of medical services, reflecting a decline in faith in the efficacy of medical care. With its massive purchasing power, the government knows it has the power to change medicine; now, because of the crisis in costs, it also has the will."[136]

Nursing Services

Nursing services contribute approximately 40 percent of the hospital's direct patient care costs and, as such, are extremely vulnerable to budget reductions. With labor costs accounting for 60 percent of total hospital expenses, "the nursing department is a prime target for work-force reductions."[137]

Rate setters have considered nursing services as part of the institution's room and board charges and no hospital cost center for nursing services has evolved. Under DRGs, nursing costs are integral to the value derived. Debate continues over the merits of the system adopted, which does not account for nursing intensity of services or patient needs.[138] It is argued that patients with certain diagnoses require greater nursing resources than others—for example, acute myocardial infarction, hernia surgery, coma—and that parallel nursing assessments of resource use should accompany each DRG.

Nurses are being implored to justify their roles and functions and to develop "managerial tools to identify nursing resource use based on a patient classification system compatible with DRGs." If not, their budget resources could be used as a "slush fund" and "raped" and "used to cross subsidize other departments. Registered nurses will perform tasks which could be effectively delegated to ancillaries."[139-141]

Opposition by American Nurses Association (ANA) to the DRG system of payment hinges on several areas, including the favoritism accorded surgical over nonsurgical treatments.Nurses have directed their support toward the "severity of illness" alternative index which does recognize the more intense nursing resource use warranted by the patients' condition. The ANA president also calls for more nursing autonomy as a profession and for cost containment by a "reduction of statutory control of the medical profession over consumer access to nursing services in the hospital, to special services in the community, and to visiting nurse and home health services."[142]

In New Jersey, a study to quantify nursing time spent on patient care by DRG incorporated and assigned relative values to the time to determine the cost. These Relative Intensity Measures (RIMs)—actually a RIM is one minute of nursing resource use—distinguish the intensity of resources consumed by each patient and demonstrate how essential the nursing component is to total patient care.[143] But objections have been raised to this methodology:

> RIMs are relative, not absolute measures of nursing resource use, which means the reality of current care, and do not purport to measure any ideal investment of resources.[144]

> RIMs do not deal with care needs which have been identified for the patient: in many institutions, one cannot assume that care delivered equates with care needed.[145]

Several hospital nursing directors in New Jersey warn, "RIMs have a suspect database: watch them closely. They do not always include the context in which care is given. Consider using your own patient classification system, along with the RIMs as a check and balance."[146]

Nursing patient classification systems (NPCS)[147] have been around for quite some time and are mandated by the Joint Commission on Accreditation of Hospitals (JCAH): "The nursing department/service shall define, implement and maintain a system for determining patient requirements for nursing care on the basis of demonstrated patient needs, appropriate nursing intervention, and priority of care."[148]

These classification systems have had their principal use in distribution of nursing manpower on various floors, substantiating budgetary resources needed, and staff recruitment. Each hospital developed its own system, so that nursing personnel can be deployed each day or each shift as level of patient care needs change. DRGs are not sensitive to these closely concurrent variations in needs of patients within a particular DRG, since these are retrospective average scales.

Classification of patients by their dependency on nursing functions has been proposed, using the following typology:

1. Daily essential functions—usual services nurses provide to every hospitalized patient

2. Physician-dependent functions—services prescribed by physicians that nurses perform, for example, frequency of observations, medication, treatment regimens

3. Nursing independent functions—those activities which nursing judgment and diagnoses call into action, for example, support, patient/family education.[149]

Data would then be collected to determine the time these functions require per DRG case to fulfill quality nursing care practice. "The improvement of this system upon the RIM system is that it would induce improvement in actual care quality by tagging nursing care to patient need rather than to actual resources consumed—the characteristic of the RIM system."[150] Carolyne Davis, HCFA administrator, said that for DRGs,

> nurses can play a major part in insuring the success of the system. . . . nurses are integral to the success of hospitals in containing their costs under the prospective pricing system.[151]

> One of the real efficiencies is to reduce length of stay, and it's the RN who monitors the symptoms and intervenes to decrease the risk of complications. . . .[152]

> Nursing must rise to the challenge of clearly identifying nursing care resources in order to avoid continuing anonymity within the hospital budget.[153]

Conventional wisdom dictates that Medicare patients require more nursing services in a hospital because of their age and health problems. This led to a nursing differential of 8.5 percent on the hospital per diem rates since 1971. Controversy was introduced with findings from a 1977 New Jersey study of cost data from 22 hospitals and 217,000 patients, which indicated hospitals may be providing the elderly with less care than that given to younger patients.[154] Younger patients under 14 years required 133 percent more nursing care. More studies in New Jersey and elsewhere are in progress, measuring the amount of nursing care delivered, the patient's need for care, and the amount of nursing time spent supporting ancillary departments. This data will provide validation or termination of the differential.

The Director of the gerontological nurse practitioner masters' program at Seton Hall University in New Jersey is not surprised that "staff often shift their resources away from the chronically ill elderly to younger, acute care patients, because they believe the elderly can't be helped."[155] However, there are contrary results in other studies. A study conducted in Chicago, Illinois showed that 5.96 hours of nursing care a day is necessary for Medicare patients, 22 percent more than the 4.88 hour average.[156]

Nurses are exhorted to "view patients as products" and to "promote the dollar value of our productivity."[157] They are being urged to calculate the value of their care, to be more collaborative with physicians, and to publicize their work to both administrators and patients. Sharing new techniques, upgrading skills, and offering continuing education are important parts of the effort to be visible and acknowledged.

Primary care nursing is a concept that has been gaining acceptance in hospitals nationwide.[158] In a recent survey of 200 randomly selected hospitals, it was found that 46 percent had implemented primary nursing and 24 percent were planning or thinking about it. However, "with increasing cost containment measures, of which DRGs are one type, nursing administrators are doubting, even more so, their freedom to execute innovative nursing care modalities."[159] Successful professional primary nursing practice needs predominantly RN staffing. This stands in potential conflict with the cost consciousness of DRG implementation. DRG priorities look towards reducing this highly skilled staff and replacing RNs with licensed practical nurses. Some studies, however, show that primary nursing may be more cost effective and less costly than team nursing and has an impact on nurse satisfaction and level of quality of care. There are many variations among primary nursing systems and further research and evaluation studies need to be pursued to conclude that DRGs and primary nursing are compatible.

Critical care nursing[160-162] is also under scrutiny because of the high professional nurse to patient ratios. Hospitals are re-evaluating the size of these units and occupancy rates so that adjustments might be made in bed capacity and accompanying staff. Creation of newer stepdown units and the pressure for reduced length of stay has some implications on the criteria for admission to and transfer out of critical care units. It is predicted that:

- The size of intensive care units will shrink over time.

- Patients admitted will be more carefully selected.

- Patient stays in the unit will be brief, intended only to alleviate the crisis or stabilize the patient.

- Nurse staffing will be carefully screened, not only for clinical expertise, but also maturity, critical thinking ability, quick decision making, assertiveness, and patient management skills.

- Certification in critical care nursing, advanced cardiac life support, continuing education, and so on, will be essential for nurses in these units.

Pointedly, physicians and nurses make critical judgments impacting on life and death issues in critical care units. "Moral-legal questions need to be addressed now more than ever before. The majority of Medicare dollars are spent during the last days of life. Can we afford the technology we offer in critical care units?"[163]

Analysis of nursing costs that differ significantly from the standards are a prime consideraton of nurse administrators. "Cost shortfalls may result from relatively low-quality cost overruns, inefficiency or overcaring."[164] Excessive costs may result from the following reasons pertaining to nursing:[165]

- Skill mix may be too rich; more RNs than other neighboring hospitals.

- Overstaffed for the patients treated.

- Higher salaries than those of other neighboring hospitals.

- Absenteeism may be high and scheduling excessive to compensate nursing functions. Expenses may be incurred in performing housekeeping, dietary, or other non-nursing duties which should be charged to other cost centers.

Classifications of patients according to the DRG and relative nursing services provided was part of a recent study of 24,879 patient admissions at Rochester's Strong Memorial Hospital, a 714-bed teaching hospital.[166] These admissions represented 218,182 patient days of care under a primary nursing system with 92 percent registered nurses and 8 percent licensed practical nurses, nursing assistants, and technicians. Nursing acuity at four levels was assessed daily for the study period, with a standardized instrument to describe the patient's potential nursing needs. Nursing care hours were defined and measured to identify direct nursing costs assignable to specific patients.

Some of the findings are as follows:

- Average direct nursing costs in the average hospital room costs fall within the range of 18 to 24 percent. Nursing costs are currently part of the room costs (Exhibit 6-7).

- DRGs as a case-mix profile are not predictive of individual patient needs. DRGs are not homogeneous from a nursing acuity perspective (Exhibit 6-8).

Exhibit 6-7 Hospital Summary Costs for Top 22 DRGs on a Medical Unit

DRG	Average Ancillary Costs $	Average Room Costs* $	Average Direct Nursing Costs $	% Nsg Costs in Avg Room Costs
014 Spec Cerebrovascular Dis Ex. TIA	2,395	5,544	1,150	20.7
127 Heart Failure and Shock	1,408	3,189	578	18.0
468 Unrelated O.R. Proc. in MDC	3,806	4,642	996	21.5
122 AMI w/o C.V. Complication: Disch Alive	1,414	3,636	574	15.8
125 Other Circulatory Dis. w/C Cath	1,343	845	169	20.0
089 Pneumonia/Pleurisy Age ≥ 70 and/or CC	1,684	2,396	462	19.3
088 Chronic Obst. Pulmonary Disease	1,579	2,775	486	17.5
182 Gastroesophagitis/Mis: Dis Age ≥ 70 and/or CC	1,111	1,841	319	17.3
403 Lymphoma/Leukemia Age ≥ 70 and/or CC	4,570	3,303	633	19.2
415 O.R. Proc. for Infect./Parasitic Dis.	4,750	7,699	1,814	23.6
082 Respiratory Neoplasms	1,762	2,830	496	17.5
079 Resp. Infect/Inflam Age ≥ 70 and/or CC	3,477	5,756	1,148	19.9
416 Septicemia Age ≥ 18	3,250	3,460	699	20.2
121 A.M.I. w/C. V. Compl., Disch. Alive	1,864	4,481	706	15.8
296 Nutr. & Misc. Metab Dis Age ≥ 70 and/or CC	1,403	2,827	539	19.1
018 Cranial./Periph. Nerv. Dis. Age ≥ 70 and/or CC	2,237	5,267	1,023	19.4
140 Angina Pectoris	815	2,027	336	16.6
395 Red Blood Cell Disorders Age ≥ 18	1,268	1,857	298	16.0
096 Brochitis/Asthma Age ≥ 70 and/or CC	1,555	2,390	390	16.3
174 G.I. Bleed Age ≥ 70 and/or CC	1,896	2,666	537	20.1
129 Cardiac Arrest	5,886	13,019	2,378	18.3
310 Transureth. Proc. Age ≥ 70 and/or CC	2,116	3,437	642	18.7

CC = complication/comorbidity.
*N.B. Average room costs include *total* nursing costs.

Source: M. D. Sovie, M. A. Tarcinale, A. W. Vanputee, and A. E. Stunden, "Amalgam of Nursing Acuity, DRGs and Costs," *Nursing Management* 16, no. 3 (1985): 33.

- Nursing patient classification data coupled with DRGs enabled a budget prediction that reflected 87 percent of the actual adjusted expenditures.

- A higher number of nursing care hours was associated with patients age 70 or greater and/or with complications or comorbidity (Exhibit 6-9).

A "Severity of Illness Index" is another method of analyzing a specific hospital's case mix; it attempts to group patients according to the patients' resource consumption based on the severity of their illnesses. This index "does not specifically include an adjustment for the complexity/intensity of nursing care required,"[167] since nursing is only one of seven components in the scale.

Problems in determining nursing costs per DRG include inaccurate assignment of the DRG, inaccurate nursing assessments of patient needs, and allowances for the differences between the care needed and the care received by patients.

Exhibit 6-8 DRGs with > 100 Patient Days with Highest Nursing Intensity as Measured by Nursing Patient Classification, Categories 3 and 4

DRG		Total Adm.	Total Pt. Days	Nursing Acuity Category Percent Pt. Days in Each				Percent Days in Cat. 3 & 4
				1	2	3	4	
077	O.R. Proc. on Resp. Sx x Maj. Chest w/o CC	8	209	5.7	2.4	7.2	84.7	91.9
385	Neonates Died/Transferred	146	2290	--	1.1	17.2	80.9	98.1
386	Neonates Extreme Immaturity	59	2378	--	2.9	31.3	65.6	96.9
002	Craniotomy for Trauma Age ≥ 18	35	1618	2.4	4.5	23.7	69.5	93.2
387	Prematurity w/Major Problems	125	3126	--	6.1	42.6	50.6	93.2
457	Extensive Burns	7	330	0.6	6.4	36.4	56.7	93.1
123	Acute Myocardial Infarct: Expired	39	315	5.4	5.4	19.1	70.2	89.3
027	Trauma Stupor/Coma > 1 hr	23	277	3.2	7.9	25.6	63.2	88.8
192	Minor Panc./Liver/Shunt Proc.	5	213	5.2	6.1	32.4	56.3	88.7
173	Digest Sys. Malignancy Age ≥ 70	9	174	5.7	6.9	32.8	54.6	87.4
001	Craniotomy Age ≥ 18X for trauma	127	3383	9.5	11.9	32.7	45.9	78.6
091	Pneumonia/Pleurisy Age 0-17	82	440	4.1	11.4	39.3	45.2	84.5
156	Stomach Esophageal & Duodenal Proc. Age 0-17	30	268	3.4	8.6	43.7	44.4	88.1
213	Amputations for Mscl/Connec. Tis. Disorders	16	493	3.0	11.0	42.0	44.0	86.0
415	OR Proc. for Infect/Parasitic Diseases	33	940	7.4	14.6	35.2	42.8	78.0
003	Craniotomy Age < 18	84	1133	6.5	17.2	34.4	41.8	76.2
109	Other Cardiothor Proc. w/o Pump	39	647	8.8	11.0	39.3	41.0	80.3
064	Ear/Nose/Throat Malignancy	25	281	4.3	14.6	40.6	40.6	81.2
029	Trauma Stupor/Coma < 1 hr Age 18-69	22	201	15.4	12.9	30.8	40.8	71.6
081	Resp. Infect/Inflamm. Age 0-17	14	175	3.4	12.0	46.3	38.3	84.6
074	Other ENT Diag. Age 0-17	14	169	2.4	13.0	47.3	37.3	84.6
028	Truma stupor/Coma < 1 hr Age ≥ 70 and/or CC	13	208	7.0	16.7	40.8	35.6	76.4
137	Cardiac Congenital & Valve Disorder Age 0-17	22	205	2.0	12.7	51.7	33.7	85.4
458	Non Extensive Burns w/skn graft	34	802	4.6	14.0	48.0	33.4	81.4
405	Lymphoma/Leukemia Age 0-17	39	463	5.0	14.0	46.2	34.8	81.0

Subtotal 20,738 = 9.5% of Total Patient Days in Sample

Source: M. D. Sovie, M. A. Tarcinale, A. W. Vanputee, and A. E. Studen, "Amalgam of Nursing Acuity, DRGs and Costs, *Nursing Management* 16, no. 3 (1985): 40.

Making DRGs sensitive to the severity of illness and nursing care cost components is a difficult methodologic issue on which some current research is being focused.

Karen Mitchell, editor of *Pediatric Nursing*, indicates that if nurses are vital to the survival of their institutions, they must do the following:[168]

First: Nurses must document their cost effectiveness in terms that administrators can understand, such as lengths of stay.

Second: Nurses must assume decision making power over their own practices and staffing patterns, . . . authority over their own budgets, and document their cost savings to the institution.

Exhibit 6-9 Comparative DRGs With and Without Age ≥ 70 or CC with LOS and Nursing Hours

DRG		N. Adm.	Mean LOS	LOS SD	Min LOS	Max LOS	Nsg Hours Mean	Nsg Hours SD
007	Peripheral/Cranial Nerve & Other Nervous Systems Proc. Age ≥ 70 and/or CC	23	32.6	68.3	1	285	84.5	150.1
008	Peripheral/Cranial Nerve & Other Nervous Systems Proc. Age < 70	70	4.2	3.3	1	18	20.3	17.3
024	Seizure/Headache Age ≥ 70 and/or CC	45	16.9	24.1	1	127	63.0	91.1
025	Seizure/Headache Age 18-69	61	9.6	10.2	1	73	35.6	31.7
096	Bronchitis/Asthma Age ≥ 70 and/or CC	66	8.3	9.9	2	66	38.5	70.1
097	Bronchitis/Asthma Age 18-69	82	5.3	3.1	1	20	21.1	17.7
110	Maj. Reconst Vasc Proc. Age ≥ 70 and/or CC	124	24.5	20.1	1	106	173.0	209.3
111	Maj. Reconst Vasc Proc. Age < 70	81	13.1	5.8	7	39	74.7	39.1
130	Peripheral Vasc Dis Age ≥ 70 and/or CC	69	9.6	5.8	1	27	44.5	33.0
131	Peripheral Vasc Dis Age < 70	43	8.7	8.7	1	55	31.8	20.0
148	Maj Sm/Lg Bowel Proc. Age ≥ 70 and/or CC	111	22.6	19.7	1	138	110.4	103.6
149	Maj Sm/Lg Bowel Proc. Age < 70	49	13.6	12.8	3	93	63.1	70.3
174	GI Bleed Age ≥ 70 and/or CC	67	11.0	22.5	2	185	52.9	135.4
175	GI Bleed Age < 70	36	4.5	2.5	1	12	17.5	11.5
197	Cholecystectomy w/o CDE Age ≥ 70 and/or CC	56	12.2	5.9	6	38	51.6	34.1
198	Cholecystectomy w/o CDE Age < 70	101	7.7	2.0	5	17	31.9	8.7
210	Other Hip/Femur Proc. Age ≥ 70 and/or CC	78	32.1	21.9	6	124	143.0	109.1
211	Other Hip/Femur Proc. Age 18-69	37	38.9	19.7	7	81	127.4	84.3
442	Other OR Proc. for Injury Age ≥ 70 and/or CC	65	23.8	24.7	1	123	123.2	127.1
443	Other OR Proc. for Injury Age < 70	50	12.7	14.3	1	89	73.8	116.0

CC = Complication and/or comorbidity

Source: M. D. Sovie, M. A. Tarcinale, A. W. Vanputee, and A. E. Stunden, "Amalgam of Nursing Acuity, DRGs and Costs," *Nursing Management* 16, no. 3 (1985): 38.

Third: Nurses must be discharge planners and coordinators of home health services.

Fourth: Nurses must become involved in the refining of DRGs so that hospitals may be accurately reimbursed.

Nurses are becoming involved in diversification efforts to fill empty hospital beds to generate revenue. Empty bed areas are being converted into hospice units, swing beds are being used for skilled nursing long-term care patients, and outpatient services are being expanded to provide on-site and home health care. Management can profit from the participation of nursing administrators in program planning, projections of costs and revenues, and service delivery.[169]

"Nurses must be actively involved in the consideration of the financial aspects of nursing, keeping costs to a minimum while maintaining quality care."[170] These new roles are added to the historical, traditional caregiving and ministering to patients. "Like other professionals within the hospital, nurses must add a third dimension to their humanitarian and clinical career motivations, an acute sensitivity to the business environment in which they practice their profession."[171]

Pharmacy Services

Hospital pharmacy services represent only 5 percent of hospital expenditures, but represent one third of the pharmaceutical industry sales. Most giant drug companies do not foresee any changes as a result of the DRG implementation, despite cost consciousness and stress on generics in prescribing. However, it is acknowledged that marketability of new drugs and acceptance into hospital formularies must pass tests of price competition against alternatives and utility towards reducing length of stay.[172]

Once viewed as revenue-generating services, pharmacy costs are integrated into the DRG payment and are under the scrutiny of administrators and DRG coordinators.Pharmacy costs per DRG, and cost per DRG per physician, are being analyzed under drug use review (DUR) programs to identify patients with high-cost and low-cost pharmacy needs. Patterns of physician prescribing are also being analyzed in attempts to manage under DRGs and cope with this cost center (Exhibit 6-10).

DUR focuses attention on the following:

- Necessity of prescribing
- Appropriateness of treatment including appropriateness of dose, route of administration, and drug of choice
- Alternate therapies
- Individual physician prescribing patterns.[173]

Opportunities to explore cost-effective prescribing, alternative pharmacotherapeutics, and prevailing patterns emerge from review of data on drug use and DRG. Additionally, concurrent reviews of drug profiles seek to identify potential adverse drug reactions and drug-induced disease (from adverse drug interaction). Both reactions can contribute to increasing LOS.When coupled with prospective discussions of cost-effective paradigms, these are important elements in quality patient care stimulated by the needs of cost containment.

Exhibit 6-10 DUR Report by DRG by Prescriber for the Period January 1 to March 31, 1983

Physician	No. Patients	ALOS[a]	% Var.[b]	No. Drugs per Pt.	% Var.	No. Doses per Pt.	% Var.	No. Therapeutic Classes per Pt.	% Var.	Drug Cost[c] per Pt. ($)	% Var.
MDC 01[d]											
DRG 014: Specific Cerebrovascular Disorders except TIA											
Physician A	4	12.25 ± 2.22	13.6	12.50 ± 2.65	5.0	136.50 ± 44.43	0.9	7.25 ± 0.96	(3.2)	114.92 ± 28.33	(4.9)
Physician B	2	20.50 ± 3.54	90.2	18.50 ± 0.71	55.3	186.00 ± 32.53	37.5	10.50 ± 0.71	40.2	189.00 ± 13.48	56.5
Physician C	6	10.33 ± 1.97	(4.2)	8.67 ± 2.42	(27.2)	87.67 ± 15.08	(35.2)	4.83 ± 0.75	(35.5)	67.15 ± 19.84	(44.4)
Regional norm		10.78 ± 2.09		11.91 ± 2.63		135.27 ± 20.79		7.49 ± 0.87		120.79 ± 18.42	
National norm		12.67 ± 1.83		12.07 ± 2.16		125.62 ± 18.33		6.95 ± 0.68		110.26 ± 10.89	
DRG 015: Transient Ischemic Attacks											
Physician A	4	23.00 ± 4.24	49.6	10.75 ± 2.06	22.9	142.75 ± 47.32	18.4	7.50 ± 0.58	12.4	160.80 ± 30.34	8.0
Physician B	0										
Physician C	3	16.23 ± 2.52	5.6	9.33 ± 0.58	6.6	120.00 ± 16.52	(0.5)	5.33 ± 0.58	(20.1)	152.81 ± 7.41	2.6
Regional norm		15.37 ± 3.78		8.75 ± 1.79		120.61 ± 15.73		6.67 ± 0.93		148.89 ± 17.93	
National norm		19.61 ± 4.27		7.98 ± 1.54		110.76 ± 12.88		6.01 ± 0.87		123.64 ± 10.25	

a Average length of patient stay.
b Percentage variation from regional norm.
c Drug cost at EAC to permit standardization.
d There are a total of 23 major diagnostic categories (MDCs) and 467 DRGs (DRGs 468–470 are assigned to invalid or ungroupable diagnoses); this report includes only those DRGs to which patient cases have been assigned in this hospital during the time period of the report.

Source: F. R. Curtiss, "Pharmacy Management Strategies for Responding to Hospital Reimbursement Changes," *American Journal of Hospital Pharmacy* 40, no. 9 (September 1983): 1491.

In a study of 10,550 patients—retrospectively categorized by DRGs—discharged from a 316-bed community hospital,[174] the most expensive DRGs, in terms of pharmacy services, were ranked by MDCs and DRGs. DRG 107 (coronary bypass) had the highest total pharmacy charges, as did MDC 5 (diseases and disorders of the circulatory system). DRG 105 (cardiac valve procedure with pump), which had the largest LOS and highest hospital charges per patient, is ninth in rank of total pharmacy charges. This is but one example that long LOS and high-cost hospital services may not be associated with high pharmacy costs (Exhibit 6-11 and Exhibit 6-12).

Another study of 43,969 patients discharged from 43 hospitals in the Blue Cross of Central Ohio region, and 6,121 patients from a 1,017-bed community hospital in Columbus, Ohio corroborated some of these findings and revealed commonality in 13 of the 20 DRGs in pharmacy charges.[175] However, there was an indication that correlation was significant between hospital charges and pharmacy charges as well as between length of stay and pharmacy charges (Exhibit 6-13 and Exhibit 6-14).

Caution is needed in interpreting direct relationships of expensive DRGs and expensive pharmacy costs. Nonetheless, this points out the need to review these areas, which will yield cost savings.

In many hospital pharmacy departments, relative value units (RVU) systems are in development (similar to the patient care unit system) "to measure workload and compare efficiency among sections within the department and against previous performance."[176] For most product groups and pharmacy activities, including clinical functions, workload value factors are being assigned as a base for new pharmacy charges (both direct and indirect costs) for providing each service. Rates will be adjusted annually, which reflect managerial changes, staffing levels, overhead factors, and so on.[177]

Pharmacy managers are turning their attention toward streamlining their departments. They are making changes in staffing, increasing productivity, and modernizing the processes of purchasing and inventory control. Some departments have reduced pharmacy staff, increased part-timers, and optimized the pharmacists/technician ratios, while others have found that increasing professional clinical pharmacists helps to achieve goals for the service, patients, and DRG monitoring needs. Most pharmacies have increased their automation activities, using computers for purchasing and inventory control, as well as for drug profiles for patients, screening for drug interactions and physician profiles of prescribing.[178,179]

Pharmacy inventory accounts for two-thirds of departmental expense and increasing inventory turnovers to at least 10 per year, from the average 6.7 turnovers per year, is a recommended goal to control expenses. Use of wholesalers as prime vendors and for drug-depoting has been important in reducing inventory, eliminating purchase orders, and reducing staff time.[180-182] Reducing the price

Exhibit 6-11 Distribution of the 20 Most Expensive DRGs by MDC[a]

MDC	Description of MDC	No. DRGs in MDC[b]	Total Pharmacy Charges per MDC ($)
5	Diseases and disorders of the circulatory system	7	815,208
4	Diseases and disorders of the respiratory system	4	308,723
6	Diseases and disorders of the digestive system	3	212,393
13	Diseases and disorders of the female reproductive system	2	96,978
1	Diseases and disorders of the nervous system	1	72,075
7	Diseases and disorders of the hepatobiliary system and pancreas	1	57,127
17	Myeloproliferative disorders and poorly differentiated malignancy and other neoplasms	1	55,111
14	Pregnancy, childbirth, and the puerperium	1	51,543

[a] Major diagnostic category.[6]
[b] Represents the number of DRGs to which patients with this MDC were assigned during the study period.

Source: H. F. Catania, M. I. Osama, S. L. Guasco, and P. N. Catania, "Analyzing Pharmacy Charges Using DRGs," *American Journal of Hospital Pharmacy* 41, no. 5 (1984): 922.

per unit through volume purchasing, offering discounts for prompt payment, and use of bid prices are also part of strategic plans to control drug costs.[183]

Pharmacy and Therapeutics (P & T) committees are increasing their role under DRGs by controlling drug entry and reviewing use of drugs in their respective hospital formularies. Deleting drugs and creating availability of generics and lower-cost alternative products help reduce inventory and general cost of use. Communication with physicians provides an explanation of decisions made, educates professionals, and aids in decision making for prescribing.[184] In pre-DRG days, these interventions "would be viewed as reprehensible intrusion on physician autonomy and professional prerogative."[185] As specific information is developed on unusual physician prescribing patterns, the role of the P & T Committee might be expanded to "target physicians for one-on-one discussions regarding therapeutic options." The ability to successfully modify physician prescribing behavior has shifted because of administrators' "vested interest" in the pharmacy cost center and the political backing this provides to Committee

Exhibit 6-12   Ranks of the 20 Most Expensive DRGs within Various Measures of Hospital and Pharmacy Charges

DRG	Total Pharmacy Charges per DRG	No. Patients	Rank within Each Measure			
			Pharmacy Charges per Patient	Hospital Charges per Patient	Pharmacy Charges as % of Hospital Charges	Length of Stay per Patient
107	1	8	2	2	9	4
82	2	10	8	11	3	8
148	3	15	4	5	5	3
127	4	5	14	14	15	12
88	5	13	9	7	10	10
14	6	7	13	10	16	9
96	7	11	11	12	8	14
154	8	19	3	3	4	2
105	9	20	1	1	6	1
89	10	12	12	13	7	13
197	11	14	10	9	12	11
122	12	9	15	6	19	7
182	13	2	18	20	11	18
403	14	17	6	8	2	6
132	15	4	17	15	18	16
125	16	1	20	18	20	20
354	17	3	19	16	17	15
370	18	6	16	17	13	17
110	19	18	5	4	14	5
366	20	16	7	19	1	19

Source: H. F. Catania, M. I. Osama, S. L. Guasco, and P. N. Catania, "Analyzing Pharmacy Charges Using DRGs," *American Journal of Hospital Pharmacy* 41, no. 5 (1984): 923.

Exhibit 6-13 Ranks of the Top 20 Most Expensive DRGs by Total Pharmacy and I.V. Charges for All Hospitals in the Blue Cross of Central Ohio (BCCO) Region and for Riverside Methodist Hospital (RMH) in 1982

DRG	Description	MDC	BCCO			RMH		
			No. Patients	Total Pharmacy Charges[a] ($)	Rank	No. Patients	Total Pharmacy Charges[a] ($)	Rank
468	Unrelated operating room procedure for a given MDC	...	647	515,219	1	94	73,876	2
355	Nonradical hysterectomy, age < 70 w/o C.C.[b]	13	1,197	412,722	2	112	20,388	10
373	Vaginal delivery w/o complicating diagnoses	14	4,628	360,711	3	797	50,120	3
107	Coronary bypass w/o cardiac catheterization	5	208	306,739	4	797	50,120	3
371	Cesarean section w/o C.C.	14	1,082	286,527	5	103	106,824	1
198	Total cholecystectomy w/o C.D.E.,[c] age < 70 w/o C.C.	7	660	244,298	6	204	34,605	5
						107	30,939	6
183	Esophagitis, gastroenteritis, and miscellaneous digestive diseases, age 18–69 w/o C.C.	6	1,171	213,389	7	143	15,278	17
404	Lymphoma or leukemia, age 18–69 w/o C.C.	17	185	192,789	8	33	38,670	4
149	Major small and/or large bowel procedure, age < 70 w/o C.C.	6	145	184,737	9	31	25,023	7
82	Respiratory neoplasms	4	224	164,379	10	31	12,108	20
155	Stomach, esophageal, and duodenal procedures, age 18–69 w/o C.C.	6	106	151,201	11	20	17,943	13
358	Uterus and adenexa procedure for nonmalignancy except tubal interruption	13	466	144,559	12	...	...	...
148	Major small and/or large bowel procedures, age > 69 with C.C.	6	53	138,426	13	5	17,515	14
122	Circulatory disorders with acute myocardial infarction w/o cardiovascular complications; discharged alive	5	391	136,799	14	65	13,992	18
090	Simple pneumonia and pleurisy, age 18–69 w/o C.C.	4	252	125,779	15	22	16,137	16
403	Lymphoma and/or leukemia, age > 69 with C.C.	17	42	125,066	16	5	17,111	15
243	Medical back problems	8	1,069	109,019	17	...	...	...
097	Bronchitis and asthma, age 18–69 w/o C.C.	4	314	100,750	18	...	...	...
105	Cardiac valve procedure with pump and w/o cardiac catheterization	5	28	99,522	19	13	21,641	9
197	Total cholecystectomy w/o C.D.E.,[c] age > 69 with C.C.	7	150	97,439	20	...	...	...
367	Malignancy, female reproductive system, age < 70 w/o C.C.	13	...	...	...	44	24,002	8
209	Major joint procedure	8	...	...	...	34	20,264	11
430	Psychoses	19	...	...	...	167	18,864	12
005	Extracranial vascular procedures	1	...	...	...	1	12,382	19
Total			13,018	4,110,070	...	2,046	587,682	

[a] Includes all pharmacy and i.v. charges.
[b] Without complications or comorbidity = w/o C.C.
[c] Common duct exploration = C.D.E.

Source: M. J. Magee, D. S. Pathak, T. P. Sherrin, and D. N. Schneider, "ABC Analysis of the Relationship between Pharmacy Charges and DRGs," *American Journal of Hospital Pharmacy* 42, no. 3 (1985): 573.

recommendations. One of the controversial plans is to institute strict prescribing sanctions:

- Written requests for nonformulary items
- Countersignatures for certain antibiotics
- Broad authorization for drug product selection by pharmacists.[186]

New alliances are being formed with medical education departments to help disseminate information on drug monitoring, costs, new drugs, antibiotic usage,

Exhibit 6-14   Pharmacy and Hospital Charges per Patient for the 20 Most Expensive DRGs in 1982 at Riverside Methodist Hospital

DRG	Length of Stay (days)	Mean Rank	Pharmacy Charges per Patient ($)	Mean Rank	Hospital Charges per Patient ($)	Mean Rank	Pharmacy and I.V. Charges as a Percent of Hospital Charges	Mean Rank	Pharmacy and I.V. Charges as a Percent of All Pharmacy Charges	Mean Rank
107	12.7 ± 5.5	7	1037 ± 325	5	9,961 ± 2,644	4	10.4	11	8.4	1
468	11.4 ± 12.4	12	786 ± 1865	8	4,924 ± 6,339	9	16.0	8	5.8	2
373	3.1 ± 0.9	20	63 ± 48	20	1,503 ± 432	18	4.2	19	3.9	3
404	14.3 ± 11.5	6	1172 ± 1971	4	5,010 ± 5,148	8	23.4	3	3.0	4
371	5.9 ± 2.5	17	170 ± 130	17	2,576 ± 744	16	6.6	17	2.7	5
198	8.7 ± 4.5	15	289 ± 207	14	2,759 ± 1,282	15	10.5	10	2.4	6
149	12.5 ± 4.8	8	807 ± 464	7	4,411 ± 1,490	10	18.3	5	2.0	7
367	3.6 ± 4.1	19	546 ± 344	12	1,251 ± 1,099	19	43.6	1	1.9	8
105	15.8 ± 7.2	5	1665 ± 1528	3	16,402 ± 8,675	2	10.2	12	1.7	9
355	7.9 ± 1.8	16	182 ± 151	16	2,457 ± 498	17	7.4	16	1.6	10
209	16.2 ± 9.8	4	596 ± 877	11	7,564 ± 4,623	6	7.9	15	1.6	11
430	18.2 ± 12.2	3	113 ± 110	18	3,291 ± 2,068	14	3.4	20	1.5	12
155	12.0 ± 7.4	9	897 ± 1747	6	5,254 ± 7,021	7	17.1	7	1.4	13
148	28.0 ± 17.4	1	3503 ± 4935	1	17,531 ± 22,083	1	20.0	4	1.4	14
403	21.4 ± 9.2	2	3422 ± 2679	2	14,319 ± 9,630	3	23.9	2	1.3	15
90	9.6 ± 12.6	14	734 ± 1050	10	4,078 ± 6,678	11	18.0	6	1.3	16
183	4.4 ± 3.1	18	107 ± 165	19	1,218 ± 747	20	8.8	14	1.2	17
122	10.2 ± 4.6	13	215 ± 164	15	3,857 ± 1,779	12	5.6	18	1.1	18
5	11.6 ± 6.4	10	774 ± 1304	9	7,937 ± 8,442	5	9.8	13	1.0	19
82	11.6 ± 8.9	11	391 ± 495	13	3,572 ± 3,021	13	10.9	9	0.9	20

Source: M. J. Magee, D. S. Pathak, T. P. Sherrin, and D. N. Schneider, "ABC Analysis of the Relationship between Pharmacy Charges and DRGs," *American Journal of Hospital Pharmacy* 42, no. 3 (1985): 574.

adverse reactions, drug interactions, alternate therapies, and clinical pharmacy programs.[187] Cost-effective strategies are being discussed with nursing departments concerning use of I.V. administration sets, waste of I.V. solutions, and nursing convenience/pharmacy cost issues.[188] Changes in drug distribution systems to more efficient exchange carts and reduction of multiple storage sites on the floors are all intradepartmental issues being resolved in favor of labor-saving and cost-saving methods.

Within the hospital, new professional opportunities for clinical pharmacy specialists are developing; for example, primary care pharmacist (PCP) programs assign pharmacists to nursing units to verify documentation of orders, administer medications, assure accuracy and accountability of drugs, monitor prescribing, and consult with nurses and physicians.[189] Hospitals also operate poison control centers for emergency calls from the community. Institutions have also developed collaborative arrangements for computerized data development and analysis.

In order for pharmacy departments to get back their revenue-generating position in hospitals, diversification to new services not under the DRG constraints have been intensified. Pharmacy departments are meeting needs of the patients in the community with services such as:

- Home intravenous therapy (for antibiotics and cancer chemotherapeutic agents)

- Parenteral and enteral nutrition

- Blood glucose monitoring with drug dosage adjustments

- Surgical supplies, home oxygen therapy.[190-192]

Manufacturing selective products, such as suppositories or reagents not usually available in local pharmacies, has marketability to community pharmacies as well as to physicians.[193]

Offering services to nursing homes, patients of home health agencies, HMOs, and other institutions and agencies,[194] in addition to major outpatient prescription services, provides additional opportunity for expansion into profitable areas.[195,196]

Physical Therapy and Occupational Therapy

Hospital administrators view the rehabilitation services—both physical therapy (PT) and occupational therapy (OT)—with renewed interest under the DRG system. These departments can contribute to patient care and reduction in length of stay, and can be viewed as cost centers which may be reduced with minimal quality impact.

Prior to PPS and DRG methodologies of cost containment, the physical therapy department in the hospital was considered to be revenue-generating; at least, it was a self-supporting service, separately billable to Medicare and other payers, and additional to room and board charges. Under DRG, physical therapy services are included in the total payment for the specific DRG and therefore not separately billable or able to generate revenue from inpatients.

For each DRG, PT and/or OT cost components on the average are being derived which enable administrators and therapists to evolve treatment programs and options which have financial implications. Patterns of practice for major diagnostic category (MDC) and selected DRGs are being reviewed with expectation that "winners and losers" will emerge and alteration of services may be planned for specific patients.

Recent surveys have indicated that some departments are flourishing. The number of therapists has increased so as to initiate treatment as early as possible, with a discharge orientation and plans for transition to outpatient settings, home health services, and an adaptive, supportive home environment. In these settings, the therapies have been said to contribute to the reduced length of stay and enhanced quality of patient care.[197]

Increased programming is occurring in some hospitals, involving intensive physical therapy for wound care, burns, multiple lacerations, stroke, and severe muscle strains. For a group of neurology patients treated with physical, occupational, and speech therapy, the length of stay dropped from 12 to 10 days in one hospital. New inpatient pain and stress reduction centers concentrate on offering help for chronic pain sufferers, and other new schemes are directed toward psychiatric patients and adolescents to bolster the hospital admissions and general operations in coping with DRGs. Some rehabilitation departments are evaluating certain patients prior to admission as part of streamlining pre-operative procedures; therapists are becoming part of the operating room team for post-operative casting (i.e., amputations) and have increased services in the evening and weekend—all this is expressly designed to help reduce the hospital LOS.[198]

Effects of DRGs in other hospitals have been negative—with reductions in inpatient referrals and admissions, hiring freezes and reductions in professional staff, "down substitution" of PTs to PTAs (physical therapy assistants), and out-and-out department closures. Certain patients with specific DRGs have been deemed no longer eligible for therapy services and the effect on quality of care is being questioned. It has been reported that for postoperative cardiac surgery patients, therapy services have been discontinued entirely in one hospital in Virginia.[199] With a reduced length of stay, the need for therapies in the most acute stage of the patient's illness is being questioned. Referrals may wait for the post-hospital period to be accomplished in ambulatory and home settings.

There is also some concern that referrals to therapy departments increases the LOS, during which time patients are being restored to better function. To avoid this, in some hospitals, no referral is made until after discharge.

At the Yale-New Haven Medical Center, Revian Zeleznik, director of rehabilitative services, has compiled data on DRGs with a high dollar volume or a high level of charge per patient at Yale (Exhibit 6-15).[200]

The variation on LOS is noted among those patients who did and those who did not see a physical therapist. The longer stay for those with physical therapy is postulated to be because of the therapy or because the patients are more acutely ill and therefore need the service.

Ken Davis, director of the Department of Practice of the American Physical Therapy Association, believes that "more services do not necessarily result in better care" and that "one should certainly be able to thoughtfully reduce the number of tests performed and services provided, without necessarily lowering overall quality of care." He believes that some "honest introspection" is important for "looking at physical therapy care and deciding where it is truly achieving its clinical goals and where it is not."[201]

Physical therapists are being urged "to classify and prioritize those conditions that lend themselves to physical therapy interventions and those that do not." This intraprofessional reassessment and "introspection" is spurred by DRG, cost consciousness, efficiency, and challenges by other competing professional cost centers in hospital operations. Occupational therapists are similarly being exhorted "to meet treatment goals in fewer sessions" and to "concentrate on reducing length of stay by addressing previously those problems that keep the patients in the hospital."[202] Furthermore, Susan J. Scott, Director of the Government and Legal Affairs Division of the American Occupational Therapy Association, recognizes that "documentation will need to be consistent with current computer technology," so that "evaluation and progress reports should be streamlined and adapted to fit into the hospital systems," so that "occupational therapy information will be available by DRG, which will be essential for planning and budgeting."[203] Record keeping and documentation have assumed a greater importance to substantiate and justify continued service, department integrity, and value to hospital administration. Spending more time on medical records has prompted a therapist to ask, "What are we here for—to document or treat patients?"

Accompanying this variegated pattern for inpatient hospital therapy services is the widely acclaimed expansion in hospital-based ambulatory therapy services, as a part of home health care services, in nursing homes and rehabilitation centers, in HMOs and satellites, clinics and private therapy practice. This new demand is a direct result of DRGs, reduced LOS, earlier discharge, and the needs of patients who, upon leaving the hospital, are sicker than they once were and require help toward recovery and fuller function.[204] While 42 percent of physical

Exhibit 6-15   31 DRGs with Highest Percent of Patients Who Received Physical Therapy (Yale-New Haven Medical Center)

		Received PT (% of patients)	Mean Length of Stay		First day of PT (mean)
DRG	Diagnosis		with PT	without PT	
209	Major Joint Procedures	100	20.47	—	4.52
287	Skin Grafts & Wound Debridement for Endocrine, Nutri, & Metab. Disorders	100	25.12	—	4.06
459	Non-Extensive Burns with Wound Debridement & other O.R. Procedures	100	20.50	—	.50
107	Coronary Bypass w/o Cardiac Cath.	99.54	15.06	6.10	2.38
211	Hip & Femur Procedures except Major Joint, age 18-69 w/o complication or comorbidity (CC)	97.37	18.59	24.00	7.62
121	Circulatory Disorders with Acute Myocardial Infarction (AMI) & Cardiovascular (CV) Compensation, discharged alive	92.37	14.63	8.70	5.27
210	Hip & Femur Procedures except Major Joint, age 70+ and/or CC	90.08	29.50	18.50	7.55
122	Circulatory Disorders with AMI w/o CV Comp., discharged alive	90.00	11.82	5.58	4.43
284	Skin Grafts for Skin Ulcer or Cellulitis, age under 70 w/o CC	90.00	33.44	24.50	2.61
458	Non-Extensive Burns with Skin Grafts	88.00	26.41	9.33	1.45
263	Skin grafts for Skin Ulcer or Cellulitis Age 70+ and/or CC	86.84	35.79	12.80	3.03
271	Skin Ulcers	86.36	26.72	3.25	1.72
221	Knee Procedures 70+ and/or CC	85.71	5.17	2.00	3.33
213	Amputations for Musculoskeletal System & Connective Tissue Disorders	85.00	31.00	20.67	9.65
114	Upper Limb & Toe Amputation for Circulatory System Disorders	84.62	32.64	8.00	5.45

285	Amputations for Endocrine, Nutritional and Metabolic Disorders	84.21	44.31	12.33	4.56
460	Non-Extensive Burns w/o O.R. Procedure	80.00	10.46	2.86	.82
457	Extensive Burns	72.73	34.38	6.67	4.63
4	Spinal Procedures	69.09	38.05	12.18	8.53
273	Major Skin Disorders, age under 70 w/o CC	69.07	20.54	5.53	1.33
14	Specific Cerebrovascular Disorders Except TIA	64.09	26.51	8.56	7.27
439	Skin Grafts for Injuries	63.16	15.33	5.00	5.83
214	Back & Neck Procedures, 70+ and/or CC	59.65	34.18	10.65	10.26
228	Ganglion (Hand) Procedures	56.25	2.11	1.71	1.11
2	Craniotomy for Trauma, 70+	54.29	66.95	11.81	17.42
272	Major Skin Disorders, age 70+ and/or CC	51.02	26.24	13.17	4.64
1	Craniotomy age 18+ Except for Trauma	43.72	42.45	16.71	14.46
9	Spinal Disorders & Injuries	42.86	35.33	7.00	4.67
110	Major Reconstructive Vascular Procedures age 70+ and/or CC	41.67	32.77	15.66	12.90
269	Other skin, Subcut Tiss & Breast O.R. Proc age 70+ &/or CC	24.14	16.14	7.14	9.29
3	Craniotomy age under 18	20.78	38.88	13.15	9.25

Source: T. Prescious, PPS One Year Later, *Progress Report, American Physical Therapy Association,* September 1984.

therapists are hospital-based, a noticeable shift to ambulatory care settings and private practice is anticipated as this becomes more lucrative and opportunities become more expansive.

Competition between the traditional out-of-hospital therapy services and the new emphasis on hospital-based ambulatory care therapy services have driven hospitals to marketing campaigns and innovative service delivery to lure patients. One hospital in California offers a shuttle bus service to pick up and deliver patients from their home for rehabilitative services, and others provide valet parking to those who can drive up. Special services are being designed for selected DRGs to help reduce LOS; for example, one hospital has a half-day, five-day-per-week program for brain-impaired patients so that the extensive care needed is shifted from inpatient to outpatient. Day centers are developing programs which provide six hours of extensive rehabilitation for neurology patients—those with multiple sclerosis, Parkinson's disease, strokes—for a limited four to six weeks, which allow the patient to be supported at home and reduce hospitalization needs.[205]

Therapists view the early discharges with concern since they treat patients in other institutions—skilled nursing facilities (SNFs) and rehabilitation hospitals—who appear to have been "dumped" for fiscal imperatives of the DRG systems. Return to the referral hospitals because of recurrent strokes, fainting spells, dizziness, and generalized weakness is reported to occur periodically with some patients who are unable to tolerate the intensive rehabilitative approach. Agreements between referral hospitals and rehabilitative settings have been necessary to smooth the revolving door process.

These complaints are also troublesome to the home health care therapy providers. Coordination between discharge planners, inpatient therapists, and home health care therapists is vital for continuity of care. One therapist said that just after they start "transfer training," the person is gone or they have not even learned to sit up yet and the DRG push propels them to the home environment.[206]

Hospitals are contracting to provide rehabilitative therapy services to nursing homes, institutions for the mentally retarded, cerebral palsy centers, and the like to increase revenue.This is in direct competition with private practice therapists who usually provide service to these populations.

Physician-owned physical therapy services (POPTS)[207] is a practice arrangement criticized by many physical therapists. Under this arrangement, therapists are paid by the physicians on an hourly or per-patient basis and services are billed to Medicare and other providers by the physicians. Since many patients who are discharged have prescribed "physiotherapy," private generalist physicians (not necessarily physiatrists) are competing successfully, in well-equipped offices, with hospital outpatient departments.[208] Charges to patients appear to be less in the private physician's office than with institutional billing, where many indirect costs of the hospital are added on to the bills. The private practitioners—physicians and therapists—are able to compete by offering less bureaucracy, less documentation, fewer channels; they have incentives for high productivity from which they reap proportional economic benefits. In addition, since these services are not yet under DRG-like scrutiny, there appears to be more freedom in practice.

Dietitian Services

Food-service costs and services of dietitians are included in the hospital room charges and are included as part of each DRG. Managers of these departments will start costing out their services by DRG to define each unit of service. Mean costs are expected to be differentiated for commissary costs, production, assembly, and service.

Case mix and patient stay have an effect on the food costs. Kathy Emmert, R.D., food-service director at Anne Arundel General Hospital in Annapolis, explains:

> Let's say we have a heart-attack patient. He may be on a liquid diet for the first 12 or 24 hours. But after that, he's eating from our regular menu. Compare that to an appendectomy. He checks in today and doesn't eat. Tomorrow, he's in surgery. He's probably on a soft diet the day after surgery and the next day he goes home. He hasn't eaten a single meal from our regular menu.[209]

Complicated case-mix shifts can also be complicated to staff. "We had 13 patients on tube feedings and eight on total parenteral nutrition. The dietitians were going crazy, but the kitchen wasn't so busy."[210]

Patient menus are speculated to be the last area that hospitals wish to toy with, except to improve satisfaction and acceptability. "We're still in a competitive marketplace and patient food is the biggest marketing tool the hospital has."[211] So says Ed Manley, food-service director, North Broward Medical Center, Pompano Beach, Florida. Discussions of the two-tier patient menu system provokes considerable controversy in this field. One service to "public payers" offered a nonselective or limited selection menu, and a second service for private payers who could also opt for a gourmet menu for additional charges. However, such a system has provoked the following comments: "What about consumer protection, what about civil rights? The elderly have a lot of ombudsmen. There's no way they would stand for a lower class of service for Medicare patients."[212]

Some concessions to cost controls, when the patient stays are shorter, involve shortening the menu cycle and the introduction of lighter, less expensive entrees popular with patients and less costly to the departments.

Cafeteria operations are expected to be self-supporting or revenue-generating by being available to physicians, visitors, employees, and patients; also, menu price can be competitive with local neighborhood eating facilities. Catering services will also need to be clearly costed out, as well as the usual coffee-break supplies provided to staff as a hospital employment benefit.

Dietitians point out that the DRGs have not included nutritional problems as a disease group, although in some cases, nutritional-related illness is really the principal diagnosis and cause of hospitalization. It is also expected that within shorter hospital stays, nutritional patient education prior to discharge and home visits might be valuable, along with dietitian consultations being made available, both privately and at ambulatory care centers.

Marketing of nutritional services to the general community is gaining momentum. The cost effectiveness of these professional services needs to be determined and justified in the emerging competitive marketplace. "Physicians, nurses and pharmacists increase the delivery of nutrition services as part of their practice."[213]

The American Dietetic Association has a Third-Party Reimbursement Planning Committee which is developing a technical manual for documentation of dietetic services. They are also collaborating with the American Society of Hospital Food Services Administrators to develop nutrition protocols for DRGs.[214] This changing environment for members of these associations is being recognized as a challenge for strategic action, and as a guarantee for survival as a health professional team member.

Social Work Service

One of the professional categories not mentioned by specific reference in the DRG legislation is the hospital social worker. While the role of the hospital social worker has been expanding as sensitivity to the social and environmental factors in health gains greater emphasis, there is difficulty in placing dollar signs on the benefit of these activities. Need for social work services is acknowledged, especially for the Medicare elderly population who have complicated concurrent illness and a dependence on support systems of the family and community for continued independent living.[215]

Emphasis on reduced length of stay and early discharge to home with potential supports, or to alternative institutions such as nursing homes, highlights one of the major services of social workers—the coordination of the discharge planning effort. "Inadequate discharge planning could have disastrous effects on patients and their families as well as increase chances for readmissions to the hospital."[216]

It is anticipated that hospital administrators will be most receptive to activities which enhance their overall mission. "Social workers thus have the opportunity to demonstrate that their services, rather than being a luxury, are an important element in cost containment."[217]

Research is underway in trying to clarify identifiable measureable components of the social work activity and the financial implications of productivity criteria.[218]

Moving away from counseling and psychotherapy and expanding community liaison activities and outpatient services implies greater hospital support for services without reimbursement potential. "The pessimist might doubt that a hospital working under constrained payment systems will underwrite social work beyond its walls. The optimist might note, however, that such reimbursement plans place a premium on all procedures that minimize hospital use. If hospital sponsored programs in the community can do that, they may be in a position to expand."[219]

At present, DRGs do not incorporate social work services into the units of costs for patient care. Yet, their contributions for successful implementation of the system are notable. Social work leadership is concerned. "The crux is to figure out how we can cleave to our values and roles while offering indisputably cost effective service. Where a social worker fits into DRGs . . . will depend in a large part on our own initiative in the months ahead."[220]

References

1. W. B. Nestler, "Collaboration and Cooperation:Necessary and Achievable," *The Internist* 24, No. 6 (1983):14-15.

2. "MDs Blast DRGs in Newspaper Ad," *Medical World News*, 27, No. 2 (January 27, 1986):86.

3. S. D. Carter, "Diagnosis Related Groups: How Will They Affect You?" *Minnesota Medicine* 67, No. 1 (1984):52-56.

4. F. A. Riddick, "The Doctor and the DRG," *The Internist* 24, No. 6 (1983):17-18.

5. D. Neuhauser, "A Message to Physicians," *The Internist* 24, No. 6 (1983):23-25.

6. K. Shannon, "Outpatient Surgery Up 77 Percent: Data," *Hospitals* 59, No. 10 (May 16, 1985):54.

7. C. J. Kaemmerer, "A New Reimbursement System, DRGs are Coming; Minnesota Medical Association," *Connecticut Medicine* 47, No. 11 (1983):697-699.

8. Riddick, "Doctor and DRG."

9. Ibid.

10. Carter, "Diagnosis Related Groups."

11. Kaemmerer, "New Reimbursement System."

12. Riddick, "Doctor and DRG."

13. Ibid.

14. R. D. Warnke, "We're Scoring Attendings by DRG," *Medical Economics,* November 12, 1984.

15. Ibid.

16. M. Nathanson, "Computers Crank Out DRG Cost Data, But How Valid is Information," *Modern Healthcare* 13, No. 9 (1983):160, 162, 164.

17. Ibid.

18. P. L. Grimaldi, "Physicians and the DRG Model," *The Journal of the Medical Society of New Jersey* 77, No. 4 (1980):279-281.

19. K. Hunt, "DRG--What It Is, How It Works, And Why It Will Hurt," *Medical Economics* 60, No. 18 (September 5, 1983):262-272.

20. P. Dwyer, "DRGs: Regulatory, Deregulatory Device," *Hospital Progress* 62, No. 3 (1981):26, 28, 30.

21. Grimaldi, "Physicians and DRG Model."

22. P. Levin, J. F. Silverman, and R. S. Merchant, "Diagnosis Related Groups: A New Way of Managing Hospital Revenues, Costs, Reimbursement," *Oklahoma State Medical Association* 76, No. 9 (1983):324-326.

23. L. Khan, "Meeting of the Minds: Hospital/Physician Diplomacy Crucial Under Prospective System," *Hospitals* 57, No. 6 (1983):84-86.

24. N. K. Connolly, "DRGs:Their Relationship to Hospital Practice," *Southern Medical Journal* 76, No. 9 (1983):1082-1083.

25. Nathanson, "Computers Crank Out Data."

26. J. Riffer, "DRG Payment Plan to Expand Physician Role," *Hospitals* 57, No. 8 (April 16, 1983):17.

27. Hunt, "DRG—What, How, Why."

28. "The Bottom Line: DRGs May Decide Hospital Privileges," *Medical Economics,* December 10, 1984.

29. *Mount Sinai Record* 3, No. 2 (April, 1985):1-8.

30. E. Muñoz, "Surgonomics: The Cost of Gastrointestinal Hemorrhage, the Identifier Concept," *American Journal of Gastroenterology* 80, No. 2 (1985):139-142.

31. D. Wirtschafter, "Diagnosis Related Groups. The Impact of DRGs on Medical Management," *Alabama Journal of Medical Sciences* 21, No. 1 (1984):86-95.

32. S. Lewis, "Speculations on the Impact of Prospective Pricing and DRGs," *Western Journal of Medicine* 140, No. 4 (1984):638-644.

33. "Pressure Sets Hospitals, Medical Staff at Odds," *Medical World News* 26, No. 4 (February 25, 1985):65.

34. Ibid.

35. L. F. McMahon, Jr., "Physicians and the Hospital: An Expanded Managerial Role Expected with Diagnosis Related Group Based Hospital Reimbursement," *Connecticut Medicine* 48, No. 3 (1984):167-170.

36. "Hospital Staffing Structure on the Way Out as Hospital-Physician Rivalry Grows?" *Medical World News* 25, No. 17 (September 10, 1984):14-15.

37. B. E. Spivey, "The Relation Between Hospital Management and Medical Staff Under a Prospective Payment System," *New England Journal of Medicine* 310, (April 12, 1984):984-986.

38. Bassett, "Cost-per-Case."

39. D. W. Young and R. B. Saltman, "Preventive Medicine for Hospital Costs," *Harvard Business Review* 61, No. 1 (1983):126-133.

40. "Hospital Staffing," *Medical World News.*

41. "Congress Told DRG Plan May Hurt Hospital-MD Ties," *American Medical News* 26, No. 7 (February 18, 1983):2, 12.

42. K. Sandrick, "Medical Staff-Administration Relations Under PPS," *Hospitals* 58, No. 8 (April 16, 1984):79-80, 82.

43. J. Iglehart, "Report of the Ninth Duke University Medical Center Private Sector Conference," *New England Journal of Medicine* 311, No. 3 (July 19, 1984):204-208.

44. McMahon, "Physicians and the Hospital."

45. "Doctor Cooperation Needed Under PPS," *Hospitals.*

46. M. Nathanson, "Doctors Must Master DRGs, Help Administrators Rescue Hospitals," *Modern Healthcare* 14, No. 4 (1984):108.

47. "DRGs May Enlarge Physicians' Hospital Management Role," *Internal Medicine News* 17, No. 3 (July 1, 1984):7.

48. Ibid.

49. J. Carlova, "Where Doctors Turned DRGs Into Black Ink," *Medical Economics,* Nov. 11, 1985.

50. Young and Saltman, "Preventive Medicine."

51. Iglehart, "Duke University Report."

52. M. Nathanson, "DRGs Demand Closer Cooperation Between Lab Chief, M.D.'s and CEO," *Modern Healthcare* 13, No. 9 (1983):104-106.

53. "DRG Coordinator (South Florida)," *Sunday Star-Ledger*, July 1, 1984.

54. T. Sullivan, "DRGs Spur New Player on Team," *American Medical News* 27, No. 4 (January 27, 1984):3, 13, 14.

55. Ibid.

56. "DRGs Create a New Profession—The DRG Coordinator," *Hospital Peer Review* 8, No. 2 (1983):13-15.

57. Sullivan, "DRGs Spur New Player."

58. "Prospective Payment," Hospitals.

59. Ibid.

60. Ibid.

61. Sullivan, "DRGs Spur New Player."

62. E. D. Joseph and T. G. Dehn, "A PPS Action Plan for Radiology Managers," *Hospitals* 58, No. 20 (October 16, 1984):89, 92, 94, 96.

63. R. Osborn, "Prospective Reimbursement—Its Impact on Planning in Radiology," *Radiology Management* 6, No. 4 (1984):3-7.

64. J. Keefe and W. Jollie, "Parallel Planning: A Key to Successful DRG Phase-In Management," *Radiology Management* 6, No. 1 (1984):10-15.

65. W. P. Shuman, R. S. Heilman, and E. B. Larson, "DRGs and the Radiologist As a Consultant," (editorial), *American Journal of Radiology* 143, No. 1 (1984):193-194.

66. Ibid.

67. R. L. Breckenridge, "Pathology Practice Under TEFRA and DRGs," *Pathologist* 37, No. 8 (1983):560-562.

68. Ibid.

69. M. Cherskov, "Appeals Court Rules Against Pathologists in Medicare Suit," *American Medical News* 27, No. 20 (May 25, 1984):1, 27.

70. Ibid.

71. B. L. Becker, "The Impact of DRGs on New Jersey Labs," *Medical Laboratory Observer* 16, No. 1 (1984):30-41.

72. Ibid.

73. M. Nathanson, "Labs Should Try to Cut Patients' Stay, Market Testing Services," *Modern Healthcare* 14, No. 3 (February 15, 1984):146, 148.

74. Becker, "Impact of DRGs."

75. Ibid.

76. R. M. Iammarino and R. A. Swanson, "Clinical Laboratories Making The Best of DRGs," *Post Graduate Medicine* 74, No. 4 (1983):323-326.

77. W. E. Fee, "Commentary: Diagnosis-Related Groups," *Archives of Otolaryngology* 110, No. 10 (1984):631-632.

78. Ibid.

79. L. Machol, "Payment by Diagnosis: What Will It Mean to You?" *Contemporary OB/GYN* 17, No. 2 (1981):129-132.

80. F. W. Newell, "Diagnosis-Related Groups (DRGs) and the Ophthalmologist," *American Journal of Ophthalmology* 96, No. 6 (1983):802-804.

81. M. Weinberger, M. K. Potts, and K. D. Brandt, "Diagnosis-Related Group Regulations. Implications for the Practicing Rheumatologist," *Arthritis and Rheumatism* 28, No. 2 (1985):204-209.

82. Ibid.

83. *American Association of Nurse Anesthetists*, Memo re: Prospective Payment System, Unpublished, September 16, 1983.

84. B. Gardner, "The Impact of DRGs on Surgical Practice," (Editorial), *Surgery, Gynecology and Obstetrics* 159, No. 1 (1984):75-76.

85. K. Sandrick, "Cognitive vs. Procedural Fees: The Race Is On," *Private Practice* 16, No. 5 (1984):26-27, 30-31.

86. Ibid.

87. G. S. Omenn and D. A. Conrad, "Implications of DRGs for Clinicians, Sounding Board," *The New England Journal of Medicine* 311, No. 20 (November 15, 1984):1314-1317.

88. Ibid.

89. Sandrick, "Cognitive vs. Procedural Fees."

90. Ibid.

91. J. Hadley, "How Should Medicare Pay Physicians?" Milbank Memorial Fund Quarterly, *Health and Society,* 62, No. 2: (Spring), 1984: 279-299.

92. Ibid.

93. "Plan Provides Medicare Benefits through HMO Network," *Hospitals* 58, No. 1 (January 1, 1984):54.

94. "These Doctors Think Theirs Is The Better Mousetrap," *Medical Economics,* May 13, 1985.

95. L. Frederick, "What's Coming After The Medicare Freeze," *Medical Economics*, March 18, 1985.

96. Ibid.

97. "Effects of Competition on Medicare, AMA Council on Medical Service," *Journal of American Medical Association* 249, No. 14 (April 8, 1983):1864-1868.

98. Ibid.

99. D. Lyons, "Doctors Warn Congress on Fixed Medicare Fees," *New York Times*, June 22, 1984.

100. R. Pear, "U.S. Imposes Freeze on Physicians—Medicare Fees," *New York Times*, October 1, 1984.

101. K. Hunt, "Washington Outlook: A Long Cold Year For Doctors," *Medical Economics*, January 7, 1985.

102. Pear, "U.S. Imposes Freeze."

103. "Medicare Assignment Participation 37.2 Percent by October Deadline," *Hospitals* 59, No. 10 (May 16, 1985):31.

104. "Socioeconomic Monitoring System. Medicare Assignment: Recent Trends and Participation Rates," *SMS Report* 4, No. 1 1985:1-4.

105. J.B. Mitchell, K.A. Calore, J. Cromwell, H.T. Hewes, W.B. Stason, and H. West, *Alternative Methods for Describing Physician Services Performed and Billed* (Chestnut Hill, MA: Health Economics Research, Inc. November 1983).

106. "And HCFA's Message: Excessive Hospital Admissions Unacceptable," *Medical World News* 25, No. 5 (March 12, 1984):17-18.

107. J.K. Iglehart, "Physician DRG Payment, State Rate-Setting Agendas Sought," *Hospital Progress* 65, No. 3 (1984):17, 24.

108. S. McIlrath, "More Cautiously on M.D., DRGs, Sens. Dole, Heinz Recommend," *American Medical News* 27, No. 24 (June 22, 1984):2, 10.

109. Ibid.

110. "Physician DRG Support Ebbs," *American Medical News* 27, No. 46 (December 14, 1984):10.

111. "New Opposition to Physician DRGs," *Private Practice* 16, No. 3 (1984):21-22.

112. J.D. Snyder, "Battle Looms Over DRGs for Doctors On Hospital Fees for Medicare Patients," *Internal Medicine News* 18, No. 2 (January 15-31, 1985):3, 62-63.

113. S. McIlrath, "Conferees Approve Medicare Fee Freeze," *American Medical News*, 27, No. 25 (June 29/July 6, 1984):1, 12.

114. Mitchell, et al., "Alternative Methods."

115. Snyder, "Battle Looms."

116. Ibid.

117. Frederick, "What's Coming."

118. Ibid.

119. W.C. Hsiao, and W.B. Stason, "Toward Developing a Relative Value Scale for Medical and Surgical Services," *Health Care Financing Review* 1, No. 1 (Fall, 1979):23-28.

120. Snyder, "Battle Looms."

121. "MD Group Petitions FTC to Lift RVS ban," *American Medical News* 27, No. 41 (November 2, 1984):8.

122. Ibid.

123. "FTC Downplays RVS Antitrust Problems," *Washington Report on Medicine & Health* 38, No. 43 (October 29, 1984):2.

124. "PPS for Doctors a Few Years Off," *Washington Report on Medicine & Health* 38, No. 42 (October 22, 1984):1.

125. Frederick, "What's Coming."

126. "PPS for Doctors," Washington Report on Medicine & Health.

127. "Fee Schedule With RVS Eyed by AMA Board," *American Medical News* 27, No. 41 (November 2, 1984):8.

128. "AMA Plan to HCFA Seeks RVS," *American Medical News* 28, No. 6 (February 8, 1985):20.

129. "Compulsory Use of RVS Opposed," *American Medical News* 27, No. 46 (December 14, 1984):1, 35.

130. "HHS Moves on Relative Value Scale," *Medical World News* 27, No. 6 (March 24, 1986):13-14.

131. Hunt, "Washington Outlook."

132. Hadley, "How Should Medicare Pay?"

133. K. Hunt, "Congress Draws a Fresh Bead on Your Fees," *Medical Economics*, July 11, 1983.

134. M. Freudenheim, "Cost Controls Raise Concerns on Health Care," *New York Times*, July 30, 1985.

135. Frederick, "What's Coming."

136. Ibid.

137. J. Coleman, and D.S. Smith, "DRGs: Opportunity or Crisis?" *Pediatric Nursing* 10, No. 5 (1984):321-323, 361.

138. B. Wright, "Implementing DRGs," New Jersey Nurse 14, No. 4 (1984):2.

139. "DRGs: The New Pulse of Health Policy," *Nursing & Health Care* 4, No. 4 (1983):208-209.

140. M. Chow, "Diagnosis Related Groups—A New Nationwide Reimbusement System," *California Nurse* 79, No. 1 (1983):3.

141. M.K. William, "DRGs—A Primer," Nursing Economics 1, No. 2 (1983):135-137.

142. V. Bauknecht, "ANA Opposes Using Diagnostic Groups for Calculating Payment," *The American Nurse* 15, No. 1 (1983):1, 14.

143. P.K. Jones, "DRGs—A New Challenge for Nurses," *Pennsylvania Nurse* 38, No. 8 (1983):14.

144. Chow, "Diagnostic Related Groups."

145. L.R. Piper, "Accounting for Nursing Functions in DRGs," *Nursing Management* 14, No. 11 (1983):46-48.

146. J. Feldman, "Living with DRGs" *The Journal of Nursing Administration* 14, No. 5 (1984):19-22.

147. L. Huckabay, and R. Skonieczny, "Patient Classification Systems: The Problems Faced," *Nursing & Health Care* 2, No. 2 (1981):89-102.

148. Joint Commission on Accreditation of Hospitals, *Accreditation Manual for Hospitals,* 1985, Chicago, IL, 1984.

149. Piper, "Accounting for Nursing Functions."

150. F. Shaffer, "A Nursing Perspective of the DRG World. Part 1," *Nursing & Health Care* 5, No. 1 (1984): 48-51.

151. "Academy Discusses Health Policy Changes, DRGs," *American Nurse* 15, No. 10 (1983):10, 13.

152. K. Mitchell, "DRGs: De Revenues Gone!!" (editorial), *Pediatric Nursing* 10, No. 5 (1984):317.

153. Chow, "Diagnostic Related Groups."

154. S. Laviolette, "DRG Study Challenges Medicare Differential," *Modern Healthcare* 10, No. 2 (1980):18-20.

155. Ibid.

156. Ibid.

157. J. O'Leary, "With DRGs, Blow Your Own Horn," *RN* 48, No. 4 (1985):87-88.

158. G.M. van Servellen, and M.M. Mowry, "DRGs and Primary Nursing: Are They Compatible?" *Journal of Nursing Administration* 15, No. 4 (1985):32-36.

159. Ibid.

160. M.O. Lindamood, "DRGs: Potential Effects on Critical Care Nursing," *Dimensions of Critical Care Nursing* 4, No. 2 (1985):91-99.

161. S.H. Johnson, "Implementing DRGs in Critical Care Nursing." (editorial), *Dimensions of Critical Care Nursing* 4, No. 2 (1985):67-68.

162. R.M. Haddon, E.J. Halloran, and K.W. Moyer, "Current Controversies: Dealing with DRGs," *Dimensions of Critical Care Nursing* 4, No. 2 (1985):99-102.

163. Ibid.

164. P.L. Grimaldi, "DRGs and Nursing Administration," *Nursing Management* 13, No. 1 (1982):30-34.

165. Ibid.

166. M.D. Sovie, A.W.V. Tarcivale, and E. Studen, "Amalgam of Nursing Acuity, DRGs and Costs," *Nursing Management* 16, No. 3 (1985):22-42.

167. L. Curtin, "Determining Costs of Nursing Services per DRG," *Nursing Management* 14, No. 4 (1983):16-20.

168. Mitchell, "De Revenue's Gone!!"

169. "Nurses Play Key Role in Small Hospitals' Planning," *Hospitals* 58, No. 23 (December 1, 1984):60, 64.

170. D.P. Henderson, and T.V. Sullivan, "Diagnosis Related Groups: Effects on Nursing," *Journal of Emergency Nursing* 10, No. 2 (1984):117-118.

171. R.C. Nauert, "How DRGs Will Shape the Profession of Nursing," *Issues* 5, No. 2 (1984):4-5.

172. I. Taylor, "DRGs Were Praised Despite Industry Impact," *Star-Ledger* (N.J.), February 19, 1984.

173. F.R. Curtiss, "Pharmacy Management Strategies for Responding to Hospital Reimbursement Changes," *American Journal of Hospital Pharmacy* 40, No. 9 (1983):1489-1492.

174. H. Catania, O. Ibraham, S.W. Guasco, and P. Catania, "Analyzing Pharmacy Charges Using DRGs," *American Journal of Hospital Pharmacy* 41, No. 5 (1984): 920-923.

175. M.J. Magee, D.S. Pathak, T.P. Sherrin, and D.N. Schneider, "ABC Analysis of the Relationship Between Pharmacy Charges and DRGs," *American Journal of Hospital Pharmacy* 42, No. 3 (1985):571-576.

176. D.E. Miller, "Coping with DRGs: Hospital of the University of Pennsylvania, Philadelphia," *American Journal of Hospital Pharmacy* 49, No. 9 (1983):1503-1504.

177. Ibid.

178. A.J. Vaida, "Coping with DRGs:Suburban General Hospital, Norristown, Pennsylvania," *American Journal of Hospital Pharmacy* 40, No. 9 (1983):1494-1496.

179. R.T. Turnbull and D.M. Ashby, "Coping with DRGs: Grace Hospitals, Detroit, Michigan," *American Journal of Hospital Pharmacy* 40, No. 9 (1983):1499-1500.

180. A.S. Douglas, "Planning Opportunities Seen for Pharmacists Under DRGs." *Hospitals* 58, No. 4 (February 16, 1984):66, 69.

181. J.A. Osborne, "Coping with DRGs: Baptist Medical Center of Oklahoma, Oklahoma City" *American Journal of Hospital Pharmacy* 40, No. 9 (1983):1506-1507.

182. Vaida, "Coping With DRGs."

183. Curtiss, "Pharmacy Management."

184. Vaida, "Coping With DRGs."

185. S.M. Enright, "Prospective Reimbursement and DRGs: Implications for Formulary Management," *Hospital Formulary* 18, No. 10 (1983):989-990, 999-1000.

186. Curtiss, "Pharmacy Management."

187. Vaida, "Coping With DRGs."

188. Miller, "Coping With DRGs."

189. R.W. Roberts, "Coping With DRGs: Riverside Hospital, Jacksonville, Florida," *American Journal of Hospital Pharmacy* 40, No. 9 (1983):1500-1502.

190. P. Huston, "The Pharmacist: Key Player in the Home Health Market," *Medical Marketing and Media* 20, No. 7 (1985):9-21.

191. Roberts, "Coping With DRGs."

192. W. Hittel, "DRGs for Medicare Reimbursement for Outpatient Intravenous Antibiotic Programs," *American Journal of Hospital Pharmacy* 41, No. 7 (1984):1310, 1312.

193. J.H. Upton, J.B. Crouch, and J.B. Douglas, "Coping with DRGs: The Moses H. Cone Memorial Hospital, Greensboro, North Carolina," *American Journal of Hospital Pharmacy* 40, No. 9 (1983):1496-1499.

194. Roberts, "Coping With DRGs."

195. F.R. Curtiss, "Changing the Rules of the Reimbursement Game," *American Journal of Hospital Pharmacy* 39, No. 11 (1982):1975-1977.

196. F.R. Curtiss, "Current Concepts in Hospital Reimbursement," *American Journal of Hospital Pharmacy* 40, No. 4 (1983):586-591.

197. T. Precious, "PPS One Year Later," *Progress Report. American Physical Therapy Association*, September, 1984.

198. Ibid.

199. Ibid.

200. Ibid.

201. K. Davis, "Assessing Physical Therapy Utilization in a Prospective Payment Environment," *Clinical Management* 4, No. 4:38-43.

202. S.J. Scott, "The Medicare Prospective Payment System," *American Journal of Occupational Therapy* 38, No. 5 (1984):330-334.

203. Ibid.

204. M.S. Gray, "Occupational Therapy Use Rises Under PPS," *Hospitals* 59, No. 11 (June 1, 1985):60, 62.

205. Precious, "PPS One Year Later."

206. Ibid.

207. "Two Therapists Refuse POPTS Order, Quit Hospital," *Progress Report. American Physical Therapy Association*, September, 1984.

208. "Five Percent of Physician Office Visits Referred to Physiotherapy," *Progress Report. American Physical Therapy Association*, September, 1984.

209. K. Schuster, "The DRGs are Coming . . . Cost Containment in Hospitals," *Food Management* 18, No. 8 (1983):46-50, 76-78, 82, 86-88.

210. Ibid.

211. Ibid.

212. Ibid.

213. M.B. Haschke, "DRGs: Impact and Implications for Action. President's Page." *Journal of the American Dietetic Association* 83, No. 5 (1983):584-585.

214. Ibid.

215. M.A. Caputi, and W.A. Heiss, "The DRG Revolution," *Health and Social Work* 9, No. 1 (1984):5-12.

216. "New Prosective Payment System for Medicare Suggests a Shift in Professions Hospital Role," *National Association of Social Workers News,* 1983.

217. Ibid.

218. C.J. Coulton, and N. Butler, "Measuring Social Work Productivity in Health Care," *Health and Social Work* 6, No. 18 (1981):4-12.

219. R.A. Kane, "Minding Our PPOs and DRGs," *Health and Social Work* 8, No. 2 (1983):82-84.

220. Ibid.

PART III
IMPACTS ON OTHER SECTORS OF THE HEALTH CARE INDUSTRY

CHAPTER 7
Psychiatric Care: Alternative Reimbursement Strategies

While psychiatric hospitals were excluded from the federal DRG legislation that was enacted on October 1, 1983, the bill did project the future inclusion of these hospitals within the cost containment plan. Congressional mandate calls for a report on incorporating psychiatric hospital units into the prospective payment system to be ready by December 31, 1985. A number of investigations are under way and various methodologies are being reviewed.

Existing Psychiatric DRGs

Within the ICD-9-CM classification scheme there are more than 300 entries relating to mental disorders, including alcohol and substance abuse.Using the ICD-9-CM, the federal government adopted a DRG system that contains 23 Major Diagnostic Categories and 467 specific DRGs. Only 15 of those DRGs involve mental illness, including alcohol and substance abuse. (See Exhibit 7-1 for a listing).

General hospitals with psychiatric units may apply for an exemption from the DRG program if the hospitals meet criteria established by the federal government. Otherwise, general hospitals will use the existing 15 DRGs to classify their patients.

Mental health experts contend that there is a rationale for the exclusion of psychiatric hospitals: "The exemption of psychiatric inpatient settings reflects the lower level of confidence of HCFA and the Congress that diagnosis was predictive of resource use and homogeneous clinical treatment patterns for mental illness. Psychiatric hospitals have historically been treated differently under Medicare, so the precedent is not new."[1]

Exhibit 7-1   Psychiatric DRGs in Current PPS, September 3, 1985

DRG	MDC	Title	Relative Weights	Arithmetic Mean LOS	Geometric Mean LOS	Outlier Threshold
424	19 SURG	O.R. procedures with principal diagnosis of mental illness	2.2112	22.1	15.0	32
425	19 MED	Acute adjust react + disturbances of pyschosocial dysfunction	.6097	7.6	4.8	22
426	19 MED	Depressive neuroses	.8330	11.8	7.8	25
427	19 MED	Neuroses except depressive	.7019	9.8	6.4	23
428	19 MED	Disorders of personality + impulse control	.8513	11.9	7.4	24
429	19 MED	Organic disturbances + mental retardation	.8424	11.0	7.6	25
430	19 MED	Psychoses	1.0762	15.5	10.5	28
431	19 MED	Childhood mental disorders	.8495	10.4	6.6	24
432	19 MED	Other diagnoses of mental disorders	.6969	8.1	4.9	22
433	20	Substance use and induced organic mental disorders, left AMA	.3906	4.4	2.9	16
434	20	Subst abuse, intox induce mntl syn exc depend & or oth sympt trt	.7098	8.2	5.4	22
435	20	Substance dependence, detox and/or other symptomatic treatment	.7980	10.2	6.7	24
436	20	Substance dependence with rehabilitation therapy	1.0166	14.2	9.8	27
437	20	Substance dependence, combined rehabilitation and detox therapy	1.3276	19.0	14.6	32
438		No longer valid	.0000			

Source: *Federal Register*, September 3, 1985, page 35734.

The New Jersey Experience

New Jersey's DRG system has used mental health classifications in its reimbursement system. However, changes are being contemplated that would result in "increasing the gap between those who are 'most in need' such as the chronically ill and the ability of the service system to be increasingly responsive to their needs."[2] This comment was made at a hearing before the Hospital Rate Setting Commission in New Jersey. In addition, mental health care providers pointed out that the changes were aimed at shortening the length of stay despite a policy of the state's Department of Human Services that promoted care for chronic psychiatric patients in general hospitals. It was also pointed out that the DRG system does not provide for the social and vocational services deemed essential elements of an aftercare system. However, unlike the federal government, the New Jersey system does provide funding for uncompensated care in its all-payer system. For these reasons, the mental health care providers said that the DRG changes would create a barrier to services, would discourage community health care providers from developing services for mental patients, and would increase patients' recidivism. A question was also raised about how the traditional sliding fees used by many providers would be accommodated.[3,4] Pointedly, one critic observed that "the present situation in New Jersey works against the best interest of both consumer and provider."[5]

The Maryland Experience

A study examined data on 479 cases of mental disorder admitted in 1977 and 826 cases admitted in 1980 who received care in 40 out of the 46 acute care hospitals having Maryland Blue Cross as the fiscal intermediary. Maryland uses a Guaranteed Inpatient Revenue (GIR) system that reimburses on a per-case basis. Investigators looked at the hospital charges during the index admission and for three months following the admission. Results indicated the following:

- A significant negative relation between per-case reimbursement and total hospital charges. Total hospital charges could be lower for patients reimbursed under the per-case method as opposed to the per-service method.

- A positive, but not significant, relation among per-case reimbursement, hospital charges at admission, and readmissions within the three-month follow-up.

It was noted that the per-case reimbursement stimulated a reduction in the cost of a hospital stay, but that the saving was most likely offset by the higher readmission rates and/or higher readmission charges. Researchers concluded that "the per case reimbursement does not have an impact on the total cost of mental health care over a specific time period but may change the pattern of care for mental disorders."[6]

Funding for Mental Health Care

In 1982, mental health expenditures accounted for about 15 percent of the nation's health care costs—about $40 to $50 billion. By type of facility, the costs were distributed as follows:

State and county mental hospitals	49%
General hospitals	14%
Community mental health centers	12%
Private psychiatric hospitals	7%
Veterans Administration neuropsychiatric hospitals	6%
Freestanding psychiatric outpatient clinics	6%
Residential treatment centers for emotionally disturbed children	4%
Other multiservice facilities[7]	2%

This distribution reflects the major historical role in funding mental health services by local governments. In fact, one analyst concluded that "there was better public financing for mental illness in the early days than there was for many other kinds of illness."[8] By 1900, 100 state mental hospitals were in operation and shortly thereafter mental hospitals accounted for 36 percent of all the hospital beds. World War II—with about 12 percent of draftees rejected for neuropsychiatric reasons and with the resultant psychiatric casualties of war—prompted increased federal intervention into funding mental health services. Provisions of the National Mental Health Act of 1946 allowed the federal government to allocate monies for training and research, as well as for direct aid to the states to establish psychiatric clinics. These funding efforts were followed by the community mental health centers program, Medicare, Medicaid, and the private insurance companies also expanding their financial base.

Similar to other health care funding, mental health services funding evolved from the local level to the state to the federal government. However, the consumer still pays for a substantial portion of psychiatric care from his own pocket. In fact, third-party payers are exhibiting increasing concern over the costs and some have taken measures to reduce the benefits covered. A model of mental health coverage, the Federal Employees Health Benefits Plan, has cut coverage drastically. Originally, the FEHBP paid for 80 percent of the cost. Recently, that was cut to 70 percent and then to 50 percent with a limit on visits per year.[9]

This short historical review reinforces the concept, rightfully or wrongly, that psychiatric services need to be discriminated against because of uncontrollable costs. Of course, third-party payers have emphasized that point on numerous occasions. Within this consideration of costing out mental health services, four trends have been observed that could influence any prospective payment system for psychiatric care:[10]

1. An increase in regulatory efforts by the federal government, the states, Blue Cross and Blue Shield, private insurance companies, and large industries. Regulations affect changes such as the limitations on the length of stay, restrictions on the treatments that will be reimbursed, utilization of a team approach, limitations on outpatient care, and requirements for peer review and second opinions.

2. A stimulation of a ''pro-competition'' attitude to contain health care costs. This resulted, for example, in the Preferred Provider Organization (PPO) that discounts care costs in contracting with specific groups of consumers. In addition, nonmedical mental health care providers are also fighting for equal opportunity to care for patients in all types of settings.

3. An increase in for-profit psychiatric facilities; more than 50 percent of psychiatric hospital beds are in investor-owned hospitals. This presents a major change in the manner in which mental health care is organized, delivered, and funded. Furthermore, new freestanding facilities may also deliver care to people requiring psychiatric intervention.

4. A prospective payment system in the form of the DRGs, a new method for paying for mental health care. Since the federal legislation mandates the inclusion of psychiatric hospitals, it will surely follow that mental health services delivered in long and short-stay hospitals will be covered along with outpatient care.[11]

This discussion has demonstrated that there is a long history of funding mental health care in a different manner from other health care services. Trends that affect the rest of the health care industry are also having an impact upon psychiatric care. Problems that have been inherent in mental health relating to diagnostic comparisons and treatment modalities are being magnified by the movement to contain costs using a prospective payment system.

Negative Reactions from Organized Psychiatry

''Psychiatry, of all medical specialties, is the least likely field in which diagnosis related groups (DRGs) seem a suitable method for determining resource utilization.''[12] This strong statement appeared in an editorial in a recent issue of *Medical Care* which also contained an article on the use of DRGs in psychiatry.

In addition to the overall comment about the unsuitability of DRGs for psychiatric illnesses, the authors also noted that disease characteristics and/or diagnostic labels may be overshadowed by the level of social impairment and the degree of danger to society, which may also influence decisions about length of stay and discharge.

Another article, part of a special section of the May 1984 issue of *Hospital and Community Psychiatry*, also explained that because of the nature of the system, the patients, and the providers, the treatment of mental illnesses is more complex. This article stated that the use of DRGs "is unlikely to predict length of stay and resource utilization accurately."[13]

Psychiatric News, the newspaper of the American Psychiatric Association, carried an editorial by the chairperson of its Committee on Private Practice, who is also a member of the Board of Trustees. Goldstein moved the issue even further along with remarks about the specific harm to the patient:

> The psychiatric patient is particularly vulnerable; not only are there misunderstandings about mental illness, the treatability and treatment of the patient's illness, and the selection of the appropriate provider of treatment, but also the care itself is usually dependent on the availability of third party coverage. This is controlled by business interests and government policy and the quality of care is rarely at issue. Coverage is being cut back, and the number of denials is on the rise.[14]

In an interview with the APA's chairperson of its Council on Standards of Practice and Funding Mechanisms, the issue of the implicit danger to psychiatric patients was echoed. English said, "the psychiatric patient has a special vulnerability and the chronic mentally ill patient the greatest vulnerability."[15]

Official APA Reaction

In a letter to the administrator of the federal agency implementing the DRG system, the medical director of the APA delivered that organization's comments regarding the prospective payment interim final rule of September 1, 1983. Noting the predominant concern of the association for the welfare of the patient and the quality of care, Sabshin said that the APA was troubled by the following aspects of the PPS:

- Integrity of the database
- Appropriateness of DRGs for psychiatric illness
- Interpretation of the criteria for excluded psychiatric units of general hospitals.[16]

Database Issues

According to the APA, HCFA does not wish to reveal the database. DRGs developed at Yale University were based upon 400,000 records from 332 hospitals of patients discharged in the last half of 1979. Few of the case records, no more than 10 percent, had psychiatric diagnoses. This database "is not valid for mental illness." There was no differentiation between general hospitals with psychiatric units and those without. Psychiatric patients may be discharged much earlier in hospitals with only a few psychiatric beds. In fact, the patients may be referred to a public mental health facility for care. This action tends to skew the length of stay toward lower stays in hospitals for patients with a psychiatric diagnosis.

Furthermore, the Yale researchers did not use the *Diagnostic and Statistical Manual of Mental Disorders, Third Edition* (DSM-III) in their grouping and coding process. Section 412.27(a) of the PPS regulations reinforces that point by stating that only patients with a diagnosis confirmed by the DSM-III should be treated.

This regulatory requirement raises the issue of the relation of the DSM-III to the ICD-9-CM, which was used in the DRG classifications. Staff from the National Center for Health Statistics, the Health Care Financing Administration, and the National Institute of Mental Health's Division of Biometry and Epidemiology worked together to develop a "crosswalk" for the translation of DSM-III to the DRG system. As the group examined the material, they noted that there were more conceptual differences between the DSM-II and DSM-III and similarly between the ICDA-8 and ICD-9-CM. Their conclusions about the 360 codes in the DSM-III and the ICD-9-CM are revealing:

- 282 codes had identical numbers or identical terminology or had minor terminology differences or analogous terminology.

- 53 codes had different numbers but were identical or had analogous terminology.

- Only 25 codes had identical numbers but possible conceptual differences.

Among the 25 possible conceptual distinctions are those that involve the following disparities:

Acute delirium vs. delirium

Schizoaffective disorder vs. schizophrenic disorder, schizoaffective type, unspecified

Unspecified neurotic disorder vs. unspecified mental disorder (nonpsychotic)

Other unknown and unspecified cause vs. diagnosis or condition deferred.

This working group concluded: "Although there are differences between DSM-III and ICD-9-CM, most are more apparent than real. . . . In addition, the few significant differences that do exist are resolved without great conceptual strain on either system."[18]

Furthermore, these authors state that it was not their purpose to make the DSM-III acceptable "in lieu" of the ICD-9-CM. An earlier article had indicated that point of view.[19]

Considering all of the above, the APA issued a summary statement on the data problem: "Therefore, the published lengths of stay derived from HCFA's database are factitious for psychiatric patients and must be recalculated from a sound and equitable sample."[20]

Federal DRGs were developed using data on Medicare patients. Generally, the psychiatric benefits covered under Medicare were slight and inadequate. There were simply not very many psychiatric patients included in the data pool. Valid conclusions could not really be drawn from that type of data.[21] APA's director of the Office of Economic Affairs also blasted the database: "We're convinced, based on investigations and talks with the people at Yale who invented the system, that these categories were derived from an inadequate database and had inadequate clinical input."[22,23]

Appropriateness of DRGs for Mental Illness

Questions have been raised regarding the use of a psychiatric diagnosis as a predictor of resource use, the variables that override the diagnosis, the linkage to the DSM-III, length of stay determinations, and outliers. On all these issues, the psychiatric community appears to be in agreement that the DRG system is inappropriate. A President of the National Association of VA Chiefs of Psychiatry commented: "Psychiatry may be penalized because of possible deficiencies in the scientific basis for some psychiatric DRG groupings. . . . the current DRG criteria for psychiatry are first approximations and really very inadequate."[24]

Ability to measure the severity of the psychiatric illness under the DRG method also taxes the use of diagnosis as the criteria for reimbursement. A prominent psychiatrist remarks: "Diagnosis is a notoriously poor predictor of resource utilization for psychiatric patients."[25] There are other influential elements that could affect mental health care, such as suicidal and homicidal gestures, drug abuse, and social impairment. It is possible that two paranoid schizophrenic patients without surgery or complications may require entirely different hospital stays. One may stay for a week and be referred to community services, while the other could stay in the hospital for a few months. Simply the availability of outside community support services may be the determining factor in decisions about a continuing hospital stay. This brings forward the issue of length of stay, a critical element in the DRG proposal.

Length of Stay

In answering a question about length of stay, an active APA member responded: "You have come to the core issue, because psychiatric lengths of stay are not as precise and clear as those in other branches of medicine . . . the length of stay for a patient whose diagnosis is defined in exactly the same way may vary across the country from five days to 120 days."[26]

Researchers reviewed the literature and found no significant relation between the length of stay and the psychiatric diagnosis. Upon finding that result, the investigators proceeded to examine the charts of 765 people admitted to a general hospital with a mental health problem. Length of stay predictor variables included the following:

Diagnosis change	Admission through the emergency room
Doctor group	Employment status
Presence of psychosis	Treatment with major or minor tranquilizers
Marital status variable	Presence of medical diagnosis
Sex	Discharge to home or day care.[27]

Two composite pictures emerged of a long-stay and a short-stay patient as follows:

- A short-stay patient was an employed man who was or had been married, or who was admitted through the emergency room, and who had no physical illness and did not require or receive treatment with drugs or electroshock and who was not referred to day care.

- Long length of stay correlated with treatment with major tranquilizers, antidepressants, electroshock, or with the presence of affective disorders.

Despite these composite pictures, the researchers stated: "On the basis of this study, we note that diagnosis *alone* does not predict length of stay and that many other factors contribute to the prediction (author's emphasis)."[28] Furthermore, a number of other variables were suggested as areas of investigation that would be worthwhile pursuing in additional studies:

- Relation among admission and discharge criteria, treatment goals, effectiveness, and length of stay

- Relation between the quality and quantity of psychiatric house staff and length of stay

- Relation of length of stay to referral source, distance of patients from hospital, and private and public status

- Effect of continuity of care and the availability of outpatient follow-up on length of stay

- Relation of length of stay to the number of psychiatric beds per capita and the utilization of those beds

- Geographic variables affecting the length of stay.[29]

In a rather extensive approach to the prediction of length of hospitalization for diagnostically related groups of psychiatric patients, Gordon and Gordon developed the Functional Level Equation as follows:

$$\text{Functional Level} = \frac{\underset{C}{\text{Coping Skill}} + \underset{D}{\text{Directive Power}} + \underset{E}{\text{Environmental Support}}}{\underset{A}{\text{Aggravating Stress}} \quad + \quad \underset{B}{\text{Biomedical Impairment}}}$$

This formula measures the six interacting biopsychosocial variables identified above. Rating scales are described for each of the six measurements in this article along with illustrations for various patients. This report suggests the following predictions:

High A + B scores   = inpatient psychiatric care
High C + D + E scores = respond to short term treatment
Low C + D + E scores = need longer length of stay
High A scores   = increase in length of stay[30]

Two additional formulas relate to calculation of the length of stay:

$$\text{LOS} = f \frac{A}{(C + D + E)} \quad \text{or in DSM-III terms}$$

$$\text{LOS} = fK \frac{\text{Axis IV score}}{\text{Axis V score}}$$

According to the authors, these formulas can be applied in situations where patients have similar symptoms or different diagnoses but belong to the same DRG. These observations may be useful in arriving at determinations of length of stay and in relating that to reimbursement. This approach could help to insert consideration of rational deliberations regarding the severity of mental illnesses into the DRG methodology.

A National Institute of Mental Health study came to similar misgivings about the length of stay issue in psychiatric DRGs: "It appears that length of stay is hardly a predictable phenomenon in mental health hospitals based on diagnosis, treatment, or other patient characteristics."[31]

While the numbers vary depending upon the source, the ratio seems to be fairly constant. DRG classifications for nonpsychiatric illnesses can explain 30 to 50 percent of the length of stay variations. For psychiatric DRGs, the system explains under five percent of the variation. Yet, one expert added food for thought by commenting that "little, if any, efficacy is lost by decreasing the length of stay in psychiatric inpatient care and substituting inpatient days for visits/days in alternative settings."[32] Of course, the alternatives must be available to do that and that has not always been the case.

Outliers

Another inappropriate part of the prospective payment plan as applied to psychiatric illness relates to the length of stay that exceeds expectations—the outliers. In the APA's response to the DRG rules, the statement said: "Any 'average' LOS is virtually meaningless for the mentally ill."[33] Distinctions were also made between when a patient "can" and when a patient "should" be discharged from a facility. In addition, a psychiatric care unit does not have the option of cutting ancillary care, since the overwhelming portion of the care is direct interaction and not laboratory or radiology. Therefore, the only manner in which a mental health unit can respond to economic pressure is to discharge the patient before that individual moves into the outlier classification and causes the facility to lose money.

In a study of more than 12,000 patients, Lee and Forthofer found that about 28 percent of the patients were considered as outliers, using the HCFA's criteria. For childhood mental disorders, DRG 431, more than one-half of the 406 patients fell into the outlier grouping. There were also differences among the types of hospitals with respect to the percentage of outliers; 13 percent for general hospitals, 29 percent for private mental hospitals, and 52 percent for state or county mental hospitals.[34]

Critics argue that if the outliers are removed from the groupings, the DRG system would explain variations in a similar manner to the rest of the medical care services. Length of stay for mental illness DRGs ranged from 8 to 70 days before eliminating the outliers. Afterward, the range goes from 5 to 13 days. With the outliers removed, the DRGs accounted for no more than eight percent of the variation. Researchers concluded that "it is apparent that the less than satisfactory predictive powers of DRGs observed . . . is not entirely due to the aberrant cases."[35]

A vice president of the Connecticut Hospital Association stated that "14 percent of the state's psychiatric patients would be DRG outliers and that 41 percent of the patient days in psychiatry would be for outlier patients."[36] This was explained by the fact that Connecticut has few state hospitals and the length of stay was linked to the experience of short-term hospitals. Patients who require more time in the hospital would fall into outlier classifications and cause big losses for the short-term facilities.

APA estimates that 25 percent of psychiatric inpatients are schizophrenic and another 25 percent have depressive disorders. Accordingly, patients who don't respond to the initial course of therapy could become outliers. Psychiatric experts feel that the patient response is so variable as to make that almost a truism. Brief admissions under the DRG plan could also result in the belief that that specific illness classification only requires short-term care and the allocation of funds may be decreased.

There is a fear that patients with a psychiatric DRG classification receiving care in a general hospital may be arbitrarily discharged when the length of stay cutoff is reached. That patient would be referred to a state facility for continued care: the "dumping" syndrome. "The critical building of commitment and confidence between the psychiatrist and the patient will be broken by purely fiscal, medically contraindicated transfers from the admitting hospital."[38]

A rather strong APA declaration sums up their view: "The APA states that the mentally ill must not be used as instruments of economy. The LOS mean and outliers for the psychiatry-related DRGs are unreasonably short and, from what little is known of the database, not a medically accurate representation of LOS for the seriously mentally ill."[39]

Criteria for Excluded Psychiatric Units

APA critics felt that one criterion applied to the excluded psychiatric units should be changed. HCFA rules stated that a treatment plan should be established, reviewed, and revised by a multidisciplinary team of at least a medical doctor, a psychologist, and a psychiatric nurse. According to the APA, some of its members interpreted the rule to mean that the team must be inseparable and meet each day on each patient. This criterion was revised in the final ruling which calls for an interdisciplinary team but does not specifically name the participants.[40]

Summary of Psychiatry's Reactions to DRGs

It is obvious that organized psychiatry feels that the DRG database is inadequate, that the prospective payment system is inappropriate for mental illness, that length of stay does not really apply, and that the federal government regulations need revision. While outliers could be used, the cutoff point of two standard deviations could not be applied with current lengths-of-stay determinations.

Basic concepts of psychiatry that call for the movement of patients into community care have been ignored in the DRG plan. Furthermore, organized psychiatry fears that the former mode of "dumping" patients into the tax-supported state hospital system would be revived. An APA conclusion states that "cost conciousness cannot be allowed, or encouraged, to transform patients into figures on a balance sheet."[41]

Critically, two major points need to be stressed. An overwhelming majority of mental health care providers agree on the following:

- Current psychiatric DRGs lack the predictive ability to link the diagnosis to the length of stay and thereby to the reimbursement allowance.

- State hospitals form a unique part of the mental health care system and directly affect the nature and financial support of the acute care system for psychiatric patients in voluntary and private hospitals.

On the Other Hand: Positive Reactions

Not all of organized psychiatry is completely opposed to the DRG System. In fact, one commentator points out that the popularity of the psychiatric liaison service should rise. After all, psychiatric liaison service has been shown to reduce the hospital length of stay. Pardes notes the formidable problems but also the potential opportunity. He believes that "psychiatry does far better when it tries to adapt to, rather than avoid, innovations in service delivery."[42]

Marketing Psychiatric Care

At an APA legislative meeting, a veteran executive of Kansas Blue Cross/Blue Shield spoke about additional trends that could influence the mental health care market: "Psychiatrists in the future competitive environment will probably be faced with delivering 80 to 90 percent of the care they render through contracts offered by Blue Cross, PPO's, HMO's, and Medicare and Medicaid."[43]

An editorial in *Psychiatric News* echoes that point as the author comments that "it will be increasingly necessary to market psychiatry to other organized physician practice groups in terms of its cost effectiveness."[44]

This marketing theme was expanded upon at the annual meeting of the National Association of Private Psychiatric Hospitals. A director for InterStudy, a research organization, advised psychiatric hospital personnel to define their product precisely and to market mental health. She said that the product should be marketed "as a competitive package of services at competitive prices."[45] Part of the competition can be met by greater use of a team approach to the delivery of care. Just as the physician assistant renders care, so can the other members of the mental health team. Replacement of "more expensive, intensive, but possibly less efficient care delivered by psychiatrists" with care by other team members would still maintain quality but reduce costs.[46]

Relating the market approach to the government's proposals, Walter McNerney also spoke at the same APA meeting: "There will be no place to hide (in a competitive health care industry), and you're going to have to face . . . the realization that the market is a tougher taskmaster than (government) regulators."[47]

Continuing, McNerney counseled providers to stress the outcome of psychiatric care. According to McNerney, absenteeism and accidents can be reduced and productivity can be increased as a result of intervention.[48] These types of outcomes must be documented and marketed to the purchasers of psychiatric care. There must be measures taken to counter the arguments that more money spent on care only enriches the physicians.

Another speaker at this APA legislative meeting opposed the argument that the competitive approach would result in inferior quality care. He declared that the business community "categorically rejects the notion that the competitive model in health care will ultimately lead to a deterioration in the quality of health care."[49] When expert health care providers protest that the business community ought to stick to their own businesses, the industry representatives reply that they can not afford to do that since health care costs are a large part of their working capital.

At the APA legislative meeting, Dauner warned mental health care providers not to hide behind the word "quality." He cautioned that "too many people believe that when someone throws up the issue of quality, all they're doing is protecting their own interest."[50]

Examples of Marketing

Kansas Blue Cross/Blue Shield started a Competitive Allowance Program (CAP) that extended the DRG system to include rehabilitation programs for alcoholism and drug abuse. Psychiatric hospitals are excluded at the moment, although there is consideration of expanding the area of psychiatric services. This movement is taking place within a competitive marketing concept of health care delivery.

A nonprofit organization that owned several facilities decided to switch to the for-profit status. A major factor in the decision was related to efforts to raise capital for the multihospital system. Executives of the new company are looking for growth opportunities in small urban and rural areas of states with favorable reimbursement plans for psychiatric care. Hospitals will be small with 40 to 75 beds, as compared to the more typical 125 bed facilities. In addition, the firm will initiate day care programs and prevention service in the psychiatric and rehabilitation market. Anthony F. Santore, chief executive officer of the new company, said: "I have no illusions that we'll become a big chain, but we can be a small, quality company."[51]

Toward the end of 1984, Hospital Corporation of America (HCA), America's largest for-profit hospital chain, agreed to purchase nine psychiatric hospitals containing a total of 1,117 beds for $194 million from Forum Group in Indianapolis. This addition increases HCA's total to 36 psychiatric hospitals with 4,600 beds, since the firm entered the market in December 1981. A subsidiary, HCA Psychiatric Company, runs the facilities.[52] Contrary to the example cited above, HCA is a big hospital chain expanding its interests in psychiatric care. As with all other business ventures, there must be an assumption that the company executives anticipate a return to their stockholders on this investment.

A medical director of the CareUnit Hospital System, a proprietary network of substance abuse treatment hospitals, adds a word of caution regarding the "hidden alcoholic." He predicted that DRGs could cause "a hospital to lose its shirt on the bread and butter hernia case." An alcoholic could be admitted for an elective hernia operation and go into delirium tremens after surgery, disrupt the incision, experience convulsions, and get a postoperative infection—all related to the patient's chronic drinking problem. A short hospital stay becomes a three-week stay. Thus, Pursch anticipates that DRGs may result in fewer alcoholics being diagnosed. Since it takes five to seven days to just detoxify an alcoholic and the DRG mean length of stay is about eight days, physicians will be reluctant to admit people with a primary diagnosis of alcoholism. Regarding the market aspects of this care, Pursch notes that treatment in an alcoholism hospital is about $100 to $250 per day as compared to upwards of $1,000 per day in general hospitals.[53]

Impact of DRGs on Mental Health Services

Many factors have been raised in discussions of the general impact of a prospective payment system upon the entire health care complex. While the implications for mental health care may be similar, or even the same, there may be less data available to judge some of the concerns. Four major impacts have been identified for consideration: efficiency, equity and access, quality, and practicality.[54]

Efficiency

At the root of the entire proposal is the question of whether or not the DRG system will contain the cost of mental health services. Rupp et al., reporting on experiences in Maryland, suggest that increased readmissions will result and erode savings accrued from the DRG allowances. At the moment, outpatient services for those covered by Medicare are restricted and ambulatory service cannot be substituted for inpatient care.

It has also been suggested that patients will be transferred to tax-supported facilities and increase the costs at that focal point.

Other issues revolve around filling empty beds, increasing charges to other patients to make up for lost revenue, and encouraging shorter hospitalization among various facilities.

Therefore, efficiency may work at one level or regarding one particular service, but the impact within the system may cause a bulge elsewhere that has to be compressed. Meanwhile, the data have to be collected and analyzed before the question of efficiency under a prospective payment plan can be answered.

Equity and Access

In a manner of speaking, assuring equity and access to mental health services cannot be easily separated from the issue of efficiency. Economic restrictions imposed by a flat payment DRG rate may cause a number of inequities. These inequities have existed within the mental health system previously, and skimming, patient dumping, and cost-shifting could continue to do so under the DRG plan.[55]

People who are judged to be good risks may be sought after by facilities, while the poor-risk individuals will continue to be neglected. Treatments favoring short stays and biomedical or organic orientations may win out over long-stay orientation with emphasis upon psychosocial, reconstructive-rehabilitation. Patients could be selectively admitted with an eye on the reimbursement rather than the clinical need.

Individuals requiring complicated treatment plans and extensive hospital stays have often been "dumped" into the public mental health facilities. At times, the public system has had to provide services with limited economic and human resources. A tremendous disadvantage could occur because the public hospitals would be expected to take care of patients who are unprofitable elsewhere in the mental health system.

Obviously, requiring patients who are not elderly and/or disabled to pay more for the same services is unfair. This "Robin Hood" theory could be forced upon institutions when they see that the DRG allowances simply will not cover their expense.

Inequities will probably effect most severely "the poor, those without social supports, chronic patients with complicated problems, and children who typically have longer lengths of stay."[56]

Quality

Quality of mental health services is in apparent conflict with the goal of a cost-containment effort. What will be the impact of shorter hospital stays? Could there be limited treatment, poorer outcomes, increased morbidity, and even deaths? Is there a meaningful clinical relation between DRGs and mental health services? While the DRG plan does have a peer review mechanism, the question of the goals of that peer review group may differ regarding the level or quality of care. These considerations are similar to those raised generically by all of the providers about the DRG system. Essentially, the providers are concerned that they have to keep an eye on the profit and loss column at the same time as they keep an eye on the patient's chart.

Practicality

Basically, the question is: Will the system work? While issues of practical administration cannot be completely separated from issues of efficiency, equity, and quality, if there is not ease in administration, the costs of implementation may eat up the savings accrued in the prospective payment system. Again, this impact holds true for the entire system and not for mental health services alone. However, if psychiatric hospitals continue to be excluded or require different administrative processing, the costs may be unfairly reflected in an evaluation. In addition, overhead costs may be distributed unequally and cause difficulties. Administration of the quality review program would also have to be effectively implemented. As with all programs, the paperwork should be reduced to a minimum so as not to create additional burdens for the health care system.

Implementation Issues

Since the prospective payment system is being phased in over a four-year period, the psychiatric hospitals would also have to be phased in over some time period. This allows clinicians and hospitals to learn the new system and to work out the bugs without having to rush into ill-thought-out decisions. It has been suggested that excluded psychiatric facilities may require a longer time period to allow for more gradual changes in clinical hospital practices and hospital administrative procedures.[57]

Nonpatient care costs such as capital expenditures, medical education, other professional training, and research have to be addressed. As with the overall DRG plan, those costs are now treated differently from the specific DRG allowances. Inhibition of technology advancement in psychiatry has also been raised as an issue. Will the same response hold for the delivery of mental health services? Critics respond by stating that perhaps the psychiatric hospital is not the place to conduct research. There are also questions raised about the costs of residency training and other educational activities. If those activities are not directly related to the care of the patient, should those costs be included in the DRG allowance or paid for by some other mechanism?

Another implementation issue could relate to a prospective payment plan for mental health services that may differ from the scheme used for the rest of the health care system. Psychiatric patients may use a reimbursement mechanism that combines the acute-care type DRG with one that adds in the Resource Utilization Group (RUGs) that costs out activities of daily living or a long-term care model that ties in community support activities. If this does develop, the paperwork and the administration may differ as may the on-line implementation.

DRG Research and Psychiatry

Congressional legislation mandates a report on the feasibility of adding psychiatric facilities to the DRG program by the end of 1985. A number of professional organizations and other groups are already working on projects designed to respond to the reactions from mental health care providers about the existing DRG proposal. Four basic policy questions have been identified:

1. Are DRGs an appropriate system for classifying mental disorders? Can they be modified to better predict resource utilization?

2. Are the alternatives such as negotiated contracts for per diem rates, capital financing, or the retention of cost reimbursement better than prospective payment?

3. Should psychiatric units in general hospitals continue to be exempted along with psychiatric hospitals?

4. Is exclusion from prospective payment a benefit in the short run? What about the long-term risks associated with the exclusion of psychiatric patients and psychiatric facilities from the mainstream of health care and the financing of health care services?[58]

Policymakers faced with these far-reaching questions will find similarities and differences when comparing the mental health care system with the rest of the health care complex. Perhaps their comprehension and understanding of mental health practice can be increased through their reexamination of the data. Goldman et al. summed up the situation: "We must be prepared with creative ideas and thoughtfully analyzed data if we are to strengthen our ability to serve patients with mental disorders in the mainstream of medicine and still preserve the special contributions of psychiatry."[59]

Reaction Follow-Ups

In response to the advent of the prospective payment system, the American Psychiatric Association established a task force to consider the issue and prepare a report. Six psychiatrists, a liaison member, and six staff persons are working on this project.[60]

A *DRG Catalog* has also been prepared by the APA containing bibliographic references on subjects such as history and overview, policy questions, current studies, data arguments, length of stay, and experiences in New Jersey. There are 124 citations listed in this nine-page catalog.[61]

Observers in the field have noted that the prospective payment proposals represent an opportunity as well as a potential threat.[62] It appears as if the APA is accepting the challenge in that light.

Alternative DRGs (ADRGs)

Current Psychiatric DRGs

As already cited in Exhibit 7-1, the DRG system uses 15 classifications for mental disorders including alcohol and substance abuse. Almost every one of those 15 DRGs include patients who may have short or long hospital stays. Those stays also vary considerably by hospital type and patient characteristics. Important characteristics include prior mental health care, age of patient, hospital type, treatment modality, and legal status of the patient. With respect to the length of stay, "the current DRGs are hardly homogeneous."[63]

Since length of stay is a prime ingredient of the reimbursement calculations, special attention will be directed to that factor. On examination of the current 15 DRGs, a large amount of variation can be noted. DRG 431 (childhood disorders) "has the largest amount of variation with the middle 50 percent contained between 9.8 days and 75.5 days (interquartile range = 65.7 days)."[64] In addition, the most marked LOS variation occurs between the types of hospitals.

General Patient Classification Issues

Basically, a model patient classification system should exhibit homogeneity within categories, hetrogeneity between categories, and should be administratively feasible. A brief review of those characteristics is in order before proceeding to the ADRG proposal for mental health.

Homogeneity Within Categories

Similar patients should use similar resources and result in similar costs and lengths of stay. While some outliers are to be anticipated, the number should not "exceed the general outlier rate of 5 to 6 percent expected for all DRGs."[65] For all 467 DRG classifications, the average explained variation in LOS is 30 percent. For the 15 psychiatric DRGs currently in use, only 3 percent of the LOS variation can be explained. Even with the outliers excluded (28 percent of the cases), only 7.6 percent of the LOS variation can be explained. With the type of hospital setting included in the analysis, the explainable LOS still only increases to 17.2 percent.[66]

It is apparent that controlling the hospital type and the outliers still has the federal government's existing DRG categories falling "far short of the first criterion of homogeneity."[67]

Heterogeneity Between Categories

In essence, this means that each DRG category should be distinct and different from the others. An analysis of the current 15 DRGs shows that several of the DRGs are similar in length of stay; DRGs 434, 435 and 436, DRGs 429 and 430, DRGs 426, 427 and 432. However, despite the similar lengths of stay, the federal government assigned relative weights that differ between the categories. Within the mental disorder grouping, the relative weights range from .7678 for DRG 427 (neuroses, except depressive) to 1.0525 for DRG 432 (other mental disorders). Since the relative weight is used to calculate the reimbursement, those differences are self-explanatory in reference to the bottom line. Yet, the services rendered to patients in mental health facilities consist mainly of personnel, and the resource consumption should be similar when patients stay for a similar length of time. Possibly, this problem may be related to the database used to formulate the 15 psychiatric DRGs. Expert analysts concluded: "If the current DRGs are indistinguishable within four or five sets, the criterion of heterogeneity between categories does not seem to have been met."[68]

Administrative Feasibility

Since the only classification is being made by diagnosis, there should not be too much trouble with the administration of the current DRG groupings. This appears to be the sole merit of the current psychiatric DRG groupings.

Development of ADRGs

When analysis of the current 15 psychiatric DRGs indicated the lack of homogeneity and hererogeneity required of an adequate patient classification system, an attempt was made to devise an alternative DRG proposal. Using the data from three national sample surveys conducted during 1980-1981 concerning 12,618 cases, an Automatic Interaction Detector (AID) was used to regroup the 35 psychiatric diagnostic groupings based on their relation to the length of stay. LOS is used as a proxy for cost in the development. These 35 diagnostic groups were then collapsed into five groups based on ability to explain the variation in length of stay. In further efforts to make the groups clinically coherent clusters, three of the five groups were subdivided, resulting in ten major diagnostic clusters (MDCs). Further analysis proceeded using variables related to LOS, such as treatment modality, age, marital status, legal status, patient discharge status, prior mental health episode, and referral status. Thus, a total of 22 ADRGs for mental illnesses emerged, as shown in Exhibit 7-2. This exhibit also indicates the number of cases in each ADRG as well as the mean length of stay. Evolution of the additional 12 ADRGs are shown with the decision variable indicated. Ten treatment related groups (TRGs) are detailed in Exhibit 7-3.

Application of the ADRGs to the sample of patients resulted in the ability to explain 12 percent of the LOS variance. Since there was still considerable variance in LOS between the general hospital psychiatric units (average LOS = 17.39 days), the private mental hospitals (average LOS = 29.20 days), and the state and county mental hospitals (average LOS = 88.51 days), hospital type was combined with the ADRGs. This then accounted for 21 percent of the variance in LOS.[69] ADRGs do appear to be more homogeneous than the DRGs with respect to the length of stay and subsequently with respect to reimbursement.

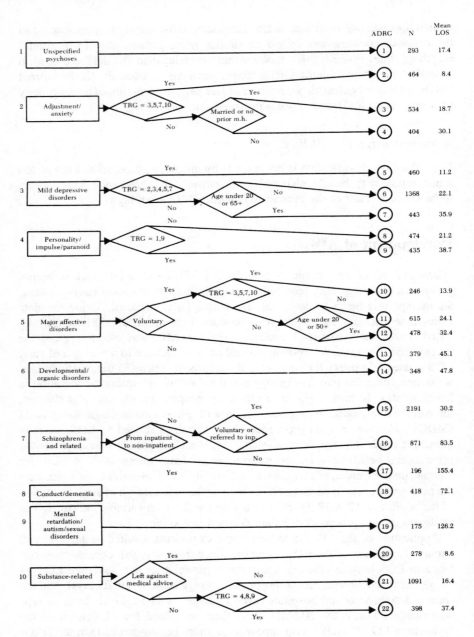

Exhibit 7-2 Alternative Diagnosis Related Groups (ADRGs)
Source: Carl Taube, Eun Sul Lee, and Ronald N. Forthofer. "DRGs in Psychiatry: An Empirical Evaluation," *Medical Care* 22 (1984): 607.

Exhibit 7-3 Treatment Related Groups (TRGs) Condensed Groupings of Treatment Categories

1. Electroconvulsive therapy or psychosurgery
2. Detoxification with training (self-care skill, social skill, activity therapies, vocational/ habilitation, or education)
3. Detoxification without training
4. No verbal therapies (individual, family/couple, or group therapy) with training
5. No verbal therapies without training
6. Individual/family therapy with training
7. Individual/family therapy without training
8. Group therapy
9. Individual/family and group therapy with training
10. Individual/family and group therapy without training

Source: E. S. Lee, and R. N. Forthofer, *Evaluation of the DHHS Proposed Diagnosis Related Groups (DRGs) for Mental Health.* An NIMH Report, September 30, 1983, p. 75.

Information that may also influence the length of stay includes the following items, many not usually found in the discharge abstract:

- Level of functioning and/or disability
- Strength of the patient's social support system
- Practice style and training of the attending psychiatrist
- Whether there is an attending psychiatrist
- Availability of appropriate referral and aftercare agencies in the community
- Treatment plan for the patient.[70]

These LOS differences and personal characteristics do constitute substantial gaps between the types of hospitals, as shown in Exhibit 7-4. Regardless of whether the DRG or the ADRG is used as the reimbursement method, there will still be a reliance upon a length-of-stay measure that is highly variable. In fact, a high-ranking official of HCFA told an audience at the annual meeting of the American Public Health Association: "Several research projects promise to improve PPS for mental problems, but none will bridge the substantial differences between state, private, and general hospital programs."[71]

Exhibit 7-4   Patient Characteristics and Length of Stay by Hospital Type

Patient Characteristics	General Hospital (N=4,611)	Private Hospital (N=5,437)	State/County Hospital (N=2,570)
Black Americans	15%	13%	24%
Not married	65	59	80
Under 20	11	16	9
Less than 12 years education	36	37	55
Veterans	11	13	19
Some prior inpatient care	71	67	81
Involuntary status	16	12	60
Medicare payment	15	16	10
Medicaid payment	23	8	8
No fee payment	3	1	45
Examples of Length of Stay in Days			
5–7 days	13%	8%	10%
16–20 days	12	10	7
45–91 days	5	9	17
92+ days	1	5	22

Source: E. S. Lee, and R. N. Forthofer, *Evaluation of the DHHS Proposed Diagnostic Related Groups (DRGs) for Mental Health*, NIMH Final Report September 30, 1983, pp. 21 and 23.

DRGs and ADRGs Compared for LOS

Continuing to use length of stay as a proxy for cost, a comparison was undertaken to determine the impact of six different predictor models on the LOS. Three were DRG models and three were ADRG models. Computer analysis revealed that the ADRGs were able to account for more of the variation than the current DRGs (See Exhibit 7-5). Comparing solely the use of DRGs versus ADRGs, it can be seen that the ADRG plan has an R-square value nearly four times greater than the DRG system alone—3 percent to almost 12 percent in predictive ability. Adding the type of hospital to the DRG and the ADRG increases predictability to 17 percent and 21 percent, respectively. Adding seven patient characteristics to the DRG and the hospital type improves accountability to 22 percent. However, just adding the HHS region variable to the ADRG and the hospital type also achieves that percentage.[72] Thus, it seems that the combination of ADRG, hospital type, and HHS region yields the same predictability as the DRG plus six additional variables. While the ADRG does present an improvement in relation to the length of stay, the bottom line is still far from producing homogeneous groupings.

Exhibit 7-5   DRG and ADRG and LOS Predictability

Predictor variables in the model	R-square	Percent	F-ratio (dfs)
DRG	0.032	3%	24.55 (14,477)
DRG,TYPE	0.172	17%	21.95 (16,477)
DRG,TYPE,REG9,TRG,V16, AGE,V36,REF,PRIOR	0.218	22	12.10 (48,477)
ADRG	0.118	12	26.30 (21,477)
ADRG, TYPE	0.207	21	24.14 (23,477)
ADRG,TYPE,REG9	0.214	21	17.99 (32,477)

TYPE = type of hospital
TRG = treatment type
AGE = age group
REF = referral status

REG9 = DHHS region
V16 = marital status
V36 = legal status
PRIOR = prior mental health care status

Source: E. S. Lee, and R. N. Forthofer, *Evaluation of the DHHS Proposed Diagnostic Related Groups (DRGs) for Mental Health*, NIMH Final Report September 30, 1983, p. 53.

ADRG Conclusions

Current DRGs account for only about three percent of the length of stay variation. "The current DRGs for mental and substance related disorders appear to be merely a convenient grouping of diagnostic codes that cannot discriminate the hospitalization pattern of mental patients."[73] Based on the study data from three national samples of more than 12,000 patients, the decision to exclude psychiatric hospitals from the Medicare prospective payment plan seems justified.

Several limitations of this study should be mentioned even though the basic facts still stand. Additional information about the following items may have been useful in the analysis:

- Severity of mental condition and functioning of patients

- Errors of measurement regarding the data on patients

- Referral patterns of patients to or from different types of facilities

- Limitations of including patients coded according to DSM-II.

"Despite these limitations, this study demonstrated that the current DRGs are not closely related to length of stay and there is a need for a new system that can better discriminate the hospitalization pattern of mental patients."[74] Two patients with the same diagnostic code could not be distinguished and their lengths of stay could not be predicted based upon the diagnosis. This implies that psychiatric classifications should not rely solely upon LOS. Other patient and/ or institution type variables should be investigated for sound criteria. Importantly, this extensive study concluded with a statement that has far-reaching implications for decision makers: "The failure to uncover important factors influencing length of stay may also suggest that length of stay in psychiatric hospitals can be easily influenced by any policy decision."[75]

Future Directions

Several ideas spring forth from the examination of the study that developed the ADRGs. Directions are suggested that may prove fruitful in the development of a classification scheme that can be linked to a reimbursement system. Consider the following proposals:

- Replicate the study using other variables, such as family or community support.
- Replicate the study using average charges instead of length of stay.
- Investigate alternatives or modifiers to the diagnostic nomenclature such as DSM-III, Axis IV, severity of psychosocial stressors, Axis V, level of adaptive functioning.
- Consider variables such as practice style, treatment philosophy, patient resistance, and demand for beds that may cause variation in length of stay far beyond the usual clinical and/or sociodemographic characteristics.[76]

Alternate classification systems suggest that an entirely different basis for prospective payment should be considered. One direction is to develop a mixed plan that includes a DRG type reimbursement for acute short-term care. Long-term care would be reimbursed under a per diem scheme. This idea has been confirmed in an unpublished report from the Veterans Administration showing that the DRGs apply to acute care and do not do as well with long-term care.[77] Another variation could use a per diem approach that might be based upon the experience of each hospital, rates for classes of hospitals, rates for classes of patients, or combinations of the above.[78]

An overlay on any of these future directions is a concern about the desirability of promoting any reimbursement plan that continues to separate psychiatry from the rest of the health care system. That concern would be further exacerbated if the reimbursement system expanded beyond merely patients covered by Medicare into an all-payer program. Therefore, any alternative reimbursement scheme could exert influence on the public-private split in mental health care delivery by either widening or closing the gap.

Legal and ethical issues are coming to the fore as the proposals for psychiatric DRGs are being considered. Can a patient or his family sue if the patient is discharged from a psychiatric facility when DRG days are used up without providing community support services? Is it possible for mental hospitals to be sued on the basis of selective admissions because they do not want high-cost DRG patients? Might there be selective referrals to transfer high-cost DRG diagnoses? These are only a few of the legal and ethical issues that may arise and are already being discussed by mental health care providers.[79]

Seeking Options

A number of studies are being initiated and discussed which involve a replication of the Yale University's group work with a different database, an exploration of the application of the DSM-III to the classification system, an episode of illness approach, or a provider unit giving care. As noted earlier, the American Psychiatric Association is also in the midst of its own study of a reimbursement system.

Acuity of illness and a DRG classification scheme for pediatric patients are on the agenda, if the National Association of Children's Hospitals and Related Institutions (NACHRI) receives the $700,000 it requested from HCFA. It is predicted that the payment system will be a hybrid of the acuity and DRG methods. This proposal aims to test the reimbursement methodology in various settings, such as community hospitals, children's hospitals, and teaching hospitals.[80]

A patient's functional status and physiology are the bases proposed by the National Association of Rehabilitation Facilities (NARF) for their classification investigations. Financial and patient data will be secured from member hospitals and the reimbursement models will also be tested at those facilities. Coopers & Lybrand of Washington, DC, a consulting firm, will conduct the study.[81]

While both of the above studies may yield information of use in consideration of a reimbursement system for psychiatric care, HHS is also awarding specific monies to examine prospective payment proposals for psychiatric care.

About $500,000 was given to the National Institute for Mental Health for comparative analysis of proposed and current patient classification methods including DRGs.[82]

With a budget projection of about $650,000 the National Association of Private Psychiatric Hospitals (NAPPH) is undertaking an investigation of alternative reimbursement methods. In summary, this study proposes to do the following:

- Develop a unique database for a psychiatric patient population, since no comparable one exists.

- Apply current case mix grouping technology to the development of a psychiatric patient classification scheme.

- Explore and model payment options and identify the factors that predict psychiatric hospital costs.

- Educate the providers of psychiatric hospital care to prospective payment concepts.[83]

Payment methods selected for this study will be based upon a per diem, per case, or combination of both. Two different measures of case mix will be tested. One includes patient and patient care factors such as age, history, nature of illness, and therapy intensity. Characteristics of the patient care unit or program will be the other sole case-mix measure. Related to the last case-mix measure is the definition of psychiatric care in this proposal that refers to nursing, social work, rehabilitative, recreational, and other services delivered to mentally ill patients in a hospital setting. Exhibit 7-6 illustrates potential variables for predicting costs.

Before specifying classification schemes, the proposal states that the DRG system is "generally understood to have less applicability to psychiatry" and the "lower reliability of the psychiatric diagnosis" is also problematical.[84]

Classification methods for review include the Commission on Professional and Hospital Activities (CPHA) list, the SysteMetrics Disease Staging system, the Optimal Case Mix Grouping approach, the AS-Score system, the Intensive Care Severity Measure (APACHE), the Patient Management Paths, the Civilian Health and Medical Plan of the Uniformed Services (CHAMPUS) study, and the HHS study. Most of the above do not meet the criteria of application to the entire group of mentally ill individuals. Most of the schemes are not even specific for mental illness. The HHS study only concerns Medicare patients and the CHAMPUS study only involves dependents of military personnel. Generalizations will be difficult from both those investigations.

Exhibit 7-6 Patient and Patient Care Characteristics for Potential Costing

- Age (children, adolescents, young adults, adults, aged). Diagnosis (alcohol disorders, drug disorders, organic-brain syndrome, depressive disorders, schizophrenia, neurosis, personality disorders, childhood disorders, transient situational disorders, social maladjustments, no mental disorder).

- Complication or comorbidity (drug dependence, alcohol dependence, potential for harm to self or others).

- Severity of condition at admission (using the SysteMetric classification or an alternative measure).

- History of psychiatric illness (previous hospitalization, previous outpatient treatment).

- Intensity of therapeutic treatment (using a ranking system reflecting combinations of interventions including psychoanalysis, individual therapy, family therapy, group therapy, and chemotherapy, as well as the activity therapies and re-entry therapies).

- Types of patient care unit (general, alcohol, child, adolescent, young adult, adult, and geriatric).

- Discharge potential (availability of appropriate community-based treatment and social and family supports).

Source: R. L. Thomas, The Development of a Prospective Payment System for Inpatient Psychiatric Care: Technical Issues and Policy Options. A Grant Proposal by the National Association of Private Psychiatric Hospitals, November 16, 1981.

DSM-III does classify people specifically for psychiatric illness. Five axes are used to evaluate and classify patients:

1. Mental disorders

2. Secondary diagnoses of personality disorders and specific developmental disorders

3. Physical disorders and conditions

4. Severity of psychosocial stressors

5. Highest level of adaptive functioning during the previous year.

This NAPPH study will employ the Rockburn Institute to collect data and to analyze; Lewin and Associates, Inc., will supervise the design, implementation of research, policy analysis, and preparation of the final report. Two advisory groups will serve to provide additional expertise: a 12-member technical advisory panel and an eight-member group to advise on policy recommendations.

Interestingly, this study aims to provide information that can be used by all health care payers.

What's Next?

Obviously, there will be further investigations and articles appearing in professional journals. In fact, *Hospital and Community Psychiatry* had another special section in the July 1985 issue that was edited by Goldman and Taube.[85-91] This section is a follow-up of the May 1984 issue with a similar section on prospective payment and psychiatry. In the latest issue, topics covered included research, length of stay, and comparisons between general hospitals with and without psychiatric units, regarding discharges, coping strategies, severity of illness, exempt units under PPS, and a plan for psychiatric payment linked to a per diem sliding scale.

In September 1985, the APA study group presented its findings and conclusions about DRGs and psychiatric patients. Their findings were similar: ". . . our analysis of the psychiatric DRGs indeed confirms that they are inadequate as a classification scheme for prospective payment. . . . implementation of a patient related case-based reimbursement system would not be appropriate at this time."[92,93] That report was followed by an APA Leadership Conference held from February 10-12, 1986, on "Prospective Payment: Implications and Issues for Psychiatry, Patient Care and the APA." In addition to reviewing the APA study on DRGs, the audience also heard evaluations of a number of other studies linked to prospective payment for psychiatric care, including the following:

National Association of Private Psychiatric Hospitals Study

National Association of State Mental Health Program Directors Study

NIMH/HCFA Study on DRGs

New Jersey DRG Experience

The Non-Exempt Hospital Psychiatric Unit Experience

AHA on PPS for Psychiatric Services

In a composite overview of the DRG studies and conclusions, Dr. Howard Goldman of NIMH derived the following major points:

- The availability of a workable reconfigured DRG or alternate classification scheme for psychiatric patients is not very likely.

- Certain hospitals, especially those with concentrations of outlier patients, would be penalized under the DRG scheme.

- There would be considerable revenue redistribution, and not necessarily in a manner consistent with policy objectives, concerning treatment of the mentally ill.

- There is considerable observed variation in patient experience (as measured by LOS) from region to region.[94]

While the APA Leadership Conference emphasized the need for further research to resolve the problems, there was also the realization that a return to cost-based reimbursement was unlikely.

There can be no doubt that mental health care services will be included within a prospective payment plan. What remains is for the equitable reimbursement methodology to be developed. A number of approaches are already underway and others will unfold as researchers test out different techniques. While psychiatry may be unique, other specialty groups have also advanced their individuality. Many of the problems cited by mental health care providers have also been noted by the rest of the health care providers. It is possible that adaptations of the DRG system may evolve that modify the reimbursement plan to resolve some of the gaps. It is also possible that psychiatric care may use the best of the DRGs, the RUGs, and the ADRGs to secure a method that truly is equitable and reliable.

References

1. C. Taube, E. S. Lee, and R. N. Forthofer, "DRGs in Psychiatry. An Empirical Evaluation," *Medical Care* 22, No. 7 (1984):597-610.

2. W. Neigher, "State Human Services Policy for the Mentally Ill and Reimbursement Structure Under DRG Funding: A Policy Analysis." St. Clare's Hospital, Denville, NJ, 1983.

3. K. M. Courey, *Testimony before N.J. Hospital Rate Setting Commission.* Denville, NJ, St. Clare's Hospital, 1982.

4. Neigher, "Policy Analysis."

5. Ibid.

6. A. Rupp, D. M. Steinwachs, and D. S. Salkever, "The Effect of *Hospital Payment Method on the Pattern and Cost of Mental Health Care,*" Hospital and Community Psychiatry 35, No. 5 (1984):456-459.

7. D. J. Scherl and J. T. English, "Current Trends in Financing Psychiatric Services: The Initial Response of Psychiatry to Prospective Payment," *Psychiatric Annals* 14, No. 5 (1984):332-339.

8. J. T. English, Z. A. Kritzler, and D. J. Scherl, "Historical Trends in the Financing of Psychiatric Services," *Psychiatric Annals* 14, No. 5 (1984):321-331.

9. Ibid.

10. Scherl and English, "Current Trends."

11. Ibid.

12. G. D. Davis and N. Breslau, "DRGs and the Practice of Psychiatry," *Medical Care* 22, No. 7 (1984):595-596.

13. H. H. Goldman, H. A. Pincus, C. A. Taube, and D. A. Regier, "Prospective Payment for Psychiatric Hospitalization: Questions and Issues," *Hospital and Community Psychiatry* 35, No. 5 (1984):460-464.

14. N. Goldstein, "Editorial," *Psychiatric News* 19, No. 9 (May 4, 1984):2, 22-23.

15. J. A. Talbott, "Prospective Payment and Psychiatry: An Interview with Joseph English, M.D.," *Hospital and Community Psychiatry* 35, No. 3 (1984):272-276.

16. M. Sabshin, *Comments on Prospective Payment Interm Final Rule by APA*, Washington, DC, October 17, 1983.

17. "Medicare Program: Prospective Payment for Medicare Inpatient Hospital Services; Final Rule," *Federal Register*, January 3, 1984.

18. J. W. Thompson, D. Green, and H. L. Savitt, "Preliminary Report on a Crosswalk from DSM-III to ICD-9-CM," *American Journal of Psychiatry* 140, No. 2 (1983):176-180.

19. A. A. Lipton and A. S. Weinstein, "Implementing DSM-III in New York State Mental Health Facilities," *Hospital and Community Psychiatry* 32, No. 6 (1981):616-620.

20. Sabshin, "Comments on Prospective Payment."

21. Talbott, "Interview with Joseph English."

22. S. Muszynski. *Prospective Payment for Psychiatric Hospitalization: The Arguments Against DRGs*, Presentation at American Public Health Association Annual Meeting, Anaheim, CA, November 13, 1984.

23. "APA to Investigate DRGs After Other Studies Show Problems," *Psychiatric News* 19, No. 7 (April 6, 1984):47.

24. T. Jemison, "Implementing DRGs: Field Reaction Differs," *U.S. Medicine* 20, No. 9 (May 1, 1984):1, 8.

25. Scherl and English, "Current Trends."

26. Talbott, "Interview with Joseph English."

27. C. Boelhouwer and M. Rosenberg, "Length of Stay: A Retrospective Computer Analysis," *Psychiatric Annals* 13, No. 8 (1983):605-611.

28. Ibid.

29. E. M. Heiman and S. B. Shanfield, "Reflections on Length of Stay," *Psychiatric Annals* 11, No. 2 (1981):155-158.

30. R. E. Gordon and K. K. Gordon, "Predicting Length of Hospital Stay of Psychiatric Patients," *American Journal of Psychiatry* 142, No. 2 (1985):235-237.

31. "APA to Investigate," *Psychiatric News* 19.

32. H. H. Goldman, *Prospective Payment for Psychiatric Hospitalization: Is Less More?* Presentation at American Public Health Association Annual Meeting, Anaheim, CA, November 13, 1984.

33. Sabshin, "Comments on Prospective Payment."

34. E. S. Lee and R. N. Forthofer, *Evaluation of the DHHS Proposed Diagnostic Related Groups (DRGs) for Mental Health*. An NIMH Report, September 30, 1983, p. 56.

35. Ibid., p. 61.

36. P. W. Brickner, "Symposium: The Potential Impact of Diagnosis Related Groups on Long Term Care," *PRIDE Institute Journal of Long-Term Home Health Care* 2, No. 4 (Fall, 1983):3-9.

37. Talbott, "Interview with Joseph English."

38. Sabshin, "Comments on Prospective Payment."

39. Ibid.

40. Ibid.

41. Ibid.

42. H. Pardes, "Prospective Payment and Psychiatry (Commentary)," *Hospital and Community Psychiatry* 35, No. 5 (1984):419.

43. "Psychiatrists Urged to Help Direct Health System Changes," *Psychiatric News* 19, No. 6 (March 16, 1984):19, 30.

44. Goldstein, "Editorial."

45. L. Punch, "Psychiatric Hospitals Told to Define Services and Sell Themselves Better," *Modern Healthcare* 14, No. 14 (1984):60.

46. Ibid.

47. Ibid.

48. Ibid.

49. Ibid.

50. "Psychiatrists Urged to Help," *Psychiatric News* 19.

51. C. Wallace, "For-Profit Psychiatric Hospital Firm Will Seek Niche in Small Urban, Rural Areas," *Modern Healthcare* 14, No. 3 (February 15, 1984):64, 66.

52. "HCA to Purchase Psychiatric Hospitals," *American Medical News* 27, No. 39 (October 19, 1984):26.

53. "Alcoholism Cover-ups Waste Health Dollars," *Hospitals* 58, No. 1 (January 1, 1984):47.

54. Goldman et al., "Questions and Issues."

55. P. Widem, H. A. Pincus, H. H. Goldman, and S. Jencks, "Prospective Payment for Psychiatric Hospitalization: Context and Background," *Hospital and Community Psychiatry* 35, No. 5 (1984):447-451.

56. Goldman et al., "Questions and Issues."

57. Ibid.

58. Ibid.

59. Ibid.

60. *Task Force on Prospective Payment,* American Psychiatric Association, Washington, DC, undated.

61. *DRG Catalog,* American Psychiatric Association, Washington, DC, undated.

62. Goldman et al., "Questions and Issues."

63. Lee and Forthofer, "Evaluation of DRGs," p. 42.

64. Ibid., p. 31.

65. C. Taube, E. S. Lee, and R. N. Forthofer, "Diagnosis Related Groups for Mental Health Disorders, Alcoholism, and Drug Abuse: Evaluation and Alternatives," *Hospital and Community Psychiatry* 35, No. 5 (1984):452-455.

66. Ibid.

67. Ibid.

68. Ibid.

69. Lee and Forthofer, "Evaluation of DRGs," p. 50.

70. Taube, Lee, and Forthofer, "DRGs in Psychiatry."

71. S. F. Jencks, *The Need for Prospective Payment of Mental Health Inpatient Costs,* Presentation at American Public Health Association Annual Meeting, Anaheim, CA, November 13, 1984.

72. Lee and Forthofer, "Evaluation of DRGs," p. 55.

73. Ibid., p. 64.

74. Ibid., p. 68.

75. Ibid., p. 69.

76. Taube, Lee, and Forthofer, "Evaluations and Alternatives."

77. C. C. Evans, F. Holden, and J. Speight, "A DRG-Based Resource Allocation System for the Veterans Administration," unpublished.

78. Taube, Lee, and Forthofer, "DRGs in Psychiatry."

79. K. H. Morgenlander, *The Legal and Ethical Impact of Psychiatric DRGs: A Facility Special Approach.* Presentation at American Public Health Association Annual Meeting, Anaheim, CA, November 14, 1984.

80. "Exempted Hospitals Want Proposals Heard," *Modern Healthcare* 14, No. 4 (1984):4.

81. Ibid.

82. "Can Payment for Psychiatric Care Be Based on DRGs?" Modern Healthcare 14, No. 5 (1984):36.

83. R. L. Thomas, "The Development of a Prospective Payment System for Inpatient Psychiatric Care: Technical Issues and Policy Options," A Grant Proposal by the National Association of Private Psychiatric Hospitals, November 16, 1983, p. 24.

84. Ibid., p. 36.

85. S. H. Fraizer, "Prospective Payment: The Vital Role of Research," *Hospital and Community Psychiatry* 36, No. 7 (1985):701.

86. R. G. Frank and J. R. Lave, "The Impact of Medicaid Benefit Design on Length of Hospital Stay and Patient Transfer," *Hospital and Community Psychiatry* 36, No. 7 (1985):749-753.

87. C. A. Taube, J. W. Thompson, B. J. Burns, P. Widem, and C. Prevost, "Prospective Payment and Psychiatric Discharges from General Hospitals With and Without Psychiatric Units," Hospital and Community Psychiatry 36, No. 7 (1985):754-760.

88. B. S. Fogel and A. E. Slaby, "Beyond Grantsmanship: Strategies for Coping With Prospective Payment," *Hospital and Community Psychiatry* 36, No. 7 (1985):760-763.

89. S. F. Jencks, H. H. Goldman, and T. G. McGuire, "Challenges in Bringing Exempt Psychiatric Services Under a PPS," *Hospital and Community Psychiatry* 36, No. 7 (1985):764-769.

90. J. E. Mezzich and S. S. Sharfstein, "Severity of Illness and Diagnosis Formulation Classifying Patients for PPS," *Hospital and Community Psychiatry* 36, No. 7 (1985):770-772.

91. R. G. Frank and J. R. Lave, "A Plan for Prospective Payment for Inpatient Psychiatric Care," *Hospital and Community Psychiatry* 36, No. 7 (1985):775-776.

92. "Findings and Conclusions of the American Psychiatric Association Study and Evaluation of the Medicare Prospective Payment System—Diagnosis Related Groups and Psychiatric Patients," Washington, D.C.: American Psychiatric Association, September 1985.

93. J. English, S. S. Sharfstein, D. J. Scherl, B. Astrachan and Muszynski. "Diagnosis Related Groups and General Hospital Psychiatry: The APA Study," *American Journal of Psychiatry* 143, No. 2 (1986):131-139.

94. "Prospective Payment" Implications and Issues for Psychiatry, Patient and the APA," Leadership Conference, Marcos Island, Florida, February 10-12, 1986. American Psychiatric Association, Washington, D.C.

CHAPTER 8
Long-Term Care Reimbursement

Despite the nonsystem features of our health care industry there have emerged financial pressures which are pushing for vertical integration, regionalization, and cooperation among various segments of service providers.

For hospitals to effectively survive the DRG trauma, the discharge planning process has been more highly developed so as to utilize alternate sources of health care in the community once the acute process has been stabilized. The length of stay in the hospital is contracted, and rehabilitation and restoration to full functional capacity as a hospital inpatient is no longer efficient, practical, or economically appropriate. Patients who are not fully well or are terminally ill and need additional support services are being discharged to long-term care facilities—skilled nursing homes, health-related facilities, home health care agencies, and hospices. Families are called upon to provide greater restorative support and to care for the terminally ill at home when alternative services are not available or suitable.

With the increase in the aged population and Medicare beneficiaries, and responsibilities for the indigent aged requiring Medicaid-financed services, and the paucity of private insurance for long-term care services, public expenditures for these services are escalating. William Read, Ph.D., Director of the American Hospital Association Office of Aging and Long-Term Care, made this comment: "The dramatic growth in the number of older adults, especially those over 75 and over 85, is having a major impact on the ability of Medicare and Medicaid to continue to subsidize health care services as we know them now,"[1] The rising cost of health care and the increasing number of the older-old mean a greater dependence on the public sector.

Hospital use by the elderly population is quite high—they are admitted more often and stay twice as long as those under 65 years. Although they are only 11 percent of the population, they consume 40 percent of the inpatient stays.[2] Hospitals will, of necessity, seek to reduce their average length of stay and discharge patients as soon as medically feasible. "Hospitals will either contract with existing nursing homes for their services or they will construct or acquire nursing homes."[3] The DRG system will spur the further growth of the nursing home industry as well as other long-term care service segments.

Four key issues have emerged and received the attention of the GAO in their February 21, 1985 report to the U.S. Senate, Special Committee on Aging.[4]

First, have Medicare patients' post-hospital needs changed? PPS creates strong incentives for hospitals to shorten patients' lengths of stay. Recent data on the use of hospitals under Medicare appear to show that the average length of stay per PPS discharge in fiscal year 1984 was 7.5 days. In comparison, the average length of stay per discharge in fiscal year 1983 (pre-PPS) was 9.5 days.[5] While reducing the length of a hospital stay may not affect a patient's need for follow-up care, at each site studied and visited the view was expressed that patients are being discharged from hospitals after shorter lengths of stay and in a poorer state of health than prior to PPS. Data provided by home health representatives in several communities show more visits per case, more cases requiring multiple visits per week, and more need for specialized services, such as I.V. therapy, catheters, and ventilator care, after the introduction of PPS.

Second, how are patients' needs being met? To the extent that Medicare patients are discharged from hospitals sooner and with greater needs for care, PPS may increase the effective demand for the post-hospital nursing home and home health services covered by Medicare. HHS has predicted that the number of persons qualifying for the Medicare skilled nursing home benefit will increase. However, the marked increase in the use of skilled nursing facilities may be precluded by such factors as the shortage of nursing home beds and the influence that state Medicaid reimbursement policies have in determining nursing homes' willingness to accept Medicare patients requiring skilled care.[6]

Where the beds in skilled nursing facilities are very scarce, any increase in Medicare skilled nursing home placements may be effectively precluded. However, with a relatively large supply of unoccupied nursing home beds, some increase in Medicare skilled nursing home placements is anticipated.

Attributing increases in home health placements to PPS may be difficult. Medicare is the major buyer of home health services, and the program's expenditures for home health services were increasing rapidly before the introduction of PPS. Between 1969 and 1980, Medicare home health expenditures grew at an average annual rate of 21.4 percent.[7] The Congressional Budget Office has projected 20 percent annual increases in Medicare home health costs for 1985-1989.[8] Determining the incremental effects of PPS on an already rapidly expanding service will involve fairly complex analysis.

Discharges of hospital patients to home health services covered by Medicare had increased, both as a result of a trend toward greater use of home health services that began before the introduction of PPS, and because of incentives created by PPS to discharge patients from the hospital more quickly. Where average length of stay has been traditionally lower than in most of the rest of the nation, hospitals and home health care agencies indicated that there do not appear to be increased discharges to home health care.

However, a data problem exists because a large proportion of monthly hospital referrals to home health care were not showing up as discharges to home health care on the hospital discharge abstracts processed by the peer review organizations.

Third, are patients having access problems? Medicare's skilled nursing facility benefit covers only skilled care and provides full payment for only the first 20 days of care. A $50 per day copayment applies from the twenty-first day to the hundredth day, after which the coverage ends. GAO has found that some nursing homes may prefer to avoid accepting Medicare patients who might become eligible for Medicaid after exhausting their Medicare benefits. This is because Medicaid reimbursement rates for skilled care are not always sufficient to cover the costs of skilled care for Medicaid patients.[9] GAO has also documented similar problems of access to nursing homes for patients whose service needs are extensive, the so-called "heavy care" patients. PPS may unintentionally increase the problem of Medicaid patients who are waiting in hospitals for nursing home beds.[10]

GAO indicates that problems of access were raised in meetings with health care providers or advocates for the elderly. Problems associated with arranging placements for patients who depend on Medicaid for reimbursement and those who require "heavy care" or the use of sophisticated "high-technology" services were mentioned. However, nursing home administrators indicate that patients who need extensive care and can afford to pay private skilled nursing facility rates do not necessarily have the problem of finding nursing home beds that patients eligible for Medicaid do.

The combination of PPS incentives for hospitals to discharge Medicare patients as soon as possible and weak incentives for nursing homes to admit some of them lead to the possibility of some inappropriate placements. Before the introduction of PPS, some patients who could not be placed in appropriate skilled-level beds remained in hospitals for considerable periods of time as so-called "back-up" patients. PPS provides stronger incentives for hospitals to discharge these patients. There is considerable speculation about what is going to happen to hospitalized Medicare patients who are difficult to place in appropriate long-term care settings.

Fourth and finally, how have long-term care costs been affected? If the introduction of PPS leads directly to a greater use of the nonhospital services that Medicare covers, including those provided by skilled nursing facilities and home health care agencies, the costs of these services will increase and thereby affect overall Medicare costs. There may be other effects on costs as well. For example, GAO has found that the use of home health care services may not be cost-effective for certain types of patients, compared to either nursing home care or hospital care.[11] Increases in the number of skilled staff employed by nursing homes and home health agencies to care for sicker patients may also mean increased costs for Medicare services.

If Medicare beneficiaries make greater use of various post-hospital services, the costs of other federally funded programs, particularly Medicaid, and of state-supported programs, insurers, and private payers may increase. Any increased use of Medicaid skilled-care or intermediate-care beds by post-hospital Medicare beneficiaries could increase the costs of the Medicaid program. The possiblity exists that out-of-pocket expenses for post-hospital care for beneficiaries and their families will also increase.

It appears that some beneficiaries are upset and confused about their Medicare benefits and how PPS has affected them. Some patients are being told, improperly, that they have to leave the hospital because their Medicare coverage has run out. Also, they sometimes do not understand why they are denied coverage for home health care or skilled nursing facility care.

It has also been pointed out that Medicare was not making appropriate adjustments to coverage rules or reimbursement amounts in response to the perceived changes in the needs of the patients. Nursing home representatives have indicated that Medicare and Medicaid reimbursement for skilled nursing home care does not meet the needs of some post-hospital patients, because either the restrictions of the rules on coverage, or variations in fiscal-intermediary determinations of coverage created problems for discharged Medicare patients.

Some problems with coverage and eligibility determination reflect a lack of clarity in the Medicare regulations and, under consistent application of those regulations, a fairly high proportion (27 percent in a 1981 study) of home health claims paid by Medicare do not meet program requirements for coverage.[12] More consistent enforcement of Medicare requirements may lead to more claims being denied and further hardships for patients in need.

Long-Term Care Components

Nursing Home Industry

Anne Bergh, a research analyst at Montgomery Securities, discussed the accelerating growth of the nursing home industry and predicted high revenue growth with concurrent margin expansion and high earnings growth. The nursing home industry is the third largest segment in health expenditures, with growth between 1970 and 1980 from $4.7 billion to $20.6 billion, and national occupancy rates are 95 percent of licensed and 68 percent of available beds. This implies a tight demand/supply situation with expectations of "an increase in private pay census or an increase in reimbursement levels.'' It is also anticipated that there will be major consolidation of nursing operations, with 50 percent of the beds in five or ten proprietary chains by 1990.[13]

With 90 percent of the nursing home industry in proprietary ownership, mergers, purchases, and public stock offerings are plentiful and the price/earning multiple quite high. The biggest corporations are Beverly Enterprises (99,990 beds), National Medical Enterprises (37,630 beds), ARA Services, Inc. (31,000 beds), and Manor Care, Inc. (10,670 beds), and the acquisitions are climbing fast.[14] "It is a highly and healthfully competitive chess game played for the right to snatch up those facilities whose owners, due to lack of economy of scale and the resulting survival capabilities, are willing to put their properties on the auction block for the highest bidder."[15]

Commenting on the problems of conglomeration and monopoly, Quentin D. Young, M.D., President, Health and Medicine Policy Research Group, has noted that there is a potential for danger and abuse in giant health industry chains:

> Once the state is largely theirs, the monopoly behavior so odious to this nation could easily be the most serious new distortion of our vast health resources . . . are harbingers of a for-profit dominance in our system of health care from birth to the grave.[16]

Building new nursing home facilities or conversion of hospital beds for long-term care are both subject to Certificate of Need (CON) regulation in most states. Because of the increasing cost of health care, certain states have increased their scope and breadth of these regulations, whereas others have suspended or waived the CON program to increase competition and attempt to be responsive to innovative programs.[17,18] There are approximately 23,000 nursing homes with 1.4 million residents and it is anticipated that by the year 2000, this might increase to 2.6 million.

Michigan has successfully restrained expenditures in long-term care through the CON program, which has kept the number of long-term care beds almost constant from 1977 to 1982 (about 41,000 beds). If access is thus reduced, one potential consequence may be longer hospital stays awaiting transfer. This penalizes hospitals under the DRG system.[19]

Recent CON law amendments in Iowa and Pennsylvania for SNFs and ICFs tie the approval of beds to the long-term plans of the Medicaid financing authorities. Wisconsin, Montana, Indiana, and Iowa also tie CON issuances to the presence of appropriations under the Medicaid program or to the number of beds potentially served by Medicaid. This attempts to assure access to facilities by Medicaid eligible patients and the indigent.

In nineteen states CON programs cover medically-oriented residential care facilities called Health Related Facilities (HRFs), 32 states cover inpatient rehabilitation facilities, eleven cover outpatient rehabilitation, 34 states use CON for home health care, and fourteen states require CON for hospice care.

Moratoriums on new approvals of beds and institutions is another method of controlling growth and costs in long-term care. Many southeastern states (Georgia, Alabama, Louisiana, Mississippi, Kentucky, South Carolina), along with other states, have expressly time-limited restrictions for months and years and enable CON programs to be assessed, evaluated, and restructured to suit the needs of the community and finances available.[20]

On March 13, 1986, a group of researchers in the Harvard Medicare Project recommended much broader coverage of nursing home care under the federal government's funding program. Proposals for long term care in the study would increase Medicare spending by $50 billion in the year 2000.[21]

Hospitals Propelled into Long-Term Care

DRG implementation and its imperatives for greater efficiency, reduced length of stay, and greater scrutiny of admissions have given hospital administrators the problem of empty beds. The usual push to greater horizontal growth—new burn units, new specialty services, has been changed to vertical growth—with diversification to long-term care services, home health, and hospice units. Hospital occupancy rates have been on a decline—76.1 percent in 1983 to 68.2 percent in October 1984, according to the American Hospital Association.[22] Responsibility for this is placed not only to the cost containment incentives, but also to increases in ambulatory surgical centers, health maintenance organizations (HMOs), and home health care agencies.

In Chicago, for example, "occupancy rates had fallen from 80 percent in 1978 to 72 percent in 1983" to 40-50 percent preliminary estimate in 1984. Conversion of 438 acute beds to long-term care beds has been requested, with anticipated average revenue of $70-$75 instead of $450 per day. This will enable some 10 percent of these Chicago hospitals to recapture revenue and sustain employment.[23]

Converting empty wings of beds into skilled long-term care beds also helps in the shift of patients to an alternate level of care, which is under unified control and therefore also maximizes the revenue from the acute hospital bed. For the patient, there is the advantage of staying with one multilevel care facility, which is less disruptive than moving to another facility. From a recent study in Colorado, there is some evidence that the quality of care is better in hospital-based nursing homes than in freestanding nursing homes, even though the case mix was more complex in the hospital-based group.[24]

However, other studies in New York State facilities indicate there is no significant correlation between hospital-based facilities and their quality of care or patient mix. There is also evidence of higher costs in the hospital-based units.[25]

Another method is to purchase existing nursing homes in the local community or build onsite new long-term care beds.[26] Two hospital chains, National Medical Enterprises (NME), which owns Hillhaven, the nation's second largest nursing home chain, and Hospital Corporation of America (HCA), which owns 18 percent of Beverly Enterprises, are finding these partnerships valuable in both segments. The Robert Wood Johnson Foundation has stimulated 24 grantees in its "Program for Hospital Initiatives in Long-Term Care." The Office of Long-Term Care and Aging of the American Hospital Association was recently established in response to this trend to give assistance to hospital leadership.[27]

The purpose of the program is to address the need for elderly persons to retain maximum independence and avoid unnecessary use of inpatient hospital and nursing home services. The program also seeks to improve the capabilities of hospital staff to care for the elderly in all areas of hospital activity, including emergency, outpatient, and long-term care services. Hospitals participating in the program will have to coordinate long-term care service with personal physicians of elderly individuals and offer a variety of services, such as home health care, homemaker services, adult day care, and nursing home care.[28]

Cost shifting from the hospitals to long-term care providers is a danger under the DRG system, where attempting to maximize hospital revenue has a ripple effect on other parts of the health care industry. Recently it was predicted that further "bundling" of payments includes "combining skilled nursing (SNF) or home health payments after an acute inpatient stay with the inpatient rates" in order to "focus the responsibility for quality care both medically and financially on one provider."[29]

Extension of DRGs to All Long-Term Care Providers

At the National Conference on Diagnosis Related Groups (DRGs) and at the National Governors' Conference hearing, Senator David Durenberger (I/R-MN) predicted an expansion of DRGs to "physicians, home health, skilled nursing, and other levels of care."[30]

The development of prospective payment systems and cost containment proposal for long-term care facilities could dampen enthusiasm and reduce revenue opportunities. But the need for early discharge and opportunity for diversification of revenue will still be the driving pressures on the hospitals.[31]

Home Health Care

Growth in the home health care industry is not necessarily attributable to it being less costly, but because hospitals are forced to discharge earlier. Spurred by the hospital's need to maximize DRG reimbursement, patients are being discharged to home before full recovery or maximum function. In fact, the one year anniversary of the "quicker and sicker" controversy was marked in the March 5, 1986 issue of *Hospitals*. Earlier, the GAO report was released by Senator Heinz, which stated that Medicare patients were released from hospitals in poorer health.[32] This creates service needs in the community to which traditional home care agencies are responsive. In addition, 600,000 patients in any given year are discharged from long-term care beds within 90 days. Of these patients, approximately 25 percent die in the nursing home, 25 percent enter hospitals with a serious illness, and 50 percent return home and may need home care or community hospice services.[33]

Along with providing skilled nursing services, physical therapy, occupational therapy, and speech therapy, home health services have expanded to include high-technology services. Agencies have diversified to provide care such as the following:[34]

Peritoneal dialysis

Care of Hickman/BROVIAC catheters for hyperalimentation or as vehicles for chemotherapy

Respirators and ventilators

Enteral tube feedings—via nasogastric tubes, gastrostomy tubes, parenteral catheters

Intravenous therapy

Apnea monitors

Insulin pumps

Estimates vary as to the potential growth of the market, now at $5-7 billion and projected to about $12-19 billion by 1990. New kinds of professionals will be needed for the more highly technical areas of service and clinical needs of patients. Agencies will need to change toward 24-hour, seven-day services, because patients will be sicker than the usual clients to whom services have been delivered at home.[35]

It is apparent that vertical integration of hospitals and home health care agencies is necessary for effective continuity of care. Agencies are being exhorted to participate actively with hospital discharge planners to identify suitable patients, to seek out alternative resources that would fit their needs, and to provide a smoother transition to the home environment.[36]

Marketing home care services to the public in this competitive market has increased consumer awareness of the availability of quality services in the home and the benefits of home care. In areas where long-term care nursing home beds are scarce, this alternative is highly attractive.

Hospitals are entering the home health care field not only because community agencies are sometimes scarce, but also for financial, organizational, and community reasons. Financially, these programs are profitable, help diversify the revenue base, retain the patient within the hospital's caring system, and result in cost efficiencies in use of the bed and at home. Organizationally, the hospital has the requisite professional staff, access to capital, managerial support services, and the ability to control the direction of professional and service components. For the community, the hospital provides an integrated, quality service for its own patients and for its referred ones.[37]

Over 900 hospitals responded that they have home care services; 548 reported hospice services in the AHA 1985 annual survey of hospitals. In another survey, three-quarters of the hospitals indicated they were planning to develop home health services in the future.[38]

Hospitals may move in this direction as a DRG coping strategy. However, options exist to contract with community home health care agencies and incorporate their professional activities into effective discharge planning. Early identification of patients who would most benefit from discharge to home care would have the greatest potential for cost saving. Such arrangements between the agency and the hospital would be of value to both. Minimum guarantees of patient referrals could assure stability for agency finances and staffing. Agencies could then adapt to the special professional components of patient care at the particular institution.[39]

Reimbursement for services to home health care agencies is under scrutiny so as to protect against a hospital shifting cost centers without totally containing its expenditures. Abt Associates has been awarded a contract by HCFA to study various methods of prospective reimbursement. Three kinds of payment methods are to be tested in the three-year prospective pay demonstration commencing on July 1, 1985 and using 120 home health agencies in ten states: California, Connecticut, Florida, Illinois, Massachusetts, Ohio, Pennsylvania, Tennessee, Texas, and Wisconsin. As spelled out in Abt documents released to prospective participants, they are:

1. Per visit: rates will be set by discipline, by agency "base year" costs. A separate rate per patient will be established to cover overhead, adjusting with the number of patients served, and paid by lump sum.

2. Per patient month: regardless of individual case severity, three different rates will be set: first month of care (higher rate); second month of care (lower rate); third month of care (lower still). If length of stay (LOS) exceeds 180 days, payment will switch to the per-visit method.

3. Per patient episode: a single, flat payment will be made for each episode of care up to 180 days in length. If length of stay (LOS) goes beyond that, payment will revert to the per-visit method.[40]

All rates will be computed on base-year costs, with some room for intensity and LOS adjustments over base year experience if there are significant changes. Once the rates are set for the first year of the demonstration, they will be "trended forward" for years two and three using HCFA's inflation factors, not incurred costs.[41]

In another study the GAO simulated a Medicare prospective payment system for home health care. Results indicated that rates would be 15 percent higher than the average costs incurred by the retrospective cost-based system.[42]

In keeping with other areas of the health system, any reimbursement system agreeable to HCFA for the Medicare beneficiaries is expected to have an impact on payments under private insurance coverage, Medicaid, and private patients.[43]

HCFA made an effort in its July 1985 rate-setting notice to curtail home care costs by limiting benefits and payments through new rate structures and new restrictive definitions of home care eligibility and allowable services. One proposal defines "homebound" to mean "bedridden" and another defines part-time and intermittent but prohibits daily skilled care. In the New Jersey Blue Cross regular home care programs, a three-day hospital stay is a prerequisite for home care services for some plan members; others who are homebound may receive services upon a physician's order. The total number of services and/or visits is also under constraints, despite the chronic nature of these conditions and illnesses.[44,45]

Shifting the burden to families, albeit with home care support, rarely considers the financial implications for the caretakers, the psychological impact, and the attendant stress and social dislocation. Burdens on the family weigh heavily on daughter or daughter-in-law, who is the "woman in the middle," providing the feeding, dressing, toileting, and comforting needs of the patient, along with nursing-type tasks.[46] While the patient may benefit from not being institutionalized, and the guilt of family members may be lessened, not all costs of care are reimbursable—not the least of which may be foregone wages of the working caregiver.[47]

One hopes that the patients do not get lost in the fast shuffle out of the hospital to home services which cannot fully meet their needs and inevitably lead to rehospitalization in the "revolving door" process.[48]

In a featured story in the February 10, 1986 issue of *Medical World News*, another facet of home health care's growing pains was noted regarding physicians. As part of the revolving door process, physicians "are often uncertain middlemen in an industry trying to work out the kinks while in the grip of a financial vise.''[49]

Hospice Care

With the final regulations for hospice care published in the *Federal Register* on December 16, 1983,[50] Medicare has entered an experiment in reimbursement for hospice care. Eligible patients need to be eligible for Part A of Medicare and certification by a physician as having a maximum of six months to live. In addition, the patient or patient's representative (if patient is incompetent) waives Medicare benefits for curative or duplicative services, in order to receive palliative benefits coverage by a hospice program.

A hospice program must satisfy the conditions of participation under Medicare in the following areas:

- A formal organizational structure and disclosure of ownership
- Administrator's and medical director's qualifications
- Written plan of care for each patient with assurances of continuation of care
- Central medical records
- Informed consent from each patient
- Interdisciplinary groups to provide and/or supervise services, i.e., medical services, nursing services, social services, occupational therapy, physical therapy, and speech-language pathology services, and so on
- Core services provided by employees of the hospice
- Bereavement and spiritual counseling
- Inservice training for employees
- Volunteer, home health aide, and homemaker services
- Provision of medical supplies, including drugs
- Arrangements and linkages with other Medicare/Medicaid participating facilities for short-term inpatient care; respite care available in an ICF

Hospices may not discharge the patient, discontinue service, or diminish service. However, the patient may revoke hospice care at any time,[51] although this compromises parts of the benefits in the remaining period.

The reimbursement rates are dependent on intensity of hospice service provision:

- Routine: $46.25 per day
- Respite: $55.33 per day
- Inpatient: $271.00 per day
- Continuous: $358.67 per day

On the average, in each hospice program the allowable cap is $6,500 per patient. Whereas some patients will use the hospice for only 30 days, others may use it for 200 days (exceeding $6,500 for the individual patient). However, the average for the total number of patients enrolled in the hospice is the basis of the reimbursement scheme and cost cap, and balance is achieved between short-stay patients and those needing longer stays.[52]

Seminars conducted by the Hospice Association of America focus on high quality hospice care in conformity with JCAH hospice standards. Emphasis is placed on assisting hospice agencies to emulate their quality assurance programs and to stress quality services.[53]

One hospice director said: "We strive to enable people to have the physical and emotional resources to remain at home for as long as possible, and if desired, to die at home amidst their loved ones."[54] Making house calls to sick and dying AIDS patients is an integral part of the services available from Bellevue Hospital Center in New York City. This is part of the trend to be supportive and to help "patients and families cope with the sadness, anger and fear that often accompany death."[55]

Physicians decry the mandate to certify a prognosis of remaining life expectancy of six months or less to meet patient eligibility criteria under Medicare. Others point out the financial concerns if the patient survives past day 210 when reimbursement is to cease. An executive of the National Hospice Organization predicted that "75 percent of hospices will not survive with Medicare's current reimbursement levels."[56]

A brief by the American Hospital Association indicates doubt that hospice care has potential for reducing total health care spending, but that "hospice care should be supported because it is a humane method of care." There is also objection to the 20 percent limit on inpatient care and other barriers which increase facility financial risk in operating hospice programs.[57]

A hospice benefit is offered by a majority of the largest employers in the U.S. as part of the company's health benefits. Among the Fortune 500 companies, 59 percent offered the hospice benefit. All insurance companies in Colorado, Maryland, Michigan, Nevada, New York and West Virginia are mandated to offer a hospice option. A model benefit has been prepared and distributed by the national Blue Cross and Blue Shield organization. One management consultant echoed the sentiments of many:

> Hospice is definitely a cost-saver if administered properly. It needs to be accepted as a means of offering humane and supportive care. For the employer and a doctor to be encouraging it for cost reasons is a ghoulish approach. Employees become apprehensive and cynical, as well they might be.[58]

Regulations currently have little incentive for nursing homes to enter the field of hospice care programs. Most nursing home industry objections concern high start-up costs, insufficient reimbursement, and specific limiting features concerning use of inpatient facilities.[59]

DRGs are not part of the reimbursement scheme for hospice care, but the hospice programs are under tight fiscal constraints. If hospice programs are not fully developed and supported as an alternative strategy for dying in the hospital, they are of limited use in freeing hospital beds and controlling health expenditures.

Prospective Rate Setting for Nursing Homes

Case Mix

Research and analysis of various components of nursing home costs has been done over the years to point out differences in providers, patient needs, services, and varieties of methods to deliver care in the institutions.[60-63]

Mechanisms for state and federal reimbursement rate setting to cover costs of patient care services in long-term care institutions has been evolving toward case-mix formulas which differ from DRGs. Use of the per diem rate in hospitals is similarly flawed in the nursing home environment, since it does not adequately reflect the intensity of service for each patient or the need for care. Diagnosis has relevance for hospitalized patients who most often have single diagnosis and predictable, computable average lengths of stay, with services more directly related to the treatment and intensity of specialized needs (i.e., surgery, X-rays, laboratory, intensive care units). Not so in the nursing homes where the nursing care service components (i.e., bathing, dressing, feeding, ambulation) are more important than the admitting diagnosis; the functional and mental status are key in determining needs for supervision, skilled care, and the potential use of resources in the institution.

Certain cost variables for institutional providers of long-term care services need attention in developing reimbursement rates.[64,65]

Geographic location: This would be used to calculate wage rate differences, but would also be used to determine patient access to care.

Newer facilities: They incur high construction costs and experience higher capital expenses.

Size of facility.

Nonprofit, government-operated, hospital-based facilities: These usually have teaching programs and experience known higher costs.

Occupancy rate: Reimbursement rates could include penalties for low occupancy to encourage admission and increase access.

Difficulties in rate setting to reimburse for the same patient care services in the proprietary and voluntary institutions need to be addressed, so that proprietary entities realize a return on equity and nonprofit organizations are compensated appropriately for their usually higher costs. Incentives need to be incorporated in payment systems so that sicker patients can gain admission despite their higher service use.[66,67] Some institutions might waste their resources or provide excessive services to patients or underutilize their resources and thereby alter their cost profiles inappropriately. Long-term care facilities are highly diverse: there are many different ownership arrangements; some facilities are free-standing while others are hospital-based long-term care units. The structure of each local community health care system results in many available options for care, each of which must be considered in determining reimbursement rates.[68,69]

One of the major reimbursement debates concerns establishment of the rate prior to the period the fee will be in effect (prospective rate setting) or after the care has been delivered (retrospective rate setting). Advocates of the prospective rate setting consider this a device to contain costs by stimulating efficiency in the delivery system, whereas the proponents of retrospective rate setting argue that the retroactive payment of costs is necessary to promote the delivery of high-quality care and to assure access to this care for Medicare and Medicaid patients. Adding relevance to this debate is the Social Security Amendment of 1983 (P.L. 98-21), which mandates a new prospective payment system for hospitals participating in Medicare.

In a study of state programs, by 1982, 33 states had adopted prospective rate setting and twelve reported retrospective rate setting. The average Medicaid payments for skilled care were always lower with the prospective method. Similar findings for the intermediate care facility rates also favored prospective rate setting. Medicaid patients had greater access and utilized more patient days.

They had somewhat greater lengths of stay where prospective rates were in effect in both skilled and intermediate facilities and no adverse effect on access was noted.[70]

The retroactive retrospective adjustments of rates covers costs of delivering services, and excesses may be passed through for further rates. With prospective rate, the institution must deliver care at the predetermined rate where inefficiencies and mismanagement are painful and costly to the institution. However, critics point to problems in quality of care, limited access to Medicaid patients, and reduction of needed services if the prospective rates are unrealistically low.[71]

Many research projects and experiments are focused on turning the payments for services into prospective payments based on case-mix. The case-mix involves three aspects.

Classifying patients into groupings that are meaningful with regard to resource needs

Estimating the relationship between patient status and resource use

Cost weights for particular resource use of patient type.

While states develop rate systems for Medicaid and the federal system mostly concentrates on Medicare, components of each of these endeavors are being incorporated for reimbursement of skilled nursing care into potential "all payer" rates for broader use.

Patient classification systems have been designed to determine appropriate placement of patients, to aid in staff resource allocations, and to help plan for care or discharge.[72-74] The major elements are

Medical diagnosis

Functional status

Mental health status

Nursing services

Problems with attempting to pay for facility care based on medical diagnosis alone is difficult because the elderly have multiple diagnoses and there is a wide range of severity of illness and therapeutic needs within each disease category.[75,76]

Attempts at diagnostic groupings (i.e., neoplasm, blood and blood-forming organ diseases, etc.), as well as individual diagnoses (i.e., stroke, hypertension), have not successfully provided enough insight into variation in facility characteristics or patient care needs. Other studies have used the medical diagnosis coupled with functional abilities, mental status, and selected risk factors (cancer, stroke, chronic renal failure, decubitus care, comatose care).[77-79]

Measures of functional status in activities of daily living (ADL) can classify disability independent of medical diagnosis. These have been found to be most useful descriptions of long-term care patients. The development and validation of these indices are described in the literature by Katz, and others have focused attention on the sequential pattern of progression of dependency in long-term care patients[80-82] (see Exhibit 8-1).

In most of the studies previously cited, the mental health status is an important variable in case-mix measures since certain patient behavior requires specific intensive staff care and resources. Those who are physically or verbally abusive, depressed, unresponsive, withdrawn and forgetful, or disruptive require additional staff attention.

Direct nursing service needs can be utilized to classify patients by listing and counting the specific services used on a daily or weekly basis. For example:

Medication	Enemas or douching
Injections	Appliances
Catheters	Oxygen and/or IPPB
Dressings	Ostomy care
Suctioning-tracheostomy care	I.V. fluids
Restorative nursing	

States such as West Virginia, Illinois, Ohio, Washington, and Maryland incorporate these and other services (decubitus ulcer care, tube feedings) in their case-mix measures used in rate setting.

The rate setting mechanisms cannot be developed until investigators research some of the necessary components: Patients need to be classified for case-mix purposes; other institutional facility factors must be identified and taken into account; and, social incentives must be incorporated into the rates to assure access for patients with high intensity service needs. While the hospital DRG system relies on relative weights that reflect the average pattern of practice and average quality of care in each DRG, this may not be acceptable for the nursing home case, where quality of care varies widely. Averages which include those facilities with poor quality of care do a disservice to facilities where care is of high quality. In addition, including superior care givers in the rates will produce an average that will reward those facilities which only provide adequate and acceptable care. One does not wish to allow facilities to profit by providing minimal care to needy patients.

Exhibit 8-1 Activities of Daily Living (ADLs) and ADL Indices Used for Case-Mix Analyses

Activities of Daily Living Variables

Feeding
Continence
Defecation
Transfer
Ambulation
Toileting
Dressing
Bathing

1. Skinner-Yett Index

ADL Variables Included:	Feeding	Continence	Ambulation	Transfer/ Dressing	Bathing
ADL Index Value:					
1	Indep————————————————————————————————→				
2	Indep————————————————————————————→				Dep
3	Indep————————————————————→			Dep	Dep
4	Indep————————→		Dep	Dep	Dep
5	Indep	Dep	Dep	Dep	Dep
6	Dep	Dep	Dep	Dep	Dep

2. Katz ADL Grades

ADL Variables Included:	Feeding	Continence	Transfer	Toileting	Dressing	Bathing
ADL Index Value:						
"A" = 1	Independent in all————————————————————————————→					
"B" = 2	Independent in 5 of 6————————————————————————→					
"C" = 3	Independent in 4 of 5————————————————→					Dep
"D" = 4	Independent in 3 of 4————————→				Dep	Dep
"E" = 5	Independent in 2 of 3——→			Dep	Dep	Dep
"F" = 6	Independent in 1 of 2		Dep	Dep	Dep	Dep
"G" = 7	Indep	Dep	Dep	Dep	Dep	Dep

3. Katz ADL Scores

ADL Variables Included:	Feeding	Continence	Transfer	Toileting	Dressing	Bathing
ADL Index Value:						
0	Independent in all 6					
1	Independent in 5 of 6; Dependent in 1					
2	Independent in 4 of 6; Dependent in 2					
3	Independent in 3 of 6; Dependent in 3					
4	Independent in 2 of 6; Dependent in 4					
5	Independent in 1 of 6; Dependent in 5					
6	Dependent in all 6					

Note: The sources of ADL Indices and the methods applied in determining variable values is described in Katz et al., 1963; Katz et al., 1976; and Skinner and Yett, 1973.

Resource Utilization Groups (RUGs)
Experiment—New York State

New York State is experimenting with a case-mix reimbursement system for long-term care facilities which is prospective in methodology, and allows for adequate reimbursement of facility needs based on characteristics of the clients in the facility. The three-year study is being conducted by the New York State Department of Health and Rensselaer Polytechnic Institute, under a grant from the Health Care Financing Administration supplemented by additional New York State funding.

The classification system is based on the work of Brant E. Fries, Ph.D. (at Rensselaer), and Leo M. Cooney, Jr., M.D. (Yale University School of Medicine), who studied 1469 patients and their resource needs in 76 Connecticut nursing homes.[83] Fries selected case mix based on the patient as a method of measure over case mix based on the facility with the belief that "It's the patients that cause the case-mix. It's the fact that different types of services are provided to particular types of patients that causes the change. Case-mix based on a facility is not a responsive measure of case-mix."[84]

In the Connecticut study, profiles of nursing home patients were collected on a variety of dimensions including demographic, social, mental, behavioral, and physical characteristics, services rendered, and activities of daily living (ADL). The areas found to be most descriptive of the patients' differences and variation in resource time were the ADLs. These activities include toileting, dressing, personal hygiene, ambulation, transferability, continence of the bowels and bladder, and feeding.[85]

Nine clusters emerged in categorizing patient needs and level of care resource use (Exhibit 8-2). The estimates of resource use closely correlated with actual observed care needs. These same ADL variables were shown to be good predictors of staff time resource use in earlier studies by McCaffree,[86,87] Flagel,[88] Swearingen,[89] Skinner and Yett,[90] and Parker.[91]

In the New York study, the RUGs categorization scheme has been expanded to 16 categories which will be validated for use and a relative value scale corresponding to these groups will be developed indicative of the total resources needed for individual patients. Payments to nursing homes will be made using a prospective formula which reflects the resource needs in accordance with their case-mix.

It is anticipated that there will be fewer "rate appeals" and sicker patients will have better access to nursing homes because of weighted rates. Noninstitutional care for patients with minimal needs will be encouraged so that some patients will be discharged or not admitted, since there is no financial incentive to keep these patients in the nursing home environment.[92]

Exhibit 8-2 RUGs Patient Classification System

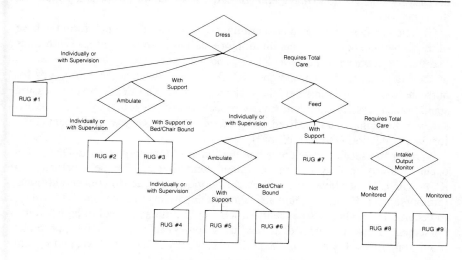

Resource Utilization Groups

Group 1: Able to dress without help or with supervision

Group 2: Able to dress only with staff support and ambulates without help or with supervision

Group 3: Able to dress only with staff support; ambulates only with staff support or is confined to bed or chair

Group 4: Requires total care for dressing; eats without help or requires supervision; and ambulates without help or with supervision

Group 5: Requires total care for dressing; eats without help or requires supervision; and ambulates only with staff support

Group 6: Requires total care for dressing; eats without help or requires supervision; and is confined to bed or chair

Group 7: Requires total care for dressing; eats only with staff support

Group 8[a]: Requires total care for dressing; requires total care in feeding; and does not have intake/output of fluids monitored

Group 9[a]: Requires total care for dressing; requires total care in feeding; and has intake/output of fluids monitored

[a]Alternate for RUG Groups 8 and 9:

Group 8A: Requires total care for dressing; eats without help or requires supervision; and on permanent placement for cognitive disabilities

Group 9A: Requires total care for dressing; eats without help or requires supervision; and on permanent placement for physical disabilities, or temporary placement for recuperation or fractures (other than hip)

Group 10A: Requires total care for dressing; eats without help or requires supervision; and on permanent placement for serious medical condition, terminal care, or temporary placement for hip fracture or cardiovascular accident.

Source: Adapted from B. E. Fries, and L. M. Cooney, *RUGs: A Patient Classification System for Long Term Care* (Troy, NY: Rensselaer Polytechnic Institute, Oct. 1983).

Dr. Fries said that in New York, where a shortage of beds exists, "It's not necessarily that we don't have enough beds, it's that we're not using the beds the right way."[93]

Questions have been raised concerning the historical data which form the base of the reimbursement, the rehabilitation orientation of some facilities (with costs that may be higher for the same RUG), and the inconsistency among reviewers of scoring patients for their assigned RUGs.[94] Special educational programs for nurse assessors are being held in various areas in New York State to assure standardized classification and review procedures for each facility.[95] The assessors will be using a standardized and pretested Patient Review Instrument (PRI) for data collection (see Exhibit 8-3).

Another foreseeable problem is that the "creep" that may occur in DRGs will occur similarly in RUGs in the facilities attempting to upgrade a patient to a RUG with a higher level of resource consumption in order to collect additional reimbursement. Facilities could also allow their patients to degenerate purposely, to become increasingly dependent, which would ultimately lead to higher reimbursement. These unprofessional, devilish schemes can be avoided by appropriate monitoring of facility case-mix experiences, quality of care reviews, and system auditing.

New York has 714 facilities with 67,500 skilled nursing beds and 26,400 intermediate care beds (exclusive of hospital long-term care beds) and the RUGs methodology will address both populations using new survey instruments tested in 52 facilities with 3427 patients and selecting additional dependent variables, such as physician services to patients, and ancillary services, such as physical therapy or occupational therapy. Patients will be classifed and grouped, and patterns of resource consumption will be refined. In terms of the DRG approach the "resource consumption" for each hospital admission diagnosis is measured in terms of length of stay (LOS).

The timetable for implementation of the reimbursement methodology will be in two steps. For 1986, the RUG data will be used for prospective case-mix indexed rates. In 1987, prospective RUG per diem rates will be in place, along with peer group averages and efficiency standards.

The first year will utilize a case-mix index (CMI) to adjust an all-inclusive operating cost per diem. The CMI will be calculated based on the RUG composition of the patient population and intensity weights associated with each RUG.

The major explicit goal of the case-mix reimbursement system is to reduce the costs of long-term care without compromising quality, and alter utilization rates to favor patients with higher care needs. By developing prior placement screening instruments for use in hospitals and communities, and by periodic reassessment of patients already in skilled care facilities, it is anticipated that by 1990 there will be 6,000 to 7,000 more skilled nursing facility beds available.

New York State Department of Health
Division of Health Care Financing

PATIENT REVIEW INSTRUMENT (PRI)
Use with separate PRI Instructions and Training Manual

I. ADMINISTRATIVE DATA

1 OPERATING CERTIFICATE NUMBER
(1—8)

2 SOCIAL SECURITY NUMBER
(9—17)

3 FACILITY IS A:
1 = HRF   2 = SNF   (18)
PRINT OFFICIAL FACILITY NAME:

11 DATE OF **INITIAL** ADMISSION: to this facility at this level of care
(HRF or SNF)
(52-59) MO.   DAY   YEAR   1 9

4 PATIENT NAME (PLEASE PRINT)

12 MEDICAID NUMBER
(60-70)

5 DATE OF PRI COMPLETION
(19-26) MO.   DAY   YEAR   1 9

13 MEDICARE NUMBER
(71-80)

6 MEDICAL RECORD NUMBER
(27-35)

14 PRIMARY PAYOR
1 = Medicaid   3 = Other
2 = Medicare   (81)

7 ROOM NUMBER
(36-40)

15 REASON FOR PRI COMPLETION:

Assessment for Reimbursement
1. Initial Assessment
2. Reassessment of Patient   (82)

8 UNIT NUMBER (Assigned by RUG II Project)
(41-42)

Utilization Review
3. Admission Review
4. Continued Stay Review
5. Discharged

9 DATE OF BIRTH
(43-50) MO.   DAY   YEAR

Assess Long Term Placement Potential
6. Patient in Hospital
7. Patient in Community

10 SEX
1 = Male
2 = Female   (51)

II. MEDICAL EVENTS

16 DECUBITUS LEVEL: ENTER THE MOST SEVERE LEVEL (0-5) AS DEFINED IN THE INSTRUCTIONS
(83)

17 MEDICAL CONDITIONS: DURING THE PAST FOUR WEEKS. READ THE INSTRUCTIONS FOR SPECIFIC DEFINITIONS.

1 = Yes   2 = No
(84-91)

A. Comatose

B. Dehydration

C. Internal Bleeding

D. Stasis Ulcer

E. Terminally Ill

F. Contractures

G. Diabetes Mellitus

H. Urinary Tract Infection

DOH-3 (rev. 3/86)

18 MEDICAL TREATMENTS: READ THE INSTRUCTIONS FOR QUALIFIERS.   1 = Yes   2 = No

A. Tracheostomy Care/Suctioning   (92-104)
(Daily — Exclude self care)

B. Suctioning — General (Daily)

C. Oxygen (Daily)

D. Respiratory Care (Daily)

E. Nasal Gastric Feeding

F. Parenteral Feeding

G. Wound Care

H. Chemotherapy

I. Transfusion

J. Dialysis

K. Bowel and Bladder Rehabilitation
(SEE INSTRUCTIONS)

L. Catheter (Indwelling or External)

M. Physical Restraints (Daytime Only)

Exhibit 8-3

III. ACTIVITIES OF DAILY LIVING (ADLs)

Answer questions 19-22 according to how each task was completed 60% of the time during the past four weeks or since admission, whichever is shorter (regardless of cause). Read the **Changed Condition Rule** and definitions in the instructions.

19 EATING: PROCESS OF GETTING FOOD BY ANY MEANS FROM THE RECEPTACLE INTO THE BODY (FOR EXAMPLE, PLATE, CUP, TUBE).

1 = Feeds self without supervision or physical assistance. May use adaptive equipment.

2 = Requires *intermittent* supervision (that is, verbal encouragement/guidance) and/or minimal physical assistance with minor parts of eating, such as cutting food, buttering bread or opening milk carton.

3 = Requires continual help (encouragement/teaching/ physical assistance) with eating or meal will not be completed.

4 = Totally fed by hand; patient does not manually participate. (Include syringe feeding.)

5 = Tube or parenteral feeding for primary intake of food. (*Not* just for supplemental nourishments.)

19 ☐ (105)

20 MOBILITY: HOW THE PATIENT MOVES ABOUT.

1 = Walks with no supervision or human assistance. May require mechanical device (for example, a walker), but not a wheelchair.

2 = Walks with intermittent supervision (that is, verbal cueing and observation). May require human assistance for difficult parts of walking (for example, stairs, ramps).

3 = Walks with *constant* one-to-one supervision and/or constant physical assistance.

4 = *Wheels* with *no* supervision or assistance, except for difficult maneuvers (for example, elevators, ramps). May actually be able to walk, but generally does not move.

5 = Is *wheeled*, chairfast or bedfast. Relies on someone else to move about, if at all.

20 ☐ (106)

21 TRANSFER: PROCESS OF MOVING BETWEEN POSITIONS, TO/FROM BED, CHAIR, STANDING, (EXCLUDE TRANSFERS TO/FROM BATH AND TOILET).

1 = Requires no supervision or physical assistance to complete necessary transfers. May use equipment, such as railings, trapeze.

2 = Requires *intermittent* supervision (that is, verbal cueing, guidance) and/or physical assistance for difficult maneuvers only.

3 = Requires one person to provide constant guidance, steadiness and/or physical assistance. Patient may participate in transfer.

4 = Requires *two* people to provide constant supervision and/or physically lift. May need lifting equipment.

5 = Cannot and is not gotten out of bed.

21 ☐ (107)

22 TOILETING: PROCESS OF GETTING TO AND FROM A TOILET (OR USE OF OTHER TOILETING EQUIPMENT, SUCH AS BEDPAN), TRANSFERRING ON AND OFF TOILET, CLEANSING SELF AFTER ELIMINATION AND ADJUSTING CLOTHES.

1 = Requires no supervision or physical assistance. May use special equipment, such as a raised toilet or grab bars.

2 = Requires *intermittent* supervision for safety or encouragement; or *minor* physical assistance (for example, clothes adjustment or washing hands).

3 = Continent of bowel *and* bladder. Requires constant supervision and/or physical assistance with major/all parts of the task, *including* appliances (i.e., colostomy, ileostomy, urinary catheter).

4 = Incontinent of bowel *and/or* bladder and is not taken to a bathroom.

5 = Incontinent of bowel *and/or* bladder, but is taken to a bathroom every two to four hours during the day and as needed at night.

22 ☐ (108)

IV. BEHAVIORS

23 VERBAL DISRUPTION: BY YELLING, BAITING, THREATENING, ETC.

1 = None during the past four weeks. (May have verbal outbursts which are not disruptive.)

2 = Verbal disruption one to three times during the past four weeks.

3 = Short-lived disruption at least once per week during the past four weeks *or predictable* disruption regardless of frequency (for example, during specific care routines, such as bathing).

4 = Unpredictable, recurring verbal disruption *at least once per week* for no foretold reason.

5 = Patient is at level #4 above, but does not fulfill the active treatment and psychiatric assessment qualifiers (in the instructions).

23 ☐ (109)

24 PHYSICAL AGGRESSION: ASSAULTIVE OR COMBATIVE TO SELF OR OTHERS WITH **INTENT FOR INJURY.** (FOR EXAMPLE HITS SELF, THROWS OBJECTS, PUNCHES, DANGEROUS MANEUVERS WITH WHEELCHAIR).

1 = None during the past four weeks.

2 = Unpredictable aggression during the past four weeks (whether mild or extreme), *but not at least once per week.*

3 = Predictable aggression during specific care routines or as a reaction to normal stimuli (for example, bumped into), regardless of frequency. May strike or fight.

4 = Unpredictable, recurring aggression at least once per week during the past four weeks for no apparent or foretold reason (that is, not just during specific care routines or as a reaction to normal stimuli).

5 = Patient is at level #4 above, but does not fulfill the active treatment and psychiatric assessment qualifiers (in the instructions).

24 ☐ (110)

Exhibit 8-3, cont.

Quality of care monitoring within the facility by the surveys and reviews of the data collected by the state agency will reinforce the use of the appropriate lowest level of care to meet the patient's existing needs.[96]

In New York State and nationally, institutional long-term care services account for 40 percent of total Medicaid expenditures. This opportunity to institute long-

25 **DISRUPTIVE, INFANTILE OR SOCIALLY INAPPROPRIATE BEHAVIOR:** CHILDISH, REPETITIVE OR ANTISOCIAL **PHYSICAL** BEHAVIOR WHICH CREATES *DISRUPTION WITH OTHERS* (FOR EXAMPLE, CONSTANTLY UNDRESSING SELF, STEALING, SMEARING FECES, SEXUALLY DISPLAYING ONESELF TO OTHERS). EXCLUDE VERBAL ACTIONS. READ THE INSTRUCTIONS FOR OTHER EXCLUSIONS.

1 = No infantile or socially inappropriate behavior, whether or not disruptive, during the past four weeks.

2 = Displays this behavior, but is not disruptive to others (for example, rocking in place).

3 = Disruptive behavior during the past four weeks, but *not* at least once per week.

4 = Disruptive behavior at least *once per week* during the past four weeks.

5 = Patient is at level #4 above, but does not fulfill the active treatment and psychiatric assessment qualifiers (in instructions).

25 ☐
(111)

26 **HALLUCINATIONS:** EXPERIENCED AT LEAST ONCE PER WEEK DURING THE PAST FOUR WEEKS. VISUAL, AUDITORY OR TACTILE PERCEPTIONS THAT HAVE NO BASIS IN EXTERNAL REALITY.

1 = Yes   2 = No

3 = Yes, but does not fulfill the active treatment and psychiatric assessment qualifiers (in the instructions).

26 ☐
(112)

V. SPECIALIZED SERVICES

27 **PHYSICAL AND OCCUPATIONAL THERAPIES:** READ INSTRUCTIONS AND QUALIFIERS. EXCLUDE REHABILITATIVE NURSES AND OTHER SPECIALIZED THERAPISTS (FOR EXAMPLE, SPEECH THERAPIST). ENTER THE LEVEL, DAYS AND TIME (HOURS AND MINUTES) PER WEEK.

A. Physical Therapy (P.T.)...

B. Occupational Therapy (O.T.)..

LEVEL

1 = Does not receive.

2 = Maintenance Program - Requires and is currently receiving physical and/or occupational therapy to help stabilize or slow functional deterioration.

3 = Restorative Therapy - Requires and is currently receiving physical and/or

occupational therapy for four or more consecutive weeks.

4 = Receives therapy, but does not fulfill the qualifiers stated in the instructions. (For example, restorative therapy given or to be given for only two weeks.)

P.T. Level ☐
(113)

P.T. Days ☐
(114)

P.T. Time ☐☐☐☐ ☐☐ ☐☐
(115-118) **HOURS MIN/WEEK**

O.T. Level ☐
(119)

O.T. Days ☐
(120)

O.T. Time ☐☐☐☐ ☐☐ ☐☐
(121-124) **HOURS MIN/WEEK**

DAYS AND TIME PER WEEK: ENTER THE CURRENT NUMBER OF DAYS AND TIME (HOURS AND MINUTES) PER WEEK THAT EACH THERAPY IS PROVIDED. ENTER ZERO IF AT #1 LEVEL ABOVE. READ INSTRUCTIONS AS TO QUALIFIERS IN COUNTING DAYS AND TIME.

28 **NUMBER OF PHYSICIAN VISITS:** ENTER ONLY THE NUMBER OF VISITS DURING THE PAST FOUR WEEKS THAT ADHERE TO THE PATIENT NEED AND DOCUMENTATION QUALIFIERS IN THE INSTRUCTIONS. EXCLUDE PSYCHIATRISTS, PHYSICIAN ASSISTANTS, AND NURSE PRACTITIONERS.

28 ☐☐
(125-126)

DIAGNOSIS

29 **PRIMARY PROBLEM:** THE MEDICAL CONDITION REQUIRING THE LARGEST AMOUNT OF NURSING TIME. THIS MAY NOT BE THE ADMISSION DIAGNOSIS BY THE PHYSICIAN.

ICD—9 Code of medical problem..

If code cannot be located, print medical name here

29 ☐☐☐.☐☐
(127-131)

30 **QUALIFIED ASSESSOR**

Assessor Identification Number (Assigned by RUG II)..

30 ☐☐☐☐☐
(132-136)

Signature of Qualified Assessor

Exhibit 8-3, cont.

term care reimbursement, based on indexing resources consumed by clusters of similar patients, has the potential for national applicability. This reimbursement scheme can reduce program costs while still satisfying the minimum standards of quality of patient care. Quality of care surveys prior to RUGs and after implementation can be useful indicators; they can be tied to state facility licensure requirements and federal program participation in Medicare and Medicaid.

Outcome-Based Reimbursement Experiments

Outcome-based reimbursement systems are being studied and proposed as alternatives to case-mix reimbursement.[97] The reimbursement scheme is related to the difference between observed and expected outcomes of care, and make the link between performance and reward both explicit and direct. One study[98] combines case mix with outcome incentives for reimbursement for Medicaid nursing home services; it was tested in 36 proprietary Medi-Cal certified nursing homes in the San Diego area. Incentive payments were designed to meet certain objectives.

An admission incentive to encourage nursing homes to admit highly dependent Medicaid patients who might otherwise be inappropriately hospitalized (dependent on case-mix criteria).

An outcome incentive to encourage nursing homes to provide care that would improve residents' outcomes (linked to maintenance or improvement goals).

A discharge incentive to encourage appropriate discharges through case management services that would free beds for more severely dependent patients (paying up to ten days of vacant bed costs for timely discharge and payments for personnel in discharge planning services).

Preliminary results indicate that admissions for the most disabled group has been higher for nursing homes with incentive payments for this component and that some patients requiring heavy care needs (including the incontinent or tube-fed) are also admitted somewhat more frequently. However, differences in patient outcomes are not large and the proportion of heavy care patients who improved, maintained, or declined was very similar for the test and control. The outcome incentive comes into play only when specific outcome goals are achieved; the treatment test facilities overall reached more goals than controls. It was also found that clarity and specificity were needed and facilities acted more on admission and outcome incentives that were most understandable to them.

Another proposed nursing home reimbursement system is based on prognosis and patient outcome and thus rests on the ability to predict patient outcome.[99] Research has been conducted on developing predictive models to pay for care linked to outcomes. Reimbursement for each patient would be calculated as the cost of caring for such a patient multiplied by a prognostic adjustment factor (PAF), where the PAF reflects the extent to which the actual outcome of care exceeds or falls short of an expected level. Since reimbursement would be based on how patient outcome at a given point in time compares to predicted outcome, the ability to develop an adequate predictive model for outcome is crucial. Two types of predictive models are being tested. The first predicts scores in various categories of functioning and the second predicts outcome as defined by death, discharge better (to community), discharge worse (to hospital), and discharge other.

Some of the negative incentives created by patient case-mix reimbursement systems may be addressed using outcome-based systems.

Administrative Issues

There are many problems in the implementation of case-mix adjusted reimbursements:

Administratively complex and costly

Frequent assessments of patients needed

Validation of data

Accuracy of medical records—over and under documentation

Inconsistencies among evaluators

Appropriateness of services

Potential abuses in patient care because of reimbursement

Incentives or disincentives

However, many states have developed compensating mechanisms specifying periodicity of assessment, validating assessment instruments, training and monitoring nurse assessors or reviewers, and using facility experience-based data and community patterns among institutions.

DRG and cost consciousness has stimulated great interest in these institutions and new patterns of reimbursement.[100]

Veterans Administration—Long-Term Care Allocations

Since mid-1983, the Department of Medicine and Surgery of the Veterans Administration (VA) has been developing a Resource Allocation System of budgeting for long-term care facilties in their system. Dr. Carleton C. Evans, director of allocation development, is the chief architect of models to measure clinical workloads at the VA. He said, "Basically, it looks at patients in long-term care settings to determine in some way the different resource requirements of different mixes of patients based on their nursing needs. Diagnosis is not a (major part) of it, though there may be some diagnostic data required . . . the variation in nursing requirements . . . determines the variation in cost."[101]

There is a Long-Term Care Patient Project currently testing two existing research models which group patients by the intensity of nursing services required. The hypothesis adopted is that "the variance in the amount of nursing care given and amount of nursing care per patient varies according to the patient's physical and functional status."[102] The models of Cameron/Knauf[103] and Fries/Cooney[104,105] are under study and testing is being carried out in the intermediate units in the VA (similar to community hospital-based skilled nursing facilities) and in facilities with nursing home beds only.

Analysis of more than 18,000 VA patient survey forms in the intermediate medical and nursing homes of physical, functional, and treatment data was further reviewed and categorized according to ADL and other variables specified in each model. Final reports are not yet available, but there is apparent preference for the Fries/Cooney model which currently is being refined in the New York State three-year RUGs experiment.[106]

This initiative imposed, on its own, allocation of resources to the huge federal system of hospitals and long-term care facilities, is directly related to the DRG push in the community sector for cost containment in the Medicare system. The VA considers the use of DRGs with a variety of weighted units as a management tool for resource allocation and not necessarily for cost containment. At the hospital and ambulatory care levels, directors will need to review cost centers, increase efficiency, and reduce length of stay, similar to the community imperatives.[107,108] With the need for alternate levels of care for veterans of all ages, expansion of long-term care residential facilities and home health care programs and conversion of empty hospital beds for long-term care is already on the drawing board.

Veterans comprise nearly half of the country's male population over 65 and a recent survey of 3,000 veterans focused on health status, economic status, and daily living arrangements so as to help plan for the needs of older veterans.[109]

Of the 28.2 million veterans, 4 million are 65 years and older; this will peak to 9 million by 1999. The fastest-growing segment, those aged 75 and older, will grow from 1 million to 4.5 million by the year 2005. It is estimated that older veterans will be entering VA hospitals for some form of medical care at the rate of more than 2.2 million per year—almost twice as many as in 1981. The potential strain on the VA system is being combatted on many fronts—with ten recently established Geriatric Research, Education, and Clinical Centers (GRECC).[110]

In addition, in 1986, 204 acute beds will be converted to nursing home beds with 2,500 more conversions expected by 1990. These conversions will reduce the VA new nursing home construction budget with savings of $62 million in 1984 and $39.2 million in 1985.[111]

The VA has had a contract nursing home program using community facilities, which will need to expand if conversions and new construction do not meet the demand. However, veterans' organizations have always demanded that veterans have their own separate facilities that cater to their special needs. Recent GAO studies, though, have revealed that costs of "new VA nursing homes are twice as expensive to build and operate as community facilities"[112] and promote the idea of more community resource use for veterans.

The enormous size of this special population and the major network of 172 hospitals, 99 nursing homes, 226 outpatient clinics, and allied programs is of such medical and managerial complexity that new ideas, such as those spurred by DRGs, have major impact. The federal imposition of DRGs on the facilities in the community is mirrored in similar restrictions and reimbursement allocation for its own federal facilities.

Exempt Long-Term Care Services or Institutions

Current regulations exempt certain services or institutions from the DRG system of prospective payment and as such appear to be an attractive new venture for those facilities with empty beds or desirous of marketing and expanding in this direction.[113] Rehabilitation hospitals, convalescent centers, and rehabilitation units of hospitals are acting as referral centers for the early-discharged patient and help keep patients at home (Exhibit 8-4).

HCFA will agree to exempt these institutions or services for two years under strict criteria and they must have been in operation for at least one year before being considered for exclusion. Documentation as to comprehensiveness and outcome orientation is important, as is appropriate equipment and staffing. Rehabilitation hospitals include neurological disorder centers and burn centers.[114]

Alcohol/drug treatment hospitals or units are exempted from DRG if they meet certain criteria of admission, have a written treatment program, a multidisciplinary approach for each patient, and a qualified nursing director and medical director. This is considered a preliminary exclusion from December 31, 1983 until October 1, 1986.[115]

Cancer hospitals with at least 50 percent of the patients having a principal diagnosis indicating neoplastic disease also are exempt from the prospective payment system. Acute hospitals or university-based medical centers with special cancer units cannot qualify for exemption in this area.[116] The impact of treating cancer in general hospitals is of concern and is reflected in the survey by the Association of Community Cancer Centers if the payment schedule is as current for the respective DRGs. The survey showed "84 percent of the oncology units in community hospitals have a higher staff/patient ratio than general medical/surgical units. A higher staff ratio equals higher cost of care."[117]

In a study at St. Barnabas Medical Center, Livingston, New Jersey, the authors commented on costs of treatment, much of which is on clinical trials or research

Exhibit 8-4 Exempt Institutions

Hospitals	
460	Psychiatric Hospitals
57	Rehabilitation Hospitals
23	Alcohol/Drug Treatment Hospitals
555	Short-stay Hospitals in Waivered States
112	Long-term Care Hospitals
42	Children's Hospitals
Units in Acute Care Hospitals	
802	Psychiatric Units
370	Rehabilitation Units
317	Alcohol/Drug Treatment Units

Source: HHS, HCFA, Background Paper, July 1985.

protocols: "It is likely that oncology programs doing research will likely need double the average DRG rate if they are to survive."[118]

Proposals on prospective pricing for currently exempt facilities are under study. The National Association of Children's Hospitals and Related Institutions (NA-CHRI) wants to compare two systems—one similar to DRGs and one more related to acuity or severity of illness, since age and acuity play an important role in pediatric care. The National Association of Rehabilitation Facilities (NARF) plans to collect financial and patient data from their member institutions to test model payment systems. NARF also has asked HCFA to study a patient classification system based on a patient's functional status and physiology.[119]

It is clear that the exemptions are temporary until the DRG system is translated effectively for various rehabilitation facilities. Most of the delay appears to be the lack of appropriate standardized classification and categorization methodology. Spokesmen from these institutions seem bent on making themselves heard, and on participating actively in the system to be adopted.

DRG Impact on Long-Term Care

Despite the growth of the long-term care field in institutions, and services responding to the complexity of care[120,121] needed for patients discharged early under stimulus of the new payment system, there is a general feeling that patients' needs are not being met appropriately.

Concern about the negative impact of the TEFRA and pursuant HCFA regulations on the nursing home section has been voiced by noted geriatrician Leslie S. Libow, M.D.: "Medicare, which has done so much for the elderly in the past, now appears to join ranks with the negative forces operating against the aged population throughout our society."[122]

He also believes that noninstitutional alternatives to care is a "false promise" because most patients in nursing homes need a level of care not available or possible in a community setting.[123]

With a contrary view, Representative Claude Pepper, Chairman of the Select Committee on Aging, Subcommittee on Health and Long-Term Care, is distressed that: "We have an official policy in this country which, contrary to the wishes of our citizens, favors institutionalization. We are spending billions of dollars to place individuals in nursing homes or a few million to take care of them at home."[124]

Since the Medicare program has restricted definitions of "skilled nursing care" or "rehabilitation care," Pepper estimates "that in excess of 5 million people are going without the home care services they need." The committee also indicated that they favored "an end to the existing bias in American health care programs in favor of institutionalization and the expansion of home care services."[125]

Other issues emerge and pose difficulties concerning the long-term care needs of patients.

Financial issues. Who will pay for care in the hospital beyond the acute DRG days while patients await alternate care services in the community or other institutions?

Placement issues. Where can patients go who are forced out of the hospital but are too ill to care for themselves?

Ethical issues. How does one resolve the conflicts between need of individuals and the needs of institutions and society?

The ethical dilemma is posed by Philip W. Brickner, M.D., Director of Community Medicine at St. Vincents Hospital in New York City: "What will short-term hospitals do when they have a patient in coma or one that is brain-dead? How can they send such people off to long-term care institutions that may have no places for them? They certainly do not want to have to absorb the cost of caring for such patients—who could live for a long time—under a fixed DRG."[126]

Testimony presented by the American Health Care Association before the U.S. Senate Finance Committee's Health Subcommittee urged reasonable long-term care financing arrangements and improved Medicare long-term care benefits. It was also proposed that individuals and families be encouraged to contribute to the cost of long-term care, and that states implement family responsibility laws. Additional incentives are proposed for individuals and families to get tax benefits and deductions for expenses paid on behalf of elderly or disabled and dependent family members.[127]

Several states are attempting to shift a greater portion of nursing home costs to relatives of Medicaid patients. Legal enforcement of relative responsibility for nursing home costs could constitute a signficiant policy change for Medicaid. The authorizing legislation specifies that state Medicaid plans may not take into account the financial responsibility of any individual for any applicant or recipient of assistance unless the applicant or recipient is the individual's spouse, child younger than twenty-one, or child older than twenty-one and also blind or disabled.

Some of the proposed state legislation would simply encourage voluntary contributions, primarily by children for their elderly parents. Such voluntary contributions are already permitted under current law, although no such payment may be deemed as income to the Medicaid recipient until actually made; therefore, it cannot be considered for the purpose of determining eligibility for Medicaid assistance.

Idaho recently passed legislation, effective October 1, 1983, which requires spouses, parents, and children of Medicaid recipients to pay as much as $3,000 a year for the recipients of nursing home care. This legislation is expected to save as much as $500,000 yearly and will include mandatory fees ranging from $35 to $250 a month. These will be derived from a sliding scale based on a relative's income minus some deductions.[128]

In these times of seeking greater financial self-support and reducing dependency, the government role is seen as being too encompassing when it is not restrictive and limiting. In comparison to these proposals, we take note of recent expansions of long-term care benefits for citizens in Canada through provincial programs. Canadian experiences in three provinces have been studied as a potential model of expanded long-term care insurance in the public sector.[129] Introducing extensive community programs including home care, homemaking, and active case management did not reduce the need for nursing home beds. "The argument for community care must rest on other grounds. A commitment to community care represents a desire to serve persons who need care and whose needs are not being met by nursing homes."[130] These public-supported programs for the elderly were introduced "not merely because the elderly have earned the benefit but because the role of society is to provide for those in need."[131] Dr. Howard R. Kelman points out that, in the American climate of resource protection and stringency under systems such as DRGs, the outlook for the allocation of increased resources to long-term care is bleak.

> The competitive clout of long-term care clients and providers when measured against population groups deemed more productive or more professionally rewarding, is weak indeed and relative to other claims against a finite resource "pie"—national defense, space exploration, farm price supports and the like . . . is scarcely considered vital, if considered at all.[132]

The likelihood of achieving significant reforms in the provision of care for long-term patients "appears dismal . . . unless such actions or policies can offer tangible promise of cost savings or containment."[133]

Basically, attempts are being made to find methodologies of fair and equitable payments to long-term care institutions for the level of care being rendered without compromising quality. In addition, incentives to increase access to care for the most frail and dependent patients with multiple illnesses and disabilities are being studied.

The federal government has begun to recognize the important role nursing homes play in making the hospital DRG system successful. As more and more attention is paid to the long-term care industry, these facilities are finding that such attention is a mixed blessing.

References

1. W. Read, "Elderly Population to Increase Dramatically by 2030," *Hospitals* 59, No. 1 (January, 1984):25-26.

2. J. A. Tedesco, "Caring for the Elderly Under Prospective Pricing," *Hospitals* 58, No. 14 (July 16, 1984):54, 59.

3. A. Bergh, "Industry Update; Industry: Nursing Homes," *Montgomery Securities,* October 14, 1983.

4. E. Chelensky, *Impacts of Medicare Prospective Payment on Post-Hospital Long-Term-Care Services.* U.S., GAO Preliminary Report (GAO/PEMD-85-8), Letter of February 21, 1985.

5. Health Care Financing Administration, *Report on PPS Monitoring Activities,* January 20, 1985, p. 4.

6. *USDHHS Report to Congress: Study of the Skilled Nursing Facility Benefit Under Medicare.* Washington, DC, January, 1985.

7. Health Care Financing Administration, *The Medicare and Medicaid Data Book, 1983.* Baltimore, MD, 1983, p. 38.

8. Congressional Budget Office, *Reducing the Deficit: Spending and Revenue Options, Part 3.* Washington, DC, February, 1984, p. 73.

9. GAO, *Improved Administration Could Reduce the Costs of Ohio's Medicaid Program.* GAO/HRD 79-98, Washington, DC, October 23, 1979, pp. 129-137.

10. GAO, *Medicaid and Nursing Home Care: Cost Increases and the Need for Services are Creating Problems for the States and the Elderly,* GAO/IPE 84-1, Washington, DC, October 21, 1983, p. 107-127.

11. GAO, *The Elderly Should Benefit from Expanded Home Health Care But Increasing These Services will not Insure Cost Reductions,* GAO/IPE 83-1, Washington, DC, December 7, 1982, pp. 26-28.

12. GAO, *Medicare Home Health Services: A Difficult Program to Control.* GAO/HRD 81-155, Washington, DC, September 25, 1981, pp. 10-17.

13. Bergh, "Industry Update."

14. "Stockwatch, as of December 7, 1984," *Contemporary Longterm Care* 8, No. 1 (1985):14.

15. W. A. Spicer, "The Man Behind the LTC Express," *Contemporary Longterm Care* 8, No. 1 (1985):39.

16. Q. D. Young, "Impact of For-Profit Enterprise on Health Care," *Journal of Public Health Policy* 5, No. 4 (1985):449-452.

17. T. J. Onusko, "Keeping Up with CON Laws," *Contemporary Longterm Care* 8, No. 1 (1985):49-51.

18. T. Lamb, "Hospitals and LTC: The Meeting of the Markets," *Contemporary Longterm Care* 8, No. 3 (1985):62-66.

19. M. G. Skrzynski, "Reimbursement Issues and Long-Term Care: Transitions," *Michigan Hospitals* 19, No. 6 (1983):7-9.

20. J. Bowe, "Conference Analyzes New Forces Shaping LTC Policies," *Today's Nursing Home* 5, No. 11 (November, 1984):142-144.

21. D. Blumenthal, M. Schlesinger and P. B. Drumheller "The Future of Medicare," *New England Journal of Medicine* 314, No. 11 (March 13, 1986): 722-728.

22. Lamb, "Hospitals and LTC."

23. Ibid.

24. P. Shaughnessy, R. Schlenker, et al. "Case Mix and Surrogate Indicators of Quality of Care Over Time in Freestanding and Hospital-Based Nursing Homes in Colorado," *Public Health Reports* 98, No. 5 (1983):486-492.

25. S. G. Ullman, "Cost Analysis and Facility Reimbursement in the Long-Term Health Care Industry," *Health Services Research* 19, No. 1 (1984):83-102.

26. C. T. Wood, "Relate Hospital Charges to Use of Services," *Harvard Business Review* 60, No. 2 (1982):123-130.

27. Lamb, "Hospitals and LTC."

28. J. Mongan, *Testimony Before the House Select Committee on Aging, on Health Cost Containment and Quality of Care*, February 26, 1985.

29. D. P. Borque, "HCFA Officials Eye Combined Payment," *American Medical News* 27, No. 4 (January 27, 1984):25.

30. "Expand DRGs, Increase Competition, Durenberger Says," *Hospitals* 58, No. 1 (January 1, 1984):30-31.

31. "Washington Perspectives—Vertical Integration: One Response to DRGs," *Washington Report on Medicine and Health* 37, No. 38 (September 26, 1983):Supplement, 4 pages.

32. "Passing Note," *Hospitals* 60, No. 5 (March 5, 1986):8.

33. Bowe, "Conference Analyzes."

34. W. S. Livergood, C. Smith, S. Hallstead, "The Impact of DRGs on Home Health Care," *Home Healthcare Nurse* 1, No. 1 (1983):29-31, 34.

35. D. F. Cuff, "Market Place: Home Health Care Stocks," *New York Times*, June 13, 1984.

36. C. Stonerock, "Special Report, The Impact of DRGs on Discharge Planning to Home Care: The New Jersey Perspective," *Upjohn Healthcare Services*, May 24, 1983.

37. J. S. Wodniak and J. Kirk, "Trend: Hospitals' Entry Into Home Health," *Caring* 3, No. 2 (1984):57-58.

38. "1985 AHA Survey," *Hospitals* 60, No. 4 (February 20, 1986):75.

39. J. C. Pyles, "Referral Arrangements Between Hospitals and Home Health Agencies," *Caring* 3, No. 2 (1984):54-56.

40. F. R. Curtiss "Financing Home Health Care Products and Services," *American Journal of Hospital Pharmacy* 43, No. 1 (1986):121-131.

41. J. Owens, Personal Correspondence, April 8, 1985.

42. USGAO, *Simulations of a Medicare Prospective Payment System for Home Helath Care*. GAO/HRD-85-110, Washington, D.C., September 30, 1985.

43. B. R. Lorenz, "Prospective Reimbursement in Health Care and Related Problems and Opportunities for Home Health Agencies," *Caring* 3, No. 2 (1984):27-28.

44. C. B. Zimmerman, "What's DRG's Impact on Home Health," *Pennsylvania Nurse* 38, No. 10 (1983):6, 8.

45. I. Taylor, "Big Growth Likely for Home Health Care," *The Star-Ledger*, (N.J.) April 8, 1984.

46. E. Brody, "Women in the Middle," *Gerontologist* 24, (1984):380-386.

47. M. R. Haug, "Home Care for the Ill Elderly—Who Benefits," *American Journal of Public Health* 75, No. 2 (1985):127-128.

48. K. S. Harlow and L. B. Wilson, "DRGs and the Community-Based Long Term Care System," Presentation to U.S. House Subcommittee on Human Resources, Committee on Education and Labor, July 30, 1985.

49. R. Trubo, "Home Health Care Encounters Growing Pains," *Medical World News* 27, No. 3 (February 10, 1986):76-88.

50. "HCFA—Medicare: Hospice Care Final Rules," *Federal Register* 48, No. 243 (December 16, 1983):56008-56036.

51. Ibid.

52. S. McLaughlin, "Regulatory Round Up: Final Hospice Regulations Published," *Caring* 3, No. 2 (February, 1984):5-8.

53. "Hospice Association to Sponsor Standards Seminar," Press release from Hospice Association of America, Washington, D.C., February 25, 1986.

54. "Brooklyn Hospice Receives Certification for Medicare," *The Jewish Week*, September 28, 1984.

55. R. Sullivan, "Bellevue Making House Calls to Help Dying AIDs Patients," *New York Times*, January 27, 1986.

56. "Long Term Care: An Industry Composite," Arthur Young International, National Health Care Group, Washington, D.C., 1985.

57. "Doubts Raised About Trial Hospice Plan," *Hospitals* 58, No. 18 (August 16, 1983):22.

58. M. Freudenheim, "Hospice Care As An Option," *New York Times*, February 4, 1986.

59. "Nursing Homes Shy Away From Hospice," *Today's Nursing Home* 5, No. 3 (1984):25.

60. H. S. Ruchlin and S. Levy, "Nursing Home Cost Analysis: A Case Study," *Inquiry* 9, No. 3 (1972):3-15.

61. H. S. Ruchlin, S. Levy, and C. Muller, "The Long-Term Care Marketplace: An Analysis of Deficiencies and Potential Reform by Means of Incentive Reimbursement," *Medical Care* 13, No. 12 (1975):979-991.

62. T. Willemain, "A Comparison of Patient Centered and Case-Mix Reimbursement for Nursing Home Care," *Health Services Research* 15, No. 14 (Winter, 1980):365-377.

63. H. L. Smith and M. D. Fottler, "Costs and Cost Containment in Nursing Homes," *Health Services Research* 16, No. 1 (Spring, 1981):17-41.

64. C. E. Bishop, "Nursing Home Cost Studies and Reimbursement Issues," *Health Care Financing Review* 1, No. 4 (Spring, 1980):47-64.

65. C. E. Bishop, "Nursing Home Cost Studies: Comments and Comparisons," *Health Services Research* 18, No. 3 (Fall, 1983):383-386.

66. W. Weissert, W. Scanlon, T. Wan, and D. Skinner, *Care for the Chronically Ill: Nursing Home Incentive Payment Experiment*, Department of Health Policy and Administration, University of North Carolina, School of Public Health, Chapel Hill, North Carolina, (Winter, 1983).

67. M. R. Meiners, G. D. Heinemann, and B. J. Jones, *An Evaluation of Nursing Home Payments Designed to Encourage Appropriate Care for the Chronically Ill: Some Preliminary Findings*. National Center for Health Services Research, Prepared for the Annual Meeting of the American Economic Association, December, 1982, New York, New York.

68. P. Shaughnessy and R. Schlenker, *Long-Term Care Reimbursement and Regulation: A Study of Cost, Case-Mix and Quality*. Working Paper 4: First-Year Analysis Report; Center for Health Services Research, University of Colorado Health Sciences Center, Denver, CO, February, 1980.

69. P. Shaughnessy, R. Schlenker, et al., "Case Mix and Surrogate Indicators of Quality of Care Over Time in Freestanding and Hospital-Based Nursing Homes in Colorado," *Public Health Reports* 98, No. 5 (1983):486-492.

70. R. J. Buchanan, "Medicaid Cost Containment: Prospective Reimbursement for Long-Term Care," *Inquiry* 20, (Winter, 1983):334-342.

71. R. J. Buchanan, "Paying for Long-Term Care: The Prospective Versus Retrospective Debate," *The Journal of Long-Term Care Administration* 9, No. 4 (Winter, 1981):43-57.

72. S. Katz, A. Ford, et al., "Studies of Illness in the Aged—The Index of ADL: A Standardized Measure of Biological and Psycholosocial Function," *Journal of the American Medical Association* 185, No. 12 (September 21, 1963):914-919.

73. S. Katz, C. Hendrick, and N. S. Henderson, "The Measurement of Long-Term Care Needs and Impact," *Health and Medical Care Services Review* 2, No. 1 (Spring, 1979).

74. K. S. Bay, P. Lealitt, and S. M. Stimson, "A Patient- Classification System: For Long-Term Care," *Medical Care* 20, No. 5 (1982):468-488.

75. M. Lawton, M. Ward, and S. Yaffe, "Indices of Health in an Aging Population," *Gerontology* 22, No. 3 (1967):334-342.

76. Shaughnessy, et al., *Long-Term Care Reimbursement*.

77. J. M. Cameron and C. A. Knauf, "Case-Mix and Resource Use in Long-Term Care," *Medical Care* 23, No. 4 (1985):296-309.

78. K. McCaffree, J. Baker, and B. Perrin, *Long-Term Care Case-Mix, Employee Time and Costs*. Final Report, Seattle, WA, Battelle Human Affairs Research Centers, February 28, 1979.

79. M. R. Meiners, G. D. Heinemann, and B. J. Jones, *The National Center for Reimbursement Study: A Progress Report*, National Center for Health Services Research. Prepared for the Annual Meeting of the American Public Health Association, November 14-18, 1982, Montreal, Canada.

80. Katz, et al., "Studies of Illness."

81. Katz, et al., "Measurement of Long-Term Care Needs."

82. D. E. Skinner and D. E. Yett, "Debility Index for Long-Term Care Patients," In R. L. Berg, ed., *Health Status Indexes*, Hospital Research and Educational Trust, Chicago, 1973.

83. B. E. Fries and L. M. Cooney, Jr., "Resource Utilization Groups. A Patient Classification System for Long-Term Care," *Medical Care* 23, No. 2 (1985):110-122.

84. A. Lawlor, "New York to Test RUGs Case-Mix Plan, Basing Reimbursement Upon Patient Needs," *Todays Nursing Home* 5, No. 7 (1984):1, 18, 20.

85. L. M. Cooney, Jr., and B. E. Fries, "Validation and Use of Resource Utilization Groups as a Case-Mix Measure for Long-Term Care," *Medical Care* 23, No. 2 (1985):123-132.

86. McCaffree, et al., "Long-Term Care Case-Mix."

87. K. McCaffree, et al., *Long-Term Care Case-Mix Compared to Direct Care Time and Costs, Final Report*, Contract #HRA-230-76-0285, Battelle Human Affairs Research Centers. February, 1979.

88. C. Flagle, et al., *Health Services in Long-Term Care*, The Johns Hopkins University and the Hospital Association of New York State

Report of USPHS Grant 5—R18-HS01250, November, 1977.

89. C. Swearingen, R. Schwartz, and J. Fisher, *A Methodology for Funding, Classifying and Comparing Costs for Services in Long-Term Care Settings*. Abt Associates, Inc. Cambridge, MA, January 15, 1978.

90. Skinner and Yett, "Debility Index."

91. R. Parker and J. Boyd, "A Comparison of Discriminate Versus a Clustering Analysis of a Patient Classification for Chronic Disease Care," *Medical Care* 12, No. 11 (1974):944-957.

92. Peat Marwick Mitchell, *Long-Term Care Practice, RUGs: A Comprehensive Review and Analysis of Resource Utilization Groups*, New York: undated report.

93. Lawlor, "New York to Test RUGs."

94. Peat Marwick Mitchell, "Long-Term Care Practice."

95. E. Kay, *New York State Case-Mix Prospective Reimbursement Project for Long-Term Care*, Communication from Southern New York Residential Health Care Facilities Association, Inc. to member facilities, August 24, 1983.

96. Personal communication, Maureen Dugan, April 8, 1986.

97. M. Stassen and C. Bishop, *Incorporating Case Mix in Prospective Reimbursement for Skilled Nursing Facility Care Under Medicare: Critical Review of Relevant Research, Background Report to HCFA (Report #1)*, Center for Health Policy Analysis and Research, Brandeis University, Waltham, MA, February, 1983 (Revised March, 1983), p. 64.

98. M. R. Meiners and R. M. Coffey, "Hospital DRGs and the Need for Long Term Care Services: An Empirical Analysis," *Health Services Research* 20, No. 3 (1985):359-384.

99. R. L. Kane, R. Bell, S. Riegler, A. Wilson, and E. Keeler, *Predicting the Outcomes of Nursing Home Patients*, The Rand Corporation, Presented at the Annual Meeting of the American Public Health Association, Montreal, Canada, November 7, 1972.

100. Stassen and Bishop, "Incorporating Case Mix."

101. T. Jemison, "U.S. Medicine Interviews Carleton C. Evans," *U.S. Medicine* 20, No. 8 (April 15, 1984):2, 21.

102. Veterans Administration, *Long-Term Care Project*. Internal Memorandum, May 30, 1984.

103. Cameron and Knauf, "Case-Mix and Resource Use."

104. Fries and Cooney, "Resource Utilization Groups."

105. Cooney and Fries, "Validation and Use."

106. Veterans Administration, *Long-Term Care Project*.

107. F. M. Holden, *Update on Resource Allocation System, Ambulatory Care Allocation Model*. Boston Development Center. Veterans Administration, Boston, MA, Draft, September 27, 1984.

108. *Three Models Used for Resource Allocation in the Veterans Administration Office of the Regional Director*, Veterans Administration, Albany, NY, May 17, 1985.

109. *The Year in Brief, The VA in 1983*. Veterans Administration. Washington, DC, February, 1984, p. 19.

110. *Medical Advances: The VA's Contribution to Health Care*. Regional Learning Resources Service. Veterans Administration, St. Louis, MO, undated.

111. A. Lawlor, "VA Hospital Beds Slated for Conversion to LTC," *Today's Nursing Home* 6, No. 3 (1985).

112. M. R. Codel, "The 1985 Legislative Outlook for Nursing Homes," *Nursing Homes* 34, No. 2 (1985):28-31.

113. "Hospitals Eye Rehabilitation Services," *Hospitals* 58, No. 12 (June 16, 1984):60, 62.

114. P. L. Grimaldi, "Final Prospective Payment Rules Contain Important Revisions," *Hospital Progress* 65, No. 3 (1984):42-43, 60.

115. Ibid., p. 60.

116. Ibid., p. 60.

117. J. M. Yasko and A. Fleck, "Prospective Payment (DRGs): What Will be the Impact on Cancer Care?" *Oncology Nursing Forum* 11, No. 3 (1984):63-72.

118. Ibid., p. 64.

119. "Exempted Hospitals Want Proposals Heard," *Modern Healthcare* 14, No. 4 (1984):41.

120. "Home Health Agency Medicare Activity Grows," *Hospitals* 59, No. 1 (January 1, 1985):25.

121. T. Turner, "Effects of DRGs on Staffing in Skilled Nursing Facilities," *The Kansas Nurse* 59, No. 11 (1984):5.

122. L. Libow, M. M. Waife, and R. W. Butler, "Threat to the Development of the Teaching Nursing Home," *Journal of the American Medical Association* 253, No. 8 (February 22, 1985):1166.

123. "Teaching Nursing Homes Will Become Major Medical Centers, Predicts Physician," *The Long-Term Care Administrator* 18, No. 18 (1984):1.

124. U.S. House of Representatives, *Building a Long-Term Care Policy: Home Care Data and Implications*, A Report by the Chairman of the Subcommittee on Health and Long-Term Care of the Select Committee on Aging, House of Representatives, Ninety-Eighth Congress, Second Session, December, 1984.

125. Ibid., p. 8.

126. P. W. Brickner, "Symposium: The Potential Impact of Diagnosis Related Groups on Long-Term Care," *PRIDE Institute Journal of Long-Term Home Health Care* 2, No. 4 (Fall, 1983):3-9.

127. American Health Care Association. "Policy Perspective," *American Health Care Association Journal* 10, No. 3 (1984):47-54.

128. Government Accounting Office, *Medicaid and Nursing Home Care: Cost Increases and the Need for Services are Creating Problems for the States and for the Elderly*. October 21, 1983, p. 101.

129. R. A. Kane and R. L. Kane, "The Feasibility of Universal Long-Term Care Benefits," *New England Journal of Medicine* 312, No. 12 (May 23, 1985):1357-1364.

130. Ibid., p. 1362.

131. Ibid., p. 1364.

132. R. Kelman, "Social Responsibility for Long-Term Care," *Aging and Society* 3, No. 1 (1983).

133. Ibid.

More than a billion physician encounters took place in outpatient settings in 1980 in the United States. Approximately 55 billion dollars was expended for ambulatory care.[1] Between 1970 and 1980, hospital outpatient costs alone rose from $1.7 billion to $9.9 billion. During that same time period, Medicare and Medicaid combined to distribute ambulatory care reimbursements that went from $282 million to $3 billion—an eleven-fold increase.[2]

At this time, DRGs do not apply to outpatient ambulatory care. DRGs currently only apply to reimbursement for patients covered by Medicare for inpatient hospital treatment. However, it is reasonable to expect the federal government and other jurisdictions to examine what additional health care services they are funding that could apply to a DRG system. Obviously the next logical progression would extend the DRG program to ambulatory care, which is covered under the Medicare program. Next, there could be a move to inpatient and ambulatory care coverage under the Medicaid program. There could also be a swing by the third-party payers to adopt the governmental system and make the coverage an all-payer system, as in some of the states with experimental waiver programs. In essence, a reimbursement system could emerge that would include all types of medical and health care services.

Shifting to Ambulatory Care

In addition, hospital administrators have considered—and some are initiating—a shift in their focus of service from inpatient services to ambulatory care services, where appropriate, to circumvent the limitations of the restrictive DRG allowance. This "gaming" has also resulted in the government's efforts to move to include ambulatory care within a DRG-like reimbursement system. A top federal government HCFA administrator envisioned increases in outpatient surgery, home health care, satellite diagnostic centers, and freestanding clinics stimulated by the demands of the DRG payments.[3] This idea was also stressed by another official who noted that hospital rate-setting may cause hospitals to provide ancillary services formerly situated in the hospital on an outpatient basis. Rubin, an HHS official, also inquired as to the net saving of that movement to ambulatory care and indicated that the result is not yet clear as to cost savings.[4]

In a June 22, 1984 issue of *American Medical News*, an article was headlined, "DRGs Seen Boosting Outpatient Care, Competition." In the article, Dr. Robert Berenson forecast that DRGs would cause a "large shift to outpatient care." He also said: "There will be some physicians who just find that they can't practice in the hospital anymore."[5] Moving from predictions to actual experience, Donald Welch, president of Adventist Health System/U.S., copes with prospective payment by increasing outpatient services not covered by the DRG system. He said: "One of the biggest things we're doing is accelerating outpatient surgery. We're doing a lot of [procedures on an outpatient basis] that we weren't doing two years ago. . . . [One Adventist hospital performs] literally hundreds of outpatient cardiac catheterizations, which we wouldn't have even thought about doing before."[6]

Double Dipping

In the shifting of services to outpatient ambulatory care, "double dipping" emerged as a tactic. Double dipping occurs when a hospital performs diagnostic tests in its own outpatient department or at an affiliated freestanding facility before the patient is admitted to the hospital. These tests can then be billed under Medicare Part B, which does not fall within the prospective payment plan. According to a hospital management expert, the double dipping strategy has "the best chance of working in a joint venture between a hospital and a physicians' group, in which the physicians run the freestanding ambulatory facility."[7] To avoid charges of "gaming," preadmission tests must be done at least 48 hours before admission.

A potential drawback of this strategy is that the IRS may look askance at the cooperative arrangements between nonprofit hospitals and proprietary freestanding diagnostic centers. Another caveat is to make sure that the testing facility will serve a large enough volume of Medicare patients to make the new operation efficient.

Shifting patients into the ambulatory care network for double dipping may also create a Catch-22 situation. Preadmission testing will unbundle those services and the overall cost for the patient's stay in the hospital will be lowered. When the federal government does its periodic adjustment of DRG rates, the allowances may be lowered to reflect the less expensive hospital costs.

Outpatient Surgery

Surgery performed on an outpatient basis will increase under the DRG system. A Day-Stay-Center at Monmouth Medical Center in Long Beach, New Jersey predicted that they would have 150 more cases per year under the DRG program.[8] That forecast came after 18 months of operation under the DRG system in New Jersey.

At a national conference entitled "Same-Day Surgery—1983," Daniel J. Sullivan, a medical consultant, advised the audience: "The current Medicare prospective system will only be applied to inpatient stays, not to outpatient services. You will still have 100 percent cost reimbursement for outpatient services; so to the extent that you can move your costs out of the inpatient to the outpatient, you can get more money back from the government."[9]

Mobile Intensive Care Unit (MICU)

In a slightly different twist, the mobile intensive care units aligned themselves within the DRG system by associating MICU costs in the indirect patient care category. In New Jersey, the Rate Setting Commission budgeted the MICU operational expenditures as part of the "pass-through" costs wherein funds are usually adequate to reimburse for actual services. This funding approach had an immediate impact on MICU units. MICUs increased from 24 in 1979 to 61 in 1982. More than 85 percent of the state's population was served by MICUs in 1982. In 1981, MICU reimbursement rates ranged from $250,000 to $300,000 per operational unit. In New Jersey, at least, advanced life support services appear to be considered an inherent part of the inpatient hospital setting.[10]

Effects of Shifting

Movement of inpatients into the outpatient flow seems to be a logical progression and is now advocated by management experts. Two effects of this shift have been noted:

1. Hospitals will get a higher reimbursement for the outpatient services they provide.

2. Hospitals will manage to keep inpatient costs below the prospective rates allowed for Medicare.[11]

Obviously, this tactic of shifting services to outpatient ambulatory care will be short-lived. Already, legislators are submitting bills to pay physicians for office-based care on a DRG-like basis. As an example, Representative Edward R. Roybal introduced the Medicare Fair Payment Act of 1984 to force physicians to accept fees set by the government as payment in full.[12]

With the tremendous volume of ambulatory care reimbursed under existing federal, state, and local government programs, cost containment must be considered all along the line. It would not be logical to assume that Medicare inpatient hospital costs will be contained without resultant efforts in the area of ambulatory care.

In an August 26, 1983 interview with Larry A. O'Day, director, Bureau of Eligibility, Reimbursement and Coverage for HCFA, he was asked about the effect of prospective payment upon outpatient utilization. O'Day responded that the system created incentives to stimulate more outpatient services such as preadmission diagnostic testing and ambulatory surgery centers. However, the next question specially dealt with reimbursement.

Q: Do you anticipate a shift in outpatient reimbursement from a reasonable cost basis to prospective payment?

A: Yes, I think there will eventually be some sort of prospective payment system for outpatients. While this is interestingly not one of the things Congress told us to study, it is, nevertheless, our highest internal priority item to study. It is certainly one of the things that we are looking at very closely. The biggest problem is finding the appropriate unit of payment.[13]

Following through on this federal government stance, several investigators have already received grant support to examine various methods of discovering the appropriate unit of payment.

Patient Classification Efforts

Most of the existing patient classifications were not designed with resource use as a fundamental concept. Therefore, the measurement of productivity is lacking and causes a wide gap in adaptation to a prospective reimbursement system.

Nevertheless, it is appropriate to cite the following examples of classifications that are relevant to a consideration of an ambulatory reimbursement plan:

- International Classification of Diseases, Ninth Edition, Clinical Modification (ICD-9-CM)[14]

- International Classification of Health Problems for Primary Care (ICHPPC)[15]

- Royal College of General Practitioners Classification of Diseases—Eighth Revision[16]

- Kaiser Clinical—Behavioral Classification System[17]

- Johns Hopkins Ambulatory Care Coding Scheme (JHACS)[18]

- NAPCRG Process Classification for Primary Care[19]

- Diagnostic Clusters[20]

- Reason for Visit Classification for Ambulatory Care[21]

- Resource Use by Episode of Care[22]

- Intensity of Care[23]

- Utilization by Frequency of Services Used[24]

Ambulatory Care Case Mix

Cost-containment efforts in the ambulatory care area assume that the provision of ambulatory care is less expensive than inpatient hospital care. If the patient is able to physically receive ambulatory care without potential harm, there would not be too much opposition to that assumption. However, the different sites where ambulatory care is rendered and the relative cost at each site make the optimal care choice more questionable for patients. Discussions about the relative merits of hospital outpatient services, neighborhood health centers, freestanding emergency services, and the private office could become heated. One recent study of three hospital clinics and three neighborhood health centers revealed that the weighted total average cost per visit in the hospital clinics was 10 dollars greater—$64.50 to $54.14. However, the range for the hospitals was $51.51 to $71.68, while the neighborhood health centers ranged from $41.46 to $86.40. One neighborhood center had a higher cost per visit than any of the three hospitals. Investigators concluded: "The results give a strong indication that the demonstration project hospital-based clinics are not more costly than the freestanding demonstration-project clinics."[25] Variables affecting their conclusion included differences in the product mix, differences in capital expenses, differences in medical case mix, differences in the comprehensiveness, and variations in the emphasis on community outreach services.

Administrators of hospital outpatient clinics claim that the patients seen in their hospital are sicker and have more social problems than people seen in private offices. Public hospitals claim that their patients are sicker and need more services than people seen at outpatient departments of the private hospitals. Both public and private nonprofit voluntary hospitals say that their patients are sicker than those individuals seen at proprietary hospitals. Apparently, hospital administrators base their reactions upon actual experience at their institutions.

Therefore, the discovery of an appropriate unit of reimbursement for ambulatory care is a complex undertaking.

Similarity of Patient Populations

Comparisons among the possible locations for the delivery of ambulatory care have considered the elements of complexity, severity, and urgency regarding the medical aspects. Social problems have been divided into major, moderate, and minor classifications. Specific disease states, such as hypertension and urinary tract infections, have been compared as to their treatment activities. Of course, the demographic background of the patient is an overlay on all the comparisons.

Lion compared patients seen by internists in private practice and patients seen by internists and residents in internal medicine working in the hospital outpatient department. She found: "Contrary to the explanation that case-mix differences are one of the reasons for the generally accepted higher cost of a visit to a hospital OPD compared with a physician in private practice, *no case-mix difference was found when a variety of measures was analyzed*" [author's emphasis].[26] Furthermore, the investigator commented that the higher costs must be explained by "hospital overhead allocation, additional hospital staff, and research and educational costs."[27]

Using data collected by Mendenhall at USC,[28,29] Lion and Altman compared case-mix differences between hospital practitioners and private physicians in general practice, family practice, internal medicine, and pediatrics—a total of 2,019 physicians and 84,598 patients. They concluded: "We find relatively minor case mix differences, with the OPD patients from 5 to 15 percent sicker than their counterparts in private practice."[30]

In addition, the researchers said that the overall difference is not very large and could not justify the much higher costs in hospital OPDs.

Another investigation examined the premise that outpatient departments affiliated with teaching hospitals see people who are medically sicker and who have more social problems. Hospital residents and staff were compared with private practitioners specializing in internal medicine, pediatrics, family practice, and general practice. Ten leading diagnoses were compared at various teaching hospitals. Social problems were classified into minor, moderate, or major. Minor social problems included anxiety, obesity, minor psychological, and medical noncompliance. Moderate problems included family problems, financial problems, housing problems, and living/situational problems. Major problems included alcoholism, drug abuse, retardation, physical disability, and major psychiatric problems.

In relation to the leading diagnoses, the investigators concluded that the "patients of urban hospital primary care units do not look too different from the private practice patients." Social problems only evoked an additional two minutes or about 8 percent additional physician time.

Even when the medical and social case-mix differences are combined, there was a sum of less than a 15 percent differential in physician time in OPDs.

Lion and Williams' conclusion follows:

> In short, it appears that hospitals must base their case for differential reimbursement primarily on other issues, such as providing access to the indigent, higher capital requirements, higher teaching and personnel costs, or other factors. Roughly, a fifth of the cost differential—no small amount, but far less than had been previously supposed—is found to be due to either medical or social case mix using the most optimistic assumptions. Therefore, although further study is needed, it is apparent that case mix is not the major reason for the differences in costs among settings.[31]

While the studies cited above tend to indicate that the ambulatory patient is similar, regardless of the setting, there are critics who will argue otherwise. Investigators cited have received government funding to engage in case mix research and that would be the rationale for the emphasis on their specific work.

Based on the premise that the populations in ambulatory care settings are reasonably similar—as shown in the investigations—the next step is to proceed toward defining appropriate units for reimbursement. Several concepts will be explored, including diagnosis clusters, episode of illness and ambulatory visit groups (AVGs), and ambulatory patient related groups (APGs).

Diagnosis Clusters

Using data from the 1977 and 1978 National Ambulatory Medical Care Survey (NAMCS), Schneeweiss et al. developed diagnosis clusters for the 96,332 diagnoses recorded by office-based physicians in all specialties. Criteria used to sort out the clusters included the following:

1. Groups that are clinically homogeneous should be identified.

2. Clusters should include the great majority of discrete diagnoses but also be precise enough to still be clinically meaningful.

3. Clinically related conditions should be grouped to decrease the effect of idiosyncratic labeling by individual practitioners.

4. Related diagnoses with high aggregate frequency but low individual frequency should be included in the clusters.

5. Clusters should be applicable to any ambulatory setting.

6. Clusters should be independent of physician specialty.[32]

Applying the guidelines to the data, 92 diagnosis clusters were constructed by a consensus of a group of clinicians including generalists and specialists. Eighty-one percent of all the ambulatory visits to office-based physicians were explained through the use of 60 of the diagnosis clusters. Using only 15 clusters, 50 percent of the ambulatory visits can be classified. Eighty-six percent of all the recorded diagnoses were covered by the 92 clusters. Listed below are the top five, middle five, and last five of the 60, and bottom five diagnosis clusters:

1. General medical examination

2. Acute upper respiratory infection

3. Pre- and postnatal care—including complicated pregnancy abortion

4. Hypertension

5. Nonpsychotic depression/anxiety/neuroses

*   *   *

44. Peripheral neuropathy/neuritis

45. Personality disorders—all

46. Viral exanthemas

47. Vertiginous syndromes

48. Glaucoma

*   *   *

56. Cholecystitis/cholelithiasis

57. Wax in ear

58. External abdominal hernias

59. Chronic cystic disease of breast

60. Malignant neoplasm of skin

*   *   *

88. Hypertrophy of tonsils or adenoids

89. Debility and undue fatigue

90. Helminthiasis, scabies, pediculosis

91. Alcoholism

92. Diseases of the nail (except infections)[33]

This methodology brings together the existing coding schemes and allows the physician to describe the same patient with identical terms. Researchers grouped together the International Classification of Diseases (ICDA-9 and ICD-9-CM) and the International Classifications of Health Problems in Primary Care (ICHPPC and ICHPPC-2) to arrive at the 92 diagnosis clusters; the investigators believe "it is possible to collapse almost any existing data into the diagnostic clusters presented here."[34]

As a tool for analyzing the content of ambulatory care, the diagnosis cluster method could also be used for prospective reimbursement for ambulatory care.

Episode of Illness

Another mechanism used in seeking the appropriate method of reimbursement for medical care is episode of illness. Within this context, all medical care inputs used to produce the output in the form of treatment can be thought of as "bundles of care," including office procedures, hospital admissions, laboratory, radiology, and drug orders for each episode.[35]

Therefore, an individual with hypertension or an upper respiratory infection would be treated over a period of time and the costs would be calculated on the episode of illness, with all services and resources included for that treatment.

There are a number of problems with this approach. While the beginning and end of an acute care episode may be relatively easy to determine, chronic care such as hypertension or diabetes may be much more troublesome. Exactly where does the continued care for long-term conditions end? What happens when the chronic patient also has an acute illness? Since Medicare patients will be older, it is quite conceivable that those individuals will be suffering from chronic problems as well as intermittent acute illnesses.

Another issue would relate to patients who will also have secondary diagnoses. In those cases, the individuals "will have care for the same condition rendered under alternate diagnoses intermixed with progress checks and check-ups."[36] Added on to that potential mix-up is the possibility that the laboratory tests will be processed independently of the ambulatory visit when the test was ordered.

A diagnosis may not, and probably is not, attached to the laboratory or other test report.

Even with the suggestion that a ceiling or maximum be placed upon the amount reimbursable for an episode of illness, there are difficulties. It may be possible to establish a number of allowable visits and diagnostic tests within a given period of time for specific conditions. However, this is a difficult task to achieve without actually evaluating a particular patient. Furthermore, the maximum tends to become a beckoning siren that draws the use of resources and services upward to meet that top reimbursement allowance. That procedure would replicate what has already occurred in the prior Medicare program under the reasonable and customary charges concept for inpatient care.

Johnson et al. reviewed a number of studies that investigated the use of an episode of care methodology. They concluded that "each approach has contributed useful information although hampered by both data limitations and conceptual difficulties."[37] In their study of an episode approach to the care and costs of obesity, Johnson et al. claimed that many limitations were overcome. Using their methodology, the researchers claimed to be able to do the following tasks:

- Identify all the different services and procedures provided through time.

- Assign the specific services and procedures rendered at a visit to a given diagnosis at that visit.

- Link contacts for care to any illness, including chronic diseases, into coherent episodes of care, even with concurrent illnesses.

- Adjust or examine results in light of coexisting illnesses with any diagnoses of interest.

- Generate and standardize costs of the services and procedures rendered during episodes.[38]

Medical care services and procedure variables included the number of doctor office visits, the number of laboratory procedures, the number of telephone or letter contacts for care, the number of radiology procedures, the number of hospital admissions, and the number of drug orders. Patient, provider, and medical care process characteristics included sex, age, physician specialty, associated morbidities, initial date of care, medical exam without illness, endocrine disease, psychologically-manifested diseases, bone and organs of movement disease, sprains and strains, hypertensive heart disease, arterial or venous-related heart disease, gastrointestinal disease, and first contact for obesity.

Using confirmed diagnoses of obesity, record data from a sample of patients at the Kaiser-Permanente Medical Care Program from September 1966 through

December 1973 were analyzed. Automatic interaction detection (AID) was used to identify the bundles of care. In their conclusion, the researchers confirmed the difficulty of utilizing an episode of illness approach with obesity as a prototype for a chronic condition: "Episodes of obesity are commonly recognized in the medical record, but few medical services are provided to address the problem, even when it is repeatedly noted and even though it is a recognized contributor to or a complicating factor for a variety of medical conditions."[39] The most striking finding was the large share of episodes, of both short and long duration, that received little or no medical care.[40]

Other researchers engaged in developing a prospective payment system for outpatient care also concluded that the episode of illness scheme was not satisfactory. They concluded: "This leaves the visit-specific basis for reimbursement as the most logical prospective payment system available for most types of ambulatory care, at least in the short term."[41]

Ambulatory Patient Related Groups (APGs) and Ambulatory Visit Groups (AVGs)

Although both APGs and AVGs have been used to label methods of reimbursement for ambulatory care, they are one and the same.[42,43] Formerly, the same Yale University investigators that developed the DRGs referred to their ambulatory system as APGs in one of their manuals. However, at a later date the AVG label was used. Currently, AVG appears to be the preferred terminology. Obviously, since the same researchers are working on AVGs as those who developed DRGs, there are bound to be similarities.

Basically, AVG development calls for patients to be classified "into groups that require similar patterns of services and consume similar quantities of resources."[44] Three basic tasks had to be accomplished to achieve that goal:

1. Identification of service and resource usage measures

2. Identification of potential classifiers

3. Development of a classification scheme.

Under the AVG scheme, as with the DRG, the measurement is concerned with resource consumption patterns. AVGs serve as cost objectives and depend on factors such as the attending physician's specialty and the age of the patient. According to Knapp, the development of a standard cost system that bears up under experience will be the true test of the proposed AVG system.[45] Limitations to the standard cost system that need resolution relate to the allocation of charges for ancillary services, to allocation of routine nursing services, and to direct and indirect costs. Again, these limitations are similar to those considered under the DRG program.

Using the data from the National Ambulatory Medical Care Survey, the Yale University investigators came up with 14 Major Ambulatory Categories (MACs) that are organ-based. Evolving out from the 14 MACs are 154 Ambulatory Visit Groups (AVGs) that are mostly based upon the primary diagnosis and related to the ICD-9-CM DRG system. Variables used in the grouping process include presenting problem, reason for visit, primary diagnosis, presence or absence of a secondary diagnosis, initial visit, follow-up visit, and patient age. Variance in physician time was the criterion used for clustering. (See Exhibit 9-1 for the list of 14 MACs and the 154 AVGs).

Exhibit 9-1   List of Major Ambulatory Categories (MACs)*

MACs	Initial Group Name	AVG
1	Infective and Parasitic Disorders	1–12
2	Endocrine, Nutritional and Metabolic Disorders	13–24
3	Mental Disorders	25–36
4	Disorders of the Nervous System	37–39
5	Disorders of the Circulatory System	40–59
6	Disorders of the Respiratory System	60–70
7	Disorders of the Digestive System	71–84
8	Disorders of the Genitourinary System	85–94
9	Disorders of the Skin and Subcutaneous Tissue	95–102
10	Disorders of the Musculoskeletal System and Connective Tissue	105–109
11	Accidents, Poisonings, and Violence	110–122
12	Disorders of the Eye	123–132
13	Disorders of the Ear	133–143
14	Other	
	Special Conditions and Exam without Sickness	144–154
	Disorders of the Blood and Blood-Forming Organs	
	Complications of Pregnancy, Childbirth, and Puerperium	
	Congenital Anomalies	
	Certain Causes of Perinatal Morbidity and Mortality Symptoms	
	Miscellaneous	

*These MACs and AVGs are being modified and the final total number in each grouping will probably be different from those in Exhibit 7-1. Nevertheless, this exhibit still is worth examining to gain an understanding of the clustering process.

Exhibit 9-1   (contd.)

List of 154 Ambulatory Visit Groups (AVGs)*

AVG	Description
1	Infective, new patient with a venereal disease.
2	Infective, new patient with a skin infection.
3	Infective, new patient without venereal disease or skin infection and without a secondary diagnosis.
4	Infective, new patient without venereal disease or skin infection and with a secondary diagnosis.
5	Infective, revisit for an old problem, without a visit for an acute problem follow-up or post operative care.
6	Infective, revisit for an old problem, with a visit for an acute problem follow-up or post operative care.
7	Infective, revisit for an old problem, with a visit for an acute problem follow-up or post operative care, and with a secondary diagnosis.
8	Infective, revisit for a new problem, age 0–12 years, with a childhood disease.
9	Infective, revisit for a new problem age 0–12 years, with other infective disorders.
10	Infective, revisit for a new problem, age 13–49 years.
11	Infective, revisit for a new problem, age 50–99 years, without a secondary diagnosis.
12	Infective, revisit for a new problem, age 50–99 years with a secondary diagnosis.
13	Endocrine or Metabolic, new patient who was not referred, without a periodic examination, with obesity.
14	Endocrine or Metabolic, new patient who was not referred, without a periodic examination, without obesity.
15	Endocrine or Metabolic, new patient who was referred or is having a periodic examination, without a secondary diagnosis.
16	Endocrine or Metabolic, new patient who was referred or is having a periodic examination, with a secondary diagnosis.
17	Endocrine or Metabolic, revisit for an old problem, without a periodic examination, with a presenting problem of weight gain, that has not been followed as a routine chronic problem.
18	Endocrine or Metabolic, revisit for an old problem, without a periodic examination, with a presenting problem of weight gain, that has been followed as a chronic problem.
19	Endocrine or Metabolic, revisit for an old problem, without a periodic examination, with a presenting problem other than weight gain, without a secondary diagnosis.
20	Endocrine or Metabolic, revisit for an old problem, without a periodic examination, with a presenting problem other than weight gain, with a secondary diagnosis.
21	Endocrine or Metabolic, revisit for an old problem, receiving a periodic examination.

Exhibit 9-1   (contd.)

22 Endocrine or Metabolic, revisit for a new problem, without a periodic examination, without diabetes.

23 Endocrine or Metabolic, revisit for a new problem, without a periodic examination, with diabetes.

24 Endocrine or Metabolic, revisit for a new problem, receiving a periodic examination.

25 Mental, new patient, who was not referred, with a presenting problem or restlessness, loneliness, nervousness or general symptoms.

26 Mental, new patient, who was not referred, with a presenting problem of anxiety, depression, obsession, or drug abuse.

27 Mental, new patient, who was not referred, with other presenting problems.

28 Mental, new patient, who was referred.

29 Mental, revisit for an old problem, not receiving psychotherapy during this visit with a presenting problem of restlessness, loneliness, nervousness or general symptoms.

30 Mental, revisit, for an old problem, not receiving psychotherapy during this visit with a presenting problem of anxiety, depression, obsessions, or drug abuse.

31 Mental, revisit, for an old problem, not receiving psychotherapy during this visit, with other presenting problems.

32 Mental, revisit for an old problem, receiving psychotherapy during this visit, with a presenting problem of restlessness, loneliness, nervousness, or general symptoms.

33 Mental, revisit for an old problem, not receiving psychotherapy during this visit, with other presenting problems.

34 Mental, revisit for a new problem, not receiving psychotherapy this visit.

35 Mental, revisit for a new problem, receiving psychotherapy during this visit, with a presenting problem of restlessness or loneliness.

36 Mental, revisit for a new problem, receiving psychotherapy during this visit, and with other presenting problems.

37 Nervous system, new patient, who was not referred.

38 Nervous system, new patient, who was referred.

39 Nervous system, revisit with either a new or old problem.

40 Circulatory, new patient, who was not referred, with a presenting problem of shortness of breath, chest pain or heart murmur.

41 Circulatory, new patient, who was not referred, without a presenting problem of shortness of breath, chest pain or heart murmur, with a diagnosis of vascular disease.

42 Circulatory, new patient, who was not referred, without a presenting problem of shortness of breath, chest pain, or heart murmur, and with a diagnosis of hypertension.

43 Circulatory, new patient, who was not referred, without a presenting problem of shortness of breath, chest pain or heart murmur, without a diagnosis of vascular diseases or hypertension.

Exhibit 9-1 (contd.)

44 Circulatory, new patient, who was referred, with a presenting problem of shortness of breath, chest pain, or heart murmur.

45 Circulatory, new patient, who was referred, with other presenting problems.

46 Circulatory, revisit for an old problem, without a periodic examination, who was not referred, without a presenting problem of chest pain or a diagnosis of hypertension, without a secondary diagnosis.

47 Circulatory, revisit for an old problem, without a periodic examination, who was not referred, without a presenting problem of chest pain or a diagnosis of hypertension, with a secondary diagnosis.

40 Circulatory, revisit for an old problem, without a periodic examination, who was not referred, with a presenting problem of chest pain, with a diagnosis of hypertension.

49 Circulatory, revisit for an old problem, without a periodic examination, who was not referred, with a presenting problem of chest pain, without a secondary diagnosis.

50 Circulatory, revisit for an old problem, without a periodic examination, who was not referred, with a presenting problem of chest pain, with a secondary diagnosis.

51 Circulatory, revisit for an old problem, without a periodic examination, who was referred.

52 Circulatory, revisit for an old problem, receiving a periodic examination.

53 Circulatory, revisit for a new problem, without a periodic examination, who was not referred, without a presenting problem of chest pain or a diagnosis of hypertension, without a secondary diagnosis.

54 Circulatory, revisit for a new problem, without a periodic examination, who was not referred, without a presenting problem of chest pain or a diagnosis of hypertension, with a secondary diagnosis.

55 Circulatory, revisit for a new problem, without a periodic examination, who was not referred, without a presenting problem of chest pain, with a diagnosis of hypertension.

56 Circulatory, revisit for a new problem, without a periodic examination, who was not referred, with a presenting problem of chest pain, without a secondary diagnosis.

57 Circulatory, revisit for a new problem, without a periodic examination, who was not referred, with a presenting problem of chest pain, with a secondary diagnosis.

58 Circulatory, revisit for a new problem, without a periodic examination, and who was referred.

59 Circulatory, revisit for a new problem, receiving a periodic examination.

60 Respiratory, new patient, who was not referred, with a visit not specified as acute, with a presenting problem of upper respiratory symptoms or infection, or for medication.

61 Respiratory, new patient, who was not referred, with a visit not specified as acute, with other presenting problems.

62 Respiratory, new patient, who was not referred, with an acute problem, with a presenting problem of upper respiratory symptoms or infection, or for medication.

Exhibit 9-1   (contd.)

63 Respiratory, new patient who was not referred, with an acute problem, with other presenting problems.

64 Respiratory, new patient who was referred.

65 Respiratory, revisit, without a periodic examination, for medication.

66 Respiratory, revisit without a periodic examination, with a presenting problem of upper respiratory symptoms or infection, including hay fever age 0–49 years.

67 Respiratory, revisit, without a periodic examination, with a presenting problem of upper respiratory symptoms or infection, including hay fever age 50–99 years.

68 Respiratory, revisit without a periodic examination, with other presenting problems, age 0–49 years.

69 Respiratory, revisit, without a periodic examination, with other presenting problems, age 50–99 years.

70 Respiratory, revisit receiving periodic examination.

71 Digestive, new patient, with a visit not specified as acute, without a secondary diagnosis.

72 Digestive, new patient, with a visit not specified as acute, with a secondary diagnosis.

73 Digestive, new patient, with an acute problem, age 0–12 years.

74 Digestive, new patient, with an acute problem, age 13–49 years.

75 Digestive, new patient, with an acute problem, age 49–99 years.

76 Digestive, revisit for an old problem, not specified as post-operative care, or acute problem follow-up.

77 Digestive, revisit for an old problem, not specified as post-operative care, requiring acute problem follow-up.

78 Digestive, revisit for an old problem, requiring post-operative care.

79 Digestive, revisit for a new problem, not specified as acute, age 0–12 years.

80 Digestive, revisit for a new problem, not specified as acute, age 13–49 years.

81 Digestive, revisit for a new problem, not specified as acute, age 50–99 years.

82 Digestive, revisit for a new problem, specified as acute problem, age 0–12 years.

83 Digestive, revisit for a new problem, specified as acute problem, age 13–49 years.

84 Digestive, revisit for a new problem, specified as acute problem, age 50–99 years.

85 Genitourinary, new patient, age 0–39 years, without a secondary diagnosis.

86 Genitourinary, new patient, age 0–39 years, with a secondary diagnosis.

87 Genitourinary, new patient, age 40–99 years, with a presenting problem of breast or gynecologic disorder.

88 Genitourinary, new patient, age 40–99 years, with other presenting problems.

89 Genitourinary, revisit for an old problem, without a periodic examination, who was not referred.

Exhibit 9-1 (contd.)

90 Genitourinary, revisit for an old problem, without a periodic examination, who was referred.

91 Genitourinary, revisit for an old problem, receiving a periodic examination.

92 Genitourinary, revisit for a new problem, with a kidney infection or cystitis.

93 Genitourinary, revisit for a new problem, without a kidney infection or cystitis, age 0–39 years.

94 Genitourinary, revisit for a new problem, without a kidney infection or cystitis, age 40–99 years.

95 Skin, new patient, without a periodic examination, with impetigo, eczema, warts or acne.

96 Skin, new patient, without a periodic examination, without impetigo, eczema, warts or acne, and with urticaria.

97 Skin, new patient, without a periodic examination, with other disorders.

98 Skin, new patient receiving a periodic examination.

99 Skin, revisit without a periodic examination, with impetigo, eczema, warts or acne, age 0–18 years.

100 Skin, revisit without a periodic examination, with impetigo, eczema, warts or acne, age 19–99 years.

101 Skin, revisit without periodic examination, with other disorders.

102 Skin, revisit receiving a periodic examination.

103 Musculoskeletal, new patient who was not referred, with a presenting problem of upper or lower extremity pain, swelling or injury.

104 Musculoskeletal, new patient who was not referred, with other presenting problems.

105 Musculoskeletal, new patient who was referred.

106 Musculoskeletal, revisit without a periodic examination, who was not referred, with arthritis or related diagnosis.

107 Musculoskeletal, revisit without a periodic examination, who was not referred, with other disorders.

108 Musculoskeletal, revisit without a periodic examination, who was referred.

109 Musculoskeletal, revisit receiving a periodic examination.

110 Accident, poisoning and violence, new patient, neither referred nor receiving periodic examination, with a presenting problem of a wound, eye injury or surgical aftercare.

111 Accident, poisoning and violence, new patient, neither referred nor receiving a periodic examination, with a presenting problem of a face, neck or back injury.

112 Accident, poisoning and violence, new patient, neither referred nor receiving a periodic examination, with other presenting problems with a diagnosis of sprain, laceration, contusion, or eye injury.

Exhibit 9-1   (contd.)

113 Accident, poisoning and violence, new patient, neither referred nor receiving a periodic examination, with other presenting problems, with other diagnosis.

114 Accident, poisoning and violence, new patient who was referred or is receiving a periodic examination, without a secondary diagnosis.

115 Accident, poisoning and violence, new patient who was referred or is receiving a periodic examination, with a secondary diagnosis.

116 Accident, poisoning and violence, revisit for an old problem, with a diagnosis of sprain, laceration, contusion or eye injury with surgical aftercare.

117 Accident, poisoning and violence, revisit for an old problem, with a diagnosis of sprain, laceration, contusion or eye injury without surgical aftercare.

110 Accident, poisoning and violence, revisit for an old problem, with other diagnosis, without an acute problem follow-up.

119 Accident, poisoning and violence, revisit for an old problem, with other diagnosis, with an acute problem follow-up.

120 Accident, poisoning and violence, revisit for a new problem, with a diagnosis of sprain, laceration, contusion or eye injury with surgical aftercare.

121 Accident, poisoning and violence, revisit for a new problem, with a diagnosis of sprain, laceration, contusion, or eye injury without surgical aftercare.

122 Accident, poisoning and violence, revisit for a new problem, with other diagnoses.

123 Eye, new patient with conjunctivitis, lid or corneal disorder.

124 Eye, new patient without conjunctivitis, lid or corneal disorders.

125 Eye, revisit for an old problem, not for post operative care, with conjunctivitis, lid or corneal disorders.

126 Eye, revisit for an old problem, not for post operative care, with refractive error.

127 Eye, revisit for an old problem, not for post operative care, with other eye disorders.

128 Eye, revisit for an old problem, recieving post-operative care.

129 Eye, revisit for a new problem, without a periodic examination, with conjunctivitis, lid or corneal disorder.

130 Eye, revisit for a new problem, without a periodic examination, with refractive error.

131 Eye, revisit for a new problem, without a periodic examination, with other disorders.

132 Eye, revisit for a new problem, receiving a periodic examination.

133 Ear, new patient, who was not referred, with a presenting problem of earache.

134 Ear, new patient, who was not referred, with a presenting problem of hearing impairment.

135 Ear, new patient, who was not referred, with other presenting problems.

136 Ear, new patient who was referred.

137 Ear, revisit for an old problem, with otitis.

Exhibit 9-1 (contd.)

138 Ear, revisit for an old problem, with otosclerosis or other hearing disturbance.

139 Ear, revisit for an old problem, with other disorders.

140 Ear, revisit for a new problem, without a periodic examination, with otitis.

141 Ear, revisit for a new problem, without a periodic examination, with otosclerosis or other hearing disturbance.

142 Ear, revisit for a new problem, without a periodic examination, with other disorders.

143 Ear, revisit for a new problem, receiving a periodic examination.

144 Other, receiving a well baby examination or child care.

145 Other, receiving a vaccination, immunization, prophylactic innoculation or sensitization.

146 Other, receiving surgical aftercare excluding orthopedic, radiation, chemotherapy, dialysis or cardiac device adjustments.

147 Other, receiving a general medical examination, and not presenting for a gynecological examination.

148 Other, receiving a general medical examination, and presenting for a gynecological examination.

149 Other, with a diagnosis of pregnancy, new patient.

150 Other, with a diagnosis of pregnancy, revisit for an old problem.

151 Other, with a diagnosis or pregnancy, revisit for a new problem.

152 Other, other diagnosis, new patient, who was not referred.

153 Other, other diagnosis, new patient, who was referred.

154 Other, other diagnosis revisit.

Source: R. B. Fetter, R. F. Averrill, J. L. Lichtenstein, and J. L. Freeman: *Ambulatory Visit Groups: A Framework for Measuring Productivity in Ambulatory Care* (New Haven, CT: Yale University, undated).

It should be noted that the National Ambulatory Medical Care Survey data is derived from visits to physicians in private practice. This raises the issue of generalization to ambulatory care delivered in hospital outpatient departments or other organized ambulatory care settings. Researchers are currently working on that problem to seek a resolution.

MACs are initially portioned by visit status into new patients and patients previously seen. If the patient has been seen before, the visit is listed as to whether the problem is a new one or linked to an existing condition. Additional portioning takes into account the patient's age, if the problem is acute or chronic, a routine exam, postoperative care, and primary and secondary diagnoses.

Exhibit 9-2 illustrates an AVG branching tree for disorders of the respiratory system. Decisions needed to determine resources and services expended in that

Exhibit 9-2

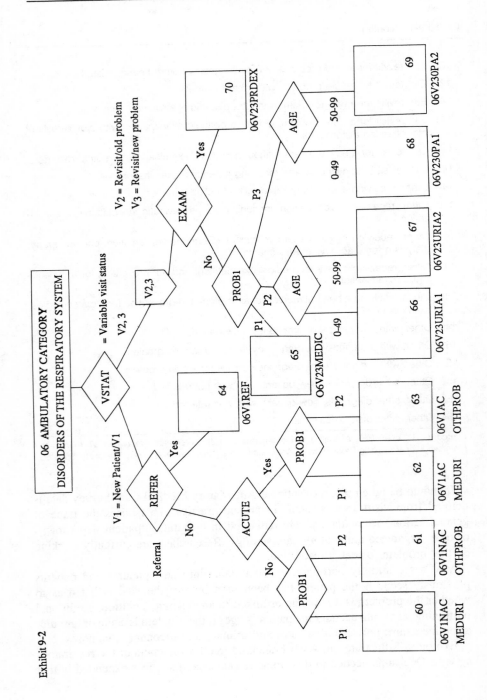

06 AMBULATORY CATEGORY
DISORDERS OF THE RESPIRATORY SYSTEM

= Variable visit status
V1 = New Patient/V1
V2 = Revisit/old problem
V3 = Revisit/new problem

Exhibit 9-2   (contd.)

AVG 60 06V1NACMEDURI

(RESP, NPT, N REF, N ACUTE, MEDICATION, URI, RE-LATED SYMP) Respiratory, new patient, who was not referred, with a visit not specified as acute, with a presenting problem of upper respiratory symptoms or infection, or for medication. *Includes*: For Medication, Nasal congestion, Sinus problem, Sneezing, Cold, Fever, Chills, Cough, Throat soreness, Symptoms referable to tonsils, Earache.

AVG 61 06V1NACOTHPROB

(RESP, NPT, N REF, N ACUTE, OTHER PROB INCLUDING HAY FEVER) Respiratory, new patient, who was not referred, with a visit not specified as acute, with other presenting problems. *Includes*: Shortness of breath, Pain in chest, Disorders of voice, Hay fever, General physical examination, Progress visit, Other presenting problems.

AVG 62 06V1ACMEDURI

(RESP, NPT, N REF, ACUTE, MEDICATION, URI RELATED SYMP) Respiratory, new patient who was not referred, with an acute problem, with a presenting problem of upper respiratory symptoms or infection, or for medication. *Includes*: Acute and same as AVG 60.

AVG 63 06V1ACOTHPROB

(RESP, NPT, N REF, ACUTE, OTHER PROB INCLUDING HAY FEVER) Respiratory, new patient who was not referred, with an acute problem, with other presenting problems. *Includes*: Same as AVG 61.

AVG 64 06V1REF

(RESP, NPT, REF) Respiratory, new patient who was referred.

AVG 65 06V23MEDIC

(RESP, OPT, NEXAM, MEDICATION) Respiratory, revisit, without a periodic examination, for medication. *Includes*: For medication.

AVG 66 06V23URIA1

(RESP, OPT, NEXAM, URI, AGE 0–49) Respiratory, revisit without a periodic examination, with a presenting problem of upper respiratory symptoms or infection, including hay fever age 0–49 years. *Includes*: Nasal congestion, Sinus problem, Sneezing, Cold, Cough, Hay fever, Throat soreness, Symptoms referable to tonsils, Earache, Chills, Fever.

AVG 67 06V23URIA2

(RESP, OPT, NEXAM, URI, AGE 50–59) Respiratory, revisit, without a periodic examination, with a presenting problem of upper respiratory symptoms or infection, including hay fever age 50–59 years. *Includes*: Same as AVG 66.

Exhibit 9-2   (contd.)

AVG 68 06V23OPA1

(RESP, OPT, NEXAM, OTHER PROB, AGE 0–49) Respiratory, revisit, without a periodic examination, with other presenting problems, age 0–49 years. *Includes*: Shortness of breath, Other disorders of respiratory rhythm and sound, Flu, Pain in chest, Asthma, Other symptoms referable to the respiratory system, NEC, Other presenting problems.

AVG 69 06V23OPA2

(RESP, OPT, NEXAM, OTHER PROB, AGE 50–99) Respiratory, revisit, without a periodic examination, with other presenting problems, age 50–99 years. *Includes*: Same as AVG 68.

AVG 70 06V23PRDEX

(RESP, OPT, EXAM) Respiratory, revisit receiving periodic examination.

Source: R. B. Fetter: "Ambulatory Patient Related Groups," *Report to HCFA*, April 1980.

ambulatory visit are indicated by the yes and no choices. AVG trees are illustrated for new patient and for a revisit.

In a study of hospital outpatient reimbursement methods, investigators cited several clear advantages for the AVG system.

1. AVGs have the potential for describing hospital outpatient case mix on a common basis.

2. Providers can be reimbursed on a per-case basis.

3. AVG system is suitable for a prospective reimbursement scheme based on the expected case mix by payer.

4. In addition to cost control, AVG allows for budgeting, case mix comparisons, utilization review, quality assurance, and planning.[46]

As to be expected, the advantages of the AVG proposal are similar to those for the DRG methodology.

Revised Ambulatory Visit Groups Classification

On February 21, 1986, more than 250 health care professionals attended a seminar, "The New ICD-9-CM Ambulatory Visit Groups Classification Scheme," sponsored by the Yale University School of Organization and Management. Principal investigator for the Yale AVG project team was Dr. Robert B. Fetter, who was also involved in the development of the original DRG classification scheme. Interest in attending the seminar was so great that the location had to be moved to larger quarters. Audience members included representatives from ambulatory care facilities, hospitals, various levels of government health programs, prepaid health care services, private physicians, health care researchers, and health care consulting firms.

Starting with an emphasis on the product of ambulatory health care and seeking to generalize to a variety of settings, the classification scheme concentrates on the visit rather than the episode. Researchers used a greatly expanded database with information from 13 settings, including one IPA, two prepaid fee-for-service group practices, three hospital emergency rooms, two hospital outpatient clinics, two ambulatory surgical centers, one large HMO group practice, and two sources of office-based physicians. On the basis of the added data and the product orientation, a revised ambulatory classification model emerged.

An initial variable relates to whether or not the reason for the ambulatory visit is linked to a body system. If not, the type of visit is classified into prevention, treatment, medicolegal problems, administrative visits, or other visits as follows:

- *Prevention* includes physical exam, well-child care, screening and surveillance, prophylactic measures.

- *Treatment* includes social problem counseling, medical counseling, rehabilitation, surgical aftercare, injections and medications, and desensitization to allergens.

- *Medicolegal* problems include rape, battered child exam, and psychiatric exam.

- *Administrative* visits include partial physical and administrative encounters.

- *Other* includes problems not classified above.

If the ambulatory visit is related to a body system, the encounter is classified into one of 19 Major Ambulatory Diagnostic Categories (MADCs). These MADCs are similar to the 23 MDCs in the DRG scheme; however, MDCs 3 and 4, 6 and 7, 19 and 20, and 21 and 22 are combined to account for the fewer groupings. The next visit variable relates to whether or not a significant CPT-4 procedure is involved and results in procedure AVGs and medical AVGs.

Procedure AVGs distinguish between the visit of a new patient and a revisit; diagnostic clusters are used for either type of patient. Clusters include many of the problems detailed in Exhibit 9-1. Most frequently, medical clusters deal with problems similar to those detailed in Exhibit 9-3, including respiratory problems, hypertension, back problems, dermatitis, ear problems, joint diseases, wounds, and fractures.

In summary, the revised ARG classification scheme builds upon the earlier plan by creating 19 MADCs and approximately 600 to 700 AVGs grouped by procedures and medical clusters. Computer software will be available to implement the new scheme.[47]

Coincidentally, an article on AVGs appeared in the February 20, 1986, issue of *Hospitals*. Karen Schneider, project director for the Yale study group, noted that AVGs are most useful for internal management controls and quality review. She also said, "It's conceivable that (AVGs) could also be used for payment, but not for a few years. I'd like to see it tested first, and all the kinks removed."[48] However, a Washington, D.C., research expert did not sense strong government interest in using AVGs for payment, but saw stronger support for an eventual capitation system. In fact, an unnamed HCFA official added, "I just don't see what this system is going to do."[49] In reponse, Richard Averill of Health Systems International argued that the capitation system trend was evident, but it could take 15 to 20 years. He countered, "What do you do in the interim, just keep reimbursement on fee-for-service, or try something different? AVGs are ready *now*."[50] [speaker's emphasis]

Hospital Outpatient Department vs. Private Practice

Some argue that hospital outpatient departments see people who are quite different from individuals seen in private offices. Severity of illness and severe social problems are often cited as characteristics of the hospital's outpatient population. However, as noted earlier, researchers have indicated that the differences between the case mix at the hospital OPD and the private office are slight.[51]

A summation of the reasons for the high cost of ambulatory visits to a hospital include the following traditional arguments:

1. Hospital OPD clients are medically sicker.

2. Hospital OPD patients are more difficult to treat because of their attendant socioeconomic problems.

3. Hospital OPD charges include inappropriate allocated overhead costs.

4. Hospital OPDs expend resources for their teaching responsibilities.

5. Hospital OPDs have higher costs due to required direct expenses such as expensive equipment and standby capacity.[52]

Generally, overhead, education, and research costs are specific hospital ambulatory costs that are not part of other types of ambulatory practice.

A 1979 study of small (under 130 beds), medium (130-299 beds), and large (over 300 beds) hospital outpatient departments calculated average nonphysician costs per OPD visit. In order, the nonphysician average visit cost was $22.11, $31.28, and $44.05. Most of the direct expenses result from salaries of technical personnel on duty in hospital OPDs—between 76 and 80 percent of the total direct costs. However, "contrary to the conventional wisdom, OPDs located in larger, presumably more complicated hospitals, do not appear to be bearing a larger portion of overhead than OPDs in smaller hospitals."[53] Analysis of research and education components of the OPD visit cost indicates some unanswered questions. "Hospitals with no teaching involvement are more expensive overall per OPD visit than those with minimal or low involvement."[54] In fact, those same investigators have a grant to study the unexplained differences. Their proposal listed three reasons for continuing the investigation:

1. Relatively little is known about how hospital OPD visits differ from those in private practice.

2. Relatively little is known about which variables are important predictors of resources used for ambulatory care, as they differ between OPDs and private practice.

3. Virtually nothing is known about how a case-mix-based reimbursement scheme will affect OPDs, compared with private practice.

Age and AVGs

Five age categories are built into the proposed AVG system. However, the highest is age 50 and over. These age breaks fail to distinguish between the under and over age 65 population, which is so important in consideration of Medicare reimbursement. It has been suggested that there should be an age break at 65 and perhaps another at 75.[55]

A comparison of the 10 top AVGs seen by internists in private practice, separated by over and under age 65, reveals that 7 out of the top 10 AVGs are the same. However, their ranking is different[56] (see Exhibit 9-3). Note that in the under age 65 listing, the number 1 and number 4 most common AVGs would be combined if the AVGs had an age 65 break. This exhibit uses age 65 as an indicator of Medicare eligibility in the comparison.

Interestingly enough, an interspecialty comparison of the content of ambulatory medical care in the United States found that 15 diagnostic clusters accounted for 50 percent of all visits. Only eight of the 28 specialties accounted for a substantial percent of the care to patients with any of the following 15 diagnoses:

Exhibit 9-3 Comparison of Top Ten AVGs—Patients 65 and Over Compared with Patients under 65 for Internists in Private Practice

Description of AVG	AVG	Patients 65 and over		Patients under 65	
		Number of cases	Mean Minutes	Number of cases	Mean Minutes
Revisit for a circulatory problem without chest pain or hypertension but with a secondary diagnosis	47	487 (1)	15.76	330 (7)	15.88
Revisit for hypertension	48	449 (2)	13.38	821 (2)	12.53
Revisit for a respiratory problem including shortness of breath, flu, and asthma in someone 50 or over	69	421 (3)	13.75	527 (4)	12.99
Revisit for circulatory problem without a secondary diagnosis	46	337 (4)	13.42	322 (8)	13.93
Revisit for arthritis	106	324 (5)	15.12	559 (3)	14.66
Revisit for nervous system problem (headaches, seizures, dizziness, head injury)	39	218 (4)	14.15	278	15.11
Revisit for a digestive system problem	76	188 (7)	14.72	467 (5)	16.71
Revisit for an endocrine problem (diabetes, thyroid) with a secondary diagnosis	20	171 (8)	14.55	298 (9)	15.89
Revisit for other diagnoses[1]	154	139 (9)	13.91	188	14.52
Previously known patient who has developed hypertension	55	124 (10)	15.97	192	16.17
Revisit for a respiratory problem including shortness of breath, flu and asthma in someone under 50	68			950 (1)	11.23
Revisit for an endocrine problem (diabetes, thyroid) with a secondary diagnosis	19			337 (6)	14.43
Revisit for a genitourinary problem	89			292 (10)	13.69
All AVGs		4,611	15.61	10,906	15.79

[1]Residual category
Source: J. Lion, M. G. Henderson, A. Malborn, M. M. Wiley, and J. Noble: "Ambulatory Visit Groups: A Prospective Payment System for Outpatient Care," *Journal of Ambulatory Management* 7, no. 4 (1984): 30–45.

General medical examination

Acute upper respiratory infection

Prenatal and postnatal care

Hypertension

Depression/anxiety

Soft-tissue injury

Medical and surgical aftercare

Ischemic heart disease

Acute sprains or strains

Otitis media

Dermatitis/eczema

Fractures and dislocations

Chronic rhinitis

Diabetes mellitus[57]

Physician Time and AVGs

Exhibit 9-3 also shows that internists spend fairly similar amounts of time with the under and over 65 age groups. "Overall, the unadjusted time for all AVGs is virtually identical."[58] In an earlier study, different investigators discovered that people over 65 used less ambulatory physician time for the same diagnoses.[59]

In a comparison of salaried internists in hospital OPDs with internists in private practice, the salaried physicians took more time with patients—18.48 to 15.40 mean minutes for all AVGs.[60] This variation also occurred when comparing seven out of the 10 most common AVGs for the physicians. A revisit for an endocrine problem (diabetes, thyroid) without a secondary diagnosis had physicians at both sites taking 15.40 minutes. On the other extreme, a revisit for a circulatory problem without a secondary diagnosis found that OPD physicians used 20.06 minutes compared to 13.67 minutes for private practice doctors. This differential was also confirmed earlier in an analysis of all 154 AVGs that indicated salaried OPD internists took about 25 percent more time to treat the same case mix.[61]

Thus, it would appear that physician encounters are affected more by the site and/or salary arrangements than by the age of the patients.

Outliers

AVGs do not include the same reimbursement procedure as the DRGs relative to patient care that takes an unusual amount of time and/or resources. Part of the problem lies in the fact that provider time is rarely measured routinely in ambulatory services. Most data on provider time comes from special studies where researchers collect the information. Currently, the AVGs range from around 9 to 47 minutes without the associated tests added into the encounter. To counter this, it has been suggested that AVGs with similar mean resources be combined into large AVGs. However, this yields medically heterogeneous groupings which may be unacceptable to physicians. In addition, there may be a need for new groupings to cover unusual circumstances.[62]

According to a research team working on AVGs, "There will, however, probably not [author's emphasis] be outlier reimbursement under an AVG-based system."[63]

AVG Implications

Cost differentials relative to elements such as the site of ambulatory care, physician salary, encounter duration, resource use, age, socioeconomic problems, and severity of illness all play a role in AVG reimbursement proposals. Except for pass-throughs for capital expenses, medical education, and outliers, the DRG inpatient reimbursement plan also avoids responding to the cost difficulties. Standardized AVGs refer to a model "average" patient.

In April 1984, policy analysts felt that AVG implementation in the near future would result in a number of winners and losers among ambulatory care providers. Predictions included the following:

1. General practitioners would be winners relative to specialists who treat patients with the same characteristics.

2. Physicians in private practice would be winners relative to hospital OPDs.

3. OPDs in small hospitals would be winners relative to OPDs in large hospitals.

4. An all-payer system would not unduly penalize practitioners with a large component of Medicare patients.

5. All of the above effects would probably be exacerbated under a scheme which might be unable to segregate or pay more for outliers.[64]

These impacts would occur because general practitioners take less time in their encounters; similarly, private practitioners take less time than salaried OPD physicians, small hospitals have lower nonphysician costs, Medicare patients do not require extra time, and outliers are not covered in AVGs.

Consistent with these policy implications is the question of how to reimburse providers taking care of high-risk individuals seen on an ambulatory basis. Specifically, hospital OPDs and inner-city public teaching hospital OPDs could suffer devastating financial strain while striving to serve Medicare and Medicaid recipients. A possible solution for high-risk ambulatory care services might be a percentage subsidy across the board rather than a quantification of the extra services provided.[65]

Ambulatory Reimbursement Motivations

These implications lead to the need to examine the motives for designing an ambulatory care reimbursement system. Consider the following imperatives:

1. A need for a rational ambulatory care reimbursement system that is consistent

2. A need for a system that will contain costs

3. A need to shift the focus of patient care away from excessive hospital use and costly subspecialty services to a primary ambulatory care setting.[66]

As of the moment, AVGs that stress time and resource use seem to be the wave of the future. Visits rather than episodes are being stressed in the search for an appropriate unit of payment.

References

1. *Physician Visits: Volume and Interval Since Last Visit, U.S., 1980,* U.S. Department of Health and Human Services, National Center for Health Statistics, Pub. No. (PHS) 83-1572, Series 10, No. 144, June 1983.

2. J. Lion, *Development of a Case Mix Based Reimbursement Method for Hospital Outpatient Departments and Free Standing Clinics,* Proposal to HCFA, October 25, 1982.

3. A. A. Lee, "How DRGs will Affect Your Hospital—And You," *RN* 47, No. 5 (1984):71-81.

4. R. J. Rubin, Remarks at Yale School of Public Health, New Haven, CT, June 3, 1983.

5. S. McIlrath, "DRGs Seen Boosting Outpatient Care, Competition," *American Medical News* 27, No. 24 (June 22, 1984):10.

6. L. Punch, "Physicians Must Alter Practice Patterns Under DRGs: Chains," *Modern Healthcare* 14, No. 3 (February 15, 1984):114, 116, 118.

7. M. Nathanson, "Double Dipping Can Hike Profits, But Advantages May Be Short-lived," *Modern Healthcare* 14, No. 3 (February 15, 1984): 154, 156.

8. "Ambulatory Surgery Units Will Increase Volume with DRGs," *Same-Day Surgery* 7, No. 7 (1983):77-79.

9. Ibid.

10. R. J. Freeman, "DRGs: A Fiscal Foundation for Advanced Prehospital Care," *Journal of Emergency Medical Services* 7, No. 10 (1982):36-39.

11. "Ambulatory Surgery," *Same-Day Surgery.*

12. "New Plan Would Make Medicare Assignment All-Or-Nothing Proposition," *Medical World News* 25, No. 8 (April 23, 1984):25.

13. "Prospective Payment—The Regulator's View: An Interview with Mr. Larry A. O'Day," *DRG Monitor* 1, No. 2 (1983):1-8.

14. *International Classification of Diseases. Ninth Revision. XX. Clinical Modification,* Commission on Professional and Hospital Activities, Ann Arbor, MI, 1978.

15. J. Froom, "The International Classification of Health Problems for Primary Care," *Medical Care* 14, No. 5 (1976):450-454.

16. R. C. Westbury and M. Tarrant, "Classification of Diseases in General Practice: A Comparative Study," *Canadian Medical Association Journal* 101, No. 10 (November 15, 1976):82-87.

17. A. V. Hurtado and M. R. Greenlick, "A Disease Classification System for Analysis of Medical Care Utilization, With a Note on Symptom Classification," *Health Services Research* 6, No. 3 (Fall, 1971):235-350.

18. D. M. Steinwachs and A. I. Mushlin, "The Johns Hopkins Ambulatory-Care Coding Scheme," *Health Services Research* 13, No. 1 (Spring 1978):36-49.

19. H. L. Tindall, L. Culpepper, J. Froom, R. A. Henderson, A. D. Richards, W. W. Rosser, and H. T. Weigert, "The NAPCRG Process Classification for Primary Care," *Journal of Family Practice* 12, No. 2 (1981):309-318.

20. R. Schneeweiss, R. A. Rosenblatt, D. C. Cherkin, C. R. Kirkwood, and L. G. Hart, "Diagnosis Clusters: A New Tool for Analyzing the Content of Ambulatory Care," *Medical Care* 21, No. 1 (1983):105-122.

21. *A Reason for Visit Classification for Ambulatory Care*, Vital and Health Statistics, Series 2, No. 78, U. S. Department of Health, Education, and Welfare, Pub. No. (PHS) 79-1352, February 1979.

22. I. Moscovice, "A Method for Analyzing Resource Use in Ambulatory Care Settings," *Medical Care* 15, No. 12 (1977):1024-1044.

23. M. Gold, "Effects of Hospital-Based Primary Care Setting on Internists' Treatment of Primary Care Episodes," *Health Services Research* 16, No. 4 (1981):383-405.

24. J. J. Kronenfeld, "Sources of Ambulatory Care and Utilization Models," *Health Services Research* 15, No. 1 (Spring 1980):3-20.

25. A. J. Lee, H. B. Wolfe, and B. Swenson, "Hospital-Based Versus Free-Standing Ambulatory Care Costs: A Comparison," *Journal of Ambulatory Care Management* 7, No. 1 (1984):25-39.

26. J. Lion, "Case-Mix Differences Among Ambulatory Patients Seen By Internists in Various Settings," *Health Services Research* 16, No. 4 (Winter 1981):407-413.

27. Ibid.

28. R. C. Mendenhall, R. A. Girard, and S. Abrahamson, "A National Study of Medical and Surgical Specialties I. Background, Purpose, and Methodology," *Journal of the American Medical Association* 240, No. 9 (September 1, 1978):848-852.

29. Ibid.

30. J. Lion and S. Altman, "Case-Mix Differences Between Hospital Outpatient Departments and Private Practice," *Health Care Financing Review* 4, No. 1 (1982):89-98.

31. J. Lion and J. L. Williams, "Medical and Socioeconomic Case Mix in Outpatient Departments," in *Ambulatory Care* by S. Altman, J. Lion, and J. L. Williams (Lexington, MA: Lexington Books), pp. 161-178.

32. Schneeweiss et al., "Diagnosis Clusters," p. 12.

33. Ibid.

34. Ibid.

35. R. E. Johnson, T. M. Vogt, and R. L. Penn, "An Episode Approach to the Care and Costs of Obesity," *Journal of Ambulatory Care Management* 7, No. 1 (1984):47-60.

36. J. Lion, M. G. Henderson, A. Malborn, M. M. Wiley, and J. Noble, "Ambulatory Visit Groups: A Prospective Payment System for Outpatient Care," *Journal of Ambulatory Management* 7, No. 4 (1984):30-45.

37. Johnson et al., "An Episode Approach."

38. Ibid.

39. Ibid.

40. Ibid.

41. Lion et al., "Ambulatory Visit Groups," p. 7.

42. R. B. Fetter, *Development of an Ambulatory Patient Classification System*, Grant application to HCFA, April 27, 1983.

43. R. B. Fetter, R. F. Averill, J. L. Lichtenstein, and J. L. Freeman, *Ambulatory Visit Groups: A Framework for Measuring Productivity in Ambulatory Care*, New Haven, CT: Yale University. Undated.

44. R. B. Fetter, *Ambulatory Patient Related Groups*, Report to HCFA, April 1980, p. 2.

45. R. E. Knapp, "The Development of Outpatient DRGs," *Journal of Ambulatory Care Management* 6, No. 2 (1983):1-11.

46. Lion, "Development of a Case Mix," p. 28.

47. F. Kavaler, personal communication. March 1986.

48. "Ambulatory Care DRGs: Yes? No? Maybe So?" *Hospitals* 60, No. 4 (February 20, 1986):70

49. Ibid.

50. Ibid.

51. Lion and Williams, "Medical and Socioeconomic Case Mix," p. 177.

52. Lion, "Development of a Case Mix," p. 4.

53. Ibid., p. 22.

54. Ibid., p. 4.

55. J. Lion, *Development of a Case Mix Based Reimbursement Method of Hospital Outpatient Departments and Free Standing Clinics*, Continuation Proposal to HCFA, January 31, 1984, p. 32.

56. Lion et al., "Ambulatory Visit Groups."

57. R. A. Rosenblatt, D. C. Cherkin, R. Schneeweiss, and L. G. Hart, "The Content of Ambulatory Medical Care in the U. S.," *The New England Journal of Medicine* 309, No. 15 (October 13, 1983):892-897.

58. Lion et al., "Ambulatory Visit Groups," p. 12.

59. E. B. Keeler, D. Solomon, J. C. Beck, R. Mendenhall, and R. Kane, "Effect of Patient Age on Duration of Medical Encounters with Physicians," *Medical Care* 20, No. 11 (1982):1101-1108.

60. Lion et al., "Ambulatory Visit Groups," p. 13.

61. Lion and Altman, "Case-Mix Differences."

62. Ibid., p. 18.

63. Ibid.

64. Ibid., p. 20.

65. Ibid., p. 21.

66. Ibid.

CHAPTER 10
Insured and Selected
Populations

While DRGs now only affect Medicare inpatients, the concept is spreading to business coalition groups, private, voluntary, and proprietary insurance companies, prepaid health plans, and other federal sectors such as the Veterans Administration and military health systems. Already, some of these sectors are experimenting with PPS/DRG as a reimbursement mechanism.

Not everybody is in agreement that the DRG system will control hospital costs. Wennberg et al. investigated just that question and found considerable variation in admission practices of physicians. According to the researchers, "Professional discretion plays an important part in determining hospitalization for most DRGs."[1] That statement ensued after the researchers looked at 30 Maine hospitals for 1980-1982. Furthermore, the authors remarked that there are many opportunities for physicians to increase admissions—especially for physicians who receive bonuses or share profits in proprietary hospitals. In conclusion, Wennberg et al. took the view that costs may not be controlled:

> In the absence of additional controls on hospital capacity or employment levels, the DRG system may well accelerate the rate of increase in per capita costs for hospital care. . . . the DRG program offers little prospect for limiting hospital costs in the absence of effective controls on use of resources.[2]

Egdahl put it even more starkly: "True cost management can come only from a hospital system shrinkage that involves loss of jobs and closings."[3]

Somers suggested trying to prevent illness as a way of controlling Medicare costs.[4,5] This approach is neither novel nor new, but little headway has been made in integrating prevention into the acute health care delivery system. Four letters to the editor responded to Somers' cost containment suggestion. One called for changing assumptions about medical insurance to stress prevention. Another noted that organized health care plans do stress prevention and Medicare now allows beneficiaries to enroll. One writer said prevention increases costs because life is extended and care is more expensive for older people. A final letter stated that costs were irrelevant if society really wanted to spend the health care dollar. Somers replied and cited the cost-effective Canadian experience where both preventive and curative medical activities are reimbursed. She asked: "How much longer can Medicare lag behind?"[6]

Throughout the nation, American companies have formed coalitions on health to tackle the problem of rising costs. Speaking on behalf of the Washington Business Group on Health, Goldbeck supported the proposed PPS at Congressional hearings. In addition, he stated that changes in the health care delivery system "represented an evolution from the giving of a benefit to the management of an asset."[7] Another corporate entity, the New Jersey Business Group on Health (NJBGH), examined the DRG-based hospital reimbursement program in that state. According to Henderson, the NJBGH's medical director, "the major purchasers of health care are very interested in being able to directly monitor what they are buying." Questions raised by the NJBGH representative concerned cost containment, cost shifting, innovation, quality of care, and operational procedures.[8]

A nationwide business group, the Business Roundtable Task Force on Health, represents about 200 of the Fortune 500 companies. This Task Force studied health care costs and reported that inflation was moderating. That decline was attributed to managerial attention to containing health care costs through restructured benefit plans, use of alternative delivery systems such as HMOs, and involvement with business coalitions.[9,10]

For 1984, the Chrysler Corporation's activities reportedly saved $58 million in medical care costs. Joseph A. Califano, Jr., a former HEW Secretary and now a Chrysler director, explained the rationale: "I believe the great hope to cut health care costs rests in an awakened, varied, competitive world of business purchasers insisting on high quality care at much lower cost."[11]

These business groups do not only concern themselves with their employees. Many companies continue their health benefit programs to retired employees and contribute as taxpayers to the governmental programs. Therefore, business health groups have raised powerful voices to influence health care delivery systems in the United States.

All-Payer Reimbursement System

Immediately before the federal PPS began on October 1, 1983, a *New York Times* editorial commented that the Administration "hopes that private insurers will negotiate similar fixed payments to protect themselves against cost shifting."[12] This logically leads to the concept of an all-payer reimbursement system. By definition, an all-payer prospective reimbursement system means that all payers, such as Medicare, Medicaid, Blue Cross, private commercial insurance carriers, and self-payers, pay for the same hospital inpatient care using the same payment method, but not necessarily the same rate.[13] As Lewis noted, under an all-payer prospective system the hospitals "must reduce costs because there is little opportunity to shift them from one payer to another."[14] Vladeck spoke about the intuitive irrationality of having different financing systems with a varied assortment of payers covering specific segments of the population. He defined the key issue as "universal access through universal financing."[15]

In discussing hospital cost shifting, Ginsburg and Sloan stated that the resolution was an all-payer hospital rate setting system. Factors involved in the consideration of adopting an all-payer system include the following:

- Containing the overall cost of health care.

- Eliminating the inequity of payment differentials.

- Funding care for indigent patients or other uncompensated care.

- Funding for capital and other related costs of health care.[16]

A prime advantage of an all-payer system lies in the fact that hospital expenditures are contained. Research strongly affirms that rate setting curtails hospital costs.[17,18] According to a report from the Health Insurance Association of America (HIAA), the Maryland Health Services Cost Review Commission saved about $124 million in Medicare and Medicaid hospital payments from 1978 to 1981. Data also showed lower annual cost increases than the national average in Maryland and New Jersey. HIAA cited the all-payer advantages in those two states.

- Slowing down the rate of increase in hospital costs for all patients

- Authorizing fair payment for all payers

- Providing incentives for hospitals to reduce utilization.[19]

When considering a statewide all-payer prospective payment plan in Connecticut, the state medical society's executive director called attention to the cost increases in New Jersey under DRGs. He also said that the first year of Massachusetts's rate setting caused the layoff of 3,000 hospital employees.[20]

Starting with Meyer calling the all-payer system "a bizarre form of cost shifting,"[21] critics point out the method's disadvantages. Meyer labeled all-payers bizarre because he felt costs were shifted back to an almost bankrupt Medicare system or to hospitals to cut services and save money. Speaking for the Federation of American Hospitals (FAH), a group of private hospitals, Bromberg delivered a "short list of adverse side effects" of an all-payer system.

1. Innovation would be stifled.

2. There would be no price competition.

3. Centralized bureaucratic preferences or political clout would influence decisions on who gets capital.

4. Consumers would have no voice in how or where resources are allocated.

5. Future patients would be short-changed because taxpayers would eventually have to bail out financially strapped hospitals that used up their cash reserve on operating expenses.

6. Evidence is strong that rate setting does not improve efficiency.

7. A system driven by the new Medicare incentives may negate the need for an all-payer system.[22]

From a management control view, Young and Saltman add more drawbacks to a state rate setting program.

- Both fixed and variable costs are included in payment rates despite the former being time-influenced and the latter being related to volume or intensity of mix of resource inputs.

- Cost variables other than case mix, volume, or price are not distinguished, leaving hospital management to control inputs per case—which is the physician's appropriate responsibility.

- Patient classification requires a system allowing for ease in management.[23]

There is an effort to resolve the arguments pro and con. Federal legislation (P.L. 98-21) requires the HHS Secretary to study and report to Congress by the end of 1985 on the application of the DRG methodology to payment by all-payers for inpatient hospital services. Meanwhile, various federal and state legislative initiatives are taking place. In addition, the February 24, 1986 issue of *Medical World News* reported that the Walter O. Boswell Memorial Hospital in Sun City, Arizona became the first hospital to voluntarily institute an all-payer DRG billing system. Simplification of billing procedures was the main motivation, along with the fact that the case load was already 85 percent Medicare patients. Furthermore, Westworld Community Healthcare, Inc., a proprietary chain of 35 rural hospitals, is experimenting with a voluntary DRG all-payer system in six of their facilities. Motivation in this case relates to an alternative to high per diem charges.[24]

State Systems

While the HIAA favored state rate setting programs, the Association did call for flexibility for the state to meet their own particular needs. Nevertheless, HIAA did derive six general characteristics of a "Fair Payment System."

1. Rules set in advance for all hospitals in the state

2. Incentives and penalties for all hospitals designed to encourage cost-effective management

3. Fair payment for all patients regardless of third-party payer (private or government) involved. [author's emphasis]

4. Payer discounts based upon objective factors that result in demonstrable cost savings to the hospital

5. Monitoring use of certain hospital services

6. Uniform cost and utilization reporting requirements for all hospitals.[25]

Under the current Medicare PPS, Maryland and New Jersey have waivers to allow them to substitute an all-payer system for the federal Medicare inpatient hospital payment mechanism. Both of the waivered states use a different form of state rate setting. Maryland's was the first all-payer program in the nation beginning in 1977. New Jersey started in January 1980 and was the prototype for the federal DRG method. Recently, the waivered states joined forces with health insurers, business, labor, and consumer organizations to push for state all-payer systems. On behalf of the Coalition of State All Payer Hospital Payment Systems, all the Congressional delegations have received information urging support. Letters noted that waivered states saved about $1 billion for Medicare in 1983. While the American Hospital Association opposes a national all-payer system, the AHA does endorse state waivers. However, the Federation of American Hospitals called state rate setting "nothing more than price controls."[26] About 16 additional states are also considering rate setting proposals.[27]

In 1984, Arizona held a referendum on hospital rate controls that experts considered a barometer for the future. Approval of the measures would establish a new state authority to set hospital rates by DRGs and to review capital expenditures. Legislation was favored and financially supported by a coalition of large industries in the state including Motorola, Sperry, and Garrett. More than $1 million was spent on advertising. Support also came from HIAA and the American Association of Retired Persons (AARP). Hospitals, hospital suppliers, and manufacturers opposed the measures and spent similar amounts on advertising. Despite early polls favoring passage of the legislation, a turnaround occurred and the proposal was defeated. Voters in North Dakota turned down similar legislation in 1978.[28]

It is still too early to tell what impact the defeat in Arizona will have on other state movements toward all-payer systems. However, on a national scale, Senator Kennedy and Representative Gephardt are proposing legislation to stimulate state all-payer mechanisms.

Federal Legislation

In February 1984, Senator Kennedy and Representative Gephardt introduced the Medicare Solvency and Health Care Financing Reform Act. This bill proposes to encourage states to develop their own hospital reimbursement mechanism including all private and government payers.[29] Opposition to the proposal was strong and swift. "Most hospital groups oppose the bill, arguing it's inequitable, would kill innovation and could lead to federal rationing of health care."[30] Owen, speaking for the American Hospital Association (AHA), said the bill turns hospitals into public utilities. A representative of FAH commented, "The tremendous geographic inequities would be my biggest complaint, although we have a long list."[31] Even those groups that support the all-payer idea have reservations about the Kennedy-Gephardt bill. Larry Gage, president of the National Association of Public Hospitals (NAPH), said he "couldn't whole-heartedly support the bill but it's on the right track."[32] Group Health Association of American expressed similar feelings. Carolyne Davis, HCFA Administrator, sought to "vigorously oppose" the bill, calling it too regulatory and a "back door" entry to national health insurance.[33]

During the 1984 presidential election campaign, several candidates proposed that the prospective payment system cover all third-party payers.[34,35] In fact, one health affairs advisor predicted that, regardless of who was elected President in 1984, the U. S. health care system will adopt an all-payer mode by 1990.[36]

Insurers and DRGs

Commercial Carriers

Considering the support for an all-payer system, are the firms providing health insurance coverage moving towards the use of PPS/DRG mechanisms? As of late 1984, a headline in *Hospitals* summed up the situation: "Insurers Slow to Use DRGs But Interested."[37] Specifically, the article noted that major commercial insurance companies were slower than Blue Cross/Blue Shield plans, although efforts are underway to investigate PPS/DRG in the future. John Moynahan, Jr., a senior vice president for Metropolitan Life Insurance Company, stated that "prospective reimbursement by the private sector will be coming down the pike. I think it's inevitable."[38] A CIGNA Corporation executive agreed that "DRG/PPS is a very good payment concept."[39] However, both insurance experts predicted that DRGs will include illness severity modifications. Carriers are slow to move because of limitations on imposing a payment system and a heavy investment in an existing claims system that works. A PPS/DRG survey revealed that most of the major commercial carriers used PPS and/or DRGs only where mandated by state law.[40]

Blue Cross/Blue Shield Plans

Compared to commercial insurers, Blue Cross/Blue Shield Companies are taking more initiatives; six use PPS and four use both PPS/DRGs in pilot programs, state-mandated, and voluntary programs.[41]

Kansas BC/BS was the first to link reimbursement to PPS/DRG[42] in a plan initiated January 1, 1984, although the company began working on the concept in mid-1982. Calling their development Competitive Allowance Program (CAP), the Kansas BC/BS listed the following potentials for the CAP:

- Injection of an element of competition in the provision of health care services

- Encouragement of hospitals and doctors to be more cost-efficient in the planning and delivery of services

- Allowing subscribers the opportunity to compare the prices of services

- Allowing the outpatient program to have a greater impact on hospital admission and length of stay

- Allowing BC/BS to contract with providers at the most cost-effective rate for services.[43]

Hospitals voluntarily contract annually with BC/BS of Kansas and are guaranteed full reimbursement up to the maximum allowable payment (MAP) for any specific DRG. Consideration is given to a hospital's peer group in calculating the payment. All 136 Kansas hospitals have signed contracts. Physicians also contract yearly and receive MAPs for specific procedures at a percentage of usual and customary charges. About 87 percent of Kansas physicians participated. A medical society representative commented: "There is some apprehension, but the changes that they actually put in might not be as bad as you think."[44] However, Goldowsky's editorial in the *Rhode Island Medical Journal* wondered if the Kansas BC/BS idea might become a prairie fire roaring out of the West to spread over the nation.[45] On the part of the Kansas Hospital Association,

Wilson felt that the institutions "are looking at the situation with guarded enthusiasm."[46]

Additional incentives in the Kansas plan allow for an on-line computerized Paperless Claims Entry System and a payment inducement as described by a BC/BS of Kansas vice president:

> We will not pay the DRG amount each time a hospital submits a bill. We will pay the hospital its charges up to the DRG amount, and then, at the end of the year, we will have a cost effectiveness settlement with the hospital. If they have, in terms of dollars, twice as many charges that are under our maximum as they have over our maximum, then we will reimburse their charges in full. This is an incentive for the hospitals to keep their charges down.[47]

BC/BS of Oklahoma also began using DRGs for payment purposes on January 1, 1984. About 107 of the 126 hospitals signed contracts to participate in the Fixed Allowance Incentive Reimbursement (FAIR) plan.[48] Hospitals are grouped into four categories by bed size, with smaller hospitals, fewer than 125 beds, being paid for 49 basic DRGs as compared with 313 DRGs for facilities with more than 375 beds. Diagnoses not falling within the DRGs are paid for on reasonble charges.[49]

Other BC/BS plans adapting a DRG mechanism include Rhode Island, Arizona,[50] and Michigan.[51] Of course, Blue Cross of New Jersey has participated in that state's all-payer system since 1980. Koehler, an executive of BC of New Jersey, reported on the impact of DRGs at a nationwide meeting in November 1983. He said:

> I must state up front that we at New Jersey Blue Cross have yet to formulate a conclusive opinion as to whether or not the DRG methodology has proven to be a significant cost containment initiative.[52]

In comparison to commercial insurers, New Jersey Blue Cross receives a 6.18 differential discount, down from 30 percent. That discount "becomes a windfall competitive advantage for Blue Cross relative to commercial insurers."[53] In dollar terms, this is considerable, since New Jersey BC is the third largest in the United States and pays out 22 percent of the state's almost $3 billion worth of health care costs. Yet, New Jersey Blue Cross does believe that the incentives to contain costs are working; admissions are down and average length of stay is shortened.[54]

At the same meeting, Mellman spoke for the Prudential Insurance Company and explained that insurance companies believe DRGs are important because costs are contained and equity in hospital pricing is achieved. In addition, he noted the impact on marketing coverage, designing plans, and the education of insurance providers, policy holders, and the general public. Finally, Mellman recommended paying increased attention to public understanding, giving the DRG system a chance to mature, and providing enough staff to the state Health Department to administer the program.[55]

Currently, BC/BS insurers are more involved in adapting PPS/DRGs into their reimbursement packages, particularly in conjunction with prepaid health care plans. Commercial insurers are taking a more conservative stance even though experts think that eventually their coverage will also reflect PPS/DRG methodology.

Long-Term Care Insurance

Private insurance for long-term care expenses is an underdeveloped field and accounts for only 1 percent of revenues in the nursing home industry at present. While about 60 percent of the Medicare-covered population has supplemental private insurance to fill the gaps in expenses (Medigap insurance), few policies cover nursing home care. The insurance industry has traditionally not offered such coverage for several reasons. It perceives itself at risk from adverse selection of policy holders; the industry lacks experience in setting premium rates for long-term care coverage; and, administrative costs would be high for these policies. However, a recent survey estimated that 40,000 persons are covered in a wide range of plans for long-term care. The major emphasis of these plans is on long-term care services below the level of skilled nursing care (such as intermediate and custodial), with few home care benefits. There are differences in allowable per diem fixed payments, waiting periods, lengths of coverage, and restrictions to control utilization—such as prior hospitalization, physician review, exclusions for mental illnesses and renewability limitations (see Exhibit 10-1).[56]

While many elderly anticipate that Medicaid will fill the gap as a "safety net," in many state programs there are restrictions which similarly restrict covered services for long-term care. The market potential for private insurance for long-term care is expected to expand in the future as the elderly population continues to grow more educated and affluent. However, the health insurance industry's current position is that "incentives inherent in Medicaid preclude development of viable private sector options" and that until Medicaid and other public programs are perceived as "unacceptable alternatives," the market in private insurance will not flourish.[57]

In fact, an Op-Ed article in the *New York Times* of January 30, 1986 suggested restricting Medicare insurance benefits to only needy senior citizens. Health and Human Services Secretary Otis R. Bowen proposed a Medicare catastrophic illness insurance policy as a purchaseable guarantee against bankruptcy.[58]

Exhibit 10-1   Long-Term Care Benefits under Selected Insurance Policies

Benefits	Policy Features		
	Fireman's Fund	Kemper	United Equitable
Skilled nursing care	Choice of up to $60/day	$20/day for days 1–100; $40/day for days 101–1095	Choice of up to $40/day
Intermediate & custodial care	Choice of up to $60/day	$10/day for less than skilled care	One-half chosen rate, up to $20
Home Care	Choice of up to $30/day	$25/day for private duty nurse	None
Waiting/Elimination deductible period	Choice of 20 or 100 days	None for skilled nursing care or private duty nurse	Choice of 0, 20 or 100 days
Length of coverage	4 years for nursing home confinement; 180 days for home health	3 years for skilled nursing care or private duty nurse; 2 years for intermediate or custodial care	4 years for skilled care; choice of 6 or 12 months for less than skilled care
Pre-existing condition period	90 days	12 months	180 days
Prior hospitalization requirement	Nursing home confinement must begin within 90 days after hospitalization of at least 3 days; custodial or intermediate care covered only after skilled care; home care covered only after 180 days in SNF	Confinement must begin within 28 days after hospitalization of 3 or more days; nonskilled care must follow 20 days of covered skilled care	Skilled care must begin within 30 days after hospitalization of at least 3 days; intermediate or custodial care must follow at least 20 days of skilled care.

Source: *Alpha Centerpiece*, May, 1984, p. 2.

A prototype policy for long-term care with a variety of alternative specifications for services covered, benefits paid, waiting period, age at time of purchase, risk selection, and so on, estimated fixed premiums at $435 annually for group coverage and $543 annually for individual protection. The "potential for relieving some of the pressure on Medicaid by encouraging greater private financing" and "more favorable tax treatments of reserves" are possible federal incentives which would stimulate a greater market in the field.[59]

The first long-term care provider offering long-term care insurance to independently living residents in their retirement community is the Otterbein Home in Lebanon, Ohio. When this nonprofit Methodist community first began offering the policy, 75 percent of the residents signed up on a voluntary basis for the premiums of $40-$80 per month. The policy became mandatory on January 1, 1985, and offers two years of nursing home care after a one-year exclusion, with no prior hospitalization necessary for residents who are in their facility at least 90 days. This policy supplements but does not duplicate Medicare or other Medigap coverage. Licensed nursing homes throughout Ohio may be utilized. This is a pilot program that eventually could expand to other nonprofit and proprietary facilities and create greater interest in long-term care by the traditional insurance companies.[60]

In an attempt to stimulate insurance activity in this area, legislation in New Jersey has been proposed, mandating that insurance companies statewide offer long-term care insurance. James Cunningham, president of the State Association of Health Care Facilities, reported that there was "lukewarm" reception by the insurance representatives at a recent public hearing.[61]

While cost-containment in long-term care reimbursement schemes are directed towards controlling expenditures in Medicaid and Medicare, private paying insurance coverage is likely to be similarly affected. All-payer rates and restrictions occurring in the wake of DRGs will affect the long-term care industry as well. The impact on quality of patient care from accessibility issues to service delivery requires continuous monitoring, if the elderly who need the greatest amount of long-term care services are to be protected and served, even when they choose private insurance alternatives.

Health Maintenance Organizations (HMOs) and Competitive Medical Plans (CMPs)

Another systems approach to the management of the delivery of health care services leads to comprehensive coverage, both ambulatory and inpatient, for Medicare beneficiaries. Bolstered by many years of experience garnered by health maintenance organizations (HMOs) and by the federal government's stimulation of competitive medical plans (CMPs), the PPS added a structural option to management variables. However, this option cuts across all classification groupings and results in the comprehensive services being offered under the banner of governmental affiliations, nonprofit and profit-making organizations. It is evident that managers considering an HMO-type mission have yet another set of environmental conditions to add to the administrative variables.

Basically, the idea stemmed from a marketplace principle. If individuals receive a specified amount of money to purchase health care, they would then shop around to get the most for their money. Providers will react in a complementary manner by offering the best package to attract customers and make their organization prosper.

However, instead of actually giving eligible individuals cash, the government issues a voucher which can only be used to contract with qualified and approved health care providers.

On January 10, 1985, final rules were published in the *Federal Register*—to take effect February 1, 1985—marking the government's push to encourage the enrollment of Medicare beneficiaries in HMOs and CMPs.[62] Secretary Heckler labeled the move "a medical milestone" and predicted "a dramatic rise in HMO enrollment . . . up by as many as 600,000 beneficiaries in the next three to four years."[63]

Prospective Reimbursement Payments

Two types of organizations are eligible to negotiate at-risk contracts with HCFA: already qualified HMOs and the newly defined CMPs. Under the contract, HMOs/CMPs receive monthly payments, in advance, for each Medicare patient enrolled, based on 95 percent of the average annual per capita cost (AAPCC) adjusted for age, sex, disability, welfare, and institutionalization. Regulations contained 36 pages of standardized AAPCC distributed by states, areas, and Medicare Part A and Part B.[64] Roughly, the national average equals about $183 a month/$2,200 per year for an AAPCC payment to an HMO/CMP. According to Christy of the American Association of Retired Persons (AARP), "There's evidence that the average operating cost of the HMO is close to 80 percent of the average fee-for-service cost."[65] Regardless, the HMO or CMP is "at risk" for providing care even if costs exceed prospective payments.

However, the negotiated contract already includes the HMO's profit, so the law says that any savings must be passed along to the Medicare patients. HMOs can opt to reduce premiums, absorb copayments and deductibles, add medical benefits, accept lower monthly HCFA payments, or utilize a combination of options. In demonstration HMO Medicare programs that saved money, enrollees received additional benefits such as preventive services, eyeglasses, hearing aids, one dollar copayments on prescriptions, and even dental services.[66]

Definitions

An HMO is defined in the *Federal Register* as "an entity that provides care in a geographic area to a group of persons who are enrolled as members."[67] Added to that is the concept that the HMO delivers an agreed-upon set of health care services for a predetermined fixed fee. Health care services are usually understood to be comprehensive and available 24 hours a day.

CMPs have many of the same characteristics as HMOs regarding the range of outpatient and inpatient services, open enrollment, out-of-area coverage, and quality assurance activities. Criteria for CMPs do appear to have enough flexibility for hospitals, physician groups, PPOs (preferred provider organizations), and health insurance companies to offer health care services to the elderly.

Major HMO Advantage

A large volume of research exists that indicates that an HMO does reduce hospitalization. A recent comparative study again confirmed that point when individuals received care from either a fee-for-service physician or from doctors at the Group Health Cooperative of Puget Sound (Washington). Independent researchers concluded that the HMO physicians "were simply practicing a different style of medicine . . . the general consistency between our results and those in the literature indicates that a less 'hospital-intensive' style of medicine than that practiced by the average physician is possible."[68] Johnson statistically confirms the less hospital-intensive style by comparing the inpatient experience of persons 65 or older in the United States and the Kaiser-Permanente HMO after the initiation of Medicare. By 1979, the U. S. rate for hospital days per 1,000 persons 65 or older was 4.182 as compared to 1.851 for the HMO patients. Calculating the less intensive hospitalization into 1995, Johnson predicts that the projected $400.9 billion deficit in the Medicare Hospital Insurance Trust Fund would turn into a projected surplus of $260.9 billion. This turnaround of $660.9 billion accrues through the expanded use of HMOs by Medicare beneficiaries.[69] Anticipated bankruptcy of the Medicare Hospital Insurance Trust Fund was one of the events that precipitated the advent of the PPS/DRG plan.

Obstacles to HMO Adoption

At the Congressional hearings prior to the adoption of the PPS, Pyle commented on the fundamental incompatibility "between internal HMO mechanisms to promote cost effective delivery of health care and an external system intended to promote cost effectiveness generally."[70] For example, HMO patients generally have shorter hospital lengths of stay and preadmission lab work is usually done at the HMO site. However, the hospital receives reimbursement for the lab work as part of the DRG payment. That is a plus for the hospital's finances but an incompatibility for the HMO. Blomquist raised a related hospital length-of-stay incompatibility in arguing about the legal aspects of the legislative mandate to exempt HMOs from DRG inpatient systems. Wording in the Social Security Act Amendments of 1983 require exemption for HMOs to negotiate directly with hospitals for inpatient coverage for their members. However, Blomquist maintains that states with waivers can bypass the intent of the exemption through "back door" regulations and frustrate meaningful bargaining. According to Blomquist, the HMO exemption has not been effective and threatens the HMO's advantage. He cites the legal case for federal preemption as he concentrates on the situation in New Jersey.[71]

Another barrier inhibits expansion by requiring that current HMO enrollees can not be converted en masse to capitated PPS payment. Two new people must be enrolled for each current member changed over to the prospective method. In addition, Holoweiko lists four other obstacles to HMO development:

1. Surveys indicate that the elderly are more satisfied with their fee-for-service physicians than younger patients.

2. Medicare beneficiaries are not centrally located in one employment site and expensive promotional campaigns may be needed to enroll individuals.

3. Many Medicare recipients reside in different locations during different seasons of the year and health care coverage would be required at the varied locations.

4. Paperwork related to enrollments, disenrollments, and budgets may hinder the government's ability to carry out its necessary functions in a timely fashion.[72]

In fact, that last impediment has already surfaced in a GAO investigation of problems in administering Medicare's HMO demonstration projects in Florida. GAO researchers found the system for coordinating hospital payments susceptible to errors and to enrollment/disenrollment problems.[73]

Reactions to HMO Promotions

Despite the potential barriers to HMO growth, there are reasons for Medicare recipients to enroll in a prepaid health care plan. These reactions are being communicated to the elderly through a number of senior citizen organizations:

- Currently, health care expenses amount to about 15 percent of an elderly person's annual income. By 1989, it is estimated the percentage will be 19, or about $2,400.

- HMO members can get comprehensive care without deductibles, coinsurance, or copayment. In addition, the Medicare members may get extra benefits if the HMO saves money on the per capita reimbursements. All of the health care services are also available with a minimum of red tape.

- Educational programs conducted by the AARP and other groups aim to develop "informed buyers" who can evaluate the worth of joining an HMO.

- Major corporations are promoting HMOs because the firms are still paying their retirees' Medicare supplemental insurance premiums and the companies regard the prepaid plan as an economical choice.[74]

This increased growth of HMOs and CMPs could affect physicians in two ways, according to HHS analysts. First, doctors could accept Medicare fees as full payment for services in areas where competing prepaid plans are enrolling Medicare beneficiaries. Secondly, physicians will have more opportunities to join plans in some type of employment arrangement.[75]

On the other hand, *Private Practice*, a journal devoted to maintaining traditional physician/patient relations, consistently denigrates HMOs. Schwartz calls it two-tier medicine in which HMO doctors provide patients with the minimum number of services necessary: fewer tests are ordered, fewer consultant referrals are made, fewer patients are hospitalized—to their detriment, operations are denied, and end-of-year bonuses are paid when physicians save money for the HMO.[76] In that same journal, Buenaflor relates his own HMO experience, recalling the numerous requests for sick notes and bogus work excuses as well as disability claims. He states that only 21 percent of people in California belong to HMOs, even though such plans have existed there for 50 years. Furthermore, he quotes a newspaper story that Kaiser Permanente HMO doctors had twice as many malpractice lawsuits as other physicians.[77] With this type of negative medical input, Schwartz anticipates that even people who belong to HMOs will use the HMO for routine service but go to the private doctor for more serious problems.[78]

In a 1985 letter to the editor, Fischer advises both physicians and patients to beware of HMOs. He warns that "the deliberate underuse of medical services to maximize profits is becoming as much a concern as is overuse."[79] Citing experiences in southern Florida HMOs, Fischer documented problems such as deceptive advertising in enrollment tactics, difficulty of disenrollment for unsatisfied patients, questionable medical care, and poor continuity of care. To correct these problems, Fischer urges medical societies to initiate public educational programs which evaluate the advantages and disadvantages of the various health care delivery systems.

The HHS got about 30,000 written complaints about the HMO final rules when chiropractors were not mandated for HMO services. All but 75 were from chiropractors and their patients. Obviously, those people want chiropractic services to be included in HMO services.

Management Trends

HHS estimates an initial increase of 400,000 to 800,000 Medicare enrollees in HMOs, with about 150 prepaid plans participating and each taking 2,700 to 5,300 patients.[80] As of June 1984, there were 133 prepaid plans providing services to 875,000 Medicare beneficiaries. Of the nationwide total of 335 prepayment plans, 210 were HMOs and served 14 million people.[81] Federal officials project that HMOs and CMPs will enroll about 10 percent of the elderly and eventually serve around 3 million Medicare recipients.

With those large estimates of membership, management-oriented health care providers expect to capture a portion of the market and make a profit while rendering quality care to the elderly. Among the groups expressing interest in Medicare HMOs are proprietary hospital chains such as Humana and Hospital Corporation of America; investor-owned hospitals belonging to the Federation of American Hospitals; Blue Cross/Blue Shield organizations; commercial insurance companies; and voluntary nonprofit hospitals being hit hard by the DRG payment program.

U.S. Health Care Systems, Inc., Blue Bell, PA, is a proprietary firm that specializes in developing HMOs. That firm has 515,000 members in HMOs in Chicago, Dallas/Fort Worth, and throughout Florida, New Jersey, and Pennsylvania. Stock market analysts forecast robust profits for HMOs. One analyst states the reason HMOs should do well in the future: "You're talking about an industry where there are no assets; you're talking about management, management, management. They're (U.S. Health Care Systems) the best in the HMO field."[82]

While some commercial HMO companies may limit their Medicare enrollees, a potential market of 30 million people eligible to choose to join an HMO offers substantial growth possibilities. Carefully considering that market will be HMO companies traded on stock exchanges, such as HealthAmerica, Maxicare Health Plans, Health Group International, Independence Health Plan, Western Health Plans, and Sierra Health Services. In a general review of the HMO situation in a *New York Times* business and health column, Freudenheim paints a rosy picture, noting that "HMO growth displays vigor."[83]

Blue Cross/Blue Shield organizations also have a keen interest in enrolling the elderly. "I predict that the vast majority of Blue Cross and Blue Shield HMO affiliates will explore the Medicare HMO option and that the vast majority will apply for participation," said Seymour Kaplan, executive director of alternate delivery systems for the national BC/BS group. That prediction is based on the fact that about 70 to 80 percent of the BC/BS HMOs are already federally qualified and therefore automatically able to enroll the elderly. A survey by *Hospitals* in January 1985 listed about 40 BC/BS HMOs throughout the U.S.[84]

Commercial insurance companies are also sponsoring HMOs, such as Prudential's Pru-Care and Aetna's CHOICE. More commercial insurance firms have developed PPOs. Yet, a 1985 survey revealed that 82 percent of the Fortune 500 companies offer their employees the option of HMO coverage.[85] Many times that option is provided by a commercial insurance carrier. Some firms offer both HMOs and PPOs. Metropolitan Life Insurance Company even has a PPO that uses DRG payments.[86]

Voluntary nonprofit hospitals are also looking into establishing HMOs. These hospitals are attracted by the ability to offer more ambulatory care and to actually reduce losses incurred via the inadequate DRG payments for inpatient care. Riffer also believes that the HMO exemption from DRG provides vertical organization benefits to the hospital sponsoring its own HMO.[87]

Social/HMO (S/HMO) Experiments

The University Health Policy Consortium at Brandeis University has proposed expansion of the concept of sharing risks and costs among a large population of enrollees in a traditional HMO, to include social services, institutional, home, and community-based chronic care services not usually covered by Medicare. Supported by a grant from HCFA and some private foundations, four test sites have been chosen which have extensive experiences with prepaid comprehensive health care service delivery and/or administration of chronic care programs for the elderly.

The monthly premiums supplement coverage by Medicare Part A and B and/ or Medicaid, to form the insurance basis for provision of comprehensive services by an S/HMO, a provider with incentives for innovation and cost saving. The exhibit of the estimated premiums and benefits displays attempts to encourage less expensive noninstitutional care (Exhibit 10-2).

Concerns have been raised concerning the marketability and attractiveness of these increased premiums for the prepayment of chronic long-term care services potentially needed in the future. The federal government views the S/HMO as additional long-term care services being provided which increase the current expenditures in this area and may lead to expansions of the Medicare program. However, the February 20, 1986, issue of *Hospitals* reported that the elderly were not knocking down doors to enroll in S/HMOs. That lack of enthusiasm was tied to a lack of selling the concept to the target audience.[88]

On the other hand, the S/HMO project may "shed light on the ability of the acute and long-term care fusion to reduce costs and improve medical care,"[89] as well as provide opportunities for longitudinal study of the aging process and effectiveness of clinical interventions in a defined population.

Exhibit 10-2   Estimated Premiums and Chronic Care Benefits of Social/HMO
Demonstration Sites*

Site	Monthly Premium	Annual Chronic Care Benefit**	Renewability of Institutional Benefit
Metropolitan Jewish Geriatric Center (MJGC), Brooklyn, NY (Elderplan, Inc.)	$29.00	$6,500 in any setting	Fully renewable
Kaiser Permanente Medical Care Program, Portland, OR (Medicare Plus II)***	$39.00	100 days nursing home care $1,000 per month home/community care	Only for new "spell of illness"
Ebenezer Society, Minneapolis, MN	$29.00	$6,250 in any setting	$6,400 lifetime limit
Senior Care Action Network (SCAN), Long Beach, CA (SCAN Health Plan)	$40.00	$7,500 in any setting	Fully renewable

*Estimated premiums and benefits are preliminary and subject to change.
**The net value of the benefits is lower due to coinsurance payments ranging from 10 to 20 percent.
***Long-term care benefits for Medicaid enrollees will be excluded from the Kaiser plan in the first year pending completion of a study of Medicaid chronic care costs outside the Social/HMO. Medicaid enrollees will receive benefits from the state Medicaid program on a fee-for-service basis during that period.
Source: *Alpha Centerpiece*, May, 1984, p. 4.

HMO Impact

HMOs, with or without the social component, might well be the wave of the future; they may be beneficial for elderly care and they may provide cost savings under Medicare. New regulations promulgated in January 1985, and effective in February 1985, allow Medicare to prepay premiums for elderly who wish to join an approved HMO.

Currently 14 million people of all ages are enrolled in 335 prepaid health plans; of these people, 875,000 are Medicare recipients. An estimated 200,000 Medicare-eligible persons are expected to enroll and receive additional benefits (such as eyeglasses, prescription drugs, or dental care) not currently covered under Medicare.[90,91]

Cost savings are anticipated by the new rate setting mechanism: "Payment will be equal to 95 percent of what Medicare estimates it would have paid all the traditional providers (hospitals and fee-for-service physicians) in the same community (or in technical parlance, the average adjusted per capita cost)."[92]

Savings are anticipated on the 5 percent not expended, although recent HCFA-supported demonstrations have not shown these savings as yet and have had problems in hospital admission rates and control of utilization. Costs of the program are expected to be $30 million in fiscal year 1985 and $65 million in fiscal year 1986.

Major objections have come from the AMA, which has requested a delay in implementation of the plan to enroll Medicare patients in the HMOs. They contend that although 28 demonstration projects have been established, "none of these demonstration projects has reported its results yet." They add, "As no demonstration project has operated on a statewide basis, we believe it is irresponsible not to ascertain the impact these regulations will have on a national scale."[93]

Incursions into the private practice of medicine and shift of patients away from the private offices is of concern as well to organized medicine. However, the HMO concept of organized patient care, emphasizing patient education, prevention, monitoring of care, and ready availability of services, has positive medical benefits for the chronically ill, elderly population. Its popularity should continue to grow as DRGs further encourage all prospective prepayment plans.

Veterans Administration

While DRGs were not envisioned for use in the federal sector, the government forestalled criticism by stimulating the use of PPS/DRG in its own facilities. Even though the Veterans Administration and the military operate under a predetermined budget, managers can still make decisions regarding allocation of resources.

In July 1982, the Veterans Administration made a decision to phase in a DRG-based resource allocation system when the 1985 appropriation was distributed.[94] This happened despite the fact that the VA is not required to use DRGs. Considering that the VA services include 172 hospitals, over 80 nursing homes, over 200 outpatient settings, and more than $6 billion in expenditures, this was an important decision. DRGs were planned for use as an internal management tool to measure length of stay, clinical practice, and clinical productivity. Using the DRG model, to be phased in over five years, the VA could allocate funds equitably related to work load.[95]

As recently as early 1984, the President's Private Sector Survey on Cost Control was particularly critical of the VA hospital system. This investigation concluded that "the average length of stay is too long and that VA hospitals are underutilized."[96] That finding was affirmed by a Government Accounting Office (GAO) study that found almost half of the VA hospital bed days are medically unnecessary.[97]

To respond to that oft-repeated type of criticism, the VA developed a Weighted Work Unit (WWU) value using the 467 DRGs, the cost distribution system, and the patient treatment files for data sources. Two weighting systems were prepared, one for teaching hospitals and one for nonteaching facilities. Salary-adjusted WWUs accounted for 90 percent of the variation in reported expenditures. "For the nation as a whole, the unit cost of producing a weighted work unit on medical, surgical, and psychiatric bed sections (after adjusting the trim points) were remarkably similar."[98]

Differences in unit costs could be attributed to regional or geographic variables. In a simulation model, the Sunbelt states gained resources at the expense of the Northeast, Mid-Atlantic and Upper Midwest.[99] This situation was confirmed in the first budget shift of VA allocations.[100]

This shift from a historical cost basis toward a reasonable average cost reflects a parallel pattern to the Medicare PPS. Hospitals may be grouped into VA peer groups and related to size and region.[101] Under this system, an inefficient hospital could be underfunded up to a ceiling of no more than 20 percent of the differences between DRG prices and facility costs.[102] For long-term care, the VA is looking at consumption-related groups instead of DRGs.[103]

A report from the VA Medical Center in Ann Arbor, Michigan analyzed 1982 discharge data from 11 affiliated general medical and surgical centers of over 500 beds in the New England census area. For each of the 470 DRGs, VA length of stay norms were calculated to determine the mean, standard deviation, and 50th, 75th and 90th percentiles. These length of stay norms are particularly useful in performing utilization review.[104] In this fashion, the VA can use the DRG system in a comparative, evaluative manner.

In the first budget allocation application of the VA's use of the DRG system, 65 hospitals lost up to $600,000, while slightly more gained up to $400,000. VA officials claim that "the new resource allocation process will prospectively fund hospitals at the VA systemwide average for work performed."[105]

Another area for potential concern was raised in reference to rehabilitation medicine services in VA hospitals. Delisa pointed out that the VA includes inpatient rehabilitation activities in its resource allocation system, even though the Medicare PPS presently excludes those services. Under the DRG-based methodology linking length of stay to acute care services, Delisa felt that rehabilitation medicine services would almost surely exceed the break-even point and produce "big DRG losers" for VA management to look askance at in the allocation process. While Delisa agreed that the VA should make rehabilitation services more efficient and effective, he remarked that the present situation did not enhance quality care and suggested that the VA also wait for DRG-type criteria for long-term care and rehabilitation to be developed, to more accurately reflect use of resources and length of stay.[106]

Military Health Care

Still another application of the DRG mechanism occurred in late 1984 when hospitals in South Carolina agreed to accept DRG reimbursement levels for care rendered to military beneficiaries. Forty-three hospitals volunteered to participate and to accept the DRG amount as the full payment.[107] South Carolina was chosen because the fiscal intermediaries are the same there and 59 of 60 hospitals already use DRGs.[108] Defense Department staff suggest that some hospitals, particularly rural hospitals, could end up receiving more money for specific DRG procedures than they would get on a cost basis.[109]

Summary

With insurance companies adopting the PPS/DRG system, the spread of pre-determined reimbursement is assured. Add in the activities of the Veterans Administration, the military, and the prepaid health plans and the nationwide impact is considerable. It is apparent that the PPS/DRG mode will include a larger and larger part of the health care industry in the future.

References

1. J. E. Wennberg, K. McPherson, and P. Caper, "Will Payment Based on Diagnosis Related Groups Control Hospital Costs?" *New England Journal of Medicine* 311, No. 5 (August 2, 1984):295-300.

2. Ibid.

3. R. H. Egdahl, "Should We Shrink the Health Care System?" *Harvard Business Review* 62, No. 1 (1984):125-132.

4. A. Somers, "Why Not Try Preventing Illness As a Way of Controlling Medicare Costs?" *New England Journal of Medicine* 311, No. 14 (September 27, 1984):853-856.

5. A. Somers, "Moderating the Rise in Health Care Costs," *New England Journal of Medicine* 307, No. 15 (October 7, 1982):944-947.

6. Letters by Bartlett, Gleason, Hellman, Webb, and reply by Somers, *New England Journal of Medicine* 312, No. 5 (January 31, 1985):319-320.

7. W. B. Goldbeck, *Testimony at U.S. Senate Finance Committee on PPS*, Washington, DC, February 17, 1983, p. 253.

8. R. R. Henderson and J. J. May, "The Business Community Looks at DRG Based Hospital Reimbursement," *Health Affairs* 2, No. 1 (Spring, 1983):38-49.

9. "Climb in Health Care Costs Subsiding," *American Medical News* 27, No. 28 (July 27, 1984):11.

10. D. E. L. Johnson, "Prospective Pay, Coalitions Broke Hospital Spending," *Modern Healthcare* 14, No. 5 (1984):28-29.

11. D. E. Rosenbaum, "Chrysler Program Saves Millions in Health Costs," *New York Times*, April 29, 1985.

12. "A New Era in Medicare," (editorial), *New York Times*, September 12, 1983.

13. S. Powills, "Proliferation of All Payer Systems," *Hospitals* 58, No. 8 (April 16, 1984):28.

14. S. Lewis, "Speculations on the Impact of Prospective Pricing and DRGs," *Western Journal of Medicine* 140, No. 4 (1984):638-644.

15. B. Vladeck, "Restricting the Financing of Health Care: More Stringent Regulation of Utilization," *Bulletin of The New York Academy of Medicine* 60, No. 1 (1984):89-97.

16. P. B. Ginsberg and F. A. Sloan, "Hospital Cost Shifting," *New England Journal of Medicine* 310, No. 14 (April 5, 1984):893-898.

17. C. Coelen and D. Sullivan, "An Analysis of the Effect of Prospective Reimbursement Programs on Hospital Expenditures," *Health Care Financing Review* 2, No. 3 (1981):1-40.

18. F. A. Sloan, "Rate Regulation As a Strategy for Hospital Cost Control: Evidence From the Last Decade," *Milbank Memorial Fund Quarterly* 61 (1981):195-221.

19. Health Insurance Association of America, Prospective Payment. *A Sound Approach to Containing Hospital Costs,* Washington, DC, undated.

20. "Connecticut Eyes Prospective Payment Plan," *American Medical News* 27, No. 17 (May 4, 1984):16.

21. J. A. Meyer, "Cost Shifting—Passing the Health Bucks," *American Medical News* 27, No. 6 (February 10, 1984):28.

22. M. O. Bromberg, Discussant in *Health Care Institution in Flux,* edited by W. Greenberg and R. M. Southby (Arlington, VA: Information Resources Press, 1984), pp. 124-125.

23. D. W. Young and R. B. Saltman, "Preventive Medicine for Hospital Costs," *Harvard Business Review* 61, No. 1 (1983):127-133.

24. "Voluntary All-Payer DRGs Get a Try," *Medical World News* 27, No. 4 (February 24, 1986):108-109.

25. Health Insurance Association of America, *Prospective Payment.*

26. J. Firshein, "All Payer Coalition Backs Medicare Waivers," *Hospitals* 58, No. 22 (November 16, 1984):38.

27. S. McIlrath, "Officials Fear Rush By Voters to All Payer Rate Setting System," *American Medical News* 27, No. 42 (November 9, 1984):1, 41.

28. Ibid.

29. "Bell Encourages States to Develop All Payer Systems," *Modern Healthcare* 14, No. 3 (February 15, 1984):38.

30. C. Wallace, "Kennedy-Gephardt Bill Meets Stiff Opposition," *Modern Healthcare* 14, No. 4 (1984):38.

31. Ibid.

32. Ibid.

33. "HCFA Administrator Blasts Kennedy-Gephardt Proposal," *Modern Healthcare* 14, No. 5 (1984):34.

34. Ibid.

35. "All-Payers System Seen by 1990," *American Medical News* 27, No. 37 (October 5, 1984):22.

36. Ibid.

37. "Insurers Slow to Use DRGs, But Interested," *Hospitals* 58, No. 19 (October 1, 1984):46, 50.

38. Ibid.

39. Ibid.

40. "PPS/DRG Scoreboard for Insurers," *Hospitals* 58, No. 20 (October 16, 1984):52.

41. Ibid.

42. "Kansas Blues Propose DRG Preferred Provider Plan," *Hospitals* 57, No. 6 (March 16, 1983):26.

43. *Blue Cross and Blue Shield of Kansas.* Competitive Allowance Program (CAP). Presentation by M. R. Dauner at BC Member Hospital Forums, Spring 1983. Memo to Kansas Physicians on CAP by G. W. Johnston, 1983. Legal Issues—Letter from Kansas Medical Society by R. T. Foster, 1983. Memo to Hospitals on CAP by R. D. Pearcy, May 16, 1983. Physician and Hospital Contracts, May and June, 1983. FYI, CAP Bulletin, June 1983. Memo to Hospitals: CAP Update by R. D. Pearcy, July 5, 1983. Policies and Procedures for Hospitals in 1984, July 1983. Memo to Physicians on Service Differential Codes and Allowances, August 1983. Memo to General Hospitals. CAP Reminders, December 15, 1983. CAP Newsletter, January 6, 1984.

44. M. E. Rust, "Kansas Blues to Use DRG Pay Plan," *American Medical News* 26, No. 23 (June 17, 1983):1, 8, 9.

45. S. J. Goldowsky, "More on DRGs," (editorial), *Rhode Island Medical Journal* 66, No. 8 (1983):303.

46. "Hospitals Wait, Wonder As Blue Cross of Kansas Prepares Its New DRG Payment

Plan," *Federation of American Hospitals Review* 16, No. 5 (1983):37-38, 40.

47. Ibid.

48. "Blues Plan Adopts DRG Pay System," *American Medical News* 27, No. 14 (April 13, 1984):7.

49. S. Powills, "Blue Cross Plans Use of DRG," *Hospitals* 58, No. 6 (March 16, 1984):20.

50. Ibid.

51. "Michigan Blues Begin Pilot DRG Prospective Pay Plan," *Modern Healthcare* 14, No. 4 (1984):11.

52. F. L. Koehler, Jr., "Impact of DRGs on Blue Cross of New Jersey," in *DRGs: The Effects in N.J. The Potential for the Nation.* HCFA Pub. No. 03170, March 1984, pp. 139-145.

53. R. J. Mellman, "Impact of DRGs on Commercial Insurance Companies," in *DRGs: The Effect in New Jersey. The Potential for the Nation,* HCFA Pub. No. 03170, March 1984, pp. 146-149.

54. Koehler, "Impact on Blue Cross."

55. Mellman, "Impact on Commercial Insurance."

56. "Long-Term Care Alternatives: Innovation in Financing Chronic Care for the Elderly," *Alpha Centerpiece,* May 1984.

57. P. R. Willging, "Viewpoint: Is a Malthusian Crisis on The Way?" *Contemporary Long-Term Care* 8, No. 2 (February, 1985):58.

58. H. Schwartz, "Medicare, Not Mediscare," *New York Times,* January 30, 1986.

59. M. R. Meiners and G. R. Trapnell, "Long-Term Care Insurance, Premium Estimates for Prototype Policies," *Medical Care* 22, No. 10 (1984):901-911.

60. "Ohio Facility Offers Long-Term Care Insurance," *Today's Nursing Home 5,* No. 8 (1984):1, 26, 27.

61. Ibid.

62. *Part V. Medicare Program: Payment to HMOs and Competitive Medical Plans: Final Rule with Comment Period,* U.S. Federal Register 50, No. 7, (January 10, 1985):1314-1418.

63. J. K. Iglehart, "Medicare Turns to HMOs," *New England Journal of Medicine* 312, No. 2 (January 10, 1985):132-136.

64. Part V. Medicare Program, U.S. *Federal Register.*

65. M. Holoweiko, "Will Fee-for-Service Lose Out?" *Medical Economics,* April 29, 1985.

66. Iglehart, "Medicare Turns to HMOs."

67. "Part V. Medicare Program," U.S. *Federal Register.*

68. W. G. Manning, A. Leibowitz, G. A. Goldberg, W. H. Rogers, and J. P. Newhouse, "A Controlled Trial of the Effect of a Prepaid Group Practice on Use of Services," *New England Journal of Medicine* 310, No. 23 (June 7, 1984):1505-1510.

69. R. L. Johnson, "A Second Opinion: The Prospects of Medicare's Hospital Insurance Trust Fund," *Hospital and Health Services Administration* 29, No. 3 (1984):7-25.

70. T. Pyle, *Testimony Before U.S. Senate Subcommittee on Health Hearings on PPS.* Washington, DC, February 17, 1983.

71. R. F. Blomquist, "HMOs and State DRG Hospital Cost Control Programs: The Need for Federal Preemption," *American Journal of Law and Medicine* 10, No. 1 (Spring, 1984):1-29.

72. Holoweiko, "Fee-for-Service."

73. U.S. General Accounting Office. *Problems in Administering Medicare's HMO Demonstration Projects in Florida.* GAO/HRD 85-48, Washington, DC, March 8, 1985.

74. Holoweiko, "Fee-for-Service."

75. K. Hunt, "Uncle Sam Is Tightening The Screws on Them—And You," *Medical Economics,* April 29, 1985.

76. H. Schwartz, "Moving Into the Era of Two-Tier Medicine," *Private Practice* 17, No. 4 (1985):32-33.

77. M. Buenaflor, "More than Dollars and Cents," *Private Practice* 17, No. 4 (1985):49.

78. Schwartz, "Two-Tier Medicine."

79. L. A. Fischer, "Medicare Turns to HMOs: A Caveat" (letter), *New England Journal of Medicine* 312, No. 17 (April 25, 1985):1131-1132.

80. Holoweiko, "Fee-for-Service."

81. "Part V. Medicare Program," U.S. *Federal Register*.

82. R. Whitestone, "U.S. Health Care Sees Robust Profits," *The Home News*, May 19, 1985.

83. M. Freudenheim, "HMO Growth Displays Vigor," *N.Y. Times*, April 16, 1985.

84. "PPS/DRG Scoreboard for Insurers," *Hospitals* 58, No. 20 (October 16, 1984):52.

85. "PPOs Gain in Popularity with Fortune 500 Firms," *Medical World News* 26, No. 8 (April 22, 1985):60.

86. "PPO to be Based on DRG Payments," *American Medical News* 28, No. 4 (January 26, 1985):22.

87. J. Rifter, "Decisions Reflect New Competition," *Hospitals* 57, No. 13 (July 1, 1983):19.

88. "Social HMOs' Problems Tied to Marketing Slips," *Hospitals* 60, No. 4 (February 20, 1986):104.

89. J. Fox, "Acute, Long-Term Care 'Merged'," *U.S. Medicine* 20, No. 19 (October 1, 1984):2, 8, 9.

90. "Medicare to Pay Health Groups in Advance," *New York Times*, January 10, 1985.

91. "Medicare Enrollees Gain 'Extras' With Shift to Prepaid Health Plans," *The Star-Ledger* (N.J.) January 10, 1985.

92. J. K. Inglehart, "Health Policy Report: Medicare Turns to HMOs," *New England Journal of Medicine* 312, No. 2 (January 10, 1985):132-136.

93. "AMA Urges Delay of Medicare Payment Plan," *American Medical News* 28, No. 11 (March 15, 1985):8.

94. C. C. Evans, F. Holden, and J. Speight, "A DRG Based Resource Allocation System for the Veterans Administration," Washington, DC, Mimeo, undated.

95. "VA to Use DRGs in '85," *American Medical News* 27, No. 17 (May 4, 1984):18.

96. "Commission Proposals Under Review," *American Medical News* 27, No. 4 (January 27, 1984):22.

97. "Half of VA's Hospital Days Unnecessary," *U.S. Medicine* 21, No. 6 (March 15, 1985):3-5.

98. Evans, Holden, and Speight, "Resource Allocation System for VA."

99. Ibid.

100. T. Jemison, "Sunbelt Prospering Under VA's DRGs," *U.S. Medicine* 20, No. 8 (April 15, 1984):1, 26, 27.

101. T. Jemison, "VA Prepares to Implement DRG Plan," *U.S. Medicine* 19, No. 23 (December 1, 1983):21.

102. Ibid.

103. "Diagnosis Groups Being Developed for VA Hospitals," *U.S. Medicine* 19, No. 16 (August 15, 1983):18.

104. *Length of Stay Statistics for Utilization Review by DRGs*, Great Lakes Regional Health Services Research and Development Field Program. Ann Arbor, MI: V.A. Medical Center, August 1, 1983.

105. Jemison, "Sunbelt Prospering."

106. J. A. Delisa, "DRGs and Rehab Medicine in the VA," *Archives of Physical Medicine and Rehabilitation* 66, No. 22 (1985):125.

107. "CHAMPUS Using DRGs in One State," *U.S. Medicine* 20, No. 17 (September 1, 1984):15.

108. "CHAMPUS Tries Tying Levels of Payment to DRG Threshold," *U.S. Medicine* 20, No. 14 (July 15, 1984):2, 9.

109. Ibid.

PART IV
REACTIONS TO AND
THE FUTURE OF PPS/DRGs

CHAPTER 11
Quality of Care:
Critical Issues

Deterioration in the quality of care is anticipated under systems of financing which are designed to respond to productivity and efficiency rather than patient needs and satisfaction. Management is rewarded for decisions by physicians and clinicians who react to pressures from utilization review committees, discharge planners, and complex computer analysis of peer profiles, rather than for diagnostic accuracy, therapeutic triumphs, and salubrious outcomes of the patients' episode of illness.

The DRG payment system changes the incentives for hospital and physician behavior. Under the previous reasonable-cost reimbursement system, there were no incentives to limit services provided by hospitals and physicians to as many patients as possible, since the more services provided, the larger the reimbursement. Under the new DRG system, Medicare pays a fixed amount per DRG; some fear this may encourage financial manipulations that ensure institutional solvency and create consequences in medical care delivery which have severe implications for quality of care.[1]

Areas of concern include appropriateness of admission, proper application of diagnostic tests, procedures and therapeutic modalities, hospital stay review in accordance with norms for the diagnosis, and accurate assignment of the DRGs for reimbursement purposes.

Medical decision-making processes that show different patterns from peer practitioners are critical elements for audit. Among the areas scrutinized are the following: alternatives to care; efficiency in the process of care delivery; increased morbidity and mortality; post-discharge experiences; readmissions; post-hospital mortality; and interinstitutional transfer review. While the HHS believes that medical ethical standards and fear of malpractice suits will inhibit undesirable behavior, physicians fear an increase of malpractice suits if patients become suspicious of patterns of practice, if they believe they have incomplete workups or treatment, or if they have unfavorable outcomes.

Hospitals are expected to limit their financial liabilities by altering their service capabilities, which leads to inadequately staffed services and curtailed acquisition of new technology unless related to cost savings. The shift from "more is better" to "less is more" focuses on cost containment[2] rather than attention to health care access and delivery; this may assault and impinge on quality of care.

Is Quality of Care Affected?

Organized representatives of physicians and of consumer groups emphasize the detriment to quality of care under the DRG system; policy makers and government officials can point to no such measurable effects of the DRGs.

In a speech at the U.S. House of Representatives' Select Committee on Aging on March 29, 1983, Charles F. Pierce, Deputy Commissioner, New Jersey State Department of Health, indicated concern that the "quality care would suffer if patients were discharged too early or used fewer tests or other resources." But, he said that "New Jersey has found no evidence that quality of care has diminished under the DRG system."[3] Patient satisfaction is similarly debated and the physician is criticized most heavily, though not in specific terms.

Chuck Hardwick, an Assemblyman for the State of New Jersey, said, "New Jersey cannot substantiate that health care quality has been maintained. With lower DRG reimbursement levels planned nationwide, maintaining high quality care will be even more difficult."[4]

In defense of the prospective pricing system, Robert J. Rubin, M.D., HHS Assistant Secretary for Planning and Evaluation, said: "We are confident in our ability to deal with rising health care costs without compromising quality."[5] He also said that government studies indicate that quality of care has not been affected in states that have regulated reimbursement.[6]

However, Alfred A. Alessi, M.D., AMA delegate from the New Jersey State Medical Society, discussed the impact of DRGs in that state. He said: "Some data indicate an increase in liability cases because patients are being discharged too early."[7]

The GAO report released by Senator John Heinz (R-PA), Chairman of the Senate Special Committee on Aging, said that many elderly patients are "being sent out into a no-care zone, without access to the health care they so urgently need."[8] The reduced length of stay in hospital has led to patients leaving the hospital "quicker and sicker."

Responding to this, Clay Mickel, a spokesman of the AHA said: "We have seen no indications . . . that the system is resulting in a serious diminution of quality."[9]

The Select Committee on Aging of the House of Representatives reviewed the report of a state-by-state survey by state nursing home ombudsmen, which indicated that patients are discharged sicker or much sicker than before the new system of payments went into effect. There was also evidence that in rural areas the skilled nursing care is not adequate to meet the needs of the discharged patients.[10]

In hearings in February 1985 on Sustaining Quality Health Care Under Cost Containment, Chairman Edward R. Roybal said: "American senior citizens are telling me that they greatly fear that cost containment is really becoming care containment." He added: "If the administration's latest cost-containment proposals are enacted, quality of care will be further jeopardized. Even now, virtually nothing is being done to ensure that quality is sustained."[11]

Dennis Siebert at HCFA insisted, "We've said in the past that we've seen no consistent evidence of sicker patients being discharged or early discharges. Peer review organizations are in place, with a specific mandate to guard against that."[12]

In addition, HCFA Administrator Carolyne Davis testified and took issue with the GAO report which was extremely negative and "cited stable mortality and readmission rates . . . a National Center for Health Statistics study of nine high volume procedures for which institutions have pooled high-technology and high-cost services shows a 13 percent decrease in mortality."[13]

Physicians at the Medical Society of New Jersey convention on May 4, 1985 claimed that their hospital payment system is having a "dire effect on the quality of care in New Jersey." There was reluctance to document these accusations for fear of potential exposure to malpractice, but they cited pressures for early discharge and intimidation concerning their pattern of practice.[14]

It is "unreal, even impossible, to expect that steep reductions can be made in projected expenditures for government health programs . . . without cutting into the quality and availability of care for the patients involved," said James H. Sammons, M.D., executive vice-president of the American Medical Association.[15]

Deep concern "on the ability of physicians and hospitals to assure the availability of high quality health care services for the Medicare" population was voiced in testimony by the American Medical Association (AMA) to the House Select Committee on Aging. There was opposition to a freeze on hospital reimbursement unless it could be shown "that access to and quality of care would not be adversely affected." Also in question were the problems inherent in the limitation of, introduction of, and availability of, medical technology because of costs.[16]

To monitor quality of care issues and the impact of the DRG system on patients, hospitals, and physicians, the AMA has instituted a DRG Monitoring Project. In a response to survey questionnaires, "37 percent were positive in stating that quality had not yet deteriorated. 63 percent stated that quality had deteriorated or that it would deteriorate over time if the PPS continued."[17] Negative responses fell into three major categories: complicated hospital stay/readmissions, early discharge, and limitations on testing. "We are afraid that budget proposals before this Congress could jeopardize the high quality of care currently available for Medicare beneficiaries and other members of our Society."[18]

The American Hospital Association's (AHA) position is that:

> While there has been no evidence that cost containment thus far has undercut quality, we are reaching the point where continued pressure for cost reductions will begin to raise quality concerns . . . if the system is manipulated simply to produce short-term budget savings, the result will be a reduced ability by hospitals to provide services to the elderly.[19]

FAH executive director Bromberg also agreed that PPS hadn't compromised quality "—at least not yet."[20]

Professor John Thompson of Yale University, one of the researchers who developed the coding system for DRGs, has some reservations about the quality issues. He said that with prospective pricing and DRGs, "we are substituting an ephemeral idea of quality of care, and changing the relationship between quality and cost in a pretty critical situation." There are implicit decisions in that specifying a price on a DRG will likely affect how care is provided under that DRG, and unfortunately, "even those who made the decisions don't understand them."[21] In fact, HHS expelled a hospital from the Medicare program in 1986 for the first time under the PRO system. That edict to the San Diego County Hillcrest Mental Health Facility stated that it "substantially failed to comply with the obligation to provide a quality of care that meets professionally recognized standards in a substantial number of cases."[22]

Monitoring Quality of Care

Peer Review Organizations (PROs)

Federal mechanisms have been mandated to monitor and assure quality of care under the DRG system. Utilization and Quality Control Peer Review Organizations (PROs) are the designated medical review entities (MREs) responsible for determining the medical necessity, appropriateness, and quality of care of Medicare admissions. As part of this responsibility, PROs also perform DRG validation. Promises and pitfalls for PROS were reviewed in a special article in the *New England Journal of Medicine* by Dans, Weiner, and Otter that concentrated on the quality of care.[23]

Contracting process.   HCFA specified the requirements for quality assurance review activities and quality of care objectives to be achieved by each PRO in contract form. Each PRO is obligated to conduct meaningful quality review and achieve significant impact on quality of care furnished to Medicare beneficiaries.[24]

All hospitals participating in Medicare are mandated to contract for review services with the PRO designated for their area as a condition of their participation in the program. The PRO review is considered as Part A hospital cost. However, the costs for the PRO program are charged directly to the Health Insurance Trust Fund and not to the program management budget, both of which previously supported PSROs. The PRO funding levels included in the FY 1985 budget are $40 million in FY 1984 and $171 million in FY 1985.[25]

Request for Proposal (RFP No. HCFA-84-015) for the program appeared February 29, 1984, and the proposals by contractors for statewide PRO activities were mandated to incorporate the specified review system components:[26]

- Admission review (medical necessity and appropriateness)

- Procedure review (to screen operating room procedures for necessity)

- Admission pattern monitoring (to determine if increased admission rates or short-stay admissions are medically necessary and appropriate)

- Outlier review (to determine whether the stay as a whole contains noncovered or medically unnecessary or inappropriate days or services)

- DRG validation (to assure that the DRG assigned is proper)

- Coverage review (to assure application of all technical and medical coverage rules to the claims made for covered services under Medicare).

Contention and controversy were part of the evolving process of establishing the PROs, as organizations vied for public recognition and for contract dollars. By June 1984, HCFA had awarded the first contract. It rejected proposals from 15 states as technically unacceptable because of the inadequacies of the database, the contractual relationships described, and the goals and objectives set. In 13 states there was only one application, which may not have met HCFA standards.

Contract bids were evaluated on a point system designed to stimulate certain organizational advantages and proposed activities. A maximum of 1,000 points rewarded objectives controlling hospital admissions and quality of care, data collection, and analysis. To stimulate participation by the medical societies and PSROs, there were additional points for experience and quality of personnel management for the proposed PRO. Criteria concerning specific norms of care against which the reviewed cases were screened and use of subcontractors were critical elements for the award by HCFA.[27]

Most of the PRO contracts (32) were awarded to professional standards review organizations (PSROs) which had been reviewing Medicare hospitalizations prior to the PRO development. However, nine medical societies were awarded contracts: Indiana, Maryland, Missouri, Nebraska, New York, North Carolina, Oklahoma, Texas, and Virginia.

In Michigan, Florida, and California, state medical societies lost the contracts to other bidders. The Michigan Medical Society was unsuccessful against the professional standards review organization group based in Ann Arbor.[28]

The Florida Medical Society lost the $15 million contract to the Tampa-based Professional Foundation for Health Care, Inc., and protested the contracting process, using the Freedom of Information Act in federal district court to obtain documents from HCFA. The contention was based on problems with the database, unrealistic objectives, and excessive targets.

The $27 million contract to California Medical Review, Inc. (CMRI) ended the three-way competition with United Foundations for Medical Care and the California Medical Association subsidiary, called the California Peer Review Organization (CPRO). The issues here involved who would have access to medical records for review, the inexperience of staff, and the variety of subcontractors.[29]

The National Capital Medical Care Foundation for the District of Columbia lost the contract to the Delmarva Foundation for Medical Care, which is a Maryland-based organization which had lost the Maryland PRO to the Maryland Medical Society. This out-of-state reviewing PRO was one of seven to gain contracts outside their geographic area:

- Washington PRO will also review Alaska.

- Montana PRO will also review Wyoming.

- New Hampshire PRO will also review Vermont.

- Rhode Island PRO will also review Maine.

- Arizona PRO will also review Hawaii and Pacific Islands of Guam and Samoa.

Two for-profit groups also were awarded contracts: The Arizona PRO (Arizona Health Services Advisory Group in Phoenix) and the Pennsylvania Peer Review Organization (PaPRO) in Camp Hill, for their respective states.[30]

Negotiations for the Idaho PRO were extremely complex; the Idaho Foundation for Medical Care (IFMC), a subsidiary of the Idaho Medical Foundation, was in contention with HCFA on estimates of hospitalization rates, goals, total costs, price for each claim, and so on. HCFA had previous problems with Idaho—one of six states where the PSRO had been a failure—and was unsuccessful in convincing another state to take on the contract or to get the modifications necessary. In the end, HCFA demanded that the Medicare intermediary, the Idaho Blue Cross and Blue Shield plan, take on the contract with a $1.3 million spending limit, and this became the only such intermediary with PRO functions.[31]

Goals and objectives. Multiple objectives, their validation, and methods of approaching and achieving the goals were in the proposals made by each PRO. Selected activities required of PROs appear in Exhibit 11-1.

Quantification of expected performance was negotiated for each PRO. Examples follow:[32,33]

- The New York contract requires the agency to reduce by 514 the number of avoidable deaths with the diagnosis of pneumococcal, aspiration, and bacterial pneumonia.

- Connecticut PRO objectives include one to reduce by 20 percent over a two-year period the number of postoperative urinary tract infections from the use of postoperative Foley catheters in six surgical procedures.

- In New Jersey, the reduction in congestive heart failure readmissions is specified in the PRO contract by potentially reducing substandard care during previous admissions.

- Tennessee (Mid-South Foundations for Medical Care PRO) proposed a 13.25 percent reduction in elective hospital admissions over two years.

- Kentucky PRO proposes a 8.1 percent reduction in admissions.

- South Carolina Medical Care Foundation proposes a 568 admission reduction involving 80 physicians specifically identified.

Specificity about the admission and mortality reduction goals incorporated into contracts (Exhibits 11-2, 11-3) has organized hospital and physician interests who protest against these targets as "quotas" and "rationing" actions. Criticism by the Federation of American Hospitals (FAH) and the AHA have surfaced.[34,35]

Attempts to diffuse charges about these state quotas have not been effective. Carolyne Davis, HCFA administrator, "insisted that the objectives should be viewed as targets and not quotas."[36]

However, Alan R. Nelson, M.D., associated with the Utah PRO, warned, "In practice, these objectives might have the effect of encouraging an overzealous PRO to deny appropriate as well as inappropriate admissions in order to meet its contract objectives."[37]

At the AMA House of Delegates meeting in Honolulu, it was agreed that the organization should work closely with the AHA "to promote a cooperative physician-hospital partnership to mitigate the adverse impact of HCFA utilization

Exhibit 11-1   Selected Activities Required of PROs

I. Selected Admission Objectives and Required Activities

A. Reduce admissions for procedures that could be performed effectively and safely in an ambulatory surgical setting or on an outpatient basis.

B. Reduce the number of inappropriate or unnecessary admissions or invasive procedures for specific DRGs.

C. Reduce the number of inappropriate or unnecessary admissions or invasive procedures by specific practitioners or in specific hospitals.

D. Review (before admission or before procedure) every elective case for five procedure-related DRGs (from a state-specific list of the top 20 procedures or procedure-specific DRGs for 1982).

E. Review admissions occurring within seven days of a discharge and deny all claims for inappropriate admissions.

F. Review every permanent cardiac pacemaker implantation or reimplantation procedure and deny payment for all that are unnecessary.

G. Review transfers from a PPS hospital to other hospitals or to specific PPS-exempt special units or swing beds.

H. Perform Admission Pattern Monitoring.

II. Quality Objectives

A. Reduce unnecessary hospital readmissions resulting from substandard care provided during the prior admission.

B. Assure the provision of medical services which, when not performed, have "significant potential" (occurrence in 5 percent or more of cases) for causing "serious patient complications" (as in the PSRO evaluation criteria noted earlier).

C. Reduce avoidable deaths.

D. Reduce unnecessary surgery or other invasive procedures.

E. Reduce avoidable postoperative or other complications.

III. Other Required Activities

A. DRG validation.

B. Review every case involving day and/or cost outliers for necessity and appropriateness of admission and subsequent care.

Source: K. N. Lohr and R. H. Brook, *Quality Assurance in Medicine* (The Rand Corporation, Santa Monica, CA, October 1984).

Exhibit 11-2 New York PRO: Inappropriate Admission Reviews

Admission Objective Area I—Reduce the number of inappropriate or unnecessary admissions or invasive procedures by specific practitioners or in specific hospitals.

Objective Statement

Reduce 7,460 inappropriate or unnecessary admissions for procedures on the Foundation's Outpatient/Ambulatory Procedures List which can be safely and effectively performed in an outpatient or ambulatory setting.

Validation

The primary concern of this objective is to identify those admissions where the procedure itself caused the admission. Therefore, the Foundation developed the following criteria to delete cases which are not part of the problem, (e.g., cases with length of stay greater than 4 days, patients over age 85, admissions where the procedure on the Outpatient Ambulatory Procedures List was not the principal procedure, and all deaths). In addition, some of the remaining procedures were eliminated from consideration as being medically necessary. The total number of the identified procedures statewide before applying the above criteria was 60,404 or 8.2% of all admissions. After applying the criteria, 1.4% or 9947 cases of all admissions were listed as questionable admissions. Those 9,947 cases will be reviewed and a 75% reduction in these admissions should be realized.

Primary Methodology

The Foundation will notify area hospitals of its intention to review, furnish them with a list of the identified procedures and provide the criteria for the review. A 100% retrospective chart review of all the identified procedures will be performed. If a physician advisor determines that either the hospitalization and/or the procedure is medically unnecessary, a denial will be made, a determination will be made regarding the waiver of liability and ultimately, sanctions initiated. If anticipated changes (i.e. reductions in unnecessary or inappropriate admissions), are not being made, the PRO will develop and implement hospital specific corrective action plans, e.g. prepayment review.

The PRO will monitor the retrospective chart review on an ongoing basis and will review milestones and intervention methodologies quarterly.

Admission Objective Area II—Reduce the number of inappropriate or unnecessary admissions or invasive procedures by specific practitioners or in specific hospitals.

Objective Statement

Reduce by 39,235 the number of unnecessary admissions for selected one and two day stays which would not be expected to require hospitalization.

Validation

The statewide norm for the percent of one and two day stays admitted to the hospital is 7.6%. The Foundation intends to focus on those hospitals which exceed this norm. In the second year of the contract a new statewide norm will be calculated and targets adjusted.

In selecting the short stays which will be reviewed the PRO relied on studies which have indicated that short stays with Class I procedures tend to be medically justifiable. Therefore, neither these cases nor those short stays with death will be reviewed. It is estimated that 53,995 cases will be reviewed at targeted hospitals as part of this objective. Note— The actual reduction for this objective is arrived at by removing those reductions achieved as part of Admission Objective I.

Exhibit 11-2   (contd.)

Primary Methodology
   The Foundation will notify area hospitals of its intention to review, furnish them with a list of the identified procedures and provide the criteria for the review. A 100% retrospective chart review of all the identified procedures will be performed. If a physician advisor determines that either the hospitalization and/or the procedure is medically unnecessary, a denial will be made. If applicable, a determination will be made regarding waiver of liability and sanctions initiated.

   If anticipated reductions in unnecessary admissions for these procedures, are not being made, the PRO will develop and implement hospital specific corrective action plans, e.g. prepayment review. The PRO will monitor the retrospective chart review on an ongoing basis and will review milestones and intervention methodologies quarterly.

Source: Empire State Medical Scientific and Educational Foundation, Inc., Lake Success, NY, 1984.

Exhibit 11-3   New York PRO: Mortality Reduction

Quality Objective Area II—Reduce avoidable deaths.

Objective Statement
   Reduce by 514 the number of avoidable deaths with the diagnosis of pneumococcal, aspiration and bacterial pneumonia.

Validation
   In 1982, there were 5,040 cases of patients over 65 years of age admitted to hospitals with the principal diagnosis of pneumococcal, bacterial or aspiration pneumonia. 1,028 (20.4%) of these patients died. Three PSRO-area studies conducted between 1982 and 1984 found that of 1,453 cases reviewed, 313 (22%) died and of these, 78 (25%) deaths were found to be preventable. Based on the 25% of deaths which were found to be avoidable in the study, 25% deaths/year for this diagnosis are preventable statewide (.25 $\times$ 1028 = 257).

Primary Methodology
   Intensive physician education on the clinical signs and symptoms of pneumonia in the elderly will begin immediately, the importance of several preventive interventions will be underscored. All pneumococcal aspiration and bacteremic mortalities will be identified for retrospective review. Findings will be compiled in generic categories by hospital and physician patterns. If patterns are identified, hospitals will be notified of the problem and required to report all admissions with the diagnosis of pneumonia on a timely basis. Concurrent review will be initiated for these identified cases. Continued failure by a provider or practitioner to meet quality standards will lead to a sanction process.

   Review findings will be monitored monthly by the PRO. In addition, objective goals and milestones will be evaluated quarterly.

Source: Empire State Medical Scientific and Educational Foundation, Inc., Lake Success, NY, 1984.

review regulations.'' In addition, they agreed to ''actively oppose HCFA's use of arbitrary admission and quality objectives in the activities of PROs,'' and to monitor PRO activities to obtain documentation to redress problems through legislative and regulatory means.[38]

AHA is supportive of effective utilization review programs and backs the use of physician-sponsored peer review to evaluate medical care provided to Medicare patients.[39]

A legal suit against HHS was instituted by the American Hospital Association on January 29, 1985, in reaction to the PRO contract's goal of reducing Medicare admissions by 1.25 million over two years. AHA President Alex McMahon contends that such numerical objectives have ''created an environment conducive to inappropriate or excessive payment denials by PROs.''

In addition, the suit challenged ''the lack of public accountability in implementing this important program'' and lack of public comment on development of goals and objectives and the contracts. The suit is considered procedural only and did not try to postpone or halt the operation of the PRO.[40,41]

Operational issues. In order to monitor performance at the hospitals within the PRO jurisdiction of prime contractors or respective subcontractors for various geographic divisions, reviews are made of random samples of hospital records. For the New York PRO the following percentage of total Medicare admissions is required:[42,43]

Admission Review	5.0%
Admission Objective	1.0%
Prepayment admission review for specified diagnoses	0.5%
Validation of diagnostic and procedural information	3.0%
Permanent cardiac pacemaker implantation	100%
Admission pattern monitoring	1.5%
Quality review target	5.7%

Reviews are performed through use of nurses for abstracting case reports with final reviews and appeal reviews by physicians. Changes are encouraged from the providers and physicians by the threat to withhold Medicare payments for services rendered—Medicare denials. Performance records of PROs will be used at the time for renegotiation of contracts and HCFA can refuse to review contracts, seek another agency, and refuse to pay for the incurred expenses.

Early results suggest that the impact of Medicare denials has been more costly to hospitals and physicians than critics feared. For the first quarter of 1985,

- New Jersey PRO denied payment to hospitals in 7 percent of the admissions reviewed.

- New York City and Long Island admissions reviews yielded 14 percent in denials, with the rest of New York State at 11 percent.[43]

HCFA officials say that the denial rate nationwide was 2.5 percent last year and that the agency would call into question any PRO that had an abnormally high denial rate. However, the vice president of reimbursement for the Hospital Corporation of America said that some of their hospitals had higher denial rates.[44]

Hospitals, in turn, are placing physicians on notice of denials of payments by Medicare, notifying them of the reasons for the denials, and educating them in appropriate criteria for patient admissions under Medicare, for appropriate documentation and participation in the utilization review process. The letter from the Director of Mount Sinai Hospital to physicians on staff urges them to become familiar with the PRO program requirements before sanctions for noncompliance are implemented (see Exhibit 11-4). Sanctions in several hospitals range from temporary suspension or limiting of admitting privileges, to permanent withdrawal of privileges, using the reappointment process of annual credential review.

If the PROs are successful in the next two years, more than one million hospital admissions will be eliminated. Some 595,000 surgeries will be shifted from the inpatient side to ambulatory settings; more than 425,000 admissions to specific hospitals will be eliminated; and 290,000 unnecessary or inappropriate admissions or procedures will be eliminated. In addition, 32,000 complications and 6,000 deaths will be averted.

Public information controversy.   Denials of Medicare payments made to hospitals eventually result in patients receiving a "letter of denial" which indicates that their insurance coverage may or will cease for their current inpatient stay. Similar letters are sent to patients when it is determined that they do not need to be in a hospital any longer and may need alternate institutional or home care. According to one patient care coordinator, "Patients, particularly the elderly, react to the letters with confusion and anger . . . they think they have insurance coverage that's going to cover the whole world, and they don't really understand the system."[45] This information to patients about their hospital stay not only brings consternation to patients but is a cause of great concern to physicians and the treasured "doctor/patient relationship."

Dr. Thomas G. Delin, vice-president of the American Medical Peer Review Association, said that the PRO objectives, though laudable, have severe medical liability implications and "are politically volatile with its presumption of widespread negligence."[46]

At the heart of the issue is the controversy over the kinds of information to be made available to the public, to consumers or patients, to hospitals, and to

Exhibit 11-4   Letter to Physicians on Medical Staff from Hospital Director, Mount Sinai Hospital, New York

Admission and patient day denials will threaten as much as $3 million of hospital revenues during 1985. Our first two monthly reviews by the PRO have resulted in the denial of 550 Medicare days, or 16.7% of the nearly 3300 patient days reviewed.

Our efforts to control this problem are focused on educating the Medical Staff with regard to:

1. The criteria used by the PRO to review Medicare admissions and to deny payments.
2. The critical need for physician documentation in the chart of why each patient day is medically necessary.
3. Your obligation to respond promptly to calls from our utilization review coordinators (RN's) and physician advisors (MD's).

In March, the Medical Board will be voting on a program of sanctions for physicians whose hospital utilization results in PRO payment denials and for physicians who fail to respond to calls from our Utilization Review Department on a timely basis. The determination of inappropriate utilization will be subject to an internal review by our physician advisors of final PRO denials.

I urge you to take this opportunity, before a sanction program is implemented, to learn more about the PRO program requirements. It is in your interest, and that of the hospital, for you to do this promptly. Quality Assurance has already made initial presentations on PRO to the staff of each program department. They will be glad to further discuss with you the review process and the criteria which apply to the diagnoses or procedures for which you admit your patients. Please feel free to contact Ms. Joan Bass, Quality Assurance administrator, for any further information you may need. Ms. Bass can be reached on extension 7981.

Thank you for your cooperation.

Source: Personal Communication, April 1985.

individual physicians about findings of the PRO. On behalf of consumers and purchasers of health care, the president of the AARP said, "Health care consumers need the type of information that will allow them to make better informed decisions. You have that information and we want it."[47]

Similar sentiments have been voiced by business coalition groups, corporate employers, and insurers in the private sector who wish to use hospital-specific and physician-specific data to help reduce risks, contain expenditures, and effectively refer and channel their employees or clients.[48]

The AMA fears that release of specific data would jeopardize the confidentiality of information obtained by the PRO.[49] Provider institutions have privacy rights as well as patients and practitioners, according to the AHA, which suggests that the massive data collection "would create a means for the federal government to establish a national dossier on all health care providers and many patients."[50]

New rules were promulgated by the federal government in April 1985, rejecting the opposition by organized groups of physicians and institutions which attempt to narrow the disclosure of information. PROs will disclose data which shows, for each hospital:

- Mortality rate for different types of surgery
- Number of patients with postoperative infections
- Average length of hospital stay
- Cost and volume of various procedures.

Hospitals and departments of hospitals will be identified but the names of individual patients and physicians will not be disclosed. In addition, before disclosing hospital specific data, hospitals will have a 30-day period to comment; these comments must be attached to the information for disclosure. Predictably, the physicians and hospitals decry these rules while business groups and unions herald the ability to get the PRO data and make quality of care a public issue.[51]

On March 11, 1986, HHS released a list of hospitals throughout the nation that had mortality rates that were higher or lower than average for a five percent sample of Medicare patients using 1983 and 1984 discharge data.[52] All assurances to the contrary, protests from the medical and health care professions were swift and to the point. Jack Owen, executive vice president of the AHA, commented: "It's the dumbest thing I've seen HHS do."[53] Dr. Sidney Wolfe of the Public Citizens Health Research Group stated: "We've been waiting for this for a long time. . . . We're not worried about misuse of the data; people are too bright to do that."[54]

Caveats and explanations were offered concerning the validity of the data and the variability in patients seen in different hospitals along with the levels of services available in specific institutions.[55-59] It was generally agreed that trends would emerge which might require specific investigation by the PRO and others. A consensus evolved that these initial data were "suggestive and not conclusive."[60]

There is some protection from liability for institutions, physicians, and others who act in accordance with standards and norms specified under the DRG assumptions even, when an early or premature discharge of a patient subsequently causes harm. The malpractice exemption in Section 1157(c) of the Social Security Act provides, "No doctor . . . and no provider . . . of health services shall be civilly liable to any person under any law of the United States or of any State . . . on account of any action taken by him in compliance with or reliance upon professionally developed norms of care and treatment applied by (a PRO) . . ." as long as the action was part of the respective professional activities and that "he exercised due care in conduct reasonably related to and resulting from actions taken in compliance with or reliance upon such norms."[61] However, malpractice suits, case law, and data have not yet had time to accumulate to offer security about the lack of risk of liability under DRG.

Super PRO

Monitoring the PRO activities of the 54 designated areas (one for each state, District of Columbia, Puerto Rico, and the Pacific Islands of Guam and Samoa) to assure their contractual compliance to the performance-based goals is to be carried out by still another contractor. HCFA wishes to assure that the increased power of the PROs (compared to the PSROs) will not be injudiciously applied. There are reports that hospitals and physicians have been angered by the insensitivity of PRO staff in written communications and the process of review. The Super PRO would oversee all PRO activities and would also evaluate and monitor the progress of the prospective payment system as a whole.

Four responses to the initial request for contractors were all turned down: American Medical Association, Michigan Health Care Review, Inc. (a former PSRO), Iowa Foundation, and National Medical Audit, Inc. in California.[62] In the second round of bidding, SysteMetrics, Inc. of Santa Barbara, California, was awarded the $2 million contract for 14 months with a $1.3 million 10-month renewal contingency.

The Super PRO will provide quarterly evaluations of the PROs and monthly reports on the "consistency" and "appropriateness" of the medical review decision process. It will also be called on to verify PRO physicians' determinations of denials.[63] Although initial review of identified records will be by nurses and other nonphysicians in the PROs, denials of payment must have a PRO physicians' approval. Participation by physicians working as consultants or reviewers is expected to enhance the effect on physicians practices.

Displeasure with the management of some of the PRO agencies has already surfaced. PROs which were not formerly PSROs have had difficulties in start-up, development of the databases, staffing, and have experienced review delays. The Pennsylvania Peer Review Organization (PaPRO), one of the two for-profit contractors, has had payments withheld by HCFA, when after the first five months there was a backlog of over 50,000 claims and major limitations of the scope of the reviews.[64] Data processing problems with the subcontractors, toll-free telephone installation delays, and personnel problems have occurred in other PROs; the PaPRO has had their operations shut down as well as the PRO in Massachusetts. In disputes over data entries, the South Carolina Medical Care Foundation (SCMCF) voluntarily initiated a cancellation of its $3.7 million contract with HCFA.[65] In other PRO areas, HCFA is considering the possibility of termination of these contracts, rebidding, and/or getting the fiscal intermediaries more involved as alternatives. By July 1986, 15 of the 54 PRO contracts will need to be renewed or rebid to continue under HCFA. Negotiations will focus on plans to address a new scope of work and concentrate on HCFA and PRO-identified problem areas.[66] The "Super PRO" agencies could continually monitor these problem areas for HCFA.

Hospital Coping Strategies Affecting Quality

Limiting Availability of Care

Hospitals are anticipated to curtail certain "expensive" services in favor of more profitable areas. While this may be done to fine-tune hospital operations to the DRG reimbursement scheme, this strategy may have a significant effect in limiting the range of services available in the community or region.

Frank Mahoney, executive director of the Area I-PSRO in Madison, New Jersey, is concerned that "some hospitals might curtail needed services to patients, thereby cutting costs and increasing profits."[67] This would limit availability of certain services or concentrate certain services in specific institutions. The afflicted patients whose illnesses are categorized by certain DRGs may have to travel longer or delay care longer, based on lack of availability of services; this impinges on the quality of their care.

Others have argued that concentrating certain diagnostic and therapeutic abilities in select institutions can heighten quality of care since staff expertise and experience have been shown to affect morbidity and mortality outcomes. Examples such as cardiac surgery, cardiac catheterization, burn centers, trauma centers, pediatric inpatient units, and so on, have been very effective in this regard.

At a 1983 press conference announcing the new PPS regulations, Medicare officials said they were convinced that the new system would not lead to a deterioration of the quality of care.

In addition, they hoped that hospitals would start "specializing in things they do most efficiently and dropping services they cannot provide as economically as another hospital." While some believe this will diminish access to some types of care, Robert Rubin, M.D., former assistant secretary of planning and evaluation for HHS, said: "Studies had shown that quality of care is improved when a hospital performs a procedure with some frequency."[68]

Citing the March 11, 1986 mortality statistics released by HHS, consumers and health professionals alike agreed that the data "clearly show that people who undergo surgery at hospitals where the procedure is performed infrequently are more likely to die."[69] Although studies have usually used open heart surgery as an indicator of this phenomenon, "the new data show for the first time that the thesis appears to be true for many other procedures as well."[70]

Edmund J. Mihalski, professional staff member of the Senate Finance Committee, is similarly concerned that "in reducing costs, potentially maximizing profits, of course, there is a real worry that hospitals would also reduce the amount of care and, therefore, the quality of care provided to their patients. . . . Hospitals could do that through early discharges, inappropriate admissions, or by simply providing less care than a patient would need."[71]

Diagnostic testing is under close scrutiny along with the newer imaging technologies: "Are CAT scans necessary in patients who have mild headaches with no unusual features? Do the 40 percent of pregnant women now being scanned by ultrasound really need this evaluation? How often is radionuclide scanning really necessary in diagnosis? How many routine chest X-rays are needed in the absence of specific indications?"[72]

Freedom to order diagnostic tests which others deem "unnecessary" and to do procedures which others deem "unnecessary" impedes a physician's clinical practice and may hinder full diagnostic workups. Physicians may be denied access for their patients and may be barred from continuing hospital privileges if they do not conform to expected norms by limiting the extent of care and ordering of tests. Quality of care may be impeded by these cost-conscious efforts:

> Therapy must not only be effective, but cost-effective. It is inherent in such a system that patients or their families be left out of the decision-making process affecting their care, because they will expect treatments or tests that the hospital will argue are unnecessary. So patients, long believing they are entitled to the best care money can buy, are unlikely to receive such care. Most patients will not even realize that when they are denied certain treatment, the cost accountant will have determined that treatment was not cost-effective and thus unnecessary. . . . Patients will grow suspicious of being denied needed care. When an exploratory operation is suddenly called off, will it be because the hospital doesn't want to pay for it?[73]

In a recent interview, Margaret Heckler commented: "An excessive degree of laboratory tests and unnecessary treatments really might protect the physician from unwarranted litigation but it does impose a very heavy burden in terms of the patient or the government, whoever might be paying the bill. So there has to be some equity between the two." She added, "The average American is becoming very concerned and anxious about affordability of health care. We desperately need to have physicians become a part of preserving quality care, including all necessary testing, while working to make medical care much more affordable."[74]

Decisions relating to use of the limited beds in intensive care units, dialysis machines, cobalt therapy, or the diagnostic technologies of CAT scanners and NMRs raise the specter of "rationing" of medical care. "For the renal patient who dies, the victim of angina in pain, the person with misdiagnosed head injuries, alternate treatments, albeit good for the budget, are not good."[75]

Dr. William B. Schwartz, professor of medicine at Tufts University and coauthor of the book *The Painful Prescription: Rationing Health Care* believes, "We've got a menu of goodies but finite resources, and we may have to ration those goodies."

He believes the era of a physician's being able to offer a patient anything that might help is over and that "the era of choosing what to forego for which patients on the basis of a benefits curve is upon us." Also, "To the extent that DRGs set dollar limits on care that won't permit the use of expensive technology for certain categories of patients, that system will be effecting a degree of rationing."[76] As an example, Dr. Schwartz cites: "A 20-year-old who sustains massive injuries in an auto accident and requires an enormous outlay of intensive care resources to live would be much higher on the benefits curve than would a 70-year-old cancer patient in the same accident."[77]

When asked if the federal policy to cover liver transplants in children but not in adults were not a form of rationing, Dr. John E. Marshall, director of the National Center for Health Services Research, acknowledged that the "government does engage in rationing, though we are not overt in admitting it."[78]

Arthur L. Caplan, an associate for the humanities at Hastings Center, in a letter to the *New York Times*, says, "There is still no single government agency that has the responsibility for deciding what treatment are and are not efficacious in the war against illness and disease. The control of health care costs requires both financial prudence and efficiency to be both morally and medically sound."[79] He also indicates, "Rationing has been present for sometime in our hospitals, as anyone who visits a crowded intensive-care unit in one of our large urban hospitals can readily attest."[80]

Extending life for those in coma or disease states known to be progressive and terminal has cost implications which posit ethical and moral dilemmas to health practitioners. John Gigliotti, executive vice-president of United Hospitals, Inc., indicates, "The issue for the elderly, is how much resource shall society dedicate to an individual in their last days. . . . From an economic point of view the marginal contribution to society from these expenditures is negligible. From a moral, ethical point of view we will remain dedicated to preserving the dignity and quality of life."[81]

Delaying Introduction of New Technology and Innovations

Medical technology has far exceeded the capabilities of most institutions to introduce these innovations in a prompt and timely manner. However, because of the reimbursement structure, hospitals will be under further constraints to delay acquisitions unless scrutinized as cost saving or more efficient. This has implications for quality of patient care because many innovations cannot pass the efficiency test but are better for patients.

Michael D'Agnes, vice-president of finance at the Medical Center of Princeton, is concerned because the hospital recently added two expensive technologies, a CAT scanner and digital radiographic equipment. That equipment can reduce the need for more hazardous arteriograms. He said, "If a hospital delays getting this equipment because of the lack of (additional) reimbursement, I think the patient suffers."[82]

Another example relates to changing medical technology, improved treatments, and the reimbursements constraints:

> A heart attack victim 30 years ago would have been treated with extensive bed care and rest. Today a recommended treatment might be open heart surgery. If the DRG reimbursement rate were defined by the less costly treatment of the past, the progress toward open heart surgery could have been slowed. The DRG concept assumes a static medical technology, while the patient and the medical community expect a dynamic and improved technology.[83]

In Los Angeles, the chief of cardiology at Cedars-Sinai Medical Center, said that "the technology intensive character of many things we [cardiologists] do" has "the label of high cost" which can, under some circumstances, have long range cost savings, for example, coronary angiography. After testing, diagnosis, and appropriate treatment, patients might return to fuller function more quickly; such technology may be a societal cost-saving measure.[84]

Controlling Infections

Nosocomial infections (those acquired by patients during a hospital stay) are responsible for increasing length of stay and costs of care. While infection rates vary between the teaching and nonteaching hospitals and are dependent on the available services and invasive surgical procedures performed, hospitals are monitoring various aspects of possible control—surgical and nursing techniques, sterilization procedures, diet, housekeeping, and environmental sanitation.

As a conservative estimate, nosocomial infections, which occur in about 5 percent of 1.8 million hospital discharges, extend a patients' stay 3 to 4 days on the average. The most common infection areas are urinary tract, postoperative wound sites, bloodstream (bacteremia), and respiratory tract.[85] A postoperative wound infection can add seven days on the average, while urinary tract adds two or three days and bacteremias, and respiratory tract infections such as pneumonia, can add up to 30 days. Infections involve additional expense to the additional hospital days, such as diagnostic tests, X-rays, tests, and pharmacy items.

Each Major Diagnostic Category (MDC) in the DRG system has additional branches for comorbidity and complications which lead to a specific DRG. Infections are considered as complications. Only 50 percent of the discharge diagnoses receive additional compensation when infections occur. The additional compensation is usually small and the hospital is not fully compensated for the extra costs of the additional days of care.

Multiple infections and complications are not compensated differently from single events if compensated additionally at all. If a patient with a stroke suffers multiple complications—aspiration pneumonia, decubitus ulcer, malnutrition—extra compensation is not available beyond the single branching of the DRG.

Discharging patients before full therapy is completed is another cause of concern for physicians treating certain diseases. "For example, the therapy of osteomyelitis, endocarditis, or pneumonia typically takes four weeks. Because the DRG for some of these infections, namely endocarditis, is 18 days, there is intense controversy regarding how long a patient should stay."[86]

Many fear that attempts to save money by early discharge of patients with osteomyelitis or endocarditis will have an adverse impact on the outcome of care. "Cure rates will be much lower, and patients are likely to have multiple admissions if they are discharged prematurely. Although this may be better economically for the hospital, it is certainly not in keeping with good medical practice."[87]

Controlling expenditures for drugs used in treating infections has taken the form of changing and narrowing available hospital formulary items, and changing protocols for care. With 50 percent of the typical hospital's pharmacy budget spent on antibiotics, appropriate monitoring of antibiotics for use and abuse is part of infection control programs. Questions arise as to the continued prophylactic use of antibiotics prior to certain surgical procedures and these discussions have been reopened for cost containment.

Limiting the availability of selected highly technological surgery or procedures to certain institutions which will have high volume will decrease the nosocomial infection rate. "One very controversial area involves studies showing that the rate of nosocomial surgical infection is directly related to the frequency of operation and, in general, the experience of the surgeon."[88]

Other surgical interventions—such as reducing operating time, analysis of clusters of cases—will also help reduce infections postoperatively and thus keep the stay within the specified DRG expectations.

While nosocomial infections are not totally avoidable when a hospital serves high-risk elderly patients and is involved with high technology and major tertiary services, surveillance and control activities are known to have a positive effect on reducing infection rates and costs. The potential impact on quality of care with reduced complications is certainly of great benefit to patients even if the stimulus is fiscal.

Altering Staffing Patterns

Restructuring staffing patterns under DRG and PPS in order to reduce unit labor costs and increase efficiency[89] stems from the reduced LOS, shifts to outpatient services, and general pressures to decrease health care costs. Besides layoffs, other staff reduction strategies include:

- Attrition
- Voluntary hours reductions
- Early retirement
- Hiring freezes
- Voluntary furloughs
- Changing benefits (for health, education, travel)
- Flexible staffing (using per diems, on calls)
- Changing staff mix
- Consolidating jobs

Cutting hospital costs by "down substitution of staff (replacing staff with less skilled staff)" has definite implications for quality of care.[90] Inadequate staffing ratios and changing the mix of professional and ancillary personnel save money. In New Jersey, many hospitals reported a decreased ratio of registered nurses to licensed practical nurses and aides despite the expectation that with increased acutely ill patients and decreased length of stay more registered nurses would be necessary to provide higher levels of quality care. Decreasing personnel ratios affect all direct patient contact services and may delay or hamper restoration to full function and even increase chances for morbidity and mortality (i.e., reduce patient education activities, increase decubitus ulcers, increase infection rate, decrease ambulation, reduce CPR response time).[91,92]

Weekday staffing on inpatient rehabilitation units—physical therapists and occupational therapists—have experienced some of these changes, as well as lesser skilled staff being substituted for the registered professionals. Reduced staffing may also be a result of successful hospital marketing of rehabilitative services on an outpatient basis that may reduce the number of inpatients.[93,94]

For support services, such as laboratory and radiology staffing, reallocation is also being made to increase efficiency in use of hospital resources to cope with the DRG constraints.

> Delays in a patient's workup should be considered poor quality care. Thus a patient who waits over a weekend for a diagnostic test because the radiology department is closed would likely consume more resources (such as a longer hospital stay) than a similar patient who has an expeditious workup. This administrative management, if it occurs to a significant degree, is likely to place a hospital in economic straits.[95]

AHA indicated that hospitals have increased layoffs by 0.5 percent and cut the number of staffed beds by 0.6 percent.[96]

Hospital personnel management departments should pay special attention to staff needs for job security, hospital concerns of fiscal equity, appropriate recruitment, and an effective methodology for reducing staff costs, while ascertaining that quality of patient care is not compromised.

Hospital Strategies Affecting Physician Autonomy and Patient Care Services

Hospital Admission Review: Barriers to Access?

The responsibility for the decision to admit a patient is primarily with the physician, along with patient and/or family consensus. Under the DRG system the admitting diagnosis incident to hospitalization for the specified admitting diagnosis will be questioned.

- Is the hospital the best locus of treatment or is an alternative arrangement possible? Alternatives may include an ambulatory surgical center, private office care, home care program, or long-term care facility.

- Has the patient had diagnostic testing and full clinical evaluation out of the hospitals, such as laboratory tests, X-rays, bone scans, consultations?

- Are these patients admitted with a specified diagnosis and condition or status likely to conform to the length of stay of the assigned DRG, or will the admission result in an "outlier" or "loser" situation? Are complications, morbidity, or mortality expected?

- Is the admitting physician a practitioner whose pattern of practice is in accord with peers who provide service to patients with a similar diagnosis, so that during this patient's admission unnecessary diagnostic and therapeutic expenditures will not be generated?

- Can the patient and hospital afford the cost of care for this episode of illness and its sequelae under the assigned DRG at this hospital or should this patient be "dumped" (transferred) into a public institution?[97]

If the answers are "No," access to care is likely to be denied those certain members of society—the poor, elderly, uninsured—with already limited access to alternative community health services, who have extensive, expensive multiple disease states and need acute medical care.[98,99]

In Kentucky, there is mandatory preauthorization for all nonemergency Medicare and Medicaid admissions. In a year's experience, 156,166 elective cases were reviewed and "only 60 cases were turned down where the attending physician felt hospitalization was necessary . . . (and) another 344 requests where the doctors involved conceded that there had been pressure from the patient or the patient's family." The intensive follow-up of these denials and other reviews makes the Kentucky PRO feel "satisfied that our preauthorization activity is not proving harmful to patients."[100]

Admissions for unnecessary outdated procedures was also curtailed. Some physicians were still doing kidney decapsulations and when notified that the procedure was obsolete the volume dropped from 60 to 4 per year.[101]

Horror stories have been cited which implicate hospitals in turning away patients needing emergency care and admission in institutions with tertiary care capability because of the financial burden it might place on the facility.

A primary care internist in North Carolina "recounts his difficulty in getting an uninsured patient with an acute traumatic neurosurgical problem admitted to a tertiary referral center . . . as he vainly tries to persuade a staff neurosurgeon at a regional university hospital to accept the patient in transfer, only to be told that the hospital administration will not allow it for economic reasons."[102]

Arnold S. Relman, M.D., points out that similar incidents are occurring throughout the United States and comments:

As economic pressures on hospitals grow and hospital managers are encouraged—or forced—to act like businessmen concerned primarily with profit margins, more and more patients will be denied access to urgently needed care . . . In such a climate we cannot expect the emergency care of indigent and uninsured patients always to be given a very high priority—and it is not.[103]

It is feared that the DRG system for Medicare patients will "ratchet down revenues that will likely force more hospital retrenchment of commitments to other payor categories, like Medicaid." This was expressed by David Kinzer, president of the Massachusetts Hospital Association. He cited California as an example of the "out-of-sight, out-of-mind" psychology toward the medical poor people who had a 22.6 percent decline in Medicaid hospital inpatient days in the first six months of 1983. "They've sort of gotten lost," Kinzer said, and indigents' care is worsening.[104]

Promoting more outpatient surgery by providing accommodating surgical suites, streamlined preadmission testing, and postoperative support have been endorsed by the AMA since 1971. Between 1979 and 1983, the AHA reports that hospital-based outpatient surgery increased 77 percent while inpatient surgery fell only 7 percent. In addition to hospital-based units, surgery may be performed in one of the 300 freestanding surgicenters.[105]

Freestanding surgicenter rates are lower than hospital outpatient surgery rates which, in turn, are lower than hospital inpatient surgery and may amount to appreciable savings.

Hospitals recognize new revenue sources and efficiency in their new units, patients enjoy the pleasant atmosphere and the knowledge that they will go home, and physicians note the efficiency, increased revenue, and patient satisfaction. Health insurers and others are pleased with the reduced cost for procedures which would ordinarily engender a hospital stay.

Dr. Alan Nelson, a member of the AMA's Board of Trustees, says, "Some procedures we all agree can be done in an outpatient setting but there are others that are a lot less clear . . . How far should we stick the patient's neck out for budgetary restraint? Should we make them take a 1 percent risk, a 5 percent risk? . . . Where's the line?"[106]

In a recent study of nonemergency inguinal hernia[107] in a Medicare male patient, the options of doing nothing, wearing a truss, having surgery performed on an inpatient or outpatient basis, and receiving anesthesia of general or local administration for that surgery were analyzed and cost implications were compared. Although doing nothing has the risk of impending incarceration and strangulation of the hernia and other morbid complications, the physicians' and hospitals' impact were also delineated.

Surgical repair generates more revenues under DRG for inpatient procedures than in a hospital-based outpatient surgical area; surgery generates more physician payment than the prescription of use of a truss; site utilized may have no fiscal implications; and anesthesiology fees are higher for general than for local anesthesia.

The quality of care issues involve surgery vs. truss, inpatient vs. outpatient surgery, increased risks in general vs. local anesthesia, risks of surgery in the elderly, and patient needs, satisfactions, and acceptance of options. These complicated and intertwined factors, not all of which have been adequately explored, relate to a variety of diseases and surgical procedures; they challenge the dichotomy between the best interests of the providers and the patients.

In addition to the emphasis on outpatient surgery, there is a shift to greater amounts of out-of-hospital diagnostic testing; these tests are not under DRG oversight since they are not hospital-based procedures.

The College of American Pathologists is concerned that "there will be a shift to remote off-site testing for hospital laboratories and we think the emphasis, being on cost rather than quality, will decrease the quality available in the clinical laboratory."[108]

Similarly, the American College of Radiology has encouraged its members to develop local "lists that identify the most expensive procedures, those that are antiquated or inappropriate and those that can be done on an outpatient basis." In addition, the development of guidelines for accepting examinations performed outside the hospital are encouraged to assure quality of procedures and consultation.[109]

Perverse admitting practices might also evolve since "there will be no incentive whatever in such a system (DRG) to care for healthier patients in less costly outpatient settings."[110] Only the most severe cases of pneumonia, for example, are admitted when there is a shortage of beds. But if availability of beds increases it would be a hospital value to admit, even for a few days, such cases. Similarly, hospitals could discharge patients prematurely in order to readmit them again under a different diagnosis.

For quality patient care, legitimate and appropriate documentation must be made by physicians in an unbiased manner, independent of the hospitals' concerns to maximize revenues. "The physician's prime ethical imperative lies with that patient and comes into conflict with an inequitable payment system" when it denies access to medical services that are deemed appropriate.[111]

Constraining Physicians' Practices

Confronting physicians with the cost impact of their decision-making actions on behalf of patients places a new emphasis on hospital-physician relationships. The once passive institution beholden to the admitting physician has become reactive, selective, and aggressive in attitude and action to maintain hospital solvency and prosperity. The punitive, fiscal consequences of unbridled expenditures for medical care has created a new dialogue where the "cost accountant will become the doctor's first consultant."[112]

Data are collected and systematically analyzed to evolve local practice patterns for each DRG, against which any physician can be measured. "Because the hospital gathers cost and length of stay data for each diagnosis, practice patterns can be compared and discussed," said the report prepared by the Hospital Research and Educational Trust of New Jersey. For example, physician profiles could be developed that indicate frequency of lab tests, X-rays, and prescriptions used for patients in a specific DRG. Physicians could also be given comparable data on practice patterns of other peer physicians, "so that they can see how well they match the norm and how they differ."[113]

From the computer printouts of patterns of practice, the physicians, "are being pointed to as winners and losers, and the latter are often being pressured by administrators, chiefs of staff, directors of medical education and the heads of clinical departments to alter their ordering and practice habits," says Emanuel Abraham, M.D., a trustee of the American Society of Internal Medicine and director of ambulatory care at Jersey Shore Medical Center, Neptune, New Jersey. He believes that physicians can cut costs while maintaining quality of care by avoiding weekend admissions for elective procedures, reducing repetitive orders for expensive lab tests or drugs, eliminating standing orders, encouraging prompt response by consultants, probing the efficacy of therapeutic procedures, and dropping ineffective or infrequently used procedures.[114]

While the effect of these stresses on physicians is not easily measured, neither is the quality of care visibly affected. However, the American Society of Internal Medicine position paper cautions against "the replacement of careful clinical judgment by tests and procedures that are quick and easy to order but may prove to be more costly in the long run."[115]

Utilization review (UR) committees within the hospital have been given additional responsibilities and muscle under the DRG system.[116] As part of the requirements for hospital participation under Medicare, the utilization review committee must consist of at least two physicians while participation by nonphysicians is encouraged but not mandated. As part of the utilization review plan, procedures need to address:

- Review of a sample of admissions
- Review of a sample of cost outliers
- Review of all length of stay (LOS) outliers

Written information of all determinations of unnecessary admissions or that a further stay is no longer necessary must be provided to the hospital, the physician, and the patient within two days after certification. The LOS outliers must be reviewed periodically and no later than seven days after the day required in the UR plan.

Structuring of the UR committee and UR plan varies in each hospital and challenges the hospital and physicians to meet compliance with the DRG programmatic goals. These are new demands set upon previously functioning committees needed for JCAH and state licensure or operating certificates. Most UR activities were related to overutilization and underutilization of services and inefficiency in the process of care and use of resources.[117,118]

Opportunities to review practitioner patterns of practice for each DRG and to compare it to others has become a computerized by-product of data on all discharges. This offers opportunities to focus review, develop standards, educate physicians, and to alter practices.[119]

Ancillary service review programs[120] have identified variation in use by physicians, and questioned need, use, and efficiency in providing diagnostic tests and certain therapeutic services. Studies and criteria for review have been reported which review the following:

Blood gases	Physical therapy
Blood cultures	Pathology specimens
GI series X-rays	Blood transfusions
Electrocardiograms	Narcotics prescriptions
Respiratory therapy	Pharmaceutical reviews

In a variety of settings—state programs, projects designed by PSROs, Blue Cross and Blue Shield plans and other insurers, and hospitals—these reviews have brought about significant alterations in pattern of use, or overusage which have cost-saving implications. Changing physician behavior involves identification, analysis, rationalization, education, administrative changes, incentives and penalties, and is well within the purview of UR activities.

John R. O'Brien, M.D., director of Quality Assurance Program at Christ Hospital, Jersey City, New Jersey, reports that the "QA Committee monitors the use of ancillary services to ensure that neither overutilization nor underutilization of services occurs. When data suggest variations in physician ordering patterns, physicians are encouraged to look closely at their practice patterns and compare them to the ordering patterns of their peers."[121]

Under this system profiles are derived and physicians confronted with peer review, utilization review, and alleged extraordinary practices (i.e., long LOS, too many lab tests). Case management is accomplished only within the constraints of "peer" and "usual" criteria with physician individuality discouraged, and patient outcome and satisfaction unmeasured.

There is ample evidence that peer pressure concerning practice pattern leads to changing length of stay in surgical as well as medical conditions. In Toledo, Ohio, the LOS variation for inguinal hernia surgery without complications revealed a six-fold difference between the lowest and highest practitioners. When this was pointed out and rescreened four months later the practices were only

12 percent above the community standard. Similarly in diabetes mellitus "excess" days ranged from 19 to 59 percent (average 39 percent) above the standard and was restudied one year later and averaged only 8 percent above.[122]

While the chief of staff believes that there is "paranoia" among the doctors about the continuing critiques, there is also cooperation evident because they do not "tell them how they *should* practice, but rather how they *are* practicing."[123]

At the Hotel Dieu Hospital in New Orleans, the president of the medical staff "plans to compile standards for the type of tests physicians should order for different diagnosis-related groups of illnesses." While the medical staff will have input into suggesting the core of tests, those who do not abide by these "menus" will have difficulties with the credential process.[124]

Concern has also been expressed that DRGs "will create pressure to adopt *cookbook medicine* or give short shrift to the unique clinical need of the individual patient."[125]

Prior approval mechanisms and second opinion requirements also interfere with the confidential nature of the patient/doctor relationship, as does the lack of assumed confidentiality of the data being amassed on particular physicians and DRGs.

In an analysis of the New Jersey DRG payment method prepared by the Health Research and Educational Trust of New Jersey, the report noted that hospitals would be able to give each physician "a profit and loss statement" on his respective patients each month and that "in the future hospitals may want to use DRGs based data as criteria for granting physician privileges and credentials."[126] If doctors are labeled "gainers" or "losers" dependent on their value to the institution, this appelation is not too secret from the patient. Who wants to be the patient of a "loser"?

The arbitrary numerical goals for reduction in hospital mortality and morbidity, as contractually set between the PRO, the hospitals, and federal government, creates a situation where "a hospital would have to send patients home to die rather than allowing them to die in the hospital."

In addition to the above, Paul W. Speer, M.D., states that "setting an arbitrary percentage by which deaths are to be reduced makes no sense whatsoever and the reduction of post-operative complications by arbitrary fiat is equally unrealistic." He also believes that imposing these goals on physicians "means relegating them to the status of workers on an assembly line who are expected to meet certain production figures."[127]

Patterns of practice are changing with cost consciousness. More testing is done outside the hospital, in the community, before admission. Physicians are selecting alternative sites for care—ambulatory surgery centers, specialty clinics, and so on, and shunting patients around depending on the financial resources and their DRGs. Dumping of the undesirable poor and elderly is occurring, with certain hospitals carrying the burden on behalf of the rest of the community.

Variations in admission rates and practice patterns have been documented among and within the same state.[128] Recent Medicare data analyses indicate hospitalizations were 74 percent higher in Boston than in New Haven, Connecticut. If the 78,000 Boston Medicare beneficiaries had the New Haven program experience, there would have been a $63 million savings in 1982. In Iowa, if all communities had the experience of the lowest community, a savings of $36 million for hospitalizations would be realized in one year.[129]

Within Maine, women have a 70 percent chance of having a hysterectomy in one area as compared to a 20 percent chance in other cities. In Iowa, prostate surgery varied from 60 percent to 15 percent among cities. Similarly, in Vermont, tonsillectomy for children ranged from 8 percent to 70 percent among hospital locations. "The variations are so great that if the low rate were appropriate, we would not have a cost containment problem in this country."[130] However, James E. Davis, M.D., of the AMA House of Delegates from Durham, North Carolina, cautions that while variations in care should be examined carefully, they may be an indication of the "failure to provide care" as well as a signal that inappropriate care had been provided. Adoption of conservative practices "could easily result in savings that amount to more than 40 percent of the current outlay for hospitals" or savings of $16 billion for 1984 Medicare payments.[131]

Hospitals are emphasizing continuing education courses and inservice classes for physicians to enlist them in fiscal responsibility and concurrence with the UR, quality assurance, and DRG monitoring activities. These are not subtle, subliminal messages but active campaigns and implied threats to continuing hospital clinical privileges and livelihood.

Wanda Bartek, ART, Director of Medical Records at Youens Memorial Hospital in Weimar, Texas, says, "Involve the medical staff. This will be a complete re-education of the medical staff. . . . Again, education is the name of the game. Educate the medical staff, hospital personnel, and community about DRGs . . . and keep the physician involved in the DRG process."[132]

Early Discharge—Premature Discharge?

Promoting appropriate lengths of stay and shorter stays requires diligence from the initial point of hospitalization. Inquiries concerning family support systems, relevant insurance coverage, plans for rehabilitation, and return to usual daily activities are important hallmarks in measuring ability to meet DRG trim points along with the standard hospital course and medical regimen.

Discharge planners, nurses, social workers, nutritionists, and other professionals form the interdisciplinary teams essential to assuring that discharge arrangements are appropriate. Will there be a family member available to take the patient home? Will the patient require outpatient physical therapy or home health care services? Is the prescribed diet understood to support the drug regimen in

cardiac disease, diabetes? Have arrangements been made for alternative institutional care, (i.e., nursing home, health-related facility, developmental center),
including application forms and visits to sites with time for patient acceptance
and family concurrence?

"We can't afford to wait until patients have been damaged to be responsive,"
contended Vita Ostrander, President-Elect of the American Association of Retired
Persons, in recent Congressional testimony. "I have already heard of cases where
too early discharge is severely straining home health care capabilities."[133]

Patients need support and preparation for living with the scars of surgery,
amputations, colostomies, appliances, and even the multiple drug prescriptions
for chronic disease. Additionally, opportunities for patient education are fore-
shortened when time is at a premium.

Discharge planning activities in hospitals have developed a "sense of urgency"
which "rushes us to the point where our thinking may be hampered by the speed
of activity," says Susan Schneberger, Director of Social Work at McLaren
General Hospital, Flint, Michigan. No longer is there requirement for a physician's order prior to the initiation of discharge planning assessments, and routine
approval for this activity is more common.

At Miami Valley Hospital, Dayton, Ohio, "30 primary DRGs that relate to
high-risk categories" have been identified for preadmission screening by the
social workers. Concern has been expressed that in decreasing lengths of stay
the follow-up activity by social workers becomes a lower priority at a time when
patients may be "going home in states of greater vulnerability."[134]

According to Warren Nestler, M.D., director of quality assurance at Overlook
Hospital in Summit, New Jersey, such hospital tactics are unlikely. "The attending physician is the only one who can discharge a patient. If a physician
elects to discharge [a patient] prematurely, that physician is stupid. It doesn't
occur."[135] However, Delegates of the American Society of Internal Medicine
(ASIM) were presented with a report on the quality of care under the DRG
system.[136] Responses from 52 physicians to a survey in *The Internist* indicated
that they had felt pressure from their hospitals to discharge patients earlier than
medically appropriate: 19 felt pressure to discharge patients earlier than medically
necessary; 20 felt pressure to discharge patients and readmit them later.

Hospital "backup" problems are complex and relate to patients who no longer
require the acute hospital setting for care and are awaiting nursing home placement.[137] It is estimated that Medicare and Medicaid pay for between 1.0 and
9.2 million "backup" days annually of inpatient hospital care when a nursing
home bed is unavailable for patients requiring only SNF or ICF care. Access to
nursing home care for backup patients is mostly a concern of Medicare and
Medicaid because research indicates that persons with private resources to pay
for nursing home care have no problem in finding a nursing home bed.

Several factors contribute to hospital backup. Probably the most important are the heavy care needs of backup patients combined with the inadequacy of the Medicaid nursing home reimbursement rate in covering the cost of their care. Several studies show that the longest-staying backup patients tended to be Medicaid-eligible, to have behavioral problems, to be incontinent and disoriented, and to suffer from addictive illnesses. The other factors that may contribute to hospital backup relate to the community availability of nursing home beds and the role of discharge planners, physicians, and families in discharging the patient to a nursing home or alternative source of care.

Resolution of these problems is complex. One approach, using the DRG system, reduces payments to hospitals for backup patients. This may, however, unfairly penalize hospitals when it is the nursing home which either refuses to admit a patient or cannot do so because it is operating at maximum occupancy. The DRG payment method may also cause problems for patients if they are discharged by hospitals too quickly to nursing homes which cannot provide the level of care they require.

Because of the DRG incentives, hospitals will attempt to place convalescent Medicare patients in scarce nursing home beds; problems in placing heavy care Medicaid backup patients may increase. Increasing reimbursement to nursing homes as an incentive to admit heavy care backup patients will not, however, insure the patients' admission if occupancy rates are high. Further, if higher payments are made to nursing homes, they should be targeted to insure that these particular patients are admitted.

It may also be difficult to discharge backup patients if families prefer to keep elderly parents in hospitals. Finally, persons eligible for Medicare SNF coverage may remain in the hospitals because no Medicare-certified SNF bed is available or they may not be able to travel a great distance to receive care.

A few states have increased Medicaid nursing home reimbursement only for patients who were discharged from hospitals and were considered to have costly care needs.

- Oregon pays more for Medicaid patients who have more intensive care needs than the average patient. In 1980, an extra $9.16 a day was paid to SNFs and an extra $7.49 was paid to ICFs for admitting heavy care patients from hospitals.

- In Massachusetts, the state intervened twice in 1982 to reimburse nursing homes with a bonus payment to admit particularly long-staying backup patients. According to state officials, these two interventions appeared to reduce the large number of backup patients substantially, although they did not believe this was a permanent solution to the problem.

- Utah has recently begun to pay a negotiated higher rate for a specified period of time for a hospitalized patient whose care costs exceed 125 percent of the SNF rate.[138]

- In 1980, Wisconsin implemented a program in three nursing homes with higher staffing and equipment requirements than regular SNFs, and a transfer agreement with a hospital. Recent review indicated that these nursing homes did not increase the level of services for the targeted patients; some of their current residents required the new, higher level of care and reimbursement. State officials indicate that the program will be discontinued or greatly modified.

While increasing the nursing home bed supply may alleviate part of the problem, many states are reluctant to allow this because it would increase Medicaid expenditures. Two studies in New York concluded that without additional patient reimbursement, additional beds would be filled by private pay and lighter care Medicaid patients rather than the difficult-to-place backup patients.[139]

Alternatively, it has been proposed that it would be less expensive to care for backup patients in empty hospital beds, especially at a reduced rate, than it would be to build new nursing homes.

Even if hospital care were cheaper than other alternatives, there is debate as to whether hospitals are the appropriate setting for chronically ill patients.

> Hospitals in Iowa, South Dakota, Texas, and Utah participated in a demonstration project which allowed acute care beds to "swing" to long-term care beds when the patient no longer required acute care. The quality of patient care was lower in swing beds compared to a group of area nursing homes judged to be of relatively high quality, although the discrepancy was not substantial. The biggest differences were for hospitalized SNF-level patients, who were more depressed, lonely, and isolated than patients classified at the same level in nursing homes.[140]

While hospital backup has led to increasing the size of the chronically ill population in hospitals, there appears to be, in general, a growing hospital population with chronic, rather than acute, illnesses. It is estimated that 38 percent of all inpatient hospital days for the elderly in 1980 were for patients with long-term or chronic illnesses.[141] A recent task force report by the Massachusetts Hospital Association concluded that, because of the challenge of meeting the needs of this growing number of older patients with chronic disabilities, acute care hospitals should begin to provide long-term care.[142]

While some hospitals are already working with the nursing home industry because they have made collaborative arrangements or have purchased nursing homes, it has also been proposed that a more viable option would be for hospitals to develop long-term care units specifically for elderly patients.

Burdens are placed on receiving families, home health care agencies, and nursing home institutions when patients are discharged too soon and need high levels of continuing skilled care beyond the usual abilities or case load of the respective care givers. Families are not easily able to cope with the terminally ill and chronically debilitated in situations where housing space is inadequate, all adults are employed, and former independent living arrangements turn into dependent ones. Agencies and institutions are not always able to cope with the skilled services needed for caring within their usual existing budgetary constraints and are reluctant to accept the placement of these very sick patients. A poignant example was presented to the House Select Committee on Aging:

> A patient is in the terminal stage of an illness. Dying of cancer and choosing not to prolong life by intravenous feedings or other drastic measures, the patient, family and physician decide to stop aggressive treatment. Because of this decision, the patient no longer meets the acute care criteria which justifies continued hospitalization. The family is faced with the decision of trying to locate a nursing home or taking the patient home to die.
>
> Transferring to a nursing home, patient and family must leave the familiar surroundings of the hospital and personnel whom they have grown to trust and who know the patient. Choosing to care for the patient at home means learning to give pain medications, plus the multitude of other needs that must be met on a 24-hour basis. Medicare-covered home care will only cover the costs of a professional nurse two or three times a week for up to two hours a day. That is, of course, if a home care nurse is available in the patient's community or if there is a nursing home close to the patient's home. Thus, what often occurs is patients on their death bed are forced to seek assistance and make monumentous decisions at a time when they are least capable of decision making. Certainly, a quality issue facing thousands of Americans each and every day.[143]

Most would agree that a "waiting" patient poses problems to busy physicians and nurses who view this patient as no longer requiring their acute care-oriented professional services. With this altered perspective, the quality of care given and received and perceived by the patient and family is altered. The persistent demands of the chronically ill in a basically hostile environment where even the level of reimbursement is challenged does not contribute to increasing function, stability, or improvements in health.

Quality of care is frequently threatened by vociferous and continuous pressures exerted by the hospital staff and, ultimately, by the physician, which results in early discharge which should be more appropriately termed "premature" discharge.

Readmissions

A study of 270,266 Medicare patients treated in the hospital between 1974 and 1977 found that 25 percent who were discharged were readmitted within two months. About 5 percent are readmitted within five days.[144] It is anticipated that under the DRG payments, the incentives are to increase readmissions.[145] Three major forces are acting to encourage more readmissions. First, with the reduced length of stay in hospital, allegations have been made that patients are being discharged prematurely for the sake of administrative processes and financial imperatives before patient readiness and full needs are met. Early discharge can lead to patients getting sick again or deteriorating at home; prompt readmission is a process called "churning." In these cases, hospitals are paid twice or more for treating one illness or injury based on multiple admissions.[146]

Incomplete treatment designated by the PRO as substandard care on the prior admission can account for some readmissions as can inadequate discharge planning.

Communities and long-term care alternative institutions are not always ready in terms of available support or direct services to cope with the sicker discharged patient. For many, readmission to a hospital is the available option which is now being further scrutinized. Does too early discharge lead to readmission at the same or other hospitals? Is there a higher morbidity (infection, complication rate, etc.) and mortality rate after discharge? Are patients being sent home to die among unprepared families to reduce the hospital mortality statistics? Does the premature discharge and medical need for readmission predispose to increased liability on the physicians and to malpractice vulnerability?

Second, many elderly patients have multiple intercurrent or simultaneous illnesses but the principal diagnosis drives the DRG payment. Hospitals are likely to encourage physicians to admit patients several times, each under separate DRGs for financial reasons.

This process is considered "unbundling" where separate diagnoses cause separate admissions (and readmissions) and separate DRG payments.

These quality issue dilemmas were cited to Congress:

- An elderly man is admitted to the hospital because of a severe case of pneumonia. Because he is weak, unable to walk, and is placed on intravenous feedings, he also develops problems with voiding. A catheter is placed in his bladder. As he recovers, the catheter is removed but problems with voiding persist. An examination reveals he needs to have prostate surgery to correct the voiding problem. The dilemma becomes: Should he be sent home and return to the hospital at a later time for prostate surgery? If the prostate surgery is performed during the same hospitalization as the pneumonia, the hospital will only be paid for the pneumonia diagnosis. If the man can be sent home and return at a later date for the surgery, the hospital will receive reimbursement for the prostate operation.

• A patient with severe arthritis needs to have a joint replacement on both hips. The hospital will only be reimbursed for the cost of one hip replacement. The dilemma becomes: Should the patient have one hip replacement done at separate times necessitating two admissions, two surgeries, two convalescant periods. Or should both hips be replaced during one hospitalization which would cause the hospital a loss of reimbursement? Physicians, in cases like this, are pulled between the choices confronting them.[147]

Third, empty hospital beds have the effect of becoming a beacon for readmissions. With scarcity and difficulty in getting patients into the hospital, a variety of medical care services were called upon to support care at home. This restraint is no longer operable and patients who may have been previously treated conservatively at home may be readmitted more easily. Physician compensation is also greater for the hospital visits, required to be daily, than for the home visit which may or may not be needed as frequently.

In a Readmission Project in three counties in New Jersey (Essex, Hudson, and Union), the rates of readmission were compared for Medicare, Medicaid, and Blue Cross of New Jersey hospitalizations for selected DRGs. The DRG system did not appear to have any effect on readmission rates. In addition, the Medicare death rates for selected DRGs did not deviate substantially from the death rates of the entire Medicare population in the area. Early discharge was not then significantly linked to readmission or ultimately death.[148]

This study was challenged by Dr. Alfred Alessi, past president of the Medical Society of New Jersey, who objected to the use of the seven days indicator for readmissions, instead of 30 days, because early discharge complications may emerge later.[149]

Hospital utilization review committees and the PRO have, as their objectives, to keep these readmissions under scrutiny to reduce unnecessary readmissions (see Exhibit 11-5). Recent criticism is noted: "The cruelest jargon of the '80s, a favorite of insurers, is unnecessary hospital readmissions. What they are saying is debatable, but what they are doing is attempting to kill off Mr. Jones on the first admission to save on the cost of his dying on a second admission."[150]

Exhibit 11-5   New York PRO: Unnecessary Readmissions

Quality Objective Area I—Reduce unnecessary hospital readmissions resulting from substandard care provided during the prior admission.

Objective Statement
   Reduce the number of unnecessary readmissions resulting from substandard care provided during the prior admission by 50%. This will result in the reduction of 4,610 admissions over the two-year period.

Validation
   Readmissions within 30 days of prior hospitalization account for 74,354 cases/year in New York State. The PRO projected unnecessary admissions based on a special review of 1,558 readmissions which was conducted by eleven PROs in the State in 1984. Of the 1,558 readmissions, 97 (6.2%) resulted from substandard care provided during the prior admission. Applying the results of the study to all readmissions in New York State, 4,610 readmissions were unnecessary due to substandard care. The PRO then determined that a 50% reduction in total number each year was appropriate.

Primary Methodology
   The PRO will initially notify area hospitals to review these cases and provide them with the criteria to be used in the review. A random sample of 25% of all readmissions within 30 days will be reviewed retrospectively. The completed worksheets of these reviews will be automated and data profiles will be generated by hospitals, diagnosis, and procedure. If specific patterns of problem readmissions are identified, the PRO will focus review accordingly. For specific hospitals or physicians found to be prematurely discharging patients, pre-discharge review will be implemented. Continued failure by a provider or practitioner to meet quality standards will lead to a sanction process.

   Review findings will be monitored by the PRO. In addition, objective goals and milestones will be evaluated quarterly.

Source: New York PRO: Empire State Medical Scientific and Educational Foundation, Inc., Lake Success, NY, 1984.

The Jury Is Out

A verdict is awaited which considers patients' interests in light of the preliminary effects of DRGs. Among these effects are reduced length of stay, cost containment through efficiencies in hospital management, and patient and physician dissatisfactions. Federal officials barrel along with new rules and regulations to close apparent loopholes and clarify areas for uniform application among the states. In these times of greater emphasis on deregulation, competition, and free market forces, the hospital and health industry faces greater scrutiny, controls, regulations, and monitoring. Whether the end justifies the means in terms of fulfilling the health service needs of the chronically ill, the frail and fragile elderly, and others under this system is yet to be determined.

Quality of care for these Medicare patients will have an impact on all age patients under all types of reimbursement, insurance, or private pay. All-payer rates will emerge under similar constraints of any federal program developed for one specific population—Medicare—if costs can be brought into acceptable limits without adverse consequences.

Risks of continued reductions in access and availability of hospital care with limited appropriate alternatives has a cumulative effect on the aging population as well as others. The variations in practice patterns which have emerged on study indicate the need to develop a consensus within the medical profession and among health care givers regarding what is appropriate and necessary care to guard quality. Patients must be protected from the abuse of overtreatment and undertreatment.

The human price of delayed availability of new innovations and technology is not easily measured and neither is the impact of rationing and the allocation of scarce resources away from the elderly and terminally ill.

The great hope for assuring quality of care rests on the PRO. New instruction manuals for the PROs were issued in April 1985 by HCFA. The following items are included:

- Clarification of timing requirements for initiating and completing review activities

- Reduction of required review levels for day and cost outlier cases to a 50 percent sample instead of 100 percent

- Hospital no longer having to collect and maintain pacemaker warranty information

- Physician attestation effective April 1 requiring full name signature on medical records—handwritten—and dates with changes on narrative diagnostic information similarly countersigned

- Clarification of physician acknowledgement requirement that the physician has received penalty notice

- Reduction of sample size for DRG validation for small hospitals

- Extension of time for PRO to notify hospitals of on-site DRG validation visits 24 hours to two working days.[151]

These areas and others are under review and additional manual instructions are being developed to cover sanctions, admission patterns, monitoring, and PRO data.

However, the AARP is not that sanguine that PROs will be effective enough in protection from the negative effects of the DRG systems. The AARP cautions that "Of great importance socially and medically is the potential for harm that cannot be justified by the cost savings achieved."[152] They point to the complaints of early discharge, lack of community alternative facilities and services, premature discharge leading to readmissions, and fears of "underprovision of services." In addition, they note that "The quality of care issue is the potential Achilles' heel of the prospective payment system. . . . If quality suffers, public support for cost containment will quickly erode."[153]

HCFA emphasizes the potential for increased quality of care under PPS and DRG[154] with regional planning occurring, with inappropriate admissions reduced, with targets for reductions in unnecessary procedures, complications, and avoidable deaths. They point to the PRO as well as other mechanisms to monitor and assure quality:

- PRO reviews extended to the new Medicare HMO program

- Survey and Certification Programs for Medicare-participating hospitals and institutions in cooperation with state survey and certification agencies and the Joint Commission on Accreditation of Hospitals

- Swing-bed programs in rural areas to enable SNF patients to have access to empty hospital beds converted for their needs (about 300 rural hospitals are participating).

In addition, several HCFA research proposals are funded to evaluate the impact of the new DRG system.

Another major problem with early discharge is the discontinuity of care. Entrants to nursing homes, home health programs, and other settings usually leave their private physician and enter new medical care relationships with scant transfer information. "Our health care system lets people down by not cumulating, distilling and organizing their medical data and making sure it travels with them."[155]

The pressure on physicians to discharge patients before they are ready engenders fears of liability: "In the recent era of malpractice suits, the medical profession's response was to leave no stone unturned in treating a patient. Now that strategy won't work, because the physician will be accountable to the hospital for costs. For many physicians, it will be a moral and ethical dilemma."[156] While physicians are being exhorted to "brush up on business principles in response to new Medicare regulations," it is not clear that the best interest of patients will be served thereby. "Pressed on one side by the necessity of limiting costs, and on the other by the fear of legal liability . . . , the physician today finds little guidance, no statutory protection, and now precious little professional security in attempting to decide what is truly in his or her patient's best interest."[157]

There is a growing recognition of the changing relationship between hospitals and physicians in a duality that constrains the physician's activities and interposes judgments between the physician and the patient under threat of disassociation and loss of hospital privileges. While each have been under respective review of accrediting and licensure entities, the DRG system brings these interactions into closer focus and carries enough fiscal clout to be effective. One can only wonder whether physicians will continue to practice and participate in Medicare under these constraints. Will the competition of excessive physician manpower supply create compliant supplicants of hospitals staffs? Will physicians compromise their knowledge, education, and skill for the new ethics and new morality of cost containment and efficiency? Will there be measurable harmful effects on quality of patient care?

Perhaps it is the appropriate role of a medical student to light the way of our future health system: "New consensus must be based on different assumptions: that health care is a right, not a commodity; that hospitals provide human services, not product lines; and that physicians and nurses are healers, not accountants."[158]

References

1. J. Lundy, *Prospective Payments for Medicare Inpatient Hospital Services,* Issue Brief No. 1B83171, Library of Congress, Congressional Research Service, April 2, 1984.

2. D. Pointer and M. Ross, "DRG Cost-per-Case Management," *Modern Healthcare* 14, No. 3 (February 15, 1984):109-110, 112.

3. C. Pierce, *The New Jersey Experience with DRG Reimbursement.* Delivered before U. S. House of Representatives, Select Committee on Aging, March 23, 1983.

4. C. Hardwick, "DRGs Spawn New Medical Team," *Private Practice* 15, No. 11 (1983):24.

5. "DRG Pricing Plan Won't Compromise Quality:Rubin," *Hospitals* 58, No.8 (April 16, 1983):23.

6. R. J. Rubin, *Remarks AMA,* 11th Annual Leadership Conference, Chicago, IL, February 18, 1983.

7. J. T. Prior, "Three New Acronyms: PPS, DRG, PRO," *New York State Journal of Medicine* 84, No. 3 (1984):102-103.

8. M. Scherf, "Medicare Discharging Elderly Earlier, Study Says," *Staten Island Advance,* Feburary 26, 1985.

9. Ibid.

10. "New Medicare System Seen Hurting Patients," *The News Tribune,* March 30, 1985.

11. E. R. Roybal, *Opening statement,* U. S. House of Representatives, Select Committee on Aging, Hearings on Sustaining Quality Health Care Under Cost Containment, February 26, 1985.

12. "New Medicare System," *The News Tribune.*

13. "PPS Improving Quality of Care: Davis," *Hospitals* 59, No. 8 (April 16, 1985):47.

14. J. Whitlow, "Jersey MDs Call Hospital Pay Plan Bad Medicine," *The Sunday Star-Ledger,* May 5, 1985.

15. N. Rucker, "Hospital Cut-Backs Hurt Quality: MDs," *Modern Healthcare* 14 No. 5 (1984):50.

16. J. D. Davis, *The Provision of Health Care for the Elderly,* Statement of the AMA to the Select Committee on Aging, U. S. House of Representatives, February 26, 1985.

17. *AMA's DRG Monitoring Project and the Prospective Pricing System,* Report of the AMA Board of Trustees. Chicago, IL, December 1984.

18. Ibid.

19. J. Mongan, "Health Cost Containment and Quality of Care," Testimony on Behalf of the American Hospital Association before the House Select Committee on Aging, February 26, 1985.

20. "Prospective Payment's Been Compatible With Quality So Far," *Medical World News* 27, No. 4 (February 24, 1986):24,26.

21. E. Friedman, "DRG Creator Says PPS May Reduce Quality of Care," *Hospitals* 58, No. 23 (December 1, 1984):30-31.

22. "HHS Expels Hospitals from Medicare Program," *Medical World News* 27, No. 6 (March 24, 1986):9.

23. P. E. Dans, J. P. Weiner and S. E. Otter. "Peer Review Organization. Promises and Pitfalls," *New England Journal of Medicine* 313, No. 18 (October 31, 1985):1131-1137.

24. C. Kelly, HCFA *Legislative Summary, Prospective Payment Provisions,* Title VI of the Social Security Amendments of 1983 (P.L. 98-21), June 1, 1983.

25. J. O'Sullivan, *Medicare,* Issue Brief 1B84052, Library of Congress, Congressional Research Services, June 6, 1984.

26. *Federal Register: Part III Medicare and Medicaid Programs: Peer Review Organizations; Final Rules.* 50(74):15312-15374, April 17, 1985.

27. J. Fochtman, "DRG Rules Debut," *Medical Marketing and Media* 18, No. 11 (1983):4, 6, 8.

28. "HCFA Awards 3 More Contracts on PROs," *American Medical News* 27, No. 40 (October 26, 1984):24.

29. S. McIlrath, "CMA Subsidiary Loses in State PRO Bidding," *American Medical News* 27, No. 37 (October 5, 1984):10.

30. "Bids Sought for PRO Monitor Groups," *American Medical News* 27, No. 44 (November 23, 30, 1984):1, 42.

31. "Most PRO Contracts Approved, HCFA Says," *American Medical News* 27, No. 41 (November 2, 1984):1, 23.

32. J. Brinkley, "In Hospital Surgery to be Reduced by Contracts to Save on Medicare," *New York Times,* December 14, 1984.

33. S. McIlrath, "New PROs Threaten Rationing: Hospitals," *American Medical News* 27, No. 29 (August 3, 1984):2, 32, 33.

34. "Playing the PRO Game: Is Anyone Winning?" *Medical World News* 26, No. 8 (April 22, 1985):51.

35. S. McIlrath, "PRO Goals Defended by HCFA," *American Medical News* 27, No. 30 (August 10, 1984):1, 16, 17.

36. Ibid.

37. Ibid.

38. "Changes in PRO Program to be Sought," *American Medical News* 27, No. 46 (December 14, 1984):9.

39. Mongan, *Testimony.*

40. J. Finn, "PRO Implementation Problems Prompt AHA Lawsuit," *Hospitals* 59, No. 5 (March 1, 1985):30-31.

41. S. McIlrath, "AHA Meet Demands PRO Rules," *American Medical News* 28, No. 6 (February 8, 1985):2, 55.

42. H. M. Feder, *Utilization Review: A PRO/ Planning Affair,* Address at American Health Planning Association Annual Meeting, Washington, DC, July 10, 1984.

43. "New IPRO Medicare Review Activities Under PPS," *Island Peer Review Organization News,* Rego Park, N.Y. (Spring 1986):2, 5.

44. "Playing the PRO Game," *Medical World News.*

45. "Health Coverage Facing Closer Scrutiny," *Sunday Home News,* April 15, 1985.

46. "PROs Tackle Contracts as HHS Reps. Race Medicare Deadline," *Medical World News* 25, No. 17 (September 10, 1984):24-25.

47. A. Owens, "Peer Reviewers are Ready to Sell Your Track Record," *Medical Economics,* June 11, 1984.

48. Ibid.

49. "PRO Proposal Jeopardizes Confidentiality," *American Medical News* 27, No. 27 (July 20, 1984):4.

50. C. Mickel, "Peer Review Laws; Policy Questions Raised," *Hospitals* 58, No. 1 (January 1, 1984):30.

51. R. Pear, "U. S. Consumers See Medicare Data on Health Care Quality," *New York Times,* April 16, 1985.

52. "List of Hospitals That Are Above or Below Average U.S. Mortality Rates," *New York Times,* March 12, 1986.

53. J. Brinkley "U.S. Releasing Lists of Hospitals With Abnormal Mortality Rates," *New York Times,* March 12, 1986.

54. Ibid.

55. S. McIlrath "Hospitals Rap Release of Mortality Rate Data," *American Medical News* 29, No. 11 (March 21, 1986):1, 29.

56. R. Sullivan "U.S. Cites 27 New York Hospitals in Medicare Deaths," *New York Times,* March 12, 1986.

57. M. J. Patterson and R. Cohen "Health Officials Dispute U.S. Mortality Study," *Star-Ledger* (Newark, N.J.), March 13, 1986.

58. J. T. Ward "Muhlenberg Officials Mad About Release of Death Data," *Home News* (East Brunswick, N.J.), March 13, 1986.

59. R. DePeri "Center Disputes Report on Medicare Patient Mortality," *Daily Targum* (New Brunswick, N.J.), March 14, 1986.

60. J. Brinkley "U.S. Releasing Lists . . ." March 12, 1986.

61. A. Gosfield, "The Arrival of PROs: Anticipating the Challenges," *G&S Notes* 3, No. 6 (1984):1-6.

62. "HCFA Reopen Bids for Super PRO," *American Medical News* 28, No. 12 (March 22, 1985):17.

63. "Bids Sought," *American Medical News.*

64. S. McIlrath, "Pennsylvania PRO Target of Medicare Corrective Action," *American Medical News* 28, No. 11 (March 15, 1985):1, 40, 44.

65. "Review Body Cancels Federal Contract," *American Medical News* 28, No. 42 (November 8, 1985):1, 42.

66. S. McILrath "New Rules for 15 PROs Bidding for Renewal," *American Medical News* 29, No. 3 (January 17, 1986):1, 27.

67. "Diagnosis Related Groups (DRGs) May Present Threat to Quality of Care," *Hospital Peer Review* 7, No. 11 (November 1982):142-4.

68. S. McIlrath, "New Rates Published, $1.5 Billion Saving Sought from DRG," *American Medical News* 26, No. 34 (September 15 1983):1, 10-11.

69. J. Brinkley "Hospital Death Data: At Least One Plus," New York Times, March 13, 1986.

70. Ibid.

71. E. Mihalski, "The New Era of Utilization Review and Quality Control; Peer Review Organizations," *Bulletin New York Academy of Medicine* 60, No. 1 (1984):43-53.

72. "From Our Correspondents, United States, Cutting the Hospital Costs," *Lancet* 2, No. 8398 (August 11, 1984):341-342.

73. Hardwick, "DRGs Spawn Team."

74. D. Williams, "Interview with Margaret Heckler," *Private Practice* 16, No. 1 (1984):57-59, 61.

75. J. F. Boyle, "Should We Learn to Say No?" *Journal of the American Medical Association* 252, No. 6 (August 10, 1984):782-784.

76. "Health Care Rationing: MD Takes Issue with Insurance, Government Officials," *Medical World News* 25, No. 14 (July 23, 1984):33-34.

77. Ibid.

78. Ibid.

79. A. Caplan, "Health Costs: Lest a 'Lifeboat' Ethic Take Hold," Letter to the Editor, *New York Times,* July 26, 1984.

80. Ibid.

81. J. Gigliotti, *Hospital Financing Under TEFRA and DRGs,* Presented to the Government Research Corporation Eighth Annual Leadership Conference on Health Policy, Washington, DC, June 16-17, 1983.

82. "Diagnosis Related Groups (DRGs) May Present Threat to Quality of Care," *Hospital Peer Review.*

83. M. Haley, "What is a DRG," *Topics in Health Care Financing* 6, No. 4 (Summer, 1980):55-61.

84. D. Branch, "Says Prospective Payment Is Undermining Health Care," *Internal Medical News* 17, No. 11 (June 1-14, 1984):54-55.

85. M. Tatge, "Hospitals May Take Shot at Paring Infections Rate to Cut Patient Stays," *Modern Healthcare* 14, No. 5 (1984):80-81.

86. "Cost Containment: An Interview with Bruce F. Farber, M.D.," *Asepsis* 7, No. 1 (First Quarter, 1985):15-19.

87. Ibid.

88. Ibid.

89. "Industry Trends, Including DRGs, Seen as Responsible for Layoffs," *Hospitals* 58, No. 22 (November 16, 1984):82.

90. P. Jones, "Financial 'Heyday' of Health Care is Past. But What About Quality Assurance Under DRGs?" *The Pennsylvania Nurse* 39, No. 7 (1984):7-8.

91. Ibid.

92. "Dealers Positioned to Smooth DRG Damage in Skin Care Field: An Interview with Dick Meer," *Medical Product Sales* 15, No. 3 (1984):48, 50-53.

93. T. Precious, "PPS One Year Later," *Progress Report*, American Physical Therapy Association, September 1984.

94. S. Scott, "The Medicare Prospective Payment System," *The American Journal of Occupational Therapy* 38, No. 5 (1984):330-334.

95. L. F. McMahon, "Diagnosis Related Groups, Prospective Payment: Effects on Medical Quality Assurance," *Evaluation and the Health Profession* 7, No. 1 (1984):25-41.

96. A. Crowe and J. Brinkley, "Medicare Rules Cut Hospital Stays, Staff," *USA Today*, July 6-8, 1984.

97. P. Ertel and R. Harrison, "Ethical and Operational Issues Concerning DRGs and the Prospective Payment System," *Topics in Health Record Management* 4, No. 3 (1984):10-31.

98. L. Glasse, "Expensive Reductions," Letter to the Editor, *New York Times*, July 26, 1984.

99. Caplan, "Health Costs."

100. R. S. Miles, "How I Became a Big Fan of Peer Review," *Medical Economics*, December 10, 1984.

101. Ibid.

102. A. Relman, "Economic Considerations in Emergency Care—What Are Hospitals For?" *New England Journal of Medicine* 312, No. 6 (February 7, 1985):372-373.

103. Ibid.

104. D. Kinzer, "Indigents Care Must Worsen Before Issue Faced," *Hospitals* 58, No. 1 (January 11, 1984):26.

105. K. Shannon, "Outpatient Surgery Up 77 Percent: Data," *Hospitals* 59, No. 10 (May 16, 1985):54.

106. Brinkley, "In Hospital Surgery."

107. D. Neuhauser and R. Pine, "DRGs and Elective Surgery: What's Best for the Provider? What's Best for the Patient?" *Medical Care* 23, No. 2 (1985):183-188.

108. Rucker, "Hospital Cut-Backs."

109. Ibid.

110. R. J. Anderson, *Testimony before the Subcommittee on Health of the Committee on Finance on the Hospital Prospective Payment System Hearing*, U.S. Senate (February 2, 1983):239-240.

111. Ertel and Harrison, "Ethical and Operational Issues."

112. Hardwick, "DRGs Spawn Team."

113. D. Lefton, "Costs Up in First Year of DRGs in Jersey," *American Medical News* 27, No. 14 (April 13, 1984):1, 32.

114. Rucker, "Hospital Cut-Backs," 89-91.

115. "ASIM Sees Threat to Patient Care in Physician DRGs," *Medical World News* 25, No. 10 (May 28, 1984):24.

116. "Part VI, Medicare Program; Prospective Payment in Medicare Inpatient Hospital Services; Final Rule," *Federal Register* 49, No. 1 (January 3, 1984):234-334.

117. A. G. Gosfield, "A Primer on Utilization Review," *DRG Monitor* 1, No. 5 (1984):1-8.

118. M. J. Andrews, "Medical Records, Medical Staff and Utilization Review—A Make or Break Triangle Under DRGs," *DRG Monitor* 1, No. 7 (1984):1-8.

119. R. L. Mullin, "Utilization Review Based on Practitioner Profiles," *Journal of Medical Systems* 7, No. 5 (1983):409-412.

120. J. M. Eisenberg, "The Use of Ancillary Services: A Role for Utilization Review," *Medical Care* 20, No. 8 (1982):849-861.

121. J. O'Brien, "Organizing QA and UR Activities Under a DRG-Based System," *Quality Review Bulletin* 9, No. 9 (September 1983):276-277.

122. A. Rosenberg, "When Peers Put the Heat on Doctors Who Overhospitalize," *Medical Economics*, September 3, 1984.

123. Ibid.

124. "Technology, Briefs, Hospitals Set to Standardize Physicians' Tests for DRGs," *Modern Healthcare* 14, No. 5 (1984):152.

125. B. Vladeck, "Medicare Hospital Payment by Diagnosis Related Groups,"

Annals of Internal Medicine 100, No. 4 (1984):576-591.

126. Lefton, "Costs Up."

127. P. W. Spear, "Health Rhetoric That Happens to Kill People," *New York Times,* August 7, 1984.

128. J. E. Wennberg, K. McPherson, and P. Caper, "Will Payment Based on Diagnosis-Related Groups Control Hospital Costs?" *New England Journal* of Medicine 331, No. 5 (August 2, 1984):295-300.

129. S. McIlrath, "Regional Variations in Practice Under Study," *American Medical News* 27, No. 45 (December 7, 1984):2, 28.

130. R. Goudreau, "Study Finds Wide Differences in Medical Practices, Costs," *The Home News,* September 2, 1984.

131. S. McIlrath, "Regional Variations."

132. W. Bartek, "DRGs Maximize Your QA Strategies," *Texas Hospitals* 39, No. 1 (June 1983):24.

133. "Peer Review Organizations Need More Muscle" (News Bulletin), *American Association of Retired Persons* 25, No. 4 (April 1984).

134. "Discharge Planning Efforts Grow Under PPS," *Hospitals* 58, No. 22 (November 16, 1983):69.

135. W. B. Nestler, "Diagnosis Related Groups (DRGs) May Present Threat to Quality of Care," *Hospital Peer Review* 7, No. 11 (1982):142-144.

136. "Quality Control, Contracting Addressed," *Medical World News* 25, No. 20 (October 22, 1984):22.

137. Government Accounting Office, *Medicaid and Nursing Home Care: Cost Increases and the Need for Services are Creating Problems for the States and the Elderly,* Washington, DC, GAO/IPE-84-1, October 21, 1983.

138. B. Spitz and G. Atkinson, *Nursing Homes, Hospitals and Medicaid: Reimbursement Policy Adjustments 1981-1982,* National Governors' Association, Center for Policy Studies, Washington, DC, March 1983.

139. Finger Lakes Health Systems Agency, *Task Force Report on the Hospital Back-Up of Long-Term Care Patients,* Rochester, NY, November 1979, pp. 31-33.

140. USDHHS, HCFA, *An Evaluation of Swing Bed Experiments to Provide Long Term Care in Rural Hospitals, Volume 2,* Washington, DC, March 1981, p. 233.

141. Robert Wood Johnson Foundation, *Program for Hospital Initiatives in Long Term Care,* Princeton, NJ, November 1982.

142. E. Campion, A. Bang, and M. I. May, "Why Acute Care Hospitals Must Undertake Long Term Care," *New England Journal of Medicine* 308, No. 2 (January 13, 1983):73.

143. P. Hanson, *Testimony before the House Select Committee on Aging, Sustaining Quality Care Under Cost Containment,* February 26, 1985.

144. G. F. Anderson and E. P. Steinberg, "Hospital Readmissions in the Medicare Population," *New England Journal of Medicine* 311, No. 21 (November 22, 1984):1349-1353.

145. K. M. Magnuson, P. Manu, and R. R. Goodspeed, "Letter to the Editor," *New England Journal of Medicine* 312, No. 12 (March 21, 1985):793-794.

146. R. Young, "Creeping Fiasco in New Jersey Hospital Costs," *The Fund Reporter* 2, No. 2 (March-April 1984):1, 3.

147. Hanson, *Testimony.*

148. F. Goldschmidt, "Full PSRO Study," *State of New Jersey Department of Health,* Trenton, NJ, July 12, 1984.

149. A. Alessi, *Testimony before the Select Committee on Aging, House of Representatives,* at New Jersey's Hospital Reimbursement System Hearing, Newark, NJ, July 11, 1983.

150. R. Byrne, "Health Care Rhetoric That Happens to Kill People," *New York Times,* August 7, 1984.

151. "HCFA Issues PRO Manual Instructions," *Hospitals* 59, No. 8 (April 16, 1985):47.

152. L. Krieger, *Testimony before the U. S. House of Representatives Select Committee on Aging and the Task Force on the Rural Elderly on Sustaining Quality Under Cost Containment,* February 26, 1985.

153. Ibid.

154. M. Kappert, *Testimony by HCFA before the Task Force on Rural Elderly on Sustaining*

Quality Under Cost Containment, February 26, 1985.

155. A. Golodetz, "Good Medical Care in Nursing Homes," *American Journal of Public Health* 75, No. 3 (1985):227.

156. S. Holman, "DRGs: Forcing Physicians Into a Business Role," *Hospital Physician* 20, No. 5 (1984):102, 111.

157. D. Johnson, "Life, Death, and the Dollar Sign," *Journal of the American Medical Association* 252, No. 2 (July 13, 1984):223-224.

158. D. Dolenc and C. Dougherty, "DRGs: The Counterrevolution in Financing Health Care," *Hastings Center Report* 15, No. 3 (June 1985):19-29.

CHAPTER 12
Staring at the Ceiling:
A Patient's View
of DRGs

Most people in America are not even aware of what the initials DRG stand for. Furthermore, most people have yet to knowingly feel any impact upon themselves. Most patients/consumers are probably not even aware that the DRG system started nationally on October 1, 1983. Attention has focused almost exclusively on the impact of the DRG system on the institutions and the professionals. Yet, the ultimate, and perhaps the most devastating, impact will be upon the warm bodies of the patients/consumers who are flat on their backs staring up at the ceilings in hospitals and elsewhere.

Organized consumer groups have spoken out on the DRG system before Congressional committees and in their publications. Continuing areas of concern tend to fall within the following categories:

- Patients will be harmed because the quality of care will suffer.

- High level technology and sophisticated laboratory tests will not be used because the hospitals will not get enough DRG reimbursements to cover costs.

- Patients will be discharged too early and too sick because the institution will want to earn more money by keeping costs well under the DRG payment allowance.

- Hospitals will favor admitting patients with private insurance coverage since the institutions will earn more via that route.

- Hospitals will adopt more of a business ethic and run the facility like a factory rather than a humanitarian center.

- Patients will somehow be required to make up the dollar differential when a hospital receives less than their actual cost for caring for the patient.

- Patient advocacy will take a back seat to the profit and loss statement.

- Levels of care will seek the least common denominator of providing adequate care rather than striving for the optimal level.

Health care professionals share many of the consumer's concerns, though they may use different words to describe an issue. While a consumer may express concern about changes "harming the patient," a professional may speak of "utilization of services affecting quality." This semantic difference still results in the same end: The patient may be harmed.

Advantages and Disadvantages for Consumers

In his testimony before a U. S. Senate Subcommittee on Health, Plunkett bluntly stated the impact of the DRG plan upon the patient/consumer: "A prospective payment system, especially one based upon diagnoses groupings, would do nothing to alleviate the problem for the consumer of health services. It would not make more services available, it would not encourage alternative services, and in all likelihood would make services for many types of illnesses, injuries and diseases more difficult to come by on a timely basis."[1]

What does the implementation of a DRG reimbursement system mean to the patient/consumer? Will medical and health care differ? Will the individual be able to perceive any differences? These are the essential issues. In most instances, consumers will continue to pay about what they paid previously out of their own pockets for care. Insurance programs or governmental programs will still be paying for services. However, by setting up a budget and insisting that hospitals stay within the financial constraints, the government is having an impact on health care for the public. When you can't stay within your own household budget, what do you do? You buy fewer groceries; you spend less on leisure; you don't buy a new pair of shoes; you make do with what you have. Hospitals under the DRG program may have to do the same. When the belt is tightened, somebody feels the pinch.

Advantages and disadvantages to patients were listed in a medical society journal. Advantages included greater attention to discharge planning and alternative care programs, greater attention to effective medical procedures affecting survival, and no additional medical charges to patients beyond the DRG payment. Disadvantages included hospitals seeking to eliminate DRG categories that lose money, sicker patients being transferred to public hospitals, early discharges, and a shifting of Medicare costs to the private sector.[2]

Another respectable medical journal agreed that the length of stay could be manipulated, that ancillary services will be reduced, that care will not be as available as previously, and that out-of-pocket expenditures will increase.[3]

Considering the advantages and disadvantages, should consumers support the DRG plan?

Consumer Support

Since they have been suffering under the oppressive burden of runaway inflation for health care services, most consumers welcome any efforts to contain costs. However, the DRG program only applies to the costs of inpatient care for those covered by Medicare. A recurrent theme repeated by consumer groups calls for a system that would mandate that all payers be included in efforts to control health care costs. This would include all governmental programs, all insurance companies, and all types of care outside the hospital as well.

American Association of Retired Persons (AARP)

AARP has groups in all the states and represents millions of retired persons. In addition, AARP funds a research center and a variety of gerontology activities. As its spokesman, Christy told the U. S. Senate Subcommittee on Health that the DRG system should "cover all payors, all services and all hospitals,"[4] and while the AARP noted that DRGs offered the best chance for developing a meaningful pricing mechanism, there were comments on other aspects of the DRG plan:

- Basis of Payment—AARP said it was essential that the payment formula include a severity of illness index.

- Assignment (accepting what Medicare pays as payment in full)—AARP wanted assignment to be mandatory for hospitals and hospital-based physicians. Other health care providers should be given strong incentives to also accept assignment.

- Utilization Review—AARP wanted consumer representation and enforcement powers in a strong UR program.

- State Plans—AARP urged that states be allowed to develop alternate plans as long as the projected savings would be equal to or greater than the federal calculations.

- Legislation—AARP did not want the DRG legislation to be put on a fast track since in-depth scrutiny and deliberation might be bypassed.[5]

AARP has been a long-time supporter of a prospective payment method for controlling health care costs. In fact, AARP had urged Congress to enact such a program. DRGs offer many advantages, in AARP's opinion, but it warned a U.S. House of Representatives Subcommittee on Health to guard against DRG creep, "perhaps the most troublesome" by-product of the DRGs. "DRG creep occurs when providers 'play' the system by judging a diagnosis in order to get a patient into a higher-paying DRG category. Similarly, DRGs could encourage unnecessary surgery, because payment for the same diagnosis is higher when surgery is involved."[6] In summary, AARP felt that the prospective payment system could help stabilize the uncontrolled growth in hospital costs.[7] They also stated "that HMOs must be exempted from a DRG-based system."[8]

National Council of Senior Citizens (NCSC)

NCSC, founded about 1963, represents more than four and one-half million senior citizens through 4,500 clubs and councils in every state. It is another consumer group representing those most affected by the DRG plans—the elderly—calling for an all-payer system. Jacob Clayman, president of the NCSC, told the U.S. Senate "We believe that prospective payment should be applied toward the entire health care system. The resultant savings would benefit all purchasers of health care, including the Federal government and the Medicare beneficiaries."[9]

At the House hearings, the executive director of the NCSC hedged on the organization's support. Hutton commented that while the basic DRG concept was a good one, it was still too early to tell if or how well the program would work.[10]

Clayman also posed 13 questions to the senators illustrating the concerns of senior citizens with the DRG plan. Issues he raised related to cost-shifting, added cost-sharing by the beneficiary, multiple diagnoses, gaming the system, realistic DRG allowances, incentives to reduce costs, movement to uncovered office care, problems of inner city and rural hospitals, payments to hospitals for uncompensated care, flexibility of the states, and how HMOs will be treated.[11]

Organized Labor

Speaking for the AFL-CIO, Robert McGlotten reaffirmed the consumers' view that the cost containment system "ought to apply to all payors and include all providers, including physician services."[12] He said that organized labor supported the concept of prospective budgeting.

However, the AFL-CIO had strong comments about the suitability of DRGs and the problems associated with DRGs. While the AFL-CIO regarded the DRG plan as an improvement over current practices, McGlotten strongly stated, "We do not believe a nationwide system based on so-called diagnostic related groups (DRGs) is the best answer. We believe the jury is still out on the New Jersey system, which has been the model for this proposal. We do not know enough about the effectiveness of this approach to adopt it immediately for Medicare."[13] Problems mentioned by the AFL-CIO representative included the cost of the plan, the possible shifting of costs, the financial difficulties of the public and inner city hospitals, the control of teaching and capital costs, and the need to exempt HMOs.

These views of organized labor continue to be expressed on various aspects of the DRG reimbursement method. In an unlikely alliance, a representative of the AFL-CIO joined with a representative of the Washington Business Group on Health to support continued health planning to control capital costs. They took this position regardless of the Medicare payment method encapsulated within the DRG legislation. Both the labor and the business representative asserted that capital drives the health care system, much like the physician supply. Ignagni told a 1984 meeting of the National Health Planning and Development Council "that organized labor believes capital policy is the linchpin of any national strategy to contain the rate of health cost growth."[14] Incentives to buy, build, and expand have to be curbed to really achieve cost containment.

In addition, the AFL-CIO, the United Auto Workers, and the AARP endorsed the Kennedy-Gephardt bill to extend prospective pricing to physician's services.[15]

On a statewide level, Leo A. Brach represented the New Jersey State AFL-CIO before a Subcommittee on Health and Long Term Care that was assessing DRGs in that state. He noted his support for the DRG mechanism but expressed the hope that the method would lead to the control and decrease of all health care costs. Based on their experiences, the New Jersey State AFL-CIO developed an eight-point "Health Care Affordability Plan" to contain costs:

1. Develop a comprehensive all-payer system.

2. Institute a flexible state responsibility for the cost control process.

3. Place a ceiling on reimbursements to physicians and other professional providers.

4. Establish a set rate schedule for laboratory and X-ray services.

5. Encourage establishment of new HMOs.

6. Create a national professional advisory committee to examine new procedures and technologies and advise on their appropriateness and on fee schedules.

7. Develop stepped-up programs to meet long-term care needs.

8. Undertake continuous health education programs.[16]

In addition, a jointly sponsored Labor-Management Health Care Cost Containment Conference was convened in New Jersey. At this meeting one participant commented that health care costs were out of control because of the passive behavior of all consumers. Union members were warned that unless costs were controlled, they could expect alarming changes in health care coverage.[17]

Public Opinion

A Harris poll conducted in August 1983 found that most Americans were satisfied with the quality and availability of medical care. However, although the interviews also revealed that people wanted the latest and newest in treatment and technology, they were willing to limit options to lower costs. Americans said that "they were willing to give prospective payment under the DRGs system a try."[18]

A representative of a New Jersey hospital reported that patient satisfaction surveys have been "outstanding under the DRG system" and that no adverse effects have been noted.[19]

In essence, consumers applaud the initiation of DRGs as a beginning but they do not want the movement to stop there. Consumer groups display an understanding of the problems inherent with the DRG plan. Furthermore, there are numerous suggestions for improvement and further expansion of cost containment concepts.

Life, Death, and the Dollar Sign

Appropriately, a commentary in the Journal of the American Medical Association chillingly summed up the threat of DRGs to the patients/consumers: ". . . these proposals also have the potential to insidiously alter the factors considered in making life-and-death decisions for individual patients."[20]

While Johnson made the point that the hospital's concentration on containing costs was the incentive, the issue of medical ethics could not be overlooked. He asked which way the scale would tip in cases where the patient's outcome was dubious. Would life support systems be discouraged and discontinued when weighed against the potential financial losses? Physicians may have to negate their Hippocratic oath to "primum non nocere" (do the patient no harm); they may not be able to be impartial advocates for the patient's best interests any longer.

As has happened in the past, the groups of patients/consumers most likely affected are the ones least likely to complain, least likely to write and/or phone their legislators, and most likely to accept their fate with a grin-and-bear-it attitude. In recent years, there has been evidence of increased militancy among these groups but they have a long way to go before achieving the impact of the professional lobbying groups.

What patient groups will be the first victims of this burden of cost containment? The same groups that are now most vulnerable—the handicapped, the retarded, the chronically ill and the poor. The humanity of our profession is imperiled by the cost cutter's knife. . . . how long will it be before a tap on our shoulder comes from a concerned colleague or administrator, wondering whether a given patient in our intensive care unit may be "better off dying" in view of his or her "poor prognosis"?[21]

If this sounds callously fatalistic, consider the fact that the Medical Society of New Jersey has already asked, "Are DRGs killing patients?"[22] This question was raised during the 1983 annual meeting of the society by an assistant county medical examiner. He wondered if there was any cause and effect possibilities as he investigated patients' deaths and noted their early discharge from the hospital under New Jersey's DRG system. The situation prompted the New Jersey State Health Department to look into the problem. As of now, the investigators have not gathered any data to suggest that the DRG system resulted in any effect on discharge, death, or readmission in the cases studied.[23]

Consumer Organizations: Their Views

On February 2 and 17, 1983, the U. S. Senate Subcommittee on Health held hearings on the hospital prospective payment system. Generally, most of those appearing before the Commmittee were in favor of a prospective payment system. Some groups had reservations, some had recommendations, and some were more aggressive than others in stating their pro and con views.

William Hutton, executive director of the National Council of Senior Citizens, pointed out five possible situations where Medicare recipients could be harmed:

1. Medicare admissions could be discouraged, thus denying access to older patients.

2. Some admissions could be encouraged, whether or not hospitalization is the most appropriate site for treatment.

3. Use of ancillary services could be restricted, reducing the hospital's cost per case but denying patients the services they need to promote or enhance recovery.

4. The quality of care administered could be seriously impaired.

5. The length of hospital stay could be inappropriately shortened, seriously affecting the Medicare patient's discharge status.[24]

These harmful effects could take place when individuals having private insurance coverage might be admitted in place of people having Medicare coverage; when a hospital admits an elderly person because it is more profitable for the institution to treat that person on an outpatient basis; when physical therapy services are limited or contracted out to charge under Part B of Medicare; when hospitals reduce their personnel to save on labor costs; or when a patient has to receive post-hospital care at a nursing home instead of being discharged to their own home.

In addition to the elderly being harmed by the DRG program, Glenn M. Plunkett, representing the American Foundation for the Blind, took the consumer's worries a step further. "Our fears are that . . . the aged, disabled and blind will be adversely affected."[25] This statement was made regardless of the consideration of the type of cost containment activities undertaken by the institutions. What prevailed, in their minds, was the probable fact that the providers of health care would seek to avoid incurring financial risk. Thus, hospitals would seek out patients without complications and avoid people with multiple serious health ailments among the aged, disabled, and blind.

Robert McGlotten of the AFL-CIO also echoed that feeling in his congressional testimony. "A prospective reimbursement system for Medicare alone would give hospitals strong incentives to turn away all, or certain types of, Medicare patients."[26]

Frances Klafter spoke in strident terms for the Gray Panthers—an activist elderly group—at the Congressional hearings. "We question whether . . . the nation's elderly parents, grandparents, aunt and uncles lying ill in hospitals . . . will be assured quality health care under this proposed plan."[27] Furthermore, the Gray Panthers felt that hospitals, under the DRG plan, had economic incentives to provide only the minimum care required to earn a specific DRG payment.

Early Discharge

Concern about the inappropriate early discharge of patients from the hospital was raised by professionals as well as patients and consumer groups. In early 1981, a president of a DRG Coordinators group in New Jersey asked, "Will the patients be discharged before they are ready?"[28] Recurrent readmissions as an aftermath were also part of the question. These professionals linked the harmful effects to the patient under the rubric of the quality of care.

In an article in the *American Medical News*, it was noted that some physicians in New Jersey were also complaining about early discharges. These physicians stated that hospitals were exerting pressure on them to release patients too soon.[29] In the largest hospital area in the state, the average length of stay had fallen from more than 10 days to fewer than seven days from 1980 to 1983.

Writing in a publication of the Consumer Commission on the Accreditation of Health Services, Young commented that hospitals are able to maximize their income by putting pressure on doctors to discharge patients at the earliest possible moment. She said: "Many patients now feel pushed out of New Jersey hospitals prematurely, before adequate home care or other alternatives to hospitalization can be arranged."[30] This situation could result in "churning" admissions. Obviously, patients do not benefit from this revolving door approach to their health care. One physician said in a letter to the editor of *American Medical News* that "patients will sue when unhappy at leaving the hospital early."[31]

Service Limitations and Reductions

Consumers are familiar with the economic ramifications of market supply and demand theories. Whenever consumers purchase anything, they can see that services are reduced or limited to assure profits. If a service or product does not return a profit, the businessman must either eliminate the product or limit the production costs. Consumers fear that hospitals will do the same within the DRG system. "Hospitals will find that they will be cutting out services that lose money," said the president of the Health Research and Educational Trust regarding experiences in New Jersey.[32] Nobody would like to be in a hospital bed wondering whether every possible service was being used in their treatment regimen.

Talking about changing patterns of medical practice, *Postgraduate Medicine* noted that hospitals may do away with routine batteries of diagnostic tests upon admission, that intensive care units (ICUs) may be a prominent target for closings, and that physicians may find their treatment options severely limited.[33]

Individuals do not need an advanced degree in economics to calculate that a hospital can not stay in operation by continually losing more money than it brings in from patient care. Private charity and endowments can not always make up the deficits. What will be limited and/or reduced is what worries the consumer, particularly the consumer who is flat on his or her back in a hospital bed.

Emotional Trauma

Based on the fears expressed about the potential for patient harm, one might realistically anticipate emotional stress and strain on people entering a hospital where the DRG system is in place. With the accent on the hospital's profit and loss statement, the patient/consumer may have good cause to worry. However, James Scott, an acting deputy administrator of the Health Care Financing Administration, reassured the elderly in a speech before a 1984 meeting of the Healthcare Financial Management Association. Based on 1983 admission data for Medicare patients, a 0 percent increase actually occurred when a projected increase of 3.4 percent was expected. He stated, "So it is safe to conclude" that hospitals are not "jerking every third senior citizen they see on a street corner off to the hospital to maximize DRG payments."[34]

On the other side of the coin, Harry Schwartz vents his interpretation in a journal devoted to the private practice concept: "But I suspect many patients, especially among the elderly, are going to be very unhappy about the new style of medicine encouraged by the DRG system. What it does, after all, is reward physicians and hospitals that do the least for patients."[35]

This dilemma is somewhat akin to astronauts sitting in a capsule considering the fact that they are being sent to the moon in a technologically sophisticated vehicle built by the lowest bidders.

The Consumer Burden

A chief economist for Standard & Poors Corporation said that it may be possible to recreate a health care market economy. He started with the premise that consumers pay only a small portion of total costs and do not have the information to make rational decisions. Then, Blitzer delivered the coup de grace: "The perfect idea is cost sharing, making consumers pay a much larger part of the total."[36] This idea allows health care to get back on the track of a typical market economy. Cost sharing will reduce health care spending since people will be reluctant to spend if the real dollars come from their own pockets.

American Hospital Association proposals had suggested this idea earlier. However, a few hospital administrators objected. Interestingly, the objection was not to the merit of the suggestion but to the potential political damage. A president of a statewide hospital association voiced the fear that "adversaries will say that we want to soak the patient more."[37]

Seven points are listed by the Healthcare Financial Management Association (HFMA) in their general guidelines concerning prospectively determined prices. HFMA is an organization representing more than 21,000 individual members who are either financial managers of health care organizations or are closely associated with those activities.

According to HFMA, patient financial participation should do the following:

1. Influence demand, while not discouraging essential services.

2. Influence choice of service (i.e., encourage lower cost ambulatory or home service in preference to inpatient service).

3. Improve understanding of services provided as well as their value.

4. Permit patients to express their preferences and priorities.

5. Contribute to accurate reporting or services provided to the patient.

6. Provide essential financial resources when other priorities dictate limitations on funding by payers.

7. Permit discretion and flexibility.[38]

In addition to these points, the HFMA also listed 12 cautions and considerations regarding patient financial participation. These concerned deductible and coinsurance provisions, relating payment to type of service, geographic restrictions, poor patients, limits to patient participation, advance deposits against participation, notice of patient participation, bad debts, discretion in billing, optional patient participation, and the effect upon decisions.[39]

Final Rules on Charges to Beneficiaries

Although Medicare beneficiaries are responsible for the deductibles and coinsurance amounts under Part A, a hospital cannot charge a beneficiary for services covered under the prospective payment system. Federal government rule makers did not intend to have covered patients accrue any new liability. Final rules issued on January 3, 1984 clarified when additional charges could be billed to beneficiaries. In addition, the regulations include a number of safeguards to protect the patients against the possibility of abuse by hospitals (see Exhibit 12-1).

Evidently the federal government favors limiting the financial participation of the patient while the administrators favor that option as a means of recouping any losses incurred when services exceed DRG allowances.

Patient Flak on Cost Participation

Not only is there an effort to make sure that the hospitals do not add on additional costs to the bill, but some patients are also alert to an inequity that could take place.

An obstetrical patient in Freehold Area Hospital in New Jersey, an all-payer state, had an insurance policy that required her to pay 20 percent of the bill. She inquired as to the per diem rate and the DRG rate for herself and her new baby. Using consumer price comparison techniques, she realized that the DRG rate was higher. Acting on that information, the woman checked herself and her baby out a half-day early against medical advice. This action resulted in putting her under the minimum stay for the DRG rate and saved her $150. Fortunately, no complications occurred for either mother or baby.[40]

Another patient in New Jersey suffered a coronary insufficiency two months after losing his job and consequently lost his health insurance coverage. While he was hospitalized for three or four days, his bill came to several thousand dollars because of his DRG diagnosis. A furious patient paid and vented his anger at his doctor.[41]

Newark's Beth Israel Medical Center treated a visitor from abroad who had a heart attack at the airport. His charges at the hospital amounted to about $4,000. However, his DRG rate was $8,000. Explaining about averages and the system did not assuage the man's indignation as he left to return home.[42]

Exhibit 12-1   Allowable Hospital Charges to Medicare Beneficiaries

Hospitals may charge patients covered by the DRG system only for the following:

1. Applicable deductible and coinsurance amounts.
2. Items and services that are excluded from coverage on some basis other than custodial care, medically unnecessary items, nonphysician services by other than the hospital, exhaustion of benefits, or nonentitlement.
3. Items and services for custodial care, medically unnecessary services, and items after all of the following conditions have been met:
   a. Patient no longer requires inpatient care as determined by the hospital directly or through its utilization review committee.
   b. Attending physician agrees in writing. If physician does not agree, the hospital can seek a review by the medical care entity. That entity's agreement will serve in lieu of the physician's agreement.
   c. Beneficiary is notified in writing by the hospital or the utilization review committee that—
      (1) Inpatient care is no longer required.
      (2) Customary charges will be made beyond the second day following the date of the notice.
      (3) Medical review entity will make formal determination on the validity of the hospital's findings if the patient remains in the hospital after he or she is liable for charges.
      (4) Appeals can be made by the hospital or the beneficiary under Medicare Part A procedures.
      (5) Charges will be refunded if there is a finding that the patient required continued care beyond the point indicated by the hospital.
   d. Patients remaining in the hospital after appropriate notification and found to still need acute level of care may not be charged for the continued care until the conditions for the charges again meet the required criteria.
4. Diagnostic procedures and studies, and therapeutic procedures and courses of treatment that are excluded from coverage under medically unnecessary items and services. Although the patient requires continued inpatient hospital care, the services are furnished after the patient acknowledges in writing being informed that—
   a. Those services were not considered necessary and reasonable under Medicare by the hospital and the intermediary.
   b. Customary charges will be billed upon receipt of the services.
   c. A formal determination on the validity of the hospital's findings will be made by the intermediary if the patient receives the services.
   d. Determinations are appealable by the hospital or the beneficiary under Medicare Part A procedures.
   e. If services are found to be covered, charges will be refunded.
5. Customary charges for noncovered items and services furnished on outliers days.
6. Differential charges for a private room or other luxury service that is more expensive than is medically required and is provided for personal comfort of the patient.

Source: Federal Register. *Medical Program: Prospective Payment for Medicare Inpatient Hospital Services: Final Rule, Part VI, Section 412.42*, HHS, Health Care Financing Administration, January 3, 1984.

Increasing Consumer Awareness

In a statement giving general guidance concerning prospective determined prices, the Healthcare Financial Management Association also noted: "Education of patients is an essential corollary to the provision of alternatives and to encouraging cost effective consumer behavior."[43]

Patients/consumers often do not exercise their rights in a health care encounter. There are a variety of psychosocial rationales for this behavior. Perhaps one of the most potent reasons has to do with the fear that the health care provider will be offended and not do their best to help. In any event, the problem of educating the public about DRGs is only just beginning to receive attention.

Seminars

Eight educational seminars were held during 1984 in Florida to raise consumer awareness of DRGs and to discuss the role of consumers, aging groups, and providers under this new system. These meetings were cosponsored by the American Association of Retired Persons, Florida Aging and Adult Services Office (Department of Health Rehabilitative Services), Florida Council on Aging, Florida Department of Insurance, Florida Hospital Association, and Blue Cross/ Blue Shield of Florida. A volunteer from the AARP initiated the project with help from the Health Advocacy Services of AARP. Using a summary checklist, and how-to guide, the seminar organizer got help to review contacting sponsors, to prepare the format of the meetings, including a sample agenda, to generate publicity and to devise a timetable for tasks to implement the educational meetings.[44] Seminars have been well attended and the activity appears to be spreading to other AARP affiliates throughout the nation. More than 500 persons attended just such a program sponsored by the Monmouth County (NJ) Senior Citizen Council in early 1985.[45]

Hospital Leaflets

Community Memorial Hospital in Toms River, New Jersey provides patients with a special brochure at discharge entitled "Understanding Your Hospital Bill—What You Need to Know About DRG." This leaflet explains why the DRG system is being used at the hospital and how different payment rates are calculated; it also explains DRG terms such as length of stay, trim points, outlier, DRG rate, and controlled charges. Finally, the brochure tells patients what to look for on their bill. Patients are given the brochure on discharge because the hospital feels that that is the moment when the information is needed. It is anticipated that there will be greater comprehension and patients will learn to survive under the new system.[46] Appropriately, this patient education activity is part of a larger program that includes the medical and dental staff, trustees, and insiders.

A booklet entitled, "What Your Patients Should Know . . . About DRGs and the Prospective Payment System" was published by the American Medical Association in 1984. In question and answer form, this booklet covers an explanation of DRGs, the implications for health care costs, issues regarding the access to health care, and the impact upon the quality of health care. Physicians are advised that the booklet can be used to respond to commonly asked questions from patients. Finally, the physicians are told that the material is not meant to be a comprehensive analysis of the DRG issues.[47]

Although hospital administrators used to regard patient education as a frill, PPS has caused a resurgence in such activities. In fact, the AHA cited leaders in patient education generally and also those facilities with programs for specific target populations. It was noted that patient education programs help contain costs by reducing readmissions.[48]

Complaints

In a study of the DRG system in New Jersey, Dunham and Morone commented that patients became irate because their bill showed that the hospital collected more than the actual cost of services, depending upon the DRG assignment. "Worse, both the services and the charges were right there on the bill for the patient to see, compare, and complain about."[49] Between May 1 and July 1, 1980, the New Jersey State Health Department reported 120 inquiries from about 40,000 discharged patients. After July 1, there were only 20 inquiries from more than 140,000 discharges.[50] A decline from one complaint in 330 discharges to one in 7,000 occurred. A survey by the New Jersey Hospital Association indicated about five complaints for every 100 patients.[51]

To exacerbate the situation, the State Health Department appeared to act in a nonsympathetic manner. "An angry patient who called the Department about a bill (was told) to simply not pay it." In writing to a department official, the executive vice president of the New Jersey Hospital Association called it "unbelievable." He further said: "We can't expect cooperation from the hospitals if the Department staff does not have the courage to face up to a problem the system has created."[52] A payer appeal system was developed that gave patients the opportunity to seek justice.

It seems evident that informed consumers may have questions about hospital bills. However, management experts advise educating the top levels first before informing the line workers. Attention is being concentrated on the professionals and the institutional employees first. After that we will probably see a greater effort to resolve the complaints of the consumers through educational activities. Until that time, there will be complaints.

Consumer Cost Consciousness

A Louis Harris poll indicated that 51 percent of the public consider the cost of doctor visits unreasonable. This contrasts with only 19 percent of the physicians who held that view. In a summary of the poll, it was noted "that physicians are almost alone in thinking that doctors fees are reasonable, that the total cost of health care is satisfactory, and that this country already has a price-competitive health care system."[53]

Part of the difficulty in raising the cost consciousness levels of consumers relates to the insurance coverage situation. If consumers do not have to pay for health care services from their own pockets, then there is not a strong incentive to worry about the costs. Somebody else is paying the tab. This attitude prevails despite the realization by consumers that the costs are reflected in their insurance premiums, in their deductibles, and in their copayments. However, those increased costs are hidden in small regular paycheck deductions.

Meyer argues that the consumer should be told about the honest cost of various health care options. Then the consumer can consider the choices along with their uncompromising financial consequences and make intelligent decisions. He suggests making the system more honest, more rational, and more fair. After doing so, Meyer suggests that we ought to live with consumer choices.[54]

On the other side, there are those who question the ability of the consumer to understand the data. Cost-saving enthusiasm may lead to scrimping. It is feared that "consumers without the skilled knowledge to intelligently purchase medical care will not be able to recognize these shortcuts and scrimpings."[55]

In keeping with this concept of providing data, Representative Ron Wyden is sponsoring an amendment to direct the U. S. Public Health Service to provide technical assistance to consumers or purchaser groups desiring to create their own databases. This amendment does not call for the PHS to collect comparative price and quality information.[56]

In proposed regulations, the Health Care Financing Administration proposes that Peer Review Organizations will be able to release data on individual physician practice patterns and generalizations concerning the quality of care at a specific institution. In opposing these proposed regulations, the American Medical Association poses two severe problems:

1. A patient might avoid the most appropriate physician and misleading data could have a devastating effect on some professionals.

2. Disclosure of patient-identified information to the patient may not always be appropriate or beneficial.

As a remedy to the second point, the AMA suggests that the patient's designated representative should be a physician.[57]

In opposing Representative Wyden's amendment, the AMA maintained that "the purchase of health care services is unique and does not necessarily lend itself to easy comparison based on price or comparative utilization."[58]

This lack of consumer cost-consciousness should really not be too surprising. Research has indicated that physicians also do not know the prices of the drugs and lab tests that they order.

Rights of Patients

Several years back there was a spate of activities concerned with the rights of patients. A Bill of Rights was developed by the American Hospital Association and was followed by similar documents from a variety of sources. A Society of Patient Representatives sprang into existence and many hospitals employ a Patient Advocate or Patient Representative. At least one prestigious college offers a master's degree in patient advocacy.

Who looks out for the patient in the DRG system? This question raises some ethical issues because of the ambivalence between the need to remain financially solvent and the ethic of providing the highest quality of care. In commenting on a case study, Penticuff put it succinctly: "Health care professionals who put the institution's financial interest above the best interests of the patient have sold their ethics to the highest DRG."[59]

At a meeting of the Massachusetts Health Care Association, Dr. Arnold S. Relman, the editor of the *New England Journal of Medicine*, opposed additional financial gain for phsyicians helping hospitals turn a profit on Medicare patients. "The doctor has to be the advocate of the patient," he said.[60]

In early 1986, HCFA announced that a patient's rights letter has to be given to each Medicare patient on admission to a hospital. That letter informs patients of the legal right to challenge their presumed early discharge to the local PRO, including the phone number of the PRO to do so immediately. A headline in the March 10, 1986 issue of *Medical World News* proclaimed, "Medicare Gets Its Miranda Decision."[61]

Professional Patient Advocacy

In a presentation on "The Impact of DRGs on Patient Representation," a professional patient representative sees the advent of DRGs as an opportunity in the competitive market place.[62] However, she has to balance being the advocate of the patient with the need to justify the value of the program to a hospital administration that pays her salary. Patient representatives have to demonstrate cost-effectiveness as they increase the census, decrease length of stay, decrease liability, and increase revenue. On the other hand, the patient representative at the same time has to convince the patient that the facility is responsive to individual needs. It is a tough acrobatic act to join the hospital's bottom line of profit and loss to the patient's bottom line of quality care.

Rudnick and Shryock tell how patient representatives can "help DRGs work for you."[63] According to the authors, patient representatives may be a key hospital resource, may reduce exposure to liability, and aid in the discharge planning process. Through the hospital's use of the ambassador/hostess/ receptionist concept, the approach to patients and families is personalized. A consumer orientation and attention to consumer perceptions are stressed. Nevertheless, the patient representative is integrated into a streamlined discharge planning matrix whose goal is to shorten the length of stay. Which master does the patient representative serve?

Patient education professionals are advised that the prospective payment plan offers opportunities for them as well as their need to carefully examine prior activities. Among the opportunities for the hospital to consider are the following:

- Adding a patient education component to the preadmission testing program

- Implementing a self-care demonstration to educate patients about such things as IV catheter care at home, and thereby decrease length of stay

- Documenting impact of preoperative and cardiac counseling in reducing length of stay and inpatient resource use

- Using closed circuit TV programming for patient education and allowing nurses to respond to individual needs

- Developing outpatient classes, such as for recently discharged diabetic patients, supported by fees to cover direct costs[64]

In addition to the above, it is possible that professional patient educators may refer people to disease-specific community programs after discharge. If cost containment affects the supply of educational materials, some have suggested that the patients and family members purchase the teaching materials.

In commenting on the hospital-based health educator's responsibilities for cost-containment, Bryce-Richardson admonished that there will be more competition for the limited resources. There will have to be greater measurement of inputs such as labor, materials, and equipment, against outputs such as reduced length of stay and resources diminition. Economic analysis will be the frame of reference in the advocacy activities of the professional patient representatives.[65]

Why Respect Patients' Rights?

Basically it's good business to respect patients' rights.

Patients who are given the opportunity to participate in decisions affecting their own care appear to have better outcomes. As a bonus, these improved outcomes may even use less resources. A report of the President's Commission on the Study of Ethical Problems in Medicine, entitled *Making Health Care Decisions*,[66] stated that patients more fully involved in medical decisions recover quicker. A hospital administrator stated that "we have the means to increase the quality of care and to lower costs by taking patients' rights seriously."[67]

In the opening paragraph of an article discussing an ethical response to DRGs, the twin specters of mortality and money are neatly combined to warm the cockles of any confused administrator threatened by DRG mandates. "Taking patients' rights seriously and taking steps to see that they are respected constitutes a powerful tool for cost effective leadership of health care institutions in an era of prospective payment. Not only is it morally correct to ensure that the rights of patients are respected, it pays off."[68]

References

1. U. S. Congress, Senate Committee on Finance, Subcommittee on Health, *Hearings on Hospital Prospective Payment System, Part II*, February 17, 1983. (Plunkett 342, Christy 320, AARP 320-321, AARP 305, Clayman 294-296, McGlotten 262, Plunkett 344, McGlotten 263, Klaftner 281).

2. C. Kaemmerer, "A New Reimbursement System, DRGs are Coming," *Connecticut Medicine* 47, No. 11 (1983):697-699.

3. S. Lewis, "Speculations on the Impact of Prospective Pricing and DRGs," *Western Journal of Medicine* 140, No. 4 (1984):638-644.

4. U. S. Congress, *Hearings.*

5. Ibid.

6. "Hospital, Medical Groups React to DRG Payment," *Employee Benefit Plan Review* 37, No. 7 (1983):70, 72-73.

7. U. S. Congress, *Hearings.*

8. "Hospital, Medical Groups React," *Employee Benefit Plan Review.*

9. U. S. Congress, *Hearings.*

10. "Hospital, Medical Groups React," *Employee Benefit Plan Review.*

11. U. S. Congress, *Hearings.*

12. Ibid.

13. Ibid.

14. "Business/Organized Labor Testify at National Council Meeting," *TODAY in Health Planning* 2, No. 4 (May 14, 1984):1-2.

15. U. S. Congress, *Hearings.*

16. L. A. Brach, *Testimony Before Subcommittee on Health and Long Term Care*, Camden County College, Camden, NJ, March 30, 1984.

17. D. Warshaw, "Labor, Industry Vow to Unite on Health Costs," *Star-Ledger* (NJ), January 17, 1984.

18. J. Nelson, "What 1983 Did to Medicine," *Private Practice* 16, No. 1 (1984):15-16, 20.

19. A. A. Lee, "How DRGs Will Affect Your Hospital—And You," *RN* 47, No. 5 (1984):71-81.

20. D. E. Johnson, "Life, Death, and the Dollar Sign. Medical Ethics and Cost Containment," *Journal of the American Medical Association* 252, No. 2 (July 13, 1984):223-224.

21. Ibid.

22. "Do DRGs Hurt Patients? State Society Plans Study," *American Medical News* 26, No. 19 (May 20, 1983):3, 9.

23. F. Goldschmidt, *Full Professional Standard Organization (PRSO) Study*, New Jersey State Health Department, Trenton, NJ, July 12, 1984.

24. "Hospital, Medical Groups React," *Employee Benefit Plan Review.*

25. U. S. Congress, *Hearings.*

26. Ibid.

27. Ibid.

28. "Officials Spot Inequities in DRG Cost Control Program," *Hospital Peer Review* 6, No. 2 (1981):13-15.

29. D. Lefton, "AHA Backs DRG-Based Prospective Pay Plan," *American Medical News* 26, No. 6 (February 11, 1983):1, 27-28.

30. R. Young, "Creeping Fiasco in New Jersey Hospital Costs," *The Fund Reporter* 2, No. 2 (1984):1, 3.

31. H. C. Moss, "Planner's Haven't Learned From Mistakes, MD Says," *American Medical News* 27, No. 19 (May 18, 1984):6.

32. "Some Services May Be Cut Under New Payment System," *Hospitals* 57, No. 17 (August 16, 1983):S14.

33. C. Katz, "New Reimbursement Formulas: The Effects of DRGs and Changing Fiscal Responsibilities," *Postgraduate Medicine* 74, No. 4 (1983):107-11.

34. "Government Says DRGs Are Meeting Expectations," *American Medical News* 27, No. 19 (May 18, 1984):20.

35. H. Schwartz, "How DRGs Will Breed Medical Rationing," *Private Practice* 15, No. 10 (1983):8.

36. M. Tatge, "Prospective Pay's Just a 'Quick Fix'," *Modern Healthcare* 14, No. 5 (1984):156-158.

37. Lefton, "AHA Backs Plan."

38. Healthcare Financial Management Association, *General Guidelines Concerning Prospectively Determined Prices*, Revised, January 10, 1983.

39. Ibid.

40. C. L. Rosenberg, "Payment By Diagnosis: How the Great Experiment Is Going," *Medical Economics* 59, No. 10 (May 10, 1982):245-246, 251-257.

41. Ibid.

42. Ibid.

43. Healthcare Financial Management Association, *General Guidelines*.

44. American Association of Retired Persons, *Diagnosis Related Group Educational Seminars*, Washington, DC, 1984.

45. "Seniors Told of Medicare Changes," *The News Tribune*, Woodbridge, NJ, February 2, 1985.

46. "Demystifying DRGs," *Profiles in Hospital Marketing* 13 (First Quarter, 1984):44-47.

47. *What Your Patients Should Know. . . About DRGs and the Prospective Payment System* (Chicago: American Medical Association, May 1984).

48. "AHA Cites Leaders in Patient Education," *Hospitals* 58, No. 21 (November 1, 1984): 64, 68.

49. A. B. Dunham and J. A. Morone, *The Politics of Innovation: The Evolution of DRG Rate Regulation in New Jersey. Volume IV-A* (Princeton: Health Research and Educational Trust of New Jersey, January 1983), pp. 97-98.

50. Ibid.

51. Ibid.

52. Ibid.

53. "Poll Finds Physicians More Realistic on Health Costs Than Medical Leaders," *Medical World News* 25, No. 14 (July 23, 1984):61.

54. J. A. Meyer, "Increased Consumer Cost-Consciousness and Competition," *Bulletin of the New York Academy of Medicine* 60, No. 1 (1984):98-105.

55. Tatge, "Quick Fix."

56. J. Fochtman, "Washington Update. Health Care Cost Information Amendment Proposed," *Medical Marketing & Media* 19, No. 8 (1984):4, 6.

57. "PRO Proposal Jeopardizes Confidentiality" (editorial), *American Medical News* 27, No. 27 (July 20, 1984):4.

58. J. Fochtman, "Washington Update."

59. J. H. Penticuff, "Commentary on the Doctor, the Patient and the DRG," *Hastings Center Report* 13, No. 5 (1983):25.

60. "Should Physicians Share Hospital's Medicare Profits? Relman Says No," *Modern Healthcare* 14, No. 4 (1984):11.

61. "Medicare Gets Its Miranda Decision," *Medical World News* 27, No. 5 (March 10, 1986):29.

62. B. Miller, DRGs *Impact of Change*, Presentation at Middle Atlantic Health Congress, Atlantic City, NJ, May 23, 1984.

63. J. D. Rudnick, Jr., and M. Shyrock, "Patient Representatives and Discharge Planning. Helping DRGs Work for You," *Osteopathic Hospitals* 28, No. 2 (1984):16-20.

64. B. Giloth, "Prospective Pricing and the Implications for Patient Education," *Promoting Health* 4, No. 6 (1983):4-5, 11.

65. M. Bryce-Richardson, *What Health Educators Need to Know About DRGs*, Presentation at American Public Health Association Annual Meeting, Anaheim, CA, November 14, 1984.

66. *Making Health Care Decisions. The Ethical and Legal Implications of Informed Consent in the Patient-Practitioner Relationship. Volume One: Report.* Washington, D.C.: President's Commission for the Study of Ethical Problems in Medicine and Biomedical and Behavioral Research (October 21, 1982).

67. J. Summers, "An Ethical Response to DRGs.Respecting Patients' Rights," *Texas Hospitals* 39, No. 10 (1984):34-35.

68. Ibid.

CHAPTER 13
Gazing into the PPS/DRG Crystal Ball

Prognosticators peering into the future of the health care delivery system in the United States may perceive a murky view. That dimness could be due to a fundamental informational flaw. As Sager puts it, "We have a $300 billion health care system—and we don't know how it works."[1] Despite the lack of data about the workings of the system, the PPS/DRG mechanism has an enormous impact on the machinery of the nation's delivery of health care services. In addition, the lack of information does not halt the predictions of various possible outcomes. The same question may elicit responses that range from one end of the spectrum to the other. Exhibit 13-1 illustrates answers to the question, "What's next for DRGs?" Note that all of these health care experts gaze into the future and come up with different projections.

Nevertheless, it is informative to discover what knowledgeable people are thinking and consider how their forecasts match our own impressions. For that reason, the crystal ball predictions are sorted out and put down along with a final consensus based on a review of the literature on PPS/DRGs.

"PPS/DRG Works Fine"—One View

On October 15, 1984, about one year after PPS began, Business Week published a cover story on changing how the health care industry works.[2] A dramatic drawing on the cover illustrated the dominant theme in the change. A physician in a white coat listened with one stethoscope earpiece while holding the end piece on a patient's chest and a man in a business suit listened with the other earpiece as he used a calculator to total profits and losses. The article talks about the revolutionary changes in the health care industry. Ellwood commented on the changes: "We're watching the start of an economic transformation of the American health care system."[3] DRGs were credited with producing "startling results" in less than a year, relative to hospital admissions and length of stay. More than 130 business coalitions for health exist to monitor costs, and these

Exhibit 13-1   DRG Forecasts: From Forever to Hardly Ever

DRGs are here to stay. There will be ongoing review and modifying, but DRGs will be with us for a long time . . . We can expect to see DRGs extended to inhospital physician services and to outpatient care.[A]
>   Jay J. Nisenfeld, Kaiser Sunnyside Medical Center, Clackamas, Oregon

By 1990 we will see . . . a fourth generation of the DRG system in place for a significant minority, if not the majority, of the population.[B]
>   Stewart Altman, Ph.D., Chairman, ProPAC

Are DRGs just another potshot? . . . DRGs are another intervention . . . in a long line of federal and state legislation . . . DRG provisions will experience trouble . . . Even if DRGs have methodological weaknesses they, at least, convey a strong message.[C]
>   Walter J. McNerney, Past President, Blue Cross and Blue Shield Associations

DRGs will be scrapped in favor of a capitation system . . . DRGs will be abandoned because of "inherent rigidity" that prevents equitable application to different localities and types of facilities and the complexity of regulations that would be required to prevent gaming of the system.[D]
>   Arthur D. Little Company, Cambridge, Massachusetts in a study for the Health Insurance Association of America

DRG-type system will spread to non-Medicare patients of all ages throughout the 50 states via proposed legislation for an all payer system, to be accompanied by explosive growth in HMOs . . . Ultimately, a "voucher" system for insured patients will make DRGs obsolete.[E]
>   Jack Owen, American Hospital Association

A. J. J. Nisenfeld, "What Impact Will DRGs Have on Group Practice?" *Medical Group Management* 30, no. 5 (1983): 50–52, 56–58, 60, 62, 64.
B. "An Honest Broker for Fine-Tuning Medicare," *Hospitals* 59, no. 19 (October 1, 1984): 102, 104–105.
C. W. McNerney, "Hunting for Solutions: Are DRGs Just Another Potshot?" *The Internist* 24, no. 6 (1983): 11–12.
D. "Study Predicts Scrapping of DRGs by Medicare," *Hospitals* 59, no. 10 (May 16, 1985): 18.
E. "Hospital Admissions Down, Competition for Posts Up," *Medical World News* 26, no. 8 (April 22, 1985): 7.

groups support PPS. An accompanying editorial said it was time for a war on runaway medical costs.[4] According to Ellwood, the trend will continue because "doctors and hospitals sense that the jig is up."[5]

According to Inspector-General Kusserow of HHS, hospitals are "doing better under Medicare than anybody thought they would." At the end of 1985, he reported that hospital profit margins on Medicare rose to 14 percent in the first year of PPS/DRG operation. However, the American Hospital Association and the Federation of American Hospitals contested the above-average profits and predicted tough times ahead for hospitals under PPS.[6]

Federal Leadership Praised

In June 1985, a *New York Times* editorial praises the role of federal leadership on regulatory reform to make hospitals contain costs: "Congress and the Reagan Administration have managed an apparently humane taming of hospital cost inflation. While caution may still be in order, so is credit for a triumph of social policy."[7]

Dramatic results were cited in the editorial: admissions went from a pre-1982 1.9 percent increase annually to a 3.3 percent decline in 1984; hospital expenditures decreased from 16.2 percent yearly increases to 5.4 percent. In addition, no decline in the quality of care was observed and the public's health was not in danger. Improvement in hospital efficiency was highlighted as the big news. In closing, the editorial commented that "intelligent Federal leadership makes a powerful difference."[8]

That powerful federal leadership at work is reflected in monthly HCFA reports on Medicare PPS monitoring activities. Exhibit 13-2 illustrates the data supplied about the status of facilities, benefit payments, admission, average length of stay, and the ranking of the 25 most common DRGs by cost, discharges, and average length of stay.

Notwithstanding the adulation of the *New York Times* and *Business Week* and the federal government itself praising the merits of PPS/DRG, the cautionary note was sounded. Speaking at an Iowa BC/BS meeting on health cost issues, HCFA Administrator Davis said that DRGs are "not fine-tuned yet."[9] In agreeing, Altman, ProPAC chairman, remarked that PPS needed an overhaul to survive.[10]

Possible directions for a PPS overhaul can be implied from a listing of the reports mandated by Congress when they passed P.L. 98-21 initiating the PPS. The ProPAC report lists the topics, the due date, and the responsible governmental agency in Exhibit 13-3.

Regardless of future directions, it is unlikely that there will be a retrogression. If the PPS falls apart, we won't go back to cost-based reimbursement, according to Altman.[11] In fact, Griffith, a professor of hospital administration, said that "retrospective cost-based reimbursement was one of the two or three biggest health care policy errors of my lifetime."[12] Even the medical practitioners agree, as Hodes notes in his editorial on the new world of health care, "it is unreasonable to assume that cost-containment initiatives will stop [only with inpatient Medicare services]."[13]

"PPS/DRG Is Less Than Successful"—Another View

Responding to the *New York Times* editorial praising the leadership of the federal government, Bessey pointed out that the gains were achieved at the detriment

Exhibit 13-2

HCFA Background Paper, January 1986

Special PPS/Non-PPS Facility Status
Short Stay PPS Hospital—At the end of
the second year of PPS implementation
(September 1985), about 5,350 short-stay
general and specialty hospitals and separate cost entities were covered by the prospective payment system. This represents 80%
of all participating hospitals.

*Hospitals receiving special consideration
under PPS (as of September 1985)*—Regional referral centers 158; Cancer treatment centers 6; "Mayo Clinic" type providers
4; Sole community hospitals 359.

*Certified hospitals and units not under PPS
(as of September 1985)*
Exempted Hospitals—Psychiatric hospitals 481; Rehabilitation hospitals 68; Alcohol/
drug hospitals 28; Other long-term care hospitals 86; Children's hospitals 53; Christian
Science Sanitoria 22; Short-stay hospitals in
waivered states 545; Short-stay hospitals in
outlying areas 59.
Exception Units—Psychiatric 733; Rehabilitation 386; Alcohol/drug 326.

Benefit Payments
Cumulative FY 1985 benefit payments under PPS were $37.0 billion through Septem-
ber 1985. This was 81% of all payments for
inpatient hospital services.

Admissions
Number of Admissions—A preliminary estimate of the number of Medicare short-stay
hospital admissions during October 1984–
April 1985 is 6.5 million. This represents a

decrease of 5.2% from October 1983–April
1984.

Admission Review—Cumulatively, from
October 1983 through October 1985, 38%
of PPS admissions reported by PSROs, FIs,
and PROs have been reviewed. A total of
2.6% were denied after review.

DRG Validation—Cumulatively, from October 1983 through October 1985, 3.5 million
PPS admissions were reviewed for DRG validation purposes.

Average Length of Stay per Discharge
Based on preliminary data for FY 1985
(October 1984–September 1985), the av-
erage number of days of care per PPS bill
was 7.7 days.
The average number of days of care per
PPS bill during FY 1984 (October 1983–
September 1984) was 7.6 days.

Diagnosis Related Groups
The table shows the 25 most frequently
occurring DRGs in fiscal year 1985, their relative cost weights, the number of discharges, average length of stay, and their
fiscal year 1984 ranks. These data are preliminary and are based on bill records received and processed in central office
through October 25, 1985.
For information on number of discharges
and average length of stay for DRGS not
shown in these tables, contact the Statistical
Information Services Branch, Division of Information Analysis, (301) 594-6705.

Prospective Payment System Monitoring DRG Analysis—PPS Bills FY 85 to Date

FY85 Rank	FY84 Rank	DRG No.	Description	Relative Cost Weight	Dis- charges	Per- cent	Average Length of Stay
1	1	127	Heart Failure and Shock	1.0300	329,727	5.1	7.6
2	6	089	Simple Pneumonia and Pleurisy	1.0914	238,798	3.7	8.4
3	5	140	Angina Pectoris	0.7470	216,416	3.4	4.9

Prospective Payment System Monitoring DRG Analysis—PPS Bills FY 85 to Date (*cont'd*)

FY85 Rank	FY84 Rank	DRG No.	Description	Relative Cost Weight	Dis-charges	Per-cent	Average Length of Stay
4	2	182	Esophagitis, Gastroenteritis, Misc. Digestive Disorders	0.6121	213,102	3.3	5.5
5	4	014	Specific Cerebrovascular Disorders	1.3386	199,389	3.1	9.6
6	8	138	Cardiac Arrhythmia & Conduction Disorders	0.9200	136,476	2.1	5.5
7	10	296	Nutritional and Misc. Metabolic Disorders	0.0886	134,959	2.1	7.0
8	12	096	Bronchitis and Asthma	0.7913	130,539	2.0	6.7
9	7	243	Medical Back Problems	0.7473	115,161	1.8	6.8
10	9	088	Chronic Obstructive Pulmonary Disease	1.0304	113,866	1.8	7.5
11	11	015	Transient Ischemic Attacks	0.6604	111,566	1.7	5.1
12	14	209	Major Joint Procedures	2.2674	107,384	1.7	13.7
13	13	336	Transurethral Prostatectomy	0.9974	104,867	1.6	6.8
14	15	174	Gastrointestinal Hemorrhage	0.9185	99,924	1.6	6.5
15	3	039	Lens Procedures	0.4958	89,932	1.4	2.0
16	16	122	Circulatory Disorders w/ Acute Myocardial Infarction	1.3509	89,357	1.4	8.9
17	17	320	Kidney and Urinary Tract Infections	0.8039	87,995	1.4	7.3
18	19	468	Unrelated O.R. Procedure	2.0818	84,955	1.3	12.9
19	20	210	Hip and Femur Procedures	2.0617	76,836	1.2	13.9
20	22	121	Circulatory Disorders w/ Acute Myocardial Infarction and Cardiovascular Complications	1.8454	76,387	1.2	11.2
21	18	294	Diabetes	0.8003	75,710	1.2	7.2
22	24	087	Pulmonary Edema and Respiratory Failure	1.5368	74,265	1.2	9.1
23	23	148	Major Small and Large Bowel Procedures	2.5228	71,508	1.1	15.8
24	29	410	Chemotherapy	0.3490	65,307	1.0	3.1
25	21	082	Respiratory Neoplasms	1.1282	63,768	1.0	8.6

Exhibit 13-3   Federally-Supported PPS Studies of Medicare's PPS Mandated by Congress

Study Topic	Report due date	Agency	Status (as of February 1986)
Reports Mandated by Social Security Amendments of 1983 (Public Law 98-21):			
1983–1984 reports:			
1. Impact of Single Limits on Skilled Nursing Facilities	12/31/84	HCFA-OLP	Complete (1/85)
2. Impact of Hospital PPS on Skilled Nursing Facilities	12/31/84	HCFA-OLP	Complete (1/85)
3. Including U.S. Territory Hospitals	4/1/84	HCFA-BERC	In clearance[a]
4. Incorporating Capital Into PPS	10/14/84	ASPE	In clearance[a]
5. Annual PPS Impact Reports, 1984–87	12/31/84–87	HCFA-ORD-R	1984, Complete 1985, In process
1985 reports:			
6. Annual Report and Recommendations on PPS to the Secretary of Health and Human Services	April, Annually	ProPAC	1st Annual Complete (4/85)
7. Occupancy of Sole Community Hospitals	4/1/85	HCFA-ORD-R	In clearance[a]
8. A-B Information Transfers	4/1/85	HCFA-ORD-BPO	In clearance[a]
9. Uncompensated Care Costs	4/1/85	HCFA-ORD-R	In clearance[a]
10. Cost of Care Information to Patients	4/1/85	HCFA-ORD-R	Complete (8/85)
11. Large Rural Teaching Hospitals	4/1/85	HCFA-ORD-R	In process
12. Case-Mix Measurement: Refinements of DRGs (including severity of illness, intensity of care, and adequacy of outlier payment)	12/31/85	HCFA-ORD-R	In clearance[a]
13. Eliminating Rural-Urban Rates	12/31/85	HCFA-ORD-R	In process
14. Exempted Hospitals Report: Long-Term Care Hospitals, Psychiatric Units, Rehabilitation Units, and Pediatric Hospitals	12/31/85	HCFA-ORD-R	In clearance[a]
15. All-Payer Feasibility, Cost-Shifting	12/31/85	HCFA-ORD-R	In process
16. Impact of Admission, Volume Adjustment	12/31/85	HCFA-ORD-R	In clearance[a]
17. Physician DRGs—Including Payments for Physicians' Services to Hospital Inpatients in DRG Payment Amounts	7/1/85	HCFA-ORD-R	In clearance[a]

1986 reports:

18. Impact of State Alternatives to PPS on Medicare, Medicaid, Private Health Expenditures, and Tax Expenditures	12/31/86	HCFA-ORD-D	—

Reports Mandated by the Deficit Reduction Act (Public Law 98-369):

1984 reports:

19. Prospective Payment for Skilled Nursing Facilities	8/1/84	HCFA-OLP	Complete (1/85)
20. Prospective Payment System Wage Index Adjustments	8/18/84	HCFA-BERC	Complete (4/85)
21. Options for Prospective Payment for Skilled Nursing Facilities	12/1/84	HCFA-OLP	Complete (1/85)
22. Definition and Identification of "Disproportionate Share" Hospitals	12/31/84	HCFA-BERC/ORD	Complete (12/85)

1985 reports:

23. Urban/Rural Payment Differential	1/18/85	HCFA-ORD-R	To be included with Study 13
24. Advisability and Feasibility of Varying by DRG Proportions of Labor and Nonlabor Components of the Federal Payment Amount	1/18/85	HCFA-ORD-R	To be included with Study 13
25. Pacemaker Payment Review (Part A)	3/1/85	ProPAC	Complete (3/85)
26. Pacemaker Payment Review (Part B)	3/1/85	HCFA-BQC	In process
27. Closure and Conversion of Underutilized Hospital Facilities	3/1/85	HCFA-BERC/ORD-D	In clearance[a]
28. Certified Registered Nurse Anesthetists	7/1/85	HCFA-BERC/ORD-D	In Process
29. Hospital Specific Variance	9/1/85	HCFA-ORD-R	To be included with Study 13
30. Exceptions to Wage Index Adjustments	—	HCFA-BERC	—

Exhibit 13-3 Federally-Supported PPS Studies of Medicare's PPS Mandated by Congress *(cont'd)*

Study Topic	Report due date	Agency	Status (as of February 1986)
Reports Requested by the House Appropriations Committee Report (Report 98-911 on H.R. 6528):			
1985 reports:			
31. Effect of PPS on Clinical Trials	—	NIH/HCFA	Initial NIH-NCHSRT study expected Winter 1986
32. Annual Report on Impact of PPS on Blood Banking	—	HCFA	Expected mid-1986
33. Effects of PPS on American Health Care System	February, annually	ProPAC	1st annual complete (2/86)

aReport has been completed and is being reviewed within DHHS before being submitted to Congress.

Abbreviations: ASPE, Assistant Secretary for Planning and Evaluation; HCFA, Health Care Financing Administration; BERC: Bureau of Eligibility, Reimbursement, and Coverage; BPO: Bureau of Program Operations; BQC: Bureau of Quality Control; OLP: Office of Legislative Policy; ORD-R: Office of Research and Demonstrations, Office of Research; ORD-D: Office of Research and Demonstrations, Office of Demonstrations and Evaluations; ProPAC, Prospective Payment Assessment Commission.

Source: Personal communication by ProPAC staff with Office of Research and Demonstrations, Health Care Financing Administration, Department of Health and Human Services, Baltimore, Maryland, February 1986.

Technical Appendixes to the Report and Recommendations to the Secretary, U.S. Department of Health and Human Services, Washington, D.C.: Prospective Payment Assessment Commission, April 1, 1986, pp. 190–191.

of the public. He cited the tradeoffs for containing costs: rationing of care, compromised quality of care, and a decline in research into new techniques or technologies. To support his claims, Bessey noted the GAO investigation that reported patients being discharged in a sicker condition than previously. Furthermore, Bessey commented that health care was "cost driven, not medically driven" with hospitals having an incentive to withhold services.[14] Additional letters in response to the *New York Times* editorial also voiced doubts about the lack of research[15] and the decline in care levels.[16]

U. S. Senator John Heinz (R-PA), Chairman of the Senate Committee on Aging, based a harsh indictment on the GAO report: "Under the DRG-based system, patients are being discharged quicker and sicker and some may be being discharged prematurely. In too many cases older patients are being sent out into a no-care zone without access to the health care they so urgently need."[17]

On a local level, Kenyon accented the plight of neighborhood hospitals feeling the pinch of PPS/DRG regulations in New Jersey. These area facilities incurred declines in bed occupancy percentages serious enough to warrant the closing of patient care units and staff reductions.[18]

Rubin, having left his assistant secretary job at HHS, even said that "American physicians might be forgiven if they are experiencing some anomie."[19] Anomie is "the disorientation and anxiety people feel when norms and expectations change dramatically, denying them their usual reference points."[20]

Linking his comments to the government's proposed payment freezes, U. S. Senator David F. Durenburger (R-MN) extended the disorientation concept: "The Reagan budget sends all the wrong signals. Reducing DRG payments to hospitals tells providers, 'You can't trust government.' Doctors and nursing homes will fight being included in a DRG system when they see what's happening to hospitals."[21]

"In short, Medicare's payment system is not working," states Rahman in an op-ed article in the January 23, 1986 issue of the *New York Times*. As a practicing physician, Rahman argues that doctors and hospitals are having to deny crucial care to patients because of impending economic losses.[22] HHS Secretary Bowen responded to Rahman in a letter to the editor on February 6, 1986. Bowen, himself a physician, emphasized that "Medicare does not specify how much hospitalization a patient can receive." In concluding, Bowen noted imperfections and the need for improvement but stated that "positive results have been realized both in upholding the quality of care under Medicare and restraining unnecessary increases in healthcare costs."[23]

Indiscriminate Budget Ax

A severe critique of the DRG program made by the director of a renowned health policy think tank highlights the deficit:

> I see a tidal wave rolling in on Medicare, because the cost increases are such that the tax base just will not support the program. What barricades

have we thrown up? The diagnosis related group system—who are we kidding? Here is a system with a four-year phase-in, with exceptions, appeals, all kinds of loopholes, 467 categories that will probably turn into 967 categories, and, as I read some of the evidence, wide differences in severity within those DRG cells. I think there will be a lot of unfairness, and when we talk about adverse risk selection and encouraging people to skim the cream, look at those severity differences within the DRG cell and you will find all the incentives you want.[24]

This director also called the DRGs an incomplete cost control device, noted that admissions and preventive care weren't included, and that the physician was really "out of the picture."[25]

Even before the President's budget proposals, in April 1984, an editorial in Hospitals expressed hurt over the unfair congressional actions, "flailing away with an axe" to effect Medicare savings. Citing the needs for DRG modifications, the editorial cited problems with the severity of illness component, the impact of socioeconomic condition on health needs, the transition to a national rate, and the achievement of equity for provider and patient alike. Headlining the editorial "A Cure That Could Cripple," the closing sentence expresses the AHA's views on the workings of PPS cost-saving efforts: "To reward their [the hospitals'] actions by gutting their fiscal stability in order to achieve cosmetic, transitory relief of Medicare's problems would be cynical and destructive."[26]

Interestingly, just three months earlier, on January 1, 1984, a Hospitals editorial talked about the opportunities to avoid regulation offered by PPS despite inherent difficulties.[27] This same theme was expressed prior to the initiation of PPS, in April 1983, at an AHA National Council of Governing Boards meeting. Ross, a partner in a national accounting firm, said that "the new system will provide hospitals with incentives for greater management flexibility, innovation, planning and control."[28]

Doubts have also been raised about the ability of PPS/DRG to cover care for the indigent. Six nonprofit urban hospitals filed a lawsuit February 6, 1985, claiming that PPS "underpays hospitals that care for a disproportionate share of low-income or Medicare patients."[29] These hospitals are asking for financial relief through adjustment of DRG rates as provided for in the legislation. HCFA is contesting the rationales of the suing hospitals and impeding access to materials.[30] HCFA finally complied with the court's order at the end of 1985 and came forth with "disproportionate share" rulings, but still had no intent to make adjustments.[31]

Delay Transition Rates

A coalition group of five state hospital associations, the Catholic Health Association, the AAMC, and the NAPH are urging Congress to delay the transition of DRG rates to a uniform national rate. That action is needed to correct inequities in the PPS, according to the group.[32] While there is some division over whether or not to delay the transition phase-in, enough doubt has been raised as evidenced in earlier attempts to freeze the transition at 75 percent hospital-specific and 25 percent national.[33]

Cost Above All Else

It would appear that for every argument that PPS works, there is a contrary argument that PPS does not. Sometimes the arguments are opposite sites of the same point. However, neither side in the debate will contest the point that "currently, cost comes ahead of anything else by a very wide margin."[34] An integral part of that cost emphasis aims to cap the government's Medicare health expenditures. Griffith explains: "Most fundamental of all, the whole payment process must be 'budget neutral.' That is, payouts may increase no more than the growth in the federal budget as a whole. So there is now a distinct, explicit cap on the cost of the Medicare program which had previously been growing at rates far higher than the GNP or the rate of inflation."[35]

At issue is whether the cost containment aftermath is considered evidence that PPS works or that PPS doesn't work, producing adverse side effects. An answer to this issue has to be found at the highest levels of national policy making.

Policy Making and PPS

During the 1984 presidential election campaign, Hart, Jackson, and Mondale all favored an all-payer prospective payment system for hospital inpatient services.[36-38] Reagan had already expressed his views in his administration's operational PPS/DRG program. An all-payer system was predicted by 1990, no matter who won the election.[39]

National policy making relies heavily on information garnered through government-sponsored health services research. Friedman interviewed 18 leading researchers in this field and described the major impact of health services research on policy decisions. Rossiter identifies key operations-oriented research areas as productivity, marketing, organizational issues, and management of risk.[40] Eleven of the 18 chose the effect of changes in payment systems and the changing market as the subject area deserving the most attention.

On March 13, 1986, a group of 14 researchers in the Harvard Medicare Project spoke about the future of Medicare after a two-year study. More than 40 proposals were prepared for reform of the Medicare system. Reforms were suggested affecting beneficiaries, physicians, hospitals, and prepaid health care activities. Major proposals called for the simplification of reimbursement methods through the combination of payment to hospitals and doctors; encouragement of enrollment in prepaid health care organizations; decreasing copayments for Medicare beneficiaries; expanding coverage of long-term care and chronic illness and increasing fairness and simplicity without additional taxes. These recommendations indicated future directions for Medicare over the next 10 to 15 years and many suggestions would require enactment by Congress. Interestingly, these reform policies were based on the premise that the government continue to play a vital role in assuring access to health care and protection from a huge burden of costs to elderly people. Furthermore, the investigation had the goals of containing Medicare expenditures, ensuring fairness to the elderly, health care providers, and others and simplicity in administration of the program. Evaluation of the actual implementation of the reforms will provide some value of the policy making effect on PPS of prominent researchers.[41-43]

Another policy making investigatory group, the Prospective Payment Assessment Commission, submitted a report to Congress in February 1986 on "Medicare Prospective Payment and the American Health Care System." This report discussed the effects of PPS policies and changes in the health care system. Other areas touched on included hospital utilization, resource use and services, the quality of health care, financial consequences for hospitals, and changes in the funding of health services. In 94 pages, ProPAC fulfills its legislated obligation to advise and suggest policies to Congress and to HHS as well as the public.[44]

In sum, these experts predict that health services research will continue to be a force in influencing policy decisions. Research may be more politically sophisticated and directed away from isolated academic pursuits. Stressing the import, an executive of a large philanthropic foundation concluded: "Tinkering with the health care system is a permanent bipartisan activity in the United States, and when government wants to change the system, it needs to know how it works."[45]

Where Do We Stand?

Evaluating the plaudits and the criticisms of PPS, what can we say about where we stand today? It is informative to compare the different ways this material is presented.

Physician View

In its Medicine '84 News Wrap-Up, the *American Medical News* said that some saw PPS as a "survival of the fittest" situation with the prognosis for hospitals remaining guarded.[46] Descriptively, the comment was terse: "Scores of hospital workers lost their jobs, records clerks moved out of the basement, and hospital suppliers engaged in price wars in 1984. Data management systems grew like Topsy, hospital financial management became a growth industry, and physicians watched warily as a leaner, meaner hospital emerged out of the nation's first year under Medicare's DRGs.''[47]

Hospital View

A review of 1984 highlights in *Hospitals* declared that PPS dominated activities in Washington, D.C. during the year. Featured events included the following:

- HHS set second year DRG payment rates.

- PROs came into being amid controversy over their stated objectives.

- Passage of the Deficit Reduction Act of 1984 set more payment policy bench marks.

- ProPAC began work on DRG adjustments.

- All-payer concepts gained some Congressional support.

- More hospitals entered the home care market.

- Data processing gross expenditures doubled, with hospitals spending more on computer and software than on any other nonlabor expenditure.

- Computer software companies greatly expanded their offerings to hospitals.

- Smaller hospitals took advantage of microprocessors in their management strategies.

- Health care cost increases moderated with providers, businesses and government sharing the credit.[48-50]

Medical Care View

Medical World News featured a review of DRGs 18 months after implementation. A drawing on the cover of this issue showed a sweating physician manipulating a patient to fit into a DRG 143 bag while a glaring Uncle Sam watched. Despite the limited available data, this article tells how the DRGs stacked up.

- For-profit hospital chains appeared to be the early winners of the DRG numbers game.

- Small rural hospitals were apparent losers.

- Episodes of inpatient care did not seem to be broken down into increased separate admissions.

- Staffs were reduced as occupancy declined.

- Friction was added to the tenuous medical staff/hospital administration relationship.

- Third party payers evidenced a liking for HMOs and PPOs.

- 25 percent of the 458 new certified home health agencies in the first six months of 1984 were hospital-based.

- Hospitals developed more aggressive marketing, advertising, and promotional strategies to attract patients.[51]

In addition, this review also noted unresolved issues relating to the performance of PPS effects, the extension of DRGs to physicians, the impact on quality, the failure to account for severity, the plight of teaching hospitals, the dumping/transfer predicament, clinical research impacts, and the uncompensated care problem. Taking the unresolved issues along with the apparent effects, this review concludes that "about the only thing that can be said with certainty is that a lot of people are still uncertain."[52]

Public View

The *New York Times* featured a front page report in an April 1985 issue.[53] In seeking a balanced view, Sullivan interviewed representatives from HCFA, the AHA, and the consumer advocacy organization, the Health Research Group. Citing statistics on the number of hospital beds, admissions, and length of stay, Sullivan declared that hospital use exhibited the steepest decline in the past 20 years due to PPS, according to health officials and hospital administrators. In addition to PPS/DRG, these other factors were given for the decline in hospital use:

- A shift of one-third of inpatient surgery to hospital outpatient facilities, independent surgical centers, and doctor's office.

- Higher out-of-pocket deductibles in health insurance plans discouraged unnecessary hospitalization.

- Tough new PROs to review appropriateness and quality of care.[54]

In an article two weeks earlier, Sullivan had reported that 25 percent of the hospital beds in New York City were unused and unnecessary.[55] An AHA executive was quoted as saying there is no question that the downturn would have happened without PPS.[56] In addition, problems with dumping, Medicaid, federal freezes, premature discharge, staff cuts, and closings were also linked to PPS/DRGs.

HCFA View

In a speech to the New England Hospital Assembly on May 1, 1985, HCFA Administrator Davis highlighted the major health system gains. Specifically, she pointed out the lower inflation rate, the drop in Medicare admissions, the shortened length of stay, and the lack of problems with access or quality of care. On graduate medical education, Davis' position was that Medicare should only pay for direct costs. She also stated that Medicare will not want to pay for uncompensated charity care. Davis described the government's Medicare initiatives "as a series of nudges to turn a ship around."[57]

Legislative View

Periodically, the Congressional Research Service of the Library of Congress prepares an issue brief on Medicare and prospective payments for inpatient care. Lundy reviewed a variety of aspects for the members of Congress, including an all-payer system, expansion of PPS, reimbursement for capital expenditures, medical education payments, physician/hospital relations, technology, urban/rural differences, and the quality of care.[58] For each point, Lundy presents the pros and cons as well as the current status. Legislators are watching the PPS/DRG program carefully and are seeking information to use to respond to their constituents.

A View From Abroad

DRGs are not confined to the United States. A number of foreign countries expressed interest in applications of the methodology to control health care inflation. Even though some foreign countries may have difficulty with the data needs and the coding system, it has been reported by Health Systems International that the following nations are investigating the use of DRGs: France, Portugal, the Netherlands, Belgium, Ireland, Sweden, Finland, Austria, Switzerland, Great Britain, West Germany, and Australia.[59]

The "Wait-and-See" View

A former HCFA administrator for policy pinpointed the foundation of all the movement in the health care delivery system relative to where we stand today. Feinstein attributed the directional shifts to "enormous behavioral changes" by hospitals.[60]

Currently, there are a number of complaints about the PPS/DRG system, including concerns about the DRG wage index, reimbursement for the care for the indigent, technology development, and the possibility of de facto rationing. In a review of 1984 medicine, an oft-repeated phrase located exactly where the health care industry stands: "We've cut the fat. The real test will come when we get into the lean."[61]

Predictions for the Health Care Industry

There has been no shortage of forecasters willing to put forth their views on the future twists and turns of the health care delivery system as it reacts to the PPS/DRG program. Some predict in only one area, others group a variety of events together.

Starting with surveys of hospital chief executive officers and 2,000 hospital decision makers, then moving into specific topics and closing with the general predictions, perhaps analysts of the field can emerge with their own priority listing to match up to what seems to be a consensus.

Hospital CEOs

A 1984 national survey of more than 430 chief executive officers of hospitals revealed that strategic planning was the number one critical concern chosen by 66 percent of the respondents. Strategic planning took on a "new qualitative and financial orientation—with a vengeance"[62] and emphasized all areas of hospital operation, without the traditional concentration on bricks and mortar. Furthermore, closely following at 61 percent, 61 percent, and 51 percent, respectively, were concerns about medical staff relations, cost containment, and marketing.

CEOs were also asked what experiences future hospital administrators would need to manage institutions. More than 80 percent labeled four areas as extremely or very important: strategic planning, finance and accounting, marketing, and human resources.[63] Similarly, executives in banking and the airlines—also competitive industries—choose the same four areas.

When asked about the status of hospitals as independents or the trend to mergers in order to survive, there was a difference of opinion by size of facility. CEOs of hospitals with fewer than 200 beds split evenly with yes/no choices. Most of the CEOs of hospitals with 200-399 beds voted no and felt that they could remain independent. CEOs from hospitals with more than 400 beds voted yes and thought that multihospital arrangements were needed to survive.

Clearly, the survey showed that hospital CEOs realized the drastically realigned environment had changed their jobs. "CEOs must make the most radical shift in priorities and institutional direction the industry has ever faced."[64]

Relative to specific services, CEOs were asked about plans for expansion, additions, reductions, or eliminations in the next two years. While some variation in the rankings occurred by hospital size, it is notable that there was agreement on the specific services being considered for adding or expanding.

Service	Number of Beds		
	400+	**200-399**	**199 or less**
Home Health Service	78.3%	76.7%	64.5%
Outpatient Surgery (in-house)	68.4	75.8	73.2
Preferred Provider Organization	63.9	66.9	48.1
Outpatient Diagnosis (in-house)	57.2	54.1	48.8
Wellness and Health Promotion	56.6	56.4	52.7

These five services received the highest percentage of each grouping of hospitals. Choices by the CEOs reinforce the movement to out-of-hospital services that do not fall within the scope of the PPS/DRG at this time. Interestingly, 67 percent of the hospital CEOs felt that it is highly likely that prospective pricing will be used to reimburse for outpatient services. About the same percentage responded that physician services are most likely to be prospectively reimbursed also. In addition, almost 90 percent of the CEOs polled felt that it was highly likely that third party payers will be included in prospective pricing. "In general, CEOs recognize the beginning of a long term trend toward more 'end-result oriented' payment systems. There will be little relief in the short term."[65]

Future hospital management. According to Moran, a federal Office of Management and Budget executive, hospitals are adopting a "retail merchandising notion and going after patients directly instead of through physicians."[66] He added that community hospitals are generally moving toward "high volume, low margin operations."[67]

In line with the concept of merchandising, the *Hospitals* magazine's nine-member Publisher's Panel on Business and Finance came to a related conclusion. They felt that "the most salient message was the need to stop thinking about *hospital management* and concentrate more on *total health care* management"[68] (author's emphasis).

This panel reviewed trends and strategies for health care in the 1990s and there was consensus about the following movements:

- By the 1990s, hospitals will be cost centers, not service centers.

- Hospitals will be in the health insurance business, operating their own companies for capitation purposes.

- DRGs were seen as an interim financing tool with capitation as inevitable.

- HMO growth was forecast, with younger physicians working for hospital chains and HMOs.

- PROs will hold firmly to their stated goals and objectives for fear of losing their governmental contracts.

- Private sector will provide less uncompensated care with fewer public hospitals to pick up the slack.

- A rapid educational process will be necessary to survive the payment trends.[69]

How do the projections of health care management experts jibe with the analysis of the investment community? Abramowitz, representing the financial interests, looked at the future of the health care delivery system in 1985 and projected events over the next five years:

- Health expenditures will decelerate to approximately 8-10 percent, down from the 13-15 percent of previous growth.

- Medicare will decelerate to 7-9 percent annual growth, down from prior 18 percent increases.

- Hospitals will increase vertical integration, adding new services and redefining existing services.

- Federal government will eliminate the 1 percent addition to inflation in Medicare growth and "may even do less than that."

- Insurance copayments for health care will be the greatest growth industry in the next five years, resulting in a major trend in price sensitivity in health care.

- Hospital beds will be reduced by 1 to 3 percent yearly.

- Multihospital systems will grow rapidly with proprietary ownership raising from 8 to 13 percent.

- Fee-for-service patients will decline from 92 to 67 percent of the population with HMOs going from 6 to 11 percent of the population.

- Medicare DRG reimbursement rates will never become 100 percent national.

- Home care growth will be the second biggest trend resulting from the DRG system.[70]

Abramowitz identified the two essential future trends as insurance copayments and DRGs that reduce hospital stays. Keeping in mind his overall predictions for the 1990s, his conclusion raises ponderable questions: "To conclude, copayments will be the major driving force in the future and will dramatically reduce the demand for health care and alter the way it will be delivered. If I were a physician, I might ask myself what I am going to do in the afternoon five years from now."[71]

Capitation

Both the health care management experts and the investment analyst predicted capitation in the future. In addition, HCFA Administrator Davis, in an October 1984 speech, also foretold of Medicare DRGs leading to "a pluralistic system with the concept of capitation, either with episodic or voucher' payments for hospitals and physicians."[72] About the same time, ProPAC chairman Altman forecast a greater percentage of capitated systems by 1990.[73] In April 1985, HCFA's research director, Dobson, discussed physician payment reform at a medical association meeting. Dobson commented that capitation systems that pay for a package of services hold "enormous potential and appeal" because they control price and quantity and encourage efficiency.[74]

Surgical and Medical Care Products

More than 2,000 physicians, surgeons, nurses, and other medical department supervisors participated in a study of the effects of DRGs on the nation's health care system.[75] Since the poll was sponsored by firms concerned with surgical and medical care products, there is an emphasis on areas that concern those firms. While 15 key impacts of the DRG program were chosen by respondents, choices after the sixth dropped to under 20 percent and are not listed. Most important cost containment changes included the following:

1. Shorten patient stay (72.7%)
2. Reduce drug, devices, and other supply costs (60.0%)
3. Reduce staff (54.4%)
4. Increase in enhanced cost/accounting computer systems (48.5%)
5. Use of lower cost distributors/buying groups (42.4%)
6. Enhanced hospital marketing programs (39.4%).

To compliment the cost containment changes evoked by DRGs, hospitals adjusted their procedures in regard to surgical and medical care products. This survey showed a trend toward the following actions:

- Increased use of standardized and/or generic products and drugs
- A return trend toward more reusable supplies
- Greater emphasis on price as the key buying factor
- Leasing of large capital equipment, or leasing with option to buy

- Increased use of large buying groups

- Enhanced new product review committees.

A shifting pattern of influence regarding purchasing decisions was reported in the survey. Nearly 70 percent thought that administrators had more influence on purchases under DRGs. About 61 percent felt that nursing directors now had more influence. On the contrary, almost 43 percent responded that physicians had less influence.

Generally, this survey reported short-term gains in fostering efficiency, in encouraging more outpatient procedures, and in a heightening price competitiveness without detriment to the quality of care. However, in the long run, the analysis was a prediction of failure: "The DRG program should be viewed as a stop-gap price control scheme. In this light, such government produced schemes in the past have worked temporarily, but then become increasingly complex and eventually unravel."[76]

Both of these surveys tend to bolster the appearance of material in the professional literature and to confirm the future trends predicted by many others.

Rationing Health Care

With a merchandising approach to health care services and a capitation system that encourages underuse, is the rationing of health care an imminent prospect? According to *Private Practice*, the official publication of the Congress of County Medical Societies, the prospect is already here: "For we cannot ignore the fact that DRGs, and similar schemes, are simply ways of covertly rationing health care, without subjecting Congress to the wrath of the American electorate. The responsibility is shifted to the American medical system, which continues to serve as the scapegoat."[77]

While others have also expressed opinions that DRGs are in effect a rationing mechanism, Caper raises the basic issue regarding the long-term policy implications of the allocation of health care resources. Caper accepts the premise that the quality of care will not necessarily suffer if hospital costs are contained. Then he concludes that "physicians and hospital leaders . . . have to understand that if they think it's inappropriate for them to make decisions about the allocation of resources, then someone else will do it for them."[78]

Several articles appeared in the December 13, 1984 issue of the *New England Journal of Medicine* dealing with the rationing of health care. As an indication of concern in the health care community, eight letters to the editor appeared in the May 16, 1985 issue.[79] These letters pinpointed the conflict between a physician's obligation to the patient and the economic incentives of cost containment. In responding to the letters, Levinsky and Fuchs both note the technical ability of physicians to make the difficult decisions and to serve the best interests of their patients. Fuchs also comments that the revolutionary "change is in the method of allocation—who does the rationing and who is affected by it."[80] Thus, the future question still resides in making the allocation decisions.

Interestingly, Parsons thinks that the issue may not be as detrimental as many believe. He does predict that rationing of health care will be widespread in the United States. However, Parsons stated that even "significant" rationing won't have a negative impact upon the health status of Americans.[81]

Another related rationing argument concerns the idea that the poor would bear the brunt of any resource allocation plan. HHS has resisted pressures to provide additional funds to hospitals serving a disproportionate share of indigent patients. Responding to a federal judge's court order and Congressional pressure, Secretary Heckler issued new rules in the July 1, 1985 *Federal Register* to take effect August 1, 1985.[82,83] However, the rules were revoked in the July 31, 1985, *Federal Register*. Regardless, another court order forced HCFA to address this issue by releasing a definition of disproportionate share hospitals at the end of 1985.

Although the future of health care rationing is an uncertain one, many claim that such rationing has already begun.

Ethical and Legal Issues

At a June 1984 conference on health care, Cranford warned the audience about future difficulties in ethical areas: "You think we are encountering complex ethical dilemmas now? Wait until you see what happens under prospective pricing as the allocation of funds decreases."[84]

Cranford stated that physicians could be influenced to undertreat patients and, particularly, to discontinue treatment in the case of hopelessly ill patients. He suggests that hospitals "develop explicitly clear and publicly accountable guidelines" to confront ethical issues. To accomplish that task, Cranford recommends two ethics committees, one to resolve ethical issues, and the other to focus on the allocation of increasingly scarce resources.[85]

Of course, ethics has always been a concern of health care providers. Most professions have statements that stress the care of the patient above all else. Most professionals usually take an oath at graduation to uphold the ethics of their profession. At his inauguration as 139th President of the American Medical Association in 1984, Joseph F. Boyle alluded to the intrusion of marketing, economics, and the like into the physician/patient relationship and the ethical role of the profession:

> Our professional ethics says that we are a collegial brother and sister-hood in which our interests are mutually intertwined. A business ethic says, 'get your share, drive the other fellow to the wall.' Professional ethics says that we shall establish standards of what constitutes moral

and professional conduct; that we will care for people, regardless of the circumstances, with compassion and concern.[86]

Specifically, Boyle mentioned the dilemma of physicians being pressured to discharge patients early or not to admit certain patients. Physicians were urged to adhere to the principle of doing only what is best for the patient.[87]

Psychiatric examples.   Morgenlander and Greenwald expand the ethical and legal impact of DRGs by concentrating on specific dilemmas within the field of inpatient psychiatric care. Ethical issues are self-evident in their examples. Legally, patients and/or their families could just as easily make a case for legal malpractice, citing rationales such as abandonment, inappropriate care, and falsified records. A DRG system in a psychiatric facility could lead to the following ethical and legal dilemmas:

- An emergency admission is stabilized and transferred. Is that an appropriate discharge? Was the patient discharged because the diagnosis was economically unsuitable for that hospital?

- Using "creative diagnosing" admissions procedures can screen out unprofitable patients based upon DRGs. Is that ethical or legal?

- Inappropriate labeling of psychiatric patients could take place intentionally for economic reasons. Could that result in treatment errors and restrictions of personal freedom? Could patients enact a self-fulfilling prophecy and deteriorate to live up to the expectations of the inappropriate diagnostic label?

- Could court officials be persuaded to order involuntary commitments to fill up empty beds in government facilities?

- In view of DRG reimbursement rates, could therapy modes change from long-term psychoanalytic orientation to a "brief treatment, behavior-modification and crisis intervention approach?"

- Is the loss of staff engendered by the DRG economies to be considered legal abandonment?

- Professionals could be urged to alter a diagnoses to fit a higher DRG rate category or to misrepresent therapeutic progress in the medical records. Could that be legally negligent care and criminal falsification of medical information?

- Outpatient alternatives could be used when DRG payments run out or instead of hospitalizaiton. If the patient commits suicide, can the facility be sued for negligence? Is it ethical?

- What are complications and comorbidity for psychiatric DRGs? Are there ethical and legal ramifications of the interpretations?[88]

These examples illustrate the variety of ethical and legal situations that could arise, not only in psychiatric facilities, but in all institutions falling under PPS/DRG mechanisms.

Ethical and social responsibility.   In a lengthy and thoughtful article, Kapp covers the legal and ethical implications of health care reimbursement by DRGs. Having both a public health and a law degree, Kapp brings both viewpoints into his analysis. Basically, Kapp asks if hospitals and physicians are the most ethically appropriate actors to undertake the awesome responsibility of this new role, and what legal risks does it engender for them?[89] Social responsibility for the allocation of scarce resources is the new role that Kapp discusses. Following a discourse on whether DRGs promote efficiency or rationing, Kapp moves on to identify potential areas of liability such as inadequate level of care rendered, premature discharge, inadequate discharge planning, excessive care, inappropriate admission, and lack of informed consent. In predicting the likelihood of lawsuits, Kapp feels that talk about "the DRG malpractice bonanza are probably grossly exaggerated."[90] Yet he does expect some DRG related lawsuits, although the total number would be quite limited. In that event, Kapp debates cost containment as a legal defense and concludes that the norms of the profession would still continue to be established by physicians. To the extent that the norms of care were revised to reflect DRG restraints, the courts would abide by those changes. Using cost control as an affirmative defense would not appear to bear much weight. Kapp advises health care providers to respond to the ethical and legal challenges of DRGs through the following actions:

- Don't "game" or manipulate the system
- Avoid "disruptive acrimony" between the medical staff and hospital administration, with attention to medical by-laws clarifications regarding staff privileges
- Cooperate to build a vertically integrated health care delivery system
- Include a discussion of quality, cost, and resource allocation within the informed consent as part of enhanced physician/patient communication
- Give particular attention to medical record documentation
- Together, physicians and hospitals should reevaluate their prevailing clinical practices and procedures

- To the extent that DRGs or other health care cost control strategies pose untenable ethical consequences and unreasonable legal peril, physicians and hospitals should take part in the political process as never before.[91]

Finally, Kapp points out that when the best clinical choices are also the most cost-effective, DRGs will work. However, when the medical choices and the cost factors are at odds, ethical and legal principles must be considered to strike a balance that is equitable to all parties concerned.

In a related article in the same issue of *Law, Medicine & Health Care*, Mariner addresses the evasion of social responsibility through the use of the DRG mechanism. She pointed out that "the DRG system represents a social mechanism for rationing supposedly scarce resources."[92] This evasion occurs in the DRG methodology through the conversion of health care professionals and hospitals from provider status to rationing agents for the health care delivery system. Mariner puts the situation into perspective as she talks about the societal role in health care: "The distribution of health care is not an individual or even a collective professional responsibility, but a societal one. As such, it must be guided by principles of justice developed on a societal level."[93]

Arguing for responsible direction regarding overall resource allocations at the highest societal level, Mariner makes a telling comparison. Having physicians make those social choices would be "akin to asking parents to change the public school curriculum by refusing to help their children with their homework."[94] In a letter to the editor, Weinmann pointedly states that "private physicians will be left holding the bag," as responsibility for DRG rationing shifts from the government to the doctors.[95] That allusion to rationing was confirmed in early 1984 when a high level HHS official responded to a question about care under DRGs and predicted, "I think, to some extent, rationing will occur, although it won't be called that."[96] Mariner's point about who takes the social responsibility is highlighted in the two views expressed—one from a private practice physician, and the other from the government.

Similarly, ethical comments come into play as the use of medical technology under PPS/DRG is considered. *Business Week* reviewed the life and death choice associated with decisions about whether or not to use sophisticated technology for a specific patient. In that review, Ellwood forecasts relative to the dilemma: "We are nearing the day when we will have to confront the rationing of very high-tech, very costly procedures."[97] He goes on to say that medicine does not want to make those ethical and moral choices and neither do the bureaucrats. But Ellwood does believe that physicians will have to decide what constitutes reasonable care. Prophetically, he adds that "so far, no one is standing in line for a chance to play God."[98]

Ethical and legal implications of the PPS/DRG modalities are not being newly discovered. Even prior to the implementation of the Medicare PPS in June 1983, the concept of the conflict between the cost factors and social responsibility was elucidated clearly: "We are witnessing a rapid acceptance of the notion that health care is more nearly an economic product than a social good."[99]

Institutional Management in the Future

In considering how managers of institutions will need to operate under DRGs, Stern and Epstein start out by projecting three aspects that are likely to cause adverse consequences:

1. DRGs are assigned to patients using limited information without considering factors such as severity of illness and socioeconomic characteristics.

2. Payments based on estimates of average costs do not consider classes of hospitals and their individualistic traits.

3. Reimbursement is provided for certain types of costs and payment is made separately for costs, such as capital and educations with no provision for free care.[100]

With that foundation as to the adverse effects, the authors proceed to examine areas such as efficiency, specialization, DRG creep, volume, teaching costs, free care, technology, and capital. They arrive at a number of likelihoods as listed below:

- Administrators are likely to increase their use of staff selection to secure physicians who can practice efficiently within DRG guidelines.

- Specialization will increase as hospitals sharpen specific skills to deliver efficient and quality care at lower than DRG allowances, although distinctions between "skimming" and "specialization" may be difficult to determine.

- Honest maximization of reimbursement will be practiced along with the gaming system.

- "We expect institutions to initiate a series of 'educational,' 'feedback,' and 'administrative' interventions to encourage shorter and more frequent admissions."

- Teaching hospitals are likely to curtail access for high-cost patients and those requiring free care.

- Administrators are likely to create strategies to recoup investments in technology and capital through unbundling or similar techniques.[101]

In closing, the authors remark that there are loopholes in the DRG method that "undermine the system's ability to limit reimbursement."[102] That statement leads to theoretical considerations of organizational management principles with the DRG as the case study.

Unintended Consequences and Misplaced Goals

Recognized concepts of organizational theory were applied to the DRG experience in the United States. Principles related to decision making, displaced goals, and unintended consequences emerged after Congress was "satisfied" by the passage of the PPS/DRG methodology. This resulted in a reversal, and the means became the ends replacing the original objectives. According to an analysis by Gay and Kronenfeld: "Both of the major actors (HCFA and the hospitals) are losing sight of the goal of DRG legislation, to contain costs for the Medicare system as a whole, and are focusing on the process itself and the potential to play reimbursement games."[103] In their study of nine South Carolina hospitals, the authors found one facility able to maximize DRG payments to achieve reimbursement at 110 percent of Medicare cost. To counter overzealous enforcement of regulations, hospitals turned to computers and consultants to get the most return for their services. With the government working its side of the fence and the hospitals the other, relationships have not been the most cordial. "Instead of HCFA and the hospitals working mutually toward the goal of cost containment, distrust of each other has interfered with the attainment of this end."[104] So, to what end will the DRGs head? Citing two other articles, Gay and Kronenfeld agree that the system is moving toward "a system of capitation, with the physician becoming the gatekeeper."[105]

Bigger and Better Institutions

If a number of hospitals and HCFA have lost sight of their goals, there are also many others that know exactly where they are going in the competitive health care marketplace. Rubin, a former HHS Assistant Secretary, pointed out the rapid rise of vertical integration as a management technique. He noted that multihospital systems supplied inpatient care, outpatient care, ambulatory surgery, home health care, occupational medicine and preventive care. In March 1984, he said, "In my judgment, we have only seen the beginning of these developments."[106]

As an example of that vertical integration prediction, almost one year later newspapers announced the $6.6 billion merger of the number one hospital management chain, Hospital Corporation of America, and the number one distributor of hospital supplies, American Hospital Supply Corporation.[107,108] This merger would have been the fourth largest in U.S. corporate history. HCA owns or manages 422 facilities including hospitals and nursing homes, leases medical equipment, and handles health care insurance. AHS Co. makes and/or distributes 130,000 medical products and handles 25 percent of the national hospital supply business. With hospitals watching their costs under DRGs, AHS Co. grew only 4.2 percent in 1984 after 15 percent growth in each of the prior ten years. However, at the last minute AHS withdrew from the merger with HCA and opted to combine instead with Baxter Travenol Laboratories, another large producer of medical supplies. This new merger results in a $3.8 billion transaction and moves into an example of horizontal integration, but nevertheless, is in the same predictive vein as the trend toward bigger and better in the health care field.

According to a Standard & Poor's Corporation survey, more than 400 hospitals joined larger chains since 1980. Multihospital systems now account for more than 30 percent of all hospitals.[109]

A closing prediction about bigger and better institutions reflects another trend accelerated by DRGs: "Some analysts predict that about three-fourths of all hospitals will be part of some multihospital group--including both profit and nonprofit--by 1990."[110]

Physicians and Economics

In a 1985 editorial in the *Journal of the American Medical Association*, Ginzberg, a health economist, presented his views on what lies ahead for American physicians. He noted that physicians exhibited "concern, unease, confusion, discontent and anxiety" about the changing structure of the U.S. health care system.[111] Ginzberg felt that "the outlook for physicians has definitely taken a marked turn for the worse."[112]

Although, Ginzberg labeled his predictions "hunches," he did feel reasonably certain that some of the following forecasts would be correct:

● Hospital utilization has probably peaked, with the probability of conversions and mergers and a competition for staff appointments.

● Efforts to eliminate the usual customary and reasonable fee determination will accelerate, with physician fee freezes only the initial step.

● A radical cutback in funding for graduate medical education is likely.

● Along with the increase in HMOs and CMPs, more and more medical graduates will opt for a form of "corporate" employment instead of private practice.

● Competition between hospitals and physicians for ambulatory care dollars will heighten and the outcome is difficult to determine at this time.

- With more choices for care available to the public, physicians are likely to see fewer patients and have lower earnings.

- With the supply of physicians still increasing, earnings are certain to be reduced unless total spending for health increases or funds can be redirected from hospitals.

- Although the public is concerned about the extent of terminal care, the medical profession has not provided leadership.

- Foreign medical graduates will continue to flow into the United States and the United States schools will not curtail enrollments.[113]

Lundberg, the editor of *JAMA*, followed Ginzberg's editorial with his own thoughts about the troubles of the medical profession. He said, "We are very successful. But we are in deep trouble."[114] A goodly portion of the trouble relates to the differences between the public's and the profession's perceptions of issues as evidenced in polls. By 1984, cost was listed as the main health care problem by 68 percent of the public, as compared to only 50 percent of the physicians. In addition, only 27 percent of the public thought physicians fees were reasonable and 67 percent felt that doctors were too interested in making money. Lundberg believes that the poll results are negative enough to warrant actions to regain the public's trust. He advises physicians to affirm the best interests of patients and the public, to take a leadership position on cost containment, to accept reduced fees where warranted, to practice better management, to promote open communication with patients, and to care for the public.[115]

In reporting on both the Ginzberg and Lundberg articles in the newspapers, Knox proclaimed that the future looks grim for American's doctors.[116]

MD Payments—Freeze? DRG?

According to Schwartz, the government's freeze on Medicare fees for physicians was another grim event—the "most severe economic and political setback in modern history" for physicians.[117] Contending that the government broke an implicit agreement to hold off on any legal action if the AMA undertook a voluntary freeze, Schwartz labeled the Congressional mandatory freeze "a last minute act of treachery."[118] Furthermore, he noted that Congress expected to enact a DRG fee system for physicians. A bill to extend PPS to physician fees drew support from the AFL-CIO, the American Association of Retired Persons, and the United Auto Workers, but not from the medical societies.[119]

HCFA Administrator Davis stated that it is unlikely that anything will happen regarding Medicare physician payments before October 1986, even though that task is a top priority for the agency. Congress is to receive reports on alternatives such as relative value scales, bundling services, and capitation systems. However, HCFA "will recommend clustering services in one payment formula; setting predetermined rates; and offering providers incentives to participate."[120] A majority of physicians appear to favor the use of relative value scales. HCFA's research director, Dobson, said that RVS seem more "equitable and rational" than physician DRGs, but the volume of services is not controlled and there' is no consensus on how to assign values.[121]

Concern about physician payments was colorfully expressed by Congressman Wyden (D-OR) when he said that the Medicare legislation is "a gun without bullets."[122] That comment implies that hospital costs cannot be controlled without directly dealing with the attending physician who controls the volume of inpatient services. That concern was examined further as National Center for Health Services Research investigators Gabel and Rice reported that freezing physician payments will not curtail health care costs, but will limit access to care.[123,124] Doctors counter the freeze and/or payment reduction by increasing the number and complexity of services for patients. In California, under a limited reimbursement system, services to Medicare patients increased from 8 to 15 percent. In addition, this study revealed that physicians are less likely to care for public program patients under restricted payment modes. Several measures were suggested by the authors to control costs while altering the fee-for-service payment mechanism:

- Increase reimbursement rates for medical services while freezing or reducing payments for other services.

- Reduce hospital admissions by freezing or cutting physician reimbursement for hospital visits and surgery while increasing payment for office and home visits.

- Contract selectively with groups of doctors to provide all Medicare and Medicaid services and referrals.[125]

Fee-For-Service Death Knell

Regardless of whether there is a freeze or imposition of physician DRGs, Parsons, a state medical society president, sees doctors in dire straits: "The DRG program is the death knell for traditional fee-for-service medicine as well as for freedom of choice of provider for patients."[126]

In addition, Parsons could not decide whether to label the after effects as "dynamic tension" or "war" resulting from the drastic changes in traditional medical care. Whittington picks up on that conflict, particularly the DRG strategy to induce hospital administrators to align themselves with the federal government. "One shudders to think what may happen in the years ahead as the natural political, economic, humanitarian and social alliance between the American hospital system and medicine is fragmented."[127] He claimed that DRGs are destined to divide and rule and explained that position with the following example: "The job of telling the doctor he must discharge his patient, or threatening to revoke his staff privileges because he keeps patients beyond the allotted time or utilizes too many expensive services, won't be handled by a bureaucrat, but by a representative of the hospital administration."[128] Not only are currently practicing physicians being affected by the economics of cost containment, but future generations of doctors will also be affected as PPS reforms graduate medical education funding, too.

Graduate Medical Education

In 1983, Kovener and Palmer interviewed health care financial management experts about the impending implementation of the Medicare PPS. They reported that "some believe it is likely that the new system will be modified to eliminate the teaching cost pass-through."[129]

As predicted, the federal government plans to freeze direct medical education payments for accredited teaching activities and cut by 50% indirect medical education payments related to additional costs incurred by having on-site residents and interns. Without changes, Medicare would pay out $1.3 billion for direct medical education costs and $1.4 billion for indirect costs in FY 1986. When PPS is fully implemented, indirect education reimbursement could reach 5.5 percent of the total PPS payments.According to an AHA representative, indirect graduate medical education payments compensate teaching hospitals for severity of illness differences, case mix, and caring for the indigent.[130]

Decrying HCFA's "meat-ax approach" Representative Henry Waxman (D-CA) charged that "there does not appear to be any interest, recognition, or concern about the implications for patient care, physician supply, or teaching hospitals."[131]

Speaking for HCFA, Desmarais countered that "it is hard to justify continuation of our blank check policy for direct medical education." He added that in view of the budget deficit, "there is no rationale for doubling indirect payments."[132]

Congressmen were urged to hold off taking any action until the role of medical education in patient care could be precisely clarified. Relman cautioned that "if you destabilize the teaching hospitals, you cut the whole structure and its foundation."[133]

Obviously concerned about the proposed reduction, the Association of American Medical Colleges contracted with Lave to prepare a clarification of the intent of the indirect medical education adjustment in the Medicare PPS. She wrote an 11-page article on the historical development and current status of the cost reimbursement situation.[134] A major point of Lave's presentation is that indirect costs are legitimate payments for associated teaching hospital factors such as the additional testing, the increased procedures, and the entering of more notes into medical records. Lave attacks the misunderstanding that indirect medical education costs are linked solely to the ratio of residents and interns per hospital bed. To enhance equity and efficiency for all participants in PPS, Lave calls for changes in DRG classifications, in DRG price setting, in DRG wage indexes, in the use of market factors, and in the urban/rural adjustments.

Even yielding that indirect medical payments may be somewhat larger than equitable, Lave cautions that the very size of the payments, combined with a budget neutrality mentality, could have dire future consequences: "The magnitude of the payments made under the rubric of the indirect costs of medical education is likely to make the adjustment a subject of attack by other hospitals. In addition, these payments are likely to be considered as a potential source of budget savings by the Administration and Congress."[135]

Tied to direct and indirect medical education payments is the fact that many teaching hospitals also serve a large number of patients covered by Medicaid programs. It is likely that what happens in the Medicare PPS will directly affect Medicaid cost containment efforts.

Medicaid and PPS/DRG

Just as the federal government is seeking to contain Medicare costs, state governments are trying to cut Medicaid expenditures. A small number of states already have adopted DRGs for use in their Medicaid programs.[136]

Medicaid DRGs at work in New Jersey, Ohio, Pennsylvania and Utah were described in a Washington Report on Medicine and Health under the headline "States Look to DRGs for Medicaid Cure."[137] Some states made changes, but the Medicaid DRG systems are quite similar to the national model. In fact, Zimmerman concluded, "DRG payment systems can be used as a potentially powerful cost containment strategy for state Medicaid programs. . . . Although a DRG bandwagon cannot yet be discerned, it appears that DRGs can offer a state a legislatively viable and highly visible programmatic strategy for containing hospital expenditures."[138]

A symposium examined the impact of Medicare PPS on state Medicaid programs at the first federally sponsored conference on DRGs in Atlantic City, New Jersey, during November 1983. Lovecchio, an HCFA official, reported that 25 states developed alternative, generally prospective, payment systems. In the other 25 states, Medicaid programs use a retrospective reasonable cost reimbursement method. Differences relating to the phase-in period, the excluded hospitals, capital costs, outliers, and relative value weights were explained. No firm directions were supplied because the federal government believes that state hospital reimbursement systems are best determined by the state, according to Lovecchio.[139]

A representative from the New Jersey Department of Human Services evaluated the state Medicaid agency options for reimbursement. However, Russo thought that the national Medicare DRG methodology would be the most appropriate over a period of time. He lists 10 administrative concerns for Medicaid agencies such as cost reporting, information systems, bundling, phase-in, patient transfers, and hospital grouping. In addition, Russo alerts administrators to the possibility of costs being shifted to Medicaid to cover Medicare shortfalls. That is given as an incentive for Medicaid agencies to adopt Medicare DRGs.[140]

Weiland told the symposium audience about New Jersey's experience using a Medicaid DRG system. Length of stay decreased by more than one-half day. Admissions were substantially reduced by about 8 percent. Project savings from utilization review were well in excess of $2.5 million. He says that the system can work for Medicaid.[141]

From a management analyst's point of view, Clinkscale pointed out the complications that state Medicaid agencies faced in moving to a Medicare PPS/DRG model. He specifically discussed Medicaid's poor database, outdated cost reports, wage indexes, utilization review, and improbability of separating psychiatric/rehabilitation facilities for cost purposes.

Clinkscale did note that DRGs appeared to be a clean and effective tool for controlling inpatient costs. Yet, he estimated it would take at least a year to properly plan to implement a DRG system in a state Medicaid environment.[142]

While no conclusive clarion call emerged from this nationwide conference, it is illuminating that the Medicare/Medicaid DRG payment issue was included in the program. Even though the Medicaid program is state-administered, the federal government puts a substantial amount of money into the operation. It would be naive to expect that if the Medicare PPS/DRG model works, there would not be a movement to induce the states to also use the methodology.

Quality of Care

Predictions about the changes in the health care delivery system may specifically relate to components such as hospital administrators, physicians, educational programs, or Medicaid. However, underlying many of the forecasts is a concern about what is going to happen to the quality of care. It is true that PROs were created in the PPS to watch over the quality of care. In fact, at the 1985 annual meeting of the FAH, Nathanson, HCFA's director of health standards and quality, spoke about the future. He said that PROs may "toughen up reviews for premature discharges"[143] as part of the nationwide PRO goals of shifting 595,000 inappropriate inpatient admissions to outpatient services, reducing unnecessary admissions and procedures by 290,000, and reducing unnecessary admissions by special hospitals and/or physicians by 425,000.[144] However, Nathanson did project quick relief for small and rural facilities from the 60 percent average PRO reviews as compared to the 30 percent average generally.[145]

At the same meeting, lawyer Aronson expressed futuristic views about the quality standards and the reactions of physicians: "Standards fall into two categories: Too vague and general or so specific as to be laughable. Physicians will object to 'second guessing,' and PRO implementation will be done in a manner odious to physicians."[146]

In her summary for Congressmen, Lundy cautioned that PPS could affect the quality of care because PPS incentives encourage the rendering of minimal services, premature discharges, unnecessary readmissions, withholding hospitalization, and the upcoding of patients.[147] Similar sentiments on the quality of care were expressed at a hearing of the House Select Committee on Aging. Representing the AHA, Mongan warned that future "arbitrary squeezes in resources will force hospitals, particularly rural and inner city facilities, to cut deeper to the bone, and quality will suffer."[148]

Representative Edward Roybal (D-CA), Chairman of the Select Committee on Aging, charged that Medicare "cost containment" is in danger of becoming "care containment."[149] He introduced the Quality Assurance Reform Act of 1985 to mandate PRO to devote equal resources and time to monitoring quality as to cost by October 1, 1986. In addition, the act would extend PRO review to all Medicare services, including those rendered in physicians' office, in nursing homes, and home health agencies by April 1, 1988. Furthermore, the Act directs the Congressional Office of Technology Assessment to appoint a nine-member National Council on Quality Assurance. To accomplish these tasks, the act would increase PRO funding by 30 percent in 1986, 40 percent in 1987, and 50 percent in 1988 and following years with adjustments for inflation.[150]

Costs and Malpractice

Whenever cost containment is related to the quality of care, the malpractice issue arises. Predictions have been made on both sides of the fence: some say lawsuits will jump, while others disagree. Fifer puts it neatly into place, "The challenge for the hospital and the physician is to walk the fine line between cost containment and 'quality care' so that constraint in resource use does not result in patient mishap."[151] He goes on to cite research evidence on inappropriate hospital utilization, surgical rate variations, and HMO performance comparisons to make a point that it is not inevitable that curtailed costs will result in decremental quality of care. "Rather it might be concluded that physicians are able to reduce resource use without compromising care quality; that the 'best' care is indeed the cheapest care."[152]

On the other hand, Dr. C. Alton Brown, president of the Physicians Liability Insurance Company of Oklahoma, predicts that DRGs may generate more malpractice suits. He says that when patients realize that they were discharged for economic reasons, they will sue. "When you treat patients by cookbook methods or some artificial standard of care based on economics, instead of on patients' actual needs, more will become dissatisfied."[153]

Basically, the conflict will be resolved at a professional level with the aid of objective research into the health status of the population. Therefore, it is probable that there will be painstaking investigations of all the elements considered integral parts of quality care as they occur or do not occur in the PPS and the correlation with morbidity and mortality.

Technology and Quality of Care

Quality of care is often closely associated with the hospital's ability to purchase new technology and to build new facilities. An HCFA administrator, James Scott, cited several considerations relative to Medicare reimbursement. He said the agency "must decide if the technology is reasonable and necessary for wide usage and to what extent the advancement has been accepted by the medical community."[154] In addition, Scott noted that there is consideration of whether or not the technology represents a good or marginal allocation of resources to meet health care needs. In a bit of a tangent, William Roper, Jr., special assistant to the President for health policy, declared that the federal government should not be making technology decisions. He opted for having those who know best—physicians and consumers—making those decisions. His comment on the link to quality represents a common cost/quality view: "The prospective pricing system forces quality and cost tradeoffs to be made but they should not be made in Washington."[155]

Lundy informed the Congressmen of the oft-repeated forecasts that PPS will stifle innovation, substitute machines for humans, and shift technology outside the hospital. Questions about reduced staffs and the impact on quality were raised but not answered.[156] However, in all fairness, it should be acknowledged that the technology/quality relation had been receiving considerable attention prior to PPS.

Capital Expenditures and Quality

Similar to technology, possible PPS restrictions on reimbursement for capital expenditures are often linked to the quality of care. Providers argue that capital improvements through new construction or new equipment directly upgrade the quality of care. As with technology, pros and cons do not lead to an easy answer. Furthermore, the resolution may be delayed beyond the legislative mandate of

October 1, 1986, when a decision was supposed to be made on how to incorporate capital reimbursement into PPS. The HHS report, due October 1, 1984, is long overdue. Until that decision, hospitals are reluctant to invest large sums in capital expenditures until they can project their reimbursement rates and calculate the cost effectiveness. This situation could possible cause detriment to patient care. Borgue, director of the National Committee for Quality Health Care, said: "The further we get from that date [October 1, 1986], the greater the risk for uncertainty regarding those capital projects [begun before and after PPS]."[157]

Consumers and PPS/DRG

"Volumes have been written about the problems of Medicare, but almost nothing from the viewpoint of patients. What's it like for us?"[158] With that opening, a retired newspaper columnist humorously, with the bite of truth beneath the surface, explained about health care under Medicare with an obvious tie to quality. Shapiro did note the complaints about the high cost of medical care, but he had only one quarrel with the cost control program. His bone of contention dealt with the length of stay limitations. "If only four hours were allotted for a six hour operation, the patient would have to complete the final two hours of the procedure himself, in the privacy of his home."[159]

Despite the fact that the consumers are the warm bodies affected by the PPS/DRG activities, there has not been a purposeful inclusion of consumers into the efforts. That situation was highlighted at the first of a series of nationwide events to celebrate the twentieth anniversary of Medicare and Medicaid. On June 19, 1985, a three day conference on the future of Medicare and Medicaid opened in Los Angeles sponsored by HCFA and the California Health and Welfare Agency. About 1,000 people attending the opening session with a payment of a $600 registration fee at the door or $475 in advance. Most of the conference participants represented hospitals, physicians, HMOs, supply firms, and drug companies.

After heated complaints from ostracized consumer groups, the conference organizers at the last minute granted them a special registration rate of $50 to sit in on the sessions. However the $50 consumer representatives had to pledge not to eat the food provided for the $600 or $450 registrants. In a reaction to the economically prohibitive registration fee, some three dozen consumer organizations combined to form the Medicare/Medicaid Defense Project to arrange a "counterconference." More than 500 marchers prepared a giant "Prescription for America's Health Care," properly adorned with hundreds of messages to the federal government encased in medicine bottles to deliver at the conference site.

Symposiums at the conference discussed strategies for increasing competition in the nation's health care system. An assistant secretary of HHS, Charles Baker, said that the issue relates to making the health care industry more like a business and less like a national free lunch. Vita Ostrander, president of the American Association of Retired Persons, told conference attendees that "the poor, the old and the sick" must have a voice in the ongoing debate about changes in Medicare and Medicaid.[160]

PRO Data for Consumers

One of the things that consumers lack is adequate information to make reasoned choices about health services. A final rule from HCFA allows PROs to release data evaluating hospitals to the public. That PRO-collected data could include mortality rates, costs, length of stay, volume, or infection rates by hospital or hospital department. In the final rule, HCFA states that PROs "are an important source of information to aid consumers and consumer organizations in reaching informed decisions about the types of health care services that are offered."[161] In fact, on March 12, 1986, the front page of the *New York Times* declared that the federal government was releasing a list of 269 hospitals with abnormal mortality rates; 142 with higher rates and 127 with lower rates. A complete list of the hospitals, by state, was published in the newspaper.[162]

Both the AHA and the AMA argued that the hospital-specific data should be confidential since some hospitals normally treat sicker patients. Consumer groups pushed for also making physician-specific data available. HCFA rejected both arguments, but did make modifications. PRO must give hospitals 30 days to comment before disclosure and any comments must be included in information given to consumers. With this PRO hospital review data, it is likely that more consumer-generated hospital comparison material will be distributed.

Comparison Shopping

In keeping with the informed consumer concept, a number of industrial firms decided to post hospital prices to help their employees make cost conscious decisions. Since these firms spend large sums on employee health benefits, the impact could be sizable. Quaker Oats Company gave its 4,000 Chicago area employees a book listing lowest, midpoint, and highest charges at 44 hospitals for frequently needed services such as normal delivery, tonsillectomy, and cardiac catheterization. Zenith Electronic Corporation did likewise for its 7,000 employees in Glenview, Illinois. Statewide listings are published by government units in Arizona, California, Florida, Illinois, Indiana, Iowa, and Maryland. Local health business groups in Boston and Minneapolis-St. Paul publish hospital price lists, too.

Experts are still evaluating whether or not posting hospital prices saves money. Some critics contend that price is not the major incentive for the consumer. Yet

Quaker Oat reported a nearly 7 percent decline in average medical costs per employee from 1982 to 1984.[163] With individuals having to pay larger shares of the medical bills, it is likely that shopping guides listing prices will appear more frequently.

Vouchers for Health Care

President Reagan's 1984 budget proposal asked for the establishment of a voluntary voucher system.[164] Under the voucher system, a Medicare recipient could choose between using the existing program or taking a voucher valued at 95 percent of the per capita Medicare program costs and shopping around for private health insurance coverage. While the voucher concept is not new, the Medicare proposal expanded the idea beyond HMOs to include a variety of additional providers as long as the client received benefits at least as comparable as those provided by Medicare regulations.

Senator David Durenberger and Representative Richard Gephardt coined the word "Medichoice" for this version of a Medicare voucher system. Reports from Medichoice demonstration projects at Fallon Community Health Plan (Worcester, MA), Nicolett Health Plan, and SHARE (Minneapolis, MN) are all enthusiastic. Besides containing costs, these Medichoice centers stress quality assurance, utilization review, alternatives to hospitalization, sophisticated management, and patient satisfaction.[165]

Senator Durenberger pushed for the voluntary voucher because of his belief that the health care system "works better in a marketplace atmosphere than in a regulatory atmosphere."[166] Market pressures should act for the benefit of all and the Senator summed up his view: "The voluntary voucher rewards the individual patient for selecting a cost-effective health plan. And it rewards the health provider for delivering cost-effective care."[167] John Tillotson, M.D., Senator Durenberger's legislative aide for health, called the voluntary voucher the way of the future to contain total costs rather than unit costs.[168]

Variations on the voucher theme pop up in the literature from time to time. Consistently, most proposals stress the marketplace ethic as the major advantage. In the American business community, including the health care industry, the assumption is made that competition will stimulate the construction of a better mousetrap. Traditional business know-how will find ways to deliver quality health care within cost containment limitations. Within that environment, HHS moved into the arena and instituted another cost containment mechanism utilizing the voucher concept for Medicare health care coverage.

Consumer Legislation

In his Quality Assurance Reform Act of 1985, Representative Roybal (D-CA) includes two specific consumer activities. One item directs PROs to maintain

24-hour hot lines for questions and complaints from Medicare providers and beneficiaries. Another mandate directs PROs to have a five-to-seven member consumer advisory board by October 1, 1986.[169] If passed, both these consumer-oriented activities would do much to bring the "grass roots" attitudes into the health care decision-making apparatus.

Seeking "incentives to promote self-responsibility," Senator Durenberger (R-MN) introduced three proposals to broaden Medicare's role in disease prevention:

S.357 gives nonsmokers and ex-smokers a $1 monthly premium reduction for nonhospital services.

S.358 increases the deductible for nonhospital services from $75 to $100. However, nonreimbursed preventive care such as immunization, health screening, and antihypertensive medication would count in satisfying the deductible.

S.359 proposes that HHS fund five demonstration projects that would provide various preventive services such as stress reduction, dietary advice, and mental health intervention.[170]

These proposals all relate to the health promotion and disease prevention emphasis of a large number of consumer health organizations. Medicare, and other health insurance programs, traditionally have not reimbursed for "wellness" care. Durenberger echoed the consumer sentiments: "Staying well and providing suitable incentives for maintaining good health not only makes good health sense, it also makes sound economic sense."[171]

All Payers—Consumer Choice

At hearings and in continuing comments about PPS, most consumer groups have advocated that the PPS cover all payers reimbursing for services rendered to their beneficiaries. In effect, this would yield the greatest benefits to the public since total health care costs would be curtailed. PPS legislation mandates a report on that concept by December 1985 (Exhibit 13-3). A Medicare Reform Act of 1984, the Kennedy-Gephardt bill,[172] proposed that, but met stiff Congressional opposition. In an Op-Ed article in the New York Times, Marmor and Smolka review various ways to help Medicare bring health cost inflation under control. Without mentioning the words "all-payer system," the authors conclude: "The right way to secure Medicare's fiscal future is to slow rates of increase in all health care costs, not just the bills the government pays. With across-the-board cost containment, we can preserve Medicare without shifting burdens to the elderly, to private purchasers or to the general tax payer."[173]

Best Guesses and Assorted Predictions

At an April 1984 conference on Medicare and Medicaid cosponsored by the AHA and the National Health Lawyers Association, more than two dozen speakers agreed that "refinement, not restructuring, is the key to Medicare prospective pricing reform."[174] Yet, they also foresaw significant changes in PPS to assure equity and to retain the incentives to curtail costs. On the other hand, New Jersey's Health Commissioner J. Richard Goldstein, sidestepped the future of DRGs at a November 1984 national conference. He said that "there are just too many forces to successfuly prognosticate the impact on the overall health care system."[175] Another prediction in the same time period by two health care experts projected a battle. Johnson and Appel commented that "our analysis leads us to believe that hospitals will fight the system. . . . DRG payment will pit larger tertiary care hospitals with more complex cases against smaller hospitals."[176]

Whether refining, refusing to prognosticate, or fighting, the question still remains—where do we go from here? That is exactly what was asked of a panel of health care financing experts at an April 1985 meeting of the Federation of American Hospitals. Their composite answer was: "Your guess is as good as ours."[177]

Medicare Hospital Insurance Trust Fund

Since the impending bankruptcy of the Medicare Hospital Insurance Trust Fund was a major precipitating factor in the implementation of PPS, it is appropriate to start with the future of that fund. A 1982 report of the Social Security Trustees predicted insolvency of the trust fund by 1987. In 1984, the "doomsdate" moved up to 1991. Now, in its 1985 report, the Trustees report that the Medicare hospital insurance fund is solvent until 1998.[178] Credit for a projection was given to prospective pricing, low inflation rates, and high employment levels. In a cautionary tone, the report also warned that the prediction assumed a freezing of hospital DRG rates for 1986 and adjustments in the future at no more than hospital market basket inflation plus one-fourth of one percent.[179] To insure solvency for the next 25 years, the report says that either benefits will have to be reduced 19 percent or payroll contributions increased 24 percent.[180]

With the imminent danger of bankruptcy forestalled, optimism prevails and the guesses and predictions can be considered at a more leisurely pace.

A Second Revolution

At the first national HCFA-sponsored conference on PPS in November 1983, Ronald B. Milch, Chairman-Elect of the Board of Trustees of the New Jersey Hospital Association, called PPS the second revolution in the U.S. health care system, with Medicare itself being the first. Starting out with his belief that PPS is a better and more equitable reimbursement system than the traditional per diem method, Milch made a number of predictions:

- A single payer Medicare system is doomed to failure due to cost shifting.

Therefore, PPS is the forerunner for a national all-payers prospective system.

- A myth that was perpetrated over the years that hospital administrators make medical decisions now appears to be a reality.

- PPS will result in some form of vertical integration by hospitals with the appropriate reorganization structure following a corporate model.

- Mergers and closings of hospitals will be seen as survival decisions are made.

- There will be increased shifting of personnel in job changes.

- Physicians will be encouraged to practice, willingly or unwillingly, two standards of care—one for Medicare patients and one for all others.[181]

In closing, Milch raises a question that is beyond his predictive powers. He asks how we will decide whether 5 percent, 10 percent, or 20 percent of our gross national product is the appropriate amount to spend for health care. He responds that prospective payment will not answer the question.[182]

Can Health Care Costs Ever Be Controlled?

A variety of health care experts at a 1985 conference at the Washington Journalism Center were asked to respond to the question, "Can health care costs ever be controlled?" Although no overall concensus was reached, a few points did emerge as projections for PPS/DRGs:

- Managed care via HMOs, PPOs, CMPs or other types will replace the traditional fee-for-service system and integrate preadmission certification, concurrent review of cases by the insurer, and discharge planning into the service plan.

- Medicare HMO regulations will result in more structural changes in the health care system than did the DRG payment system.[183]

Some forecast the expansion of the DRG system to physician services, although others said not yet. An all-payer expansion was labeled a "back-door approach to national health insurance."[184] Physicians were advised to watch out for the steamroller if they tried to stop current trends "by putting their fingers in the dike."[185]

Unpredictable Changes

At a special FAH seminar on Medicare PPS, participants agreed that major changes are likely, but nobody was sure what they will be. Some suggested that Medicare overhaul would probably result in a capitation system. It was expected that dumping uninsured, underinsured, and indigent patients would continue. Public hospitals were expected to go from bad to worse in the money-deficit situation. Conflicting forecasts also related to capital cost reimbursement, PPS expansion, unspent other monies, case-mix index, upgrading, and the quality of care. "Other speakers generally agreed that reimbursement rules could change dramatically—and perhaps unpredictably."[186]

Senior PPO Best Bet

Griffith, a professor of hospital administration, predicted that the DRG system "will be gamed in every possible way," and that a universal all-payer extension of DRGs could be ruled out. He then projects the following four criteria for an ideal Medicare payment system:

1. Encourages outpatient care instead of hospitalization

2. Encourages a continuing provider/patient relationship

3. Encourages residential rather than institutional living

4. Encourages living wills and power-of-attorney to avoid unnecessary expenditures in terminal illness.[187]

While Griffith felt that the Social Health Maintenance Organization came close to meeting his criteria, he did opt for a new entity. "I believe the answer lies in a blend of capitated and fee-for-service care like some of the PPOs." He called it a Senior PPO.[188]

OMB, Not HCFA, Change Force

At a meeting of the National Health Lawyer Association and AHA, a former HCFA official commented that future changes in PPS will be dictated by costs. Oday added that quality of care or stability of the health care system may not necessarily be considerations: "And the Office of Management and Budget, not HCFA, is the force driving the cost cutting debate."[189]

Linking cost to future directions for the PPS/DRG model then logically brings us to the federal legislative doorstep, since the elected representatives control the federal pursestrings with their appropriation powers.

Legislative Forecasts

Predictions by federal legislators carry some weight because these are the people who will actually be enacting changes in PPS/DRG. Obviously, there are many pressures on elected representatives to act in favor of their constituents, so it will be illuminating to gather the comments.

In April 1984, Representative Ron Wyden (D-OR), a member of the House Subcommittee on Health, pinpointed a number of "warts on the system" as "sure bets" for Congressional action in 1985.[190] Specifically, he expected action on physicians' fees to fold reimbursement into DRGs. In addition, Wyden anticipated curtailed payments for mycotic toenail procedures, reduced surgical fees for pacemaker implants, and equalization of Medicare blood test fees for those paid by private patients.[191]

Hospital Legislative Predictions

Lesparre, an AHA official located in Washington, DC, reviewed the legislative future of PPS/DRG at the beginning of 1985 with a focus on the hospitals. He noted that predictions are "broad and sometimes wild."[192] However, Lesparre did start with the consensus that PPS is working. Moving from that agreement, Lesparre analyzes legislative actions proposed by various federal legislators and comes up with the following possible changes:

- There will be no precipitous rush toward a legislated all-payer system, since opponents fear a link to a national health insurance scheme.

- Congress can be expected to balk at further cuts on payments to hospitals.

- Advocates are pushing for a "complexity index" to predict resource use and possibly end the urban/rural distinction.

- An end to the direct graduate medical education pass-through is predicted within two years, to be replaced with a medical education block grant based on the number of filled intern and residency positions in hospitals.

- Proposals call for incentives to the states to develop hospital cost containment plans since "we cannot stop with a Medicare-only system of DRGs."

- "Physicians must be brought into the picture of cost containment" because "the blank check isn't going to go along forever under Part B."

- A means test for Medicare beneficiaries will be under consideration.

- Congress will address the ethical policies and procedures of the delivery of health care.

- Proponents will push for adequate evaluation of technology, claiming that Medicare could save $20 billion, without lowering quality, if new technologies are tested thoroughly.

- Political sensitivities will cause many issues to stay on the back burner.

- Perceptions in Congress of the tie between health care issues and the rest of the economy have never been sharper.[193]

Key Legislative Agendas

Political comments on Medicare PPS appear frequently from all sides of Congress and from both the Senate and the House. In the Senate, the Finance Committee, the Health Subcommittee, and the Select Committee on Aging have been particularly vocal.

With Senator Robert Dole (D-KN) moving over to become Majority Leader, Senator Robert Packwood replaced him as Chairman of the Finance Committee. In an extensive interview with Edward Mihalski, the Committee's chief health staff person, McIlrath collected his predictions for Medicare changes in 1985-1986. Mihalski felt that Medicare reform will not be a front-burner issue in Congress, but still noted the following legislative agenda items:

- Congress may mitigate the effect of a proposed freeze on DRG rates for hospitals in 1986.

- Legislators may favor halting the PPS phase-in of a national DRG rate.

- Although alternatives to the proposed freeze on direct medical education costs may emerge, it is unlikely that cuts for indirect medical education costs will be scaled back.

- Legislators are moving toward agreement on increasing Medicare beneficiary cost sharing.

- Effects of hospital DRGs will be evaluated with a view toward extension of PPS to other Medicare and Medicaid reimbursed facilities such as nursing homes.

- Legislators express interest in replacing the fee-for-service payment program but there is not consensus on what the replacement should be or how the Congressional vote would go.[194]

Despite these avowed legislative intentions, Mihalski does caution that "if there is a climate created to race down a track to deficit reduction, the little pieces are not going to be as important as getting the whole thing done. We are not going to have a chance to fine-tune all these proposals as much as we would like to."[195]

Senator David Durenberger (R-MN) is Chairman of the Senate Subcommittee on Health and has been quite active in talking about Medicare PPS activities. In a speech to a nationwide meeting on DRGs in November 1983, the Senator remarked that "American medicine is in the midst of a revolution driven by cost."[196] He went on to make the following forecasts:

- We must expand the present DRG payment to include physicians, home health care, skilled nursing facilities, hospice care, and other levels of care.

- By the time Congress is ready to undertake a serious national debate about the bankruptcy of Medicare, a solution based on vouchers will be more acceptable and attractive.

- I expect that the DRG system will greatly stimulate the development of competitive medical plans.

- It is inappropriate to expect Medicare patients or private patients to carry the cost of medical education or care for the indigent.

- Cost constraints may very well force rationing decisions.

- Refinements in the DRG system itself—like a severity adjustment—will be necessary.[197]

In a March 1985 speech at an FAH meeting, Senator Durenberger recommended changes in Medicare's PPS to affect incentives for both providers and consumers. Importantly, the Senator continues to hold to earlier views on the specific items that he cited again.

- Expand PPS to all providers.

- Eliminate urban/rural price differences.

- Restructure Medicare to include prevention and lifestyle premiums.

- Use copayments as a means to cover catastrophic illness costs.

- Establish a means test for Medicare beneficiaries.

- Eliminate tax law distinctions between for-profit and nonprofit hospitals.[198]

Another important legislator is Senator John Heinz (R-PA), who is a member of the Health Subcommittee and Chairman of the Special Committee on Aging. In a November 1984 interview, he presented his views on Medicare. Starting with the fact that Medicare reform is his "highest priority," the Senator went on to cover the following points:

- We cannot stop with a Medicare-only system of DRGs. . . . we run a substantial risk of creating a two-class system of health care, perhaps even within the same hospital.

- Many of us support the rapid development of state systems to control costs across the board.

- Cost shifting may be an even more potent force in getting Congress to act than the insolvency of Medicare.

- I would not rule out a Medicare means test for beneficiaries.

- I think it fair to say that the current way we reimburse physicians is entirely outmoded, it is inequitable to many physicians, and distorts health care delivery decisions.

- Ultimately, many of us in Congress are attracted to the notion of prepaid health care . . . like HMOs in which physicians negotiate directly with the organization responsible for providing care.[199]

These legislative forecasts, in combination with similar voicings in the House committees, combine to send out a powerful message to the health care delivery system. It is apparent that Congress is not finished with its efforts to affect health care cost containment measures.

Sextet of Sure-Bet Predictions

Based on a review of the tremendous volume of literature on the PPS/DRG method of containing the costs of health care, a sextet of sure-bet predictions emerge in a major trend toward consensus. However, even "sure-bet" predictions may be affected by unforeseen events. This is not to hedge the projections or to protect the authors. Nevertheless, the number of predictions has been limited to the following sure bets for the future:

1. Cost containment is here to stay with a prospective payment, or more accurately, a prospective pricing, format that will expand to other governmental health care programs and balloon out into an all-payer system for inpatient and outpatient care.

2. DRGs will be modified, probably with a severity index, but a patient classification mechanism related to pricing will remain a fundamental com-

ponent of a cost pricing mechanism and include RUGs for long term care, AVGs for ambulatory care, ADRGs for psychiatric care, or other compatible classification models.

3. Multifacility health care systems will continue to grow at a rapid pace, both nonprofit and proprietary, with an emphasis on vertical integration through mergers and purchasing of financially distressed institutions to effect a single entity offering comprehensive care.

4. A business-oriented approach to health care, including marketing and merchandising strategies, will intensify and integrate physicians and other health care providers into a cohesive management team to achieve financial viability for the facility.

5. De facto ethical and legal rationing decisions will be made as patients are discharged "quicker and sicker" to rapidly growing alternative services such as home health care and hospices or even to no care.

6. In true American enterprise style, a variety of commercial firms, all types of health care consultants, and a broad spectrum of professional organization task forces will act in concert with the chief executive leadership of institutions and health care agencies to spend many hours attempting to maintain their excellent track record of beating the system.

Food for Future Thought

In essence, two major forces emerge among the concepts proposed to contain health care costs. One side argues forcefully that the free marketplace competition applied to the health care industry will curtail expenditures. The other side argues, just as forcefully, that governmental regulation limiting spending and overseeing the industry is the only way to contain health care costs. A June 1985 advertisement in the New York Times, paid for by the Health Insurance Association of America, offered an opinion on competition vs. regulation in health care. Carl J. Schramm, director of the Center for Hospital Finance and Management at Johns Hopkins Medical Institutions, came to a conclusion on this issue: "Neither competition nor regulation will operate as a deus ex machina and it is high time that the debate begins about real solutions that will necessarily incorporate both competitive and regulatory aspects."[200]

So now we have a combination of regulation and competition suggested. Even with the combination, the powerful juggernaut of the medical-industrial-complex may cast the biggest shadow of all over the nation's health care delivery system. In keeping with the gist of the sextet of predictions, it is thought-provoking to conclude this book with comments from Paul Ellwood, a physician who has been an active health policy innovator. Ellwood's remarks came about in reaction to a July 5, 1985 announcement that private, for-profit hospital chains were now offering health insurance to the public. He said:

> We're witnessing the industrialization of medicine. . . . We're going to end up with the majority of health care in the U.S. delivered by 10 to 15 corporations. These will be the "supermeds" replacing individual physicians, staffs, clinics, hospitals and insurance companies.[201]

References

1. E. Friedman, "Those Wonderful People Who Brought You DRGs," *Hospitals* 58, No. 5 (March 1, 1984):81-82, 85-86, 88.

2. "The Corporate Rx for Medical Costs," *Business Week*, No. 2864 (October 15, 1984):138-141, 144-146.

3. Ibid.

4. "Time for a War on Runaway Medical Costs," *Business Week*, No. 2864 (October 15, 1984):202.

5. "Time for a War," *Business Week*.

6. "Hospitals Earn Profits Under Medicare Limits," *Newark Star-Ledger*, November 26, 1985.

7. "Health and Federal Leadership," *New York Times*, June 12, 1985.

8. Ibid.

9. M. Rust, "DRGs Need Fine-Tuning: Dr. Davis," *American Medical News* 27, No. 40 (October 26, 1984):2, 28.

10. E. Friedman, "PPS Needs Overhaul to Survive: Altman," *Hospitals* 58, No. 22 (November 16, 1984):33.

11. Ibid.

12. J. R. Griffith, *DRG's—What's Next? Two Views*, Mt. Sinai School of Medicine, Department of Health Care Management, New York, May 3, 1984, p. 16.

13. B. L. Hodes, "The PPS, DRGs, and the New World of Health Care," *Archives of Ophthalmology* 103, No. 2 (1985):185-186.

14. E. C. Bessey, "High Cost of Change to Future Health Care," (letter), *New York Times*, June 19, 1985.

15. T. H. D. Mahoney, "Discharging Elderly Patients Quicker and Sicker," *New York Times*, June 25, 1985.

16. F. S. Primich, "Appalling Intrusion," *New York Times*, June 25, 1985.

17. "PPS Shortchanging Medical Patients?" *Medical World News* 26, No. 6 (March 25, 1985):17.

18. D. Kenyon, "Area Hospitals Feel Pinch," *The News Tribune*, Woodbridge, N.J., May 25, 1985.

19. R. J. Rubin, *DRG's—What's Next? Two Views*, Mt. Sinai School of Medicine, Department of Health Care Management, New York, April 2, 1984, p. 4.

20. Ibid.

21. K. Hunt, "Uncle Sam is Tightening the Screws on Them—and You," *Medical Economics*, April 29, 1985.

22. F. Rahman, "Medicare Makes a Wrong Diagnosis," *New York Times*, January 23, 1986.

23. O. R. Bowen, "How Medicare Hospital Reimbursement Works," (Letter to Editor), *New York Times*, February 6, 1986.

24. J. A. Meyer, "Increased Consumer Cost-Consciousness and Competition," *Bulletin of the New York Academy of Medicine* 60, No. 1 (1984):98-105.

25. Ibid.

26. "A Cure That Could Cripple," *Hospitals* 58, No. 7 (April 1, 1984):14.

27. "1984: Orwell's Nightmare and Current Realities," *Hospitals* 58, No. 1 (January 1, 1984):10.

28. J. Riffer, "DRG Payment Plan to Expand Physician Role," *Hospitals* 57, No. 8 (April 16, 1983):17.

29. D. Burda, "Disproportionate Share Lawsuit Against HHS Gains Hospital

Plaintiff," *Hospitals* 59, No. 8 (April 16, 1985):34.

30. "HHS Will Not Comply With Data Request in Redbud Case: Davis," *Hospitals* 59, No. 10 (May 16, 1985):13.

31. "HCFA Takes Action That Resembles Inaction on Disproportionate Share," *Hospitals* 60, No. 2 (January 20, 1986):25.

32. "Hospital Groups Unite to Press for One-Year Delay in DRG Phase-In," *Hospitals* 59, No. 8 (April 16, 1985):40.

33. C. Wallace, "Medicare Delay Bill Splinters Industry," *Modern Healthcare* 14, No. 5 (1984):28, 30.

34. Griffith, "DRG's—What's Next?", p. 17.

35. Ibid.

36. "Democratic Presidential Candidates Hold Similar Positions on Health Care Reform," *TODAY in Health Planning* 7, No. 11 (May 31, 1984):2.

37. S. McIlrath, "Health Policies of Candidates Are Outlined," *American Medical News* 27, No. 19 (May 18, 1984):1, 20.

38. "Gary Hart: Prospective Pay Should Cover All Third Parties," *Modern Healthcare* 14, No. 5 (1984):33.

39. "All-Payers System Seen by 1990," *American Medical News* 27, No. 37 (October 5, 1984):22.

40. Friedman, "Those Wonderful People."

41. Harvard Medicare Project, *Medicare: Coming of Age, A Proposal for Reform* (Cambridge, Ma.: Division of Health Policy Research and Education, Harvard University, 1986).

42. D. Blumenthal, et al., "The Future of Medicare," *New England Journal of Medicine* 314 (March 13, 1986):722-728.

43. P. Young, "Harvard Study Calls for Sweeping Revamp of the Medicare Program," *Newark Star-Ledger*, March 13, 1986.

44. Prospective Payment Assessment Commission, *Medicare Prospective Payment and the American Health Care System. Report to Congress* (Washington, D.C., February 28, 1986).

45. Friedman, "Those Wonderful People."

46. S. McIlrath, "DRGs Make Hospital Stretch Their Dollars," *American Medical News* 28, No. 1 (January 4, 1985):30.

47. Ibid.

48. J. Finn and C. Mickel, "PPS Dominated Activity in Washington, D.C.," *Hospitals* 58, No. 24 (December 16, 1984):36, 38.

49. J. Riffer, "PPS Prompts Home Care Rise; Few Hospice Benefit Takers," *Hospitals* 58, No. 24 (December 16, 1984):54.

50. K. Shannon, "PPS Information Needs Cause Dramatic Computer Surge," *Hospitals* 58, No. 24 (December 16, 1984):67.

51. J. Kelly and C. Bankhead, "DRGs: How Are They Stacking Up?" *Medical World News* 26, No. 5 (March 11, 1985):80-103.

52. Ibid.

53. R. Sullivan, "Decline in Hospital Use Tied to New U.S. Policies," *New York Times*, April 16, 1985.

54. Ibid.

55. R. Sullivan, "About 25% of Beds in Hospitals in City are Empty, State Reports," *New York Times*, April 2, 1985.

56. R. Sullivan, "Decline in Hospital Use."

57. B. Jacques, "Davis Highlights Major Health System Gains," *Hospitals* 59, No. 9 (May 1, 1985):26.

58. J. P. Lundy, *Medicare: Prospective Payments for Inpatient Hospital Services*, Congressional Research Service, Library of Congress, Issue Brief No. IB83171, Updated, Washington, D.C., March 6, 1985.

59. "DRGs Spark Interest Abroad for Planning," *Hospitals* 59, No. 11 (June 1, 1985):33, 35.

60. "DRG Prices Expected to be Revised Based on '84 Data," *Hospitals* 59, No. 7 (April 1, 1985):28.

61. McIlrath, "DRGs Make Hospital Stretch."

62. W. B. Moore, "Survey Shows CEOs' Priorities are Changing," *Hospitals* 58, No. 24 (December 16, 1984):71-77.

63. Ibid.

64. Ibid.

65. W. B. Moore, "CEOs—Plan to Expand Home Health, Outpatient Services," *Hospitals* 59, No. 1 (January 1, 1985):74-77.

66. "DRG Prices Expected to be Revised Based on '84 Data," *Hospitals* 59, No. 7 (April 1, 1985):28.

67. Ibid.

68. M. R. Traska, "Panel: Payment Changes Push Hospitals to Consider Capitation Mechanisms," *Hospitals* 59, No. 9 (May 1, 1985):46, 48, 50.

69. Ibid.

70. K. Abramowitz, "New Health Service Economics," *Bulletin of the New York Academy of Medicine* 61, No. 1 (1985):31-36.

71. Ibid.

72. Rust, "DRGs Need Fine-Tuning."

73. "An Honest Broker for Fine-Tuning Medicare," *Hospitals* 58, No. 19 (October 1, 1984):102-105.

74. J. Firshein, "Medicare Physician Payment Reform Unlikely Before October 1986: Davis," *Hospitals* 59, No. 11 (June 1, 1985):31-32.

75. Gordon Publications, Inc., *The Gordon DRG Report*. Randolph, NJ, November 1984.

76. P. W. Patterson and J. A. Pfuelb, "How Health Care's Buyers and Sellers Are Adapting to DRGs," *Medical Marketing & Media* 20, No. 6 (1985):12-18.

77. H. C. Whittington, "DRGs Destined to Divide and Rule," *Private Practice* 17, No. 6 (1985):51-52.

78. "Medical Practice: Why Does It Vary So Much?" *Hospitals* 59, No. 5 (March 11, 1985):88, 90.

79. "Letters to the Editor," *New England Journal of Medicine* 312, No. 20 (May 16, 1985):1330-1333.

80. V. R. Fuchs, "Response to Letters to the Editor," *New England Journal of Medicine* 312, No. 20 (May 16, 1985):1332-1333.

81. Friedman, "Those Wonderful People Who Brought You DRGs."

82. R. Pear, "Medicare Payments Raised for Hospitals Serving Poor," *New York Times*, July 2, 1985.

83. "Part VI: Medicare Program; Court Ordered Regulations Regarding Prospective Payment Amount and Administrative Review: Interim Rule," *Federal Register* 50, No. 126 (July 1, 1985):27208-27212.

84. T. Shahoda, "PPS to Spur Ethical Dilemmas: Speaker," *Hospitals* 58, No. 12 (June 16, 1984):22.

85. Ibid.

86. "Dr. Boyle Stresses Ethical Challenges," *American Medical News* 27, No. 25 (June 29/July 6, 1984):1, 33.

87. Ibid.

88. K. H. Morgenlander and D. E. Greenwald, "The Legal and Ethical Impact of Psychiatric DRGs: A Facility-Specific Approach." Presentation at the Annual Meeting of the American Public Health Association, Anaheim, CA, November 14, 1984.

89. M. B. Kapp, "Legal and Ethical Implications of Health Care Reimbursement by DRGs," *Law, Medicine & Health Care* 12, No. 6 (1984):245-253, 278.

90. Ibid.

91. Ibid.

92. W. K. Mariner, "DRGs: Evading Social Responsibility?" *Law, Medicine & Health Care* 12, No. 6 (1984):243-244.

93. Ibid.

94. Ibid.

95. R. L. Weinmann, "Who Holds the Bag?" (letter), *Medical World News* 26, No. 2 (January 28, 1985):52.

96. Rubin, "DRGs—What's Next?"

97. "The Life and Death Choices Created by Medical Technology," *Business Week*, No. 2864, October 15, 1984, pp. 144-145.

98. Ibid.

99. J. K. Iglehart, "Medicare Begins Prospective Payment of Hospitals," *New England Journal of Medicine* 308, No. 23 (June 9, 1983):1428-1432.

100. R. S. Stern and A. M. Epstein, "Institutional Responses to Prospective Payment Based on DRGs," *New England Journal of Medicine* 312, No. 10 (March 7, 1985):621-627.

101. Ibid.

102. Ibid.

103. E. G. Gay and J. J. Kronenfeld, *Unintended Consequences, Organizational Theory, and the Policy Process: The DRG Example*, Presentation at the Annual Meeting of the American Public Health Association, Anaheim, CA, November 1984.

104. Ibid.

105. Ibid.

106. Rubin, "DRGs—What's Next?"

107. T. S. Purdum, "Hospital Company and No. 1 Supplier Plan Huge Merger," *New York Times*, April 1, 1985.

108. C. Timberlake, "Health Care Firms Map $6.6 Billion Merger," *Star-Ledger* (N.J.) April 2, 1985.

109. Purdum, "Hospital Company and No. 1 Supplier Plan Huge Merger."

110. Ibid.

111. E. Ginzberg, "What Lies Ahead for American Physicians: One Economist's Views," *Journal of the American Medical Association* 253, No. 19 (May 17, 1985):2878-2879.

112. Ibid.

113. Ibid.

114. G. D. Lundberg, "Medicine—A Profession in Trouble?" *Journal of the American Medical Association* 253, No. 19 (May 17, 1985):287-288.

115. Ibid.

116. R. A. Knox, "Future Looks Grim for America's Doctors, Economist Says," *The Home News*, Woodbridge, NJ, May 19, 1985.

117. H. Schwartz, "Congress Gives MDs Cold Shoulder," *Private Practice* 16, No. 8 (1984):21.

118. Ibid.

119. S. Smith, "Bill to Extend DRG to Physicians Endorsed by Unions, Aged But Not by Medical Societies," *Internal Medicine News* 17, No. 11 (June 1-14, 1984):6-7.

120. Firshein, "Medicare Payment Reform Unlikely."

121. Ibid.

122. W. R. Fifer, "DRGs and Doctors," *Pennsylvania Medicine* 87, No. 1 (1984):28-33.

123. J. R. Gabel and T. H. Rice, "Reducing Public Expenditures for Physician Services: The Price of Paying Less," *Journal of Health, Politics, Policy and Law* 9, No. 4 (1985):595-609.

124. "MDs Answer Reimbursement Cuts by Ordering More Tests," *Medical Marketing and Media* 20, No. 6 (1985):59.

125. Ibid.

126. E. Friedman, "PPS Called Death Knell for Traditional Medical Care," *Hospitals* 59, No. 7 (April 1, 1985):2.

127. H. G. Whittington, "DRGs Destined to Divide and Rule," *Private Practice* 17, No. 6 (1985):51-52.

128. Ibid.

129. R. R. Kovener and M. D. Palmer, "Implementing the Medicare PPS," *Healthcare Financial Management* 37, No. 9 (1983):74-78.

130. J. Firshein, "Medical Education Payments Decried," *Hospitals* 59, No. 9 (May 1, 1985):39.

131. Ibid.

132. Ibid.

133. Ibid.

134. J. R. Lave, *The Medicare Adjustment for the Indirect Costs of Medical Education: Historical Development and Current Status*. Association of American Medical Colleges, Washington, DC, January 1985.

135. Ibid., p. 11.

136. "Many States Seeking to Cut Medicaid Costs," *New York Times*, October 14, 1984.

137. "States Look to DRGs for Medicaid Cure," *Washington Report on Medicine and Health*, May 28, 1984.

138. D. Zimmerman, *DRGs and the Medicaid Program*. Intergovernmental Health Policy Project, Washington, DC, 1984.

139. A. C. Lovecchio, "Issues and Options for Medicaid Hospital Reimbursement As a Result of the Medicare DRG System," in *DRGs: The Effect in N.J. The Potential for the Nation*, USDHHS, HCFA Pub. No. 03170, March 1984, pp. 175-179.

140. T. N. Russo, "The Impact of Medicare's PPS on State Medical Agencies," in *DRGs: The Effect in N.J. The Potential for the Nation*, USDHHS, HCFA Pub. No. 03170, March 1984, pp. 171-174.

141. E. Weiland, "The Impact of DRGs on Payers. A Medicaid Prospective," in *DRGs: The Effect in N.J. The Potential in the Nation*, USDHHS, HCFA Pub. No. 03170, March 1984, pp. 136-138.

142. R. M. Clinkscale, "The Impact of Medicare's PPS on State Medicaid Programs," in *DRGs: The Effect in N.J. The Potential for*

the Nation, USDHHS, HCFA Pub. No. 03170, March 1984, pp. 180-182.

143. J. E. Mistarz, "Peer Review Priorities, Problems Outlined," *Hospitals* 59, No. 7 (April 1, 1985):26.

144. Ibid.

145. Ibid.

146. Ibid.

147. Lundy, *Medicare: Prospective Payment*.

148. C. Mickel, "Medicare Freeze Forseen Lowering Qualify of Care, Jeopardizing Access," *Hospitals* 59, No. 7 (April 1, 1985):31-32.

149. J. Fochtman, "House Bill Focuses on Quality," *Medical Marketing and Media* 20, No. 6 (1985):8-9.

150. Ibid.

151. W. R. Fifer, "DRGs and Doctors," *Pennsylvania Medicine* 87, No. 1 (1984):28-33.

152. Ibid.

153. S. Wingrove, "Rampant Litigation Ups the Ante," *Private Practice* 17, No. 2 (1985):29-32.

154. T. Shahoda, "Consensus Lacking on How to Pay for Technology Under Medicare," *Hospitals* 59, No. 7 (April 1, 1985):28.

155. Ibid.

156. Lundy, *Medicare: Prospective Payment*.

157. J. E. Mistarz, "Delay Forseen in PPS Capital Inclusion," *Hospitals* 59, No. 7 (April 1, 1985):30.

158. E. Shapiro, "Blame Old Age, Not Medicare," *New York Times*, January 3, 1985.

159. Ibid.

160. S. Blakeslee, "Coast Parley on Medicare and Medicaid Opens Amid Protests," *New York Times*, June 20, 1985.

161. J. Fochtman, "Hospital Data to be Public Information," *Medical Marketing and Media* 20, No. 6 (1985):9.

162. J. Brinkley, "U.S. Releasing Lists of Hospitals with Abnormal Mortaility Rates," *New York Times*, March 12, 1986.

163. M. Freundenheim, "Posting Prices of Hospitals," *New York Times*, April 2, 1985.

164. J. E. Fox, "DRG System in '84 Budget for Medicare," *U.S. Medicine* 19, No. 4 (February 15, 1983):1, 30.

165. "Medichoice Offers A Way Out of DRG Payment Plan," *Hospital Peer Review* 8, No. 7 (1983):89-90.

166. C. Mickel, "Expand DRGs, Increase Competition, Durenberger Says," *Hospitals* 58, No. 1 (January 1, 1984):30-31.

167. Ibid.

168. "For Profits' Meeting Examines DRG System, Capital Options," *Hospital Progress* 65, No. 4 (1984):20-21.

169. Fochtman, "Hospital Data."

170. C. Holden, "Getting Health Promotion into Medicare," *Science* 227, No. 4691 (March 8, 1985):1183.

171. Ibid.

172. C. Wallace, "Kennedy-Gephardt Bill Meets Stiff Opposition," *Modern Healthcare* 14, No. 4 (1984):38.

173. T. R. Marmor and E. Smolka, "How to Help Medicare," *New York Times*, January 3, 1985.

174. J. Finn, "Adjustments Needed to Fine-Tune Prospective Pricing," *Hospitals* 58, No. 9 (May 1, 1984):31.

175. J. R. Goldstein, "New Jersey: Past and Present," in *DRGs: The Effect in N.J. The Potential for the Nation*, USDHHS, HCFA Pub. No. 03170, March 1984, p. 217-218.

176. A. N. Johnson and G. L. Appel, "DRGs and Hospital Case Records: Implications for Medicare Case Mix Accusary," *Inquiry* 21, (Summer, 1984):128-134.

177. C. Bankhead, "PPS:Best Guesses of What's Ahead," *Medical World News* 26, No. 8 (April 22, 1985):24-25.

178. J. Fochtman, "Medicare Won't Go Bust Until 1998," *Medical Marketing and Media* 20, No. 6 (1985):8.

179. J. Finn, "HHS Extends Medicare Trust Fund Solvency Projections," *Hospitals* 59, No. 9 (May 1, 1985):40.

180. "Insuring Medicare's Future Beyond 1988," *Medical World News* 26, No. 8 (April 22, 1985):100.

181. R. B. Milch, "Future Implications of Prospective Payment," in *DRGs: The Effect in N.J. The Potential for the Nation*, USDHHS, HCFA Pub. No. 03170, March 1984, pp. 219-220.

182. Ibid., p. 220.

183. "Fee-for-Service: Last Rites?" *Medical World News* 26, No. 5 (March 11, 1985):65, 68.

184. Ibid.

185. Ibid.

186. Bankhead, "Best Guesses."

187. Griffith, "DRGs—What's Next?"

188. Ibid.

189. Finn, "HHS Extends Medicare."

190. Ibid.

191. Ibid.

192. M. Lesparre, "Washington in 1985: Focus on Saving Medicare," *Hospitals* 59, No. 1 (January 1, 1985):68-70, 72-73.

193. Ibid.

194. S. McIlrath, "Medicare Pay to MDs on Mihalski Agenda," *American Medical News* 28, No. 10 (March 8, 1985):2, 34.

195. Ibid.

196. D. Durenberger, "The Role of the DRG Program in Federal Policy and Medicare's PPS," in *DRGs: The Effect in N.J. The Potential for the Nation*, USDHHS, HCFA Pub. No. 03170, March 1984, pp. 1-3.

197. Ibid.

198. T. Shahoda, "Durenberger Suggests Ways to Revamp, Enhance PPS," *Hospitals* 59, No. 7 (April 1, 1985):26, 28.

199. "Senator John Heinz Speaks Out on Medicare," *Hospitals* 58, No. 22 (November 16, 1984):102, 104.

200. C. J. Schramm, "Point of View. Competition vs. Regulation in Health Care," *New York Times*, June 20, 1985.

201. M. Tolchin, "Private Hospitals Are Now Offering Health Insurance," *New York Times*, July 5, 1985.

GLOSSARY

AAHC Association of Academic Health Centers

AAMC American Association of Medical Colleges

AARP American Association of Retired Persons

Abstract/Discharge Abstract/Discharge Face Sheet A summary of the admission which is prepared at the time of the patient's discharge from the hospital. Information contained on the abstract includes demographic data, payment source, length of stay, principal diagnosis, secondary diagnoses or complications, procedures performed, services provided, and other relevant material.

ACCC Association of Community Cancer Centers

ACHA American College of Hospital Administrators

ACPs Ambulatory Condition Packages

ADL Activities of Daily Living

ADRGs Alternate Diagnosis Related Groups

AHA American Hospital Association

AHPA American Health Planning Association

AHS Associated Hospital Systems

AID Automatic Interaction Detector

ALOS Average Length of Stay

AMA American Medical Association

AMA American Management Association

AMI Acute Myocardial Infarction

AMI American Medical International

AMPRA American Medical Peer Review Association

AMRA American Medical Records Association

ANA American Nurses Association

Ancillary Services Hospital services other than room and board and professional services such as X-ray, drug, laboratory, or other services not itemized separately.

APA American Psychiatric Association

APGs Ambulatory Patient Related Groups

ART Accredited Record Technician

ASG Admission Severity Group

ASIM American Society of Internal Medicine

AUTOGRP Automatic Grouping System

AVGs Ambulatory Visit Groups

BC/BS Blue Cross/Blue Shield

Budget Neutrality Legislative requirement that Medicare payment for total inpatient operating costs to hospitals under the prospective payment system during fiscal year 1984 and 1985 should be neither greater nor less than the estimate of what would have been paid under the law in effect (the Tax Equity and Fiscal Responsibility Act) prior to enactment of prospective payment.

CAP Competitive Allowance Program

CAP College of American Pathologists

Capital Costs Costs associated with the use of capital facilities and equipment, including depreciation and interest expense.

Capitation A method of payment for health services in which an individual or institutional provider is paid a fixed, per capita amount for each person served without regard to the actual number or nature of services provided to each person.

Case Mix Relative frequency of admissions of various types of patients reflecting different needs for hospital resources. Measurements of case mix include diagnoses, severity of illness, utilization of resources and hospital characteristics.

Case-Mix Index A measure of the costliness of cases treated by a hospital relative to the cost of the national average of all Medicare hospital cases, using diagnosis related group weights as a measure of the relative costliness of cases.

CAT Computerized Axial Tomography

CBO Congressional Budget Office

CCU Coronary Care Unit

CEO Chief Executive Officer

CHAMPUS Civilian Health and Medical Plan of the Uniformed Services

Classification Act or process of systematically arranging in groups or categories according to established criteria.

Clinical Culture Provider practice behavior that stresses using all available resources in an intensive patient care regimen.

CME Continuing Medical Education

CMP Competitive Medical Plan

Coinsurance A form of cost sharing whereby the insured pays a percentage of the total cost.

Comorbidity A preexisting condition that will, because of its presence with a specific principal diagnosis, increase length of stay by at least one day in about 75 percent of cases.

Complication A condition that arises during the hospital stay that prolongs length of stay by at least one day in approximately 75 percent of cases.

CON Certificate of Need

Copayment A form of cost sharing whereby the insured pays a specific amount at the point of consumption, e.g., $10 per visit.

Cost Accounting Financial procedures to directly identify exact costs of specific resources utilized for health care services to specific patients.

Cost Based Reimbursement A method of paying for services based on the costs incurred by a provider to furnish those services.

Cost Sharing General set of financing arrangements whereby the consumer must pay some out of pocket costs to receive care, either at the time of initiation of care, or during the time of the provision of health care services, or both.

Cost Shifting Movement of deficit costs from undercompensated patient care activities to other payers having adequate coverage.

COTH Council of Teaching Hospitals

CPHA Commission on Professional and Hospital Activities

CPI Consumer Price Index

CPPs Collapsed or Recombined Procedures Packages

CPR Customary-Prevailing-Reasonable

CPT-4 Current Procedural Terminology, Fourth Edition

CRNA Certified Registered Nurse Anesthetist

DAF Discretionary Adjustment Factor

Direct Medical Education Costs Costs of approved education programs that providers engage in to enhance the quality of care in an institution including nursing schools, medical education, and paraprofessional training.

Disease Staging A classification system for grouping patients based upon clinical evaluation of the severity of illness.

Disproportionate Share Unusually heavy volume of uncompensated services rendered by facilities to Medicare, low income, and indigent individuals.

Distinct Part Unit A hospital unit that first meets the general criteria to qualify as a distinct part unit, and then meets the specific criteria to qualify as a psychiatric or rehabilitation unit.

DNR Do Not Resuscitate

DRG Diagnosis-Related Group

DRG Creep The artificial inflating of diagnoses to obtain higher payment for the hospital.

DRG Weight An index number which reflects the relative resource consumption associated with each diagnosis related group.

DSM-111 Diagnostic and Statistical Manual of Mental Disorders, Third Edition

DUR Drug Use Review

ER Emergency Room

ESRD End Stage Renal Disease

Exempt Hospitals and Units Childrens', long term care (average length of stay over 25 days), rehabilitation, and psychiatric hospitals are specifically excluded from the prospective payment system. Distinct part subunits, psychiatric, and rehabilitation of acute care hospitals are exempted. Hospitals in U.S. territories, alcohol or drug abuse treatment units of acute hospitals, federal hospitals, and Christian Science sanatoria are also exempted. Cancer treatment and research facilities may receive an exemption from the HHS Secretary.

FAH Federation of American Hospitals

Fair Payment System Term used to describe a system where all insurers are included in a prospective payment plan to avoid cost shifting.

Fee-for-Service A method of paying for medical care on a retrospective basis by which each service actually received by an individual bears a related charge.

Fiscal Intermediary A public or private agency or organization selected by the providers of health care that enters into an agreement with HHS under the Hospital Insurance Program of Medicare in order to pay claims and perform other functions on behalf of such providers.

FTC Federal Trade Commission

FY Fiscal Year

Gaming Abuse of the DRG system such as having multiple admissions for the same patient for the same illness.

GAO U.S. Government Accounting Office

GIR Guaranteed Inpatient Revenue

GPMP Generalized Patient Management Pathways

GRECC Geriatric Research, Education and Clinical Centers of the VA

Grouper A computer program used by the intermediary to assign discharges to the appropriate DRG using information abstracted from the inpatient bill.

HBP Hospital Based Physician

HCA Hospital Corporation of America

HCFA Health Care Financing Administration

HCUP Hospital Cost and Utilization Project

HFMA Healthcare Financial Management Association

HHA Home Health Agency

HHS U.S Department of Health and Human Services

HI Hospital Insurance Trust Fund

HIAA Health Insurance Association of America

HIMA Health Industry Manufacturing Association

HMO Health Maintenance Organization

Horizontal Integration Health care institutional expansion to group together similar facilities providing similar services.

Hospital Market Basket The set of goods and services purchased by hospitals.

Hospital Market Basket Index Constructed by specifying the inputs that hospitals purchase and combining inputs into components; by determining a weight for each component that represents its share of total hospital expenses; and by identifying measures of price changes for each component. Overall change in the price of the market basket is computed by multiplying each component's price change by its weight and summing across all components.

HRET Health Research and Educational Trust of New Jersey

HRF Health Related Facility

HSA Health Systems Agency

HSCRC Health Services Cost Review Commission

IAS Inflation Adjustment System

ICD-9-CM International Classification of Diseases—9th Revision—Clinical Modification

ICF Intermediate Care Facility

ICHPPC International Classification of Health Problems in Primary Care

ICU Intensive Care Unit

Indirect Medical Education Costs Additional services and test procedures performed on patients because the hospital is a teaching institution.

IOM Institute of Medicine

IPA Independent Practice Association

IV Intravenous

JCAH Joint Commission on the Accreditation of Hospitals

KCF Key Clinical Findings

LOS Length of Stay

LTC Long Term Care

MAC Maximum Allowable Cost

MAC Major Ambulatory Category

MADCs Major Ambulatory Diagnostic Categories

MAP Maximum Allowable Payment

Maximization Manipulation of data to optimize hospital reimbursement.

MCR Medicare Cost Report

MDCs Major Diagnostic Categories

Medi-Cal Medicaid in California

Medichoice A system allowing individuals to choose their own health care provider using vouchers as payment.

MEDISGRPS Medical Illness Severity Grouping System

MEDPAR Medicare Provider Analysis and Review

MEI Medicare Economic Index

MERB MAC Exception Review Board

MeSH Medical Staff and Hospital

MICU Mobile Intensive Care Unit

MIRA Medicare Incentive Reform Act

MRE Medicare Review Entity

MRG Management Related Groups

MSA Metropolitan Statistical Area

NACHRI National Association of Childrens Hospitals and Related Institutions.

NAPH National Association of Public Hospitals

NAPPH National Association of Private Psychiatric Hospitals

NARF National Association of Rehabilitation Facilities

NCAB National Cancer Advisory Board

NCQHC National Committee for Quality Health Care

NCSC National Council of Senior Citizens

NECMA New England County Metropolitan Area

NIMH National Institute of Mental Health

NJBGH New Jersey Business Group on Health

NME National Medical Enterprises

NPCS Nursing Patient Classification System

NRC Nursing Resource Cluster

NSAIDS Non-Steroidal Anti-Inflammatory Drugs

NYCHHC New York City Health and Hospitals Corporation

NYPHRM New York Prospective Hospital Reimbursement Methodology

OMB Office of Management and Budget

OPD Outpatient Department

OT Occupational Therapy

OTA U.S. Congress, Office of Technology Assessment

Outlier Cases which have an extremely long length of stay (day outlier) or extraordinarily high costs (cost outlier) when compared to most discharges classified in the same DRG.

OVPs Office Visit Packages

PAS Professional Activity Study

Pass Throughs In a per case payment system, pass throughs are elements of hospital cost that are paid on the basis of cost-based reimbursement of reasonable charges.

PBCS Planning, Budgeting, and Control System

PCB Preliminary Cost Base

PCP Primary Care Pharmacist

PCRS Prospective Capital Reimbursement System

PCU Patient Care Unit

Per Diem Reimbursement calculated on total hospital expenditures divided by the total bed days to arrive at a cost per hospital day.

Per Case Reimbursement Reimbursement for medical care on a case basis instead of the traditional fee-for-service method.

PERT Program Evaluation and Review Technique

PMC Patient Management Categories

POPTS Physician Owned Physical Therapy Services

PPGP Prepaid Group Practice

PPO Preferred Provider Organization

PPS Prospective Payment System

PRI Patient Review Instrument

Primary Procedure Principal operating room procedure performed on a given patient.

Principal Diagnosis That condition which after study is determined to be the reason chiefly responsible for occasioning the admission of the patient to the hospital.

Principal Procedure Procedure that is the one most related to the principal diagnosis or the one which was performed for definitive treatment rather than performed for diagnostic or exploratory purposes, or was necessary to treat a complication. If only one procedure is performed, it is considered the principal procedure.

PRO Professional Review Organization

Product Line Management terminology used to describe the outputs of the hospital in industrial terms.

ProPAC Prospective Payment Assessment Commission

Proxy Payment Term used to designate the funding given to teaching hospitals to compensate for educational activities related to patient care services.

PSRO Professional Standards Review Organization

PT Physical Therapy

P&T Pharmacy and Therapeutics Committee

PTF Patient Treatment File

QA Quality Assurance

Rebundling of Hospital Payment Payment to hospitals for inpatient services which were formerly paid to other suppliers under separate billing. This relates to movement from Part B back into Part A hospital costs.

Recalibration Adjustment of all DRG weights to reflect changes in relative resource use associated with all existing DRG categories and/or the creation or elimination of DRG categories.

Reclassification Adjustment of certain DRG categories to reflect the creation or elimination of DRG categories or movements of certain diagnostic or procedure codes from one DRG category to another. After reclassification, the resulting categories may need to be reweighted.

Retrospective Cost Based Reimbursement A payment method in which hospitals are paid their incurred costs of treating patients after the treatment has occurred.

Revenue Bonds A public investment financing mechanism used by hospitals to raise money for capital expenditures.

RIMs Relative Intensity Measures

RMP Regional Medical Program

RN Registered Nurse

RNI Resource Need Index

RRA Registered Records Administrator

RUGs Resource Utilization Groupings

RVS Relative Value Scale

RVU Relative Value Unit

S/HMO Social Health Maintenance Organization

SCH Sole Community Hospital

SDS Same Day Surgery

Secondary Diagnosis Problems and important symptoms both related and un-related to the principal diagnosis, which either exist at the time of the patient's admission or develop and are treated during hospitalization.

Section 223 A section of the Social Security Act which set an upper amount on total inpatient operating costs per discharge reimburseable under Medicare.

Severity of Illness Refers to the relative level of loss of function and mortality caused by a particular illness.

SHARE Standard Hospital Accounting and Rate Evaluations

SHUR Systemwide Hospital Uniform Reporting

SMSA Standard Metropolitan Statistical Area

SNF Skilled Nursing Facility

Sole Community Provider One of a group of hospitals which by reason of factors such as isolation, absence of other hospitals, weather or travel conditions is the sole source of inpatient hospital services reasonably available to Medicare beneficiaries within a geographic area.

S/PPO Senior Preferred Provider Organization

SPPs Special Procedure Packages

SPU Strategic Program Unit

Step Down Care Movement of patients from hospital care units to services such as nursing homes and home health care.

TEFRA Tax Equity and Fiscal Responsibility Act of 1982

TLC Tender Loving Care

Transfer Defined as the movement of a patient from one inpatient area or unit to another area or unit of the hospital, from the care of a hospital paid under prospective payment to the care of another such hosptial, or from the care of a hospital under prospective payment to the care of a hospital in an approved statewide cost control program.

TRG Treatment Related Groups

Trim Points Length of stay or cost cutoff points that separate patients with unusually long lengths of stay or unusually high costs from ''normal'' cases within each DRG. Patients exceeding the trim points are considered outliers.

UB-82 Uniform Billing Form 82

UCR Usual, Customary, and Reasonable

UHDDS Uniform Hospital Discharge Set

Unbundling Billing under Part B for nonphysician services to hospital inpatients which are furnished to the hospital by an outside supplier or another provider.

Updating Factor Adjustment of the base year cost data for inflation.

UR Utilization Review

VA Veterans Administration

Vertical Integration Health care institutional expansion to provide a comprehensive array of health care services under a single sponsorship.

Voucher Document specifying a financial allowance that allows individuals to choose their own health care provider who then agrees to accept that amount as full payment for services rendered.

Wage Index Labor-related portion of the hospital's federal payment rates multiplied by an urban or rural wage index that represents local hospital wages. Index is related to geographic areas and urban/rural classifications.

WGBH Washington Business Group on Health

WWU Weighted Work Unit

INDEX

Italicized numbers indicate exhibits.